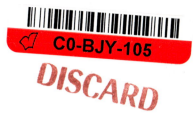

# CRC SERIES IN NUTRITION AND FOOD

Editor-in-Chief

## Miloslav Rechcigl, Jr.

**Handbook of Nutritive Value of Processed Food**
Volume I: Food For Human Use
Volume II: Animal Feedstuffs

**Handbook of Nutritional Requirements in a Functional Context**
Volume I: Development and Conditions of Physiologic Stress
Volume II: Hematopoiesis, Metabolic Function, and Resistance to Physical Stress

**Handbook of Agricultural Productivity**
Volume I: Plant Productivity
Volume II: Animal Productivity

**Handbook of Naturally Occurring Food Toxicants**

**Handbook of Foodborne Diseases of Biological Origin**

**Handbook of Nutritional Supplements**
Volume I: Human Use
Volume II: Agricultural Use

## HANDBOOK SERIES

**Nutritional Requirements**
Volume I: Comparative and Qualitative Requirements

**Nutritional Disorders**
Volume I: Effect of Nutrient Excesses and Toxicities in Animal and Man
Volume II: Effect of Nutrient Deficiencies in Animals
Volume III: Effect of Nutrient Deficiencies in Man

**Diets, Culture Media, Food Supplements**
Volume I: Diets for Mammals
Volume II: Food Habits of, and Diets for Invertebrates and Vertebrates — Zoo Diets
Volume III: Culture Media for Microorganisms and Plants
Volume IV: Culture Media for Cells, Organs and Embryos

# CRC Handbook of Nutritional Supplements

## Volume I
## Human Use

Editor

**Miloslav Rechcigl, Jr.**
Nutrition Adviser and Chief
Research and Methodology Division
Agency for International Development
U.S. International Development Cooperation Agency
Washington, D.C.

*CRC Series in Nutrition and Food*

Editor-in-Chief
Miloslav Rechcigl, Jr.

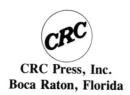

**CRC Press, Inc.**
**Boca Raton, Florida**

**Library of Congress Cataloging in Publication Data**
Main entry under title:

Handbook of nutritional supplements.

(CRC series in nutrition and food)
Includes bibliographies and index.
Contents: v. 1. Human use -- v. 2. Agricultural use.
1. Food additives. 2. Feed additives. 3. Feeds.
4. Dietary supplements. I. Rechcígl, Miloslav.
II. Series.
TX553.A3H34   1983      664'.6        82-17803
ISBN 0-8493-3969-3 (v. I)
ISBN 0-8493-3970-7 (v. II)

Direct all inquiries to CRC Press, Inc., 2000 Corporate Blvd., N.W., Boca Raton, Florida, 33431.

© 1983 by CRC Press, Inc.

International Standard Book Number 0-8493-3969-3 (Volume I)
International Standard Book Number 0-8493-3970-7 (Volume II)

Library of Congress Card Number 82-17803
Printed in the United States

# PREFACE
## CRC SERIES IN NUTRITION AND FOOD

Nutrition means different things to different people, and no other field of endeavor crosses the boundaries of so many different disciplines and abounds with such diverse dimensions. The growth of the field of nutrition, particularly in the last 2 decades, has been phenomenal, the nutritional data being scattered literally in thousands and thousands of not always accessible periodicals and monographs, many of which, furthermore, are not normally identified with nutrition.

To remedy this situation, we have undertaken an ambitious and monumental task of assembling in one publication all the critical data relevant in the field of nutrition.

The *CRC Series in Nutrition and Food* is intended to serve as a ready reference source of current information on experimental and applied human, animal, microbial, and plant nutrition presented in concise, tabular, graphical, or narrative form and indexed for ease of use. It is hoped that this projected open-ended multivolume compendium will become for the nutritionist what the *CRC Handbook of Chemistry and Physics* has become for the chemist and physicist.

Apart from supplying specific data, the comprehensive, interdisciplinary, and comparative nature of the *CRC Series in Nutrition and Food* will provide the user with an easy overview of the state of the art, pinpointing the gaps in nutritional knowledge and providing a basis for further research. In addition, the series will enable the researcher to analyze the data in various living systems for commonality or basic differences. On the other hand, an applied scientist or technician will be afforded the opportunity of evaluating a given problem and its solutions from the broadest possible point of view, including the aspects of agronomy, crop science, animal husbandry, aquaculture and fisheries, veterinary medicine, clinical medicine, pathology, parasitology, toxicology, pharmacology, therapeutics, dietetics, food science and technology, physiology, zoology, botany, biochemistry, developmental and cell biology, microbiology, sanitation, pest control, economics, marketing, sociology, anthropology, natural resources, ecology, environmental science, population, law politics, nutritional and food methodology, and others.

To make more facile use of the series, the publication has been organized into separate handbooks of one or more volumes each. In this manner the particular sections of the series can be continuously updated by publishing additional volumes of new data as they become available.

The Editor wishes to thank the numerous contributors many of whom have undertaken their assignment in pioneering spirit, and the Advisory Board members for their continuous counsel and cooperation. Last but not least, he wishes to express his sincere appreciation to the members of the CRC editorial and production staffs, particularly President Bernard J. Starkoff, Earl Starkoff, Sandy Pearlman, Amy G. Skallerup, John Hunter, and Janelle Sparks for their encouragement and support.

We invite comments and criticism regarding format and selection of subject matter, as well as specific suggestions for new data which might be included in subsequent editions. We should also appreciate it if the readers would bring to the attention of the Editor any errors or omissions that might appear in the publication.

**Miloslav Rechcígl, Jr.**
**Editor-in-Chief**

## PREFACE HANDBOOK OF NUTRITIONAL SUPPLEMENTS

Nutritional supplements, many of which, not too long ago, were still considered unconventional foods, are now becoming common ingredients of animal as well as human diet. The composition of different supplements may vary, ranging from single nutrients to complex formulated food mixtures to the food products that have been produced entirely synthetically. Through the ingenuity of food technology many of these products have become almost indistinguishable — in color, texture and flavor — from the traditional foodstuffs.

There is a need to keep abreast of the ever increasing number of new products that appear on the market, greatly varying in their value and potential use. The purpose of this Handbook is to provide such information, fulfilling a long felt void in this area.

The Handbook is composed of two parts, the first volume covering supplements for human use while the second volume is devoted to agriculture supplements.

The volume relating to food supplements for human use is organized on the basis of raw materials utilized in their production, as well as on the basis of target groups for which they are intended.

The volume on agriculture supplements covers various food byproducts and nutritional and other food supplements used in animal feeding. In addition, it also includes information on nutrition supplements for plants.

# THE EDITOR

**Miloslav Rechcigl, Jr.** is a Nutrition Advisor and Chief of Research and Methodology Division in the Agency for International Development.

He has a B.S. in Biochemistry (1954), a Master of Nutritional Science degree (1955), and a Ph.D. in nutrition, biochemistry, and physiology (1958), all from Cornell University. He was formerly a Research Biochemist in the National Cancer Institute, National Institutes of Health and subsequently served as Special Assistant for Nutrition and Health in the Health Services and Mental Health Administration, U.S. Department of Health, Education and Welfare.

Dr. Rechcigl is a member of some 30 scientific and professional societies, including being a Fellow of the American Association for the Advancement of Science, Fellow of the Washington Academy of Sciences, Fellow of the American Institute of Chemists, and Fellow of the International College of Applied Nutrition. He holds membership in the Cosmos Club, the Honorary Society of Phi Kappa Pi, and the Society of Sigma Xi, and is recipient of numerous honors, including an honorary membership certificate from the International Social Science Honor Society Delta Tau Kappa. In 1969, he was a delegate to the White House Conference on Food, Nutrition, and Health and in 1975 a delegate to the ARPAC Conference on Research to Meet U.S. and World Food Needs. He served as President of the District of Columbia Institute of Chemists and Councillor of the American Institute of Chemists, and currently is a delegate to the Washington Academy of Sciences and a member of the Program Committee of the American Institute of Nutrition.

His bibliography extends over 100 publications including contributions to books, articles in periodicals, and monographs in the fields of nutrition, biochemistry, physiology, pathology, enzymology, molecular biology, agriculture, and international development. Most recently he authored and edited *Nutrition and the World Food Problem* (S. Karger, Basel, 1979), *World Food Problem: a Selective Bibliography of Reviews* (CRC Press, 1975), and *Man, Food and Nutrition: Strategies and Technological Measures for Alleviating the World Food Problem* (CRC Press, 1973) following his earlier pioneering treatise on *Enzyme Synthesis and Degradation in Mammalian Systems* (S. Karger, Basel, 1971), and that on *Microbodies and Related Particles, Morphology, Biochemistry and Physiology* (Academic Press, New York, 1969). Dr. Rechcigl also has initiated a new series on *Comparative Animal Nutrition* and was Associated Editor of *Nutrition Reports International*.

# ADVISORY BOARD MEMBERS

# CONTRIBUTORS

**Wanda L. Chenoweth, Ph.D., R.D.**
Professor
Department of Food Science and Human
 Nutrition
Michigan State University
East Lansing, Michigan

**Hulda Crooks**
Research Assistant
Health Education Department
School of Health
Loma Linda University
Loma Linda, California

**Johanna T. Dwyer, D.Sc.**
Director
Frances Stern Medical Center Hospital
 and
Associate Professor
Tufts Medical School
Boston, Massachusetts

**Ray C. Frodey**
Vice President
Research and Quality Control
Gerber Production Company
Fremont, Michigan

**John J. Jonas, Ph.D.**
Consultant
Research and Development
Kraft, Inc.
Glenview, Illinois

**Catherine L. Justice, R.D., Ph.D.**
Associate Professor
Foods and Nutrition Department
Purdue University
West Lafayette, Indiana

**John M. Kinney, M.D.**
Professor of Surgery
College of Physicians and Surgeons
Columbia University
New York, New York

**John E. Kinsella, Ph.D.**
Director
Institute of Food Science
Cornell University
Ithaca, New York

**Audrey Lynne Loomis**
Computer Scientist
System Sciences Division
Computer Sciences Corporation
Silver Spring, Maryland

**Frank W. Lowenstein, M.D.D.P.H.**
Nutrition Consultant
Former Nutrition Adviser
National Center for Health Statistics
U.S. Public Health Service
Silver Spring, Maryland

**Rebecca C. McDonald, Ph.D.**
Research Chemist
National Space Technology Laboratories
National Aeronautics and Space
 Administration
NSTL Station, Mississippi

**Hisateru Mitsuda, Ph.D.**
Professor Emeritus
Kyoto University
 and
President
Department of Nutrition
Koshien University
Takarazuka-shi, Japan

**Juan M. Navia, Ph.D.**
Professor of Nutrition Sciences and
Public Health
 and
Senior Scientist
Institute of Dental Research
University of Alabama in Birmingham
Birmingham, Alabama

**Adewale Omololu, M.D., F.R.C.P.I.,
D.P.H.**
Professor
Department of Human Nutrition
University of Ibadan
Ibadan, Nigeria

**Vernal S. Packard, Ph.D.**
Professor and Extension Specialist
Department of Food Science and
 Nutrition
University of Minnesota
St. Paul, Minnesota

**Amira Srouji Pellett, Ph.D.**
Nutritionist
Baystate Medical Center
Springfield, Massachusetts

**Peter Lewis Pellett, Ph.D.**
Professor of Nutrition
Department of Food Science and
 Nutrition
University of Massachusetts
Amherst, Massachusetts

**N. W. Pirie (Retired)**
Rothamsted Experimental Station
Harpenden, Herts, U.K.

**Jerry F. Proctor, Ph.D.**
Deputy Managing Director
Tinamenor S.A.
Subsidiary of Dart and Kraft, Inc.
Pesues, Spain

**U. D. Register, Ph.D.**
Professor and Chairman
Department of Nutrition
School of Health
Loma Linda University
Loma Linda, California

**Robin M. Saunders, Ph.D.**
Research Leader
Cereals Research Unit
Western Regional Research Center
USDA-SEA-AR
Albany, California

**Virginia D. Sidwell, Ph.D. (Retired)**
Research Food Technologist
National Marine Fisheries Service
Washington, D.C.

**Paul M. Starker, M.D.**
Research Fellow
Department of Surgery
College of Physicians and Surgeons
Columbia University
New York, New York

**Mahadeva Swaminathan, D.Sc.
 (Retired)**
Chairman
Applied Nutrition and Dietetics Discipline
              and
Emeritus Scientist
Central Food Technological Research
 Institute
Mysore, India

**B. C. Wolverton, Ph.D.**
Chief
Environmental Assurance Branch
National Space Technology Laboratories
National Aeronautics and Space
 Administration
NSTL Station, Mississippi

**Arvid Wretlind, M.D.**
Visiting Professor
Department of Surgery
College of Physicians and Surgeons
Columbia University
New York, New York

**Aijiro Yamamoto, Ph.D.**
Professor
Department of Nutrition
Koshien University
Takarazuka, Japan

# TABLE OF CONTENTS

# *Nutritional Sources*
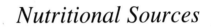

# OILSEED AND NUT PROTEINS

## M. Swaminathan

## INTRODUCTION

Protein deficiency, particularly in the diets of young children and other vulnerable groups, is one of the major nutritional problems facing the developing countries. The nature and magnitude of the "protein gap" has been discussed by the Food and Agricultural Organization (FAO) and other United Nations (UN) Agencies.[1] The most promising additional protein sources remain to be used for human consumption are the edible oilseeds, nuts, and their meals.[2,3] Nuts and oilseeds provide about 5 to 15 g of additional proteins per capita in many developing countries, where milk production and consumption are low (less than 150 g/capita/day) and milk provides less than 5 g protein per day per head.[4] A considerable amount of work has been carried out during recent years on the utilization of edible nuts and oilseeds and their meals in the preparation of supplementary foods for infants and children.[5,6] This chapter gives a summary of the available data on the chemical composition and nutritive value and the proteins of nuts and oilseeds and results of studies on the processed supplementary foods based on them.

## PRODUCTION

Data[7] regarding the production of certain oilseeds and nuts in some countries are given in Table 1. Only about 10 to 20% of the production is consumed as such in human diets, and the major portion is used for the extraction of oil. The residual oilseed meals which are rich sources of proteins, are at present, used mainly as a concentrate for cattle, swine, and poultry.

**Soybeans** — The present annual world production is over 62 million tons. Appreciable amounts are grown in some developing countries, viz., Brazil and Indonesia; the U.S. is the largest producer.

**Peanuts** — The present annual world production (peanut in shell) is over 17 million tons. Large amounts are grown in several developing countries, viz., India, Argentina, Brazil, Indonesia, and Nigeria, India being the largest producer.

**Cottonseed** — The present annual world production is over 38 million tons. Large quantities are grown in several developing countries, viz., Brazil, Burma, Mexico, India, Pakistan, U.A.R., and Sudan. The U.S. is the largest producer.

**Sesame seed** — The present annual world production is over 1.9 million tons. Appreciable quantities of sesame seed are being produced in some developing countries, viz., Mexico, India, Burma, and Sudan.

**Copra** — The present annual world production of copra is about 3.7 million tons. Copra is produced in large quantities in some developing countries, viz., Ceylon, India, Indonesia, the Philippines, and Mexico. The Philippines is the largest producer.

**Sunflower seed** — Annual world production exceeds 12 million tons. It is grown in appreciable quantities in some developing countries, viz., Argentina and Turkey. The U.S.S.R. is the largest producer.

## THE CHEMICAL COMPOSITION AND NUTRITIVE VALUE OF THE PROTEINS OF CERTAIN OILSEEDS AND NUTS

The available data regarding the chemical composition and nutritive value of the

Table 1
## PRODUCTION OF MAJOR OILSEEDS AND NUTS IN SOME COUNTRIES[7]

| | 1,000 t/year | | | | | |
|---|---|---|---|---|---|---|
| Country | Soybean | Peanut (in shell) | Cottonseed | Sesame | Copra | Sunflower seed |
| 1 | 2 | 3 | 4 | 5 | 6 | 7 |
| Africa | 77 | 4,095 | 3,573 | 510 | 151 | 284 |
| Egypt | — | 28 | 1,352 | 21 | — | — |
| Nigeria | 33 | 350 | 91 | 62 | 9 | — |
| Uganda | 36 | 170 | 254 | 17 | — | — |
| North America | 42,879 | 1,726 | 9,029 | 174 | 201 | 394 |
| Canada | 397 | — | — | — | — | 41 |
| Mexico | 375 | 49 | 898 | 150 | 145 | — |
| U.S. | 42,108 | 1,576 | 7,313 | — | — | 353 |
| South America | 5,520 | 1,075 | 3,077 | 105 | 32 | 965 |
| Argentina | 272 | 440 | 369 | — | — | 880 |
| Brazil | 5,005 | 588 | 1,883 | 2 | 1 | — |
| Colombia | 99 | 1 | 386 | 23 | 2 | — |
| Peru | 1 | 1 | 204 | — | — | — |
| Asia | 13,072 | 10,099 | 14,666 | 1,185 | 3,085 | 692 |
| Burma | 8 | 459 | 43 | 122 | — | 1 |
| Ceylon (Sri Lanka) | — | 19 | 5 | 6 | 294 | — |
| China | 11,761 | 2,698 | 6,442 | 366 | — | 70 |
| India | — | 5,798 | 3,579 | 486 | 355 | — |
| Indonesia | 529 | 505 | 5 | 6 | 660 | — |
| Japan | 118 | 97 | — | 2 | — | — |
| Pakistan | — | 54 | 1,860 | 12 | — | — |
| Philippines | 2 | 18 | — | — | 1,739 | — |
| Turkey | 7 | 44 | 1,333 | 26 | — | 560 |
| Europe | 301 | 22 | 579 | 4 | — | 2,231 |
| Bulgaria | 31 | 3 | 38 | — | — | 448 |
| France | — | — | — | — | — | 91 |
| Hungary | — | — | — | — | — | 153 |
| Italy | — | 2 | 2 | 1 | — | 26 |
| | 13 | 1 | 8 | — | — | 434 |
| Oceania | 38 | 41 | 97 | — | 271 | 102 |
| Australia | 38 | 39 | 97 | — | — | 102 |
| U.S.S.R. | 424 | 333 | 7,664 | — | — | 7,385 |
| World production | 62,311 | 17,058 | 38,686 | 1,979 | 3,741 | 12,053 |

proteins of certain oilseeds and nuts are summarized according to chemical composition and amino acid composition and nutritive value of the proteins.

### Chemical Composition

**Proteins** — Data given in Table 2 show that protein contents of different oilseeds and nuts are as follows: soybean 34.1%; peanut, 26.3%; sunflower seed, 24.0%; sesame seed, 18.6%; almond, 18.6%; cashewnut, 17.2%; and coconut (dried), 7.2%. It is evident that coconut is a poor source of protein.

**Fat** — The fat content of soybean is about 17.7% and that of other oilseeds range from 35 to 54%. Sunflower seed, soybean, safflower, and sesame seed oils are rich sources and peanut and almond oils are moderate sources, while cashewnut and coconut oils are poor sources (Table 3) of polyunsaturated fatty acids (linoleic, linolenic, and arachidonic acids).

**Carbohydrates** — Oilseeds and nuts contain varying amounts of starch, sugars, and unavailable carbohydrates such as cellulose, hemicelluloses, galactans, pentosans, etc.

## Table 2
## THE CHEMICAL COMPOSITION OF CERTAIN OILSEEDS AND NUTS[8]

| Constituent | Almond | Cashewnut | Coconut meat (dried) | Peanut kernel (without skin) | Sesame seed | Soybean seed | Sunflower seed | Whole milk powder |
|---|---|---|---|---|---|---|---|---|
| Moisture (g) | 4.7 | 5.2 | 3.5 | 5.4 | 5.4 | 10.0 | 4.8 | 2.0 |
| Protein (N × 6.25, g) | 18.6 | 17.2 | 7.2 | 26.3 | 18.6 | 34.1 | 24.0 | 26.4 |
| Fat (g) | 54.2 | 45.7 | 64.9 | 48.4 | 49.1 | 17.7 | 47.3 | 27.5 |
| Ash (g) | 3.0 | 2.6 | 1.4 | 2.3 | 5.3 | 4.7 | 4.0 | 5.9 |
| Carbohydrates total (by diff., g) | 19.5 | 29.3 | 23.0 | 17.6 | 21.6 | 33.5 | 19.9 | 38.2 |
| Crude fiber (g) | 2.6 | 1.4 | 3.9 | 1.9 | 6.3 | 4.9 | 3.8 | 0 |
| Calcium (mg) | 234 | 38 | 26 | 59 | 1160 | 226 | 120 | 909 |
| Phosphorus (mg) | 504 | 373 | 187 | 409 | 616 | 554 | 837 | 708 |
| Iron (mg) | 4.7 | 3.8 | 3.3 | 2.0 | 10.5 | 8.4 | 7.1 | 0.5 |
| Sodium (mg) | 4 | 15 | 0 | 5 | 60 | 5 | 30 | 405 |
| Potassium (mg) | 773 | 464 | 588 | 674 | 725 | 1677 | 920 | 1330 |
| Vitamin A value (IU) | 0 | 100 | 0 | 0 | 30 | 80 | 50 | 1130 |
| Thiamine (mg) | 0.24 | 0.43 | 0.06 | 0.99 | 0.98 | 1.1 | 1.96 | 0.29 |
| Riboflavin (mg) | 0.32 | 0.25 | 0.04 | 0.13 | 0.24 | 0.31 | 0.23 | 1.46 |
| Niacin (mg) | 3.5 | 1.8 | 0.6 | 15.8 | 5.4 | 2.2 | 5.4 | 0.7 |

## Table 3
### THE POLYUNSATURATED AND SATURATED FATTY ACID CONTENTS AND THE P/S RATIO OF CERTAIN COMMON OILSEED AND NUT FATS[9]

| Oil | Polyunsaturated fatty acids (%) | Saturated fatty acids (%) | Monounsaturated fatty acids (%) | P/S ratio[a] |
|---|---|---|---|---|
| Almond | 27 | 7 | 66 | 3.86 |
| Cashewnut | 8 | 18 | 74 | 0.44 |
| Coconut | 2 | 92 | 6 | 0.02 |
| Peanut | 31 | 19 | 50 | 1.63 |
| Sesame | 43 | 14 | 43 | 3.07 |
| Soybean | 64 | 18 | 18 | 3.56 |
| Sunflower seed | 53 | 12 | 35 | 4.42 |
| Butter | 3 | 10 | 27 | 0.04 |

[a]   Ratio between polyunsaturated fatty acids and saturated fatty acids.


## Table 4
### ESSENTIAL AMINO ACID CONTENTS OF THE PROTEINS OF CERTAIN OILSEEDS AND NUTS COMPARED WITH MILK PROTEINS[10]

| Amino acid | Almond | Cashewnut | Coconut meat | Peanut kernel | Sesame seed | Soybean | Sunflower seed | Cow's milk | Cottonseed |
|---|---|---|---|---|---|---|---|---|---|
| Arginine | 12.16 | 9.62 | 12.11 | 10.70 | 8.75 | 7.15 | 8.74 | 3.73 | 11.2 |
| Histidine | 2.30 | 1.98 | 1.73 | 2.43 | 1.94 | 2.38 | 2.16 | 2.69 | 2.7 |
| Isoleucine | 3.89 | 5.6 | 4.50 | 4.11 | 4.18 | 5.38 | 4.70 | 6.51 | 3.8 |
| Leucine | 6.48 | 6.98 | 6.70 | 6.08 | 7.38 | 7.71 | 6.40 | 10.02 | 5.9 |
| Lysine | 2.59 | 3.63 | 3.79 | 3.57 | 2.56 | 6.32 | 3.20 | 7.94 | 4.3 |
| Methionine | 1.15 | 1.62 | 1.76 | 0.88 | 2.80 | 1.34 | 1.63 | 2.50 | 1.4 |
| Cystine | 1.68 | 2.42 | 1.55 | 1.50 | 2.18 | 1.78 | 1.71 | 0.91 | 1.6 |
| Phenylalanine | 5.10 | 4.34 | 4.34 | 5.06 | 6.4 | 4.94 | 4.50 | 4.94 | 5.2 |
| Tyrosine | 2.75 | 3.26 | 2.53 | 3.58 | 4.12 | 3.18 | 2.38 | 5.20 | 0 |
| Threonine | 2.72 | 3.38 | 3.22 | 2.69 | 3.10 | 3.94 | 3.36 | 4.70 | 3.5 |
| Tryptophan | 0.78 | 1.16 | 0.83 | 1.10 | 1.46 | 1.38 | 1.26 | 1.44 | 1.2 |
| Valine | 5.01 | 7.30 | 5.30 | 4.98 | 3.90 | 5.25 | 4.99 | 7.01 | 4.9 |

*Note:* Expressed in g/16 g N.


**Minerals** — Oilseeds and nuts are, in general, good sources of all minerals except calcium and sodium. Phosphorus is present in them mainly as phytates. As compared with whole milk powder, they are deficient in calcium. Hence, supplementary foods based on oilseeds and nuts will have to be fortified adequately with calcium salts.

**Vitamins** — Data given in Table 2 show that, as compared with whole milk powder, oilseeds and nuts are good sources of all B-group vitamins, except riboflavin and folic acid. They do not contain vitamins A, D, C, and $B_{12}$. Hence, supplementary foods based on oilseeds and nuts will have to be fortified with these vitamins.

### Essential Amino Acid Composition and Nutritive Value of Proteins
Data regarding the essential amino acid composition of the proteins of certain oilseeds and nuts as compared with milk proteins are given in Table 4. Soy proteins are good sources of all essential amino acids except methionine. Peanut, safflower seed, and almond proteins are deficient in lysine, methionine, and threonine, while sesame

Table 5

EFFECT OF SUPPLEMENTATION WITH LIMITING AMINO ACIDS
ON THE NUTRITIVE VALUE OF OILSEED PROTEIN

| Protein source | Level of protein in diet (%) | PER | Ref. |
|---|---|---|---|
| Cottonseed | 10 | 1.66 | 142 |
| Cottonseed + lysine | 10 | 2.24 | 142 |
| Peanut flour | 10 | 1.65 | 143 |
| Peanut flour + L-lysine and DL-methionine | 10 | 2.07 | 143 |
| Peanut flour + L-lysine, DL-methionine, and DL-threonine | 10 | 2.59 | 143 |
| Sesame | 10 | 1.50 | 144 |
| Sesame + lysine | 10 | 2.91 | 144 |
| Soybean flour | 10 | 2.37 | 145 |
| Soybean flour + methionine | 10 | 3.21 | 145 |
| Soybean flour + methionine hydroxyanalogue | 10 | 3.20 | 145 |
| Sunflower seed | 10 | 1.24 | 142 |
| Sunflower seed + L-lysine HCl | 10 | 1.84 | 142 |
| Sunflower seed + L-lysine and DL-threonine | 10 | 2.16 | 142 |

and sunflower seed proteins are deficient in lysine. Cashew proteins are good sources of all essential amino acids, while coconut proteins are slightly deficient in lysine and methionine.[10] The protein efficiency ratios of nuts and oilseeds range from 1.5 to 2.3, depending on the material (Table 5).

## Amino Acid Supplementation of the Proteins of Oilseeds and Nuts

Supplementation with methionine increases markedly the protein efficiency ratio (PER) of both raw and processed soybean. The PER of methionine-fortified processed soybean is nearly equal to that of milk proteins. Highly significant increases in the PER of sesame proteins as a result of fortification with lysine have been reported.[12] Fortification of cottonseed meal with lysine increased the PER to a significant extent. Supplementation of peanut proteins with lysine, methionine and threonine increased the PER to a marked extent.[11,12]

## DELETERIOUS CONSTITUENTS PRESENT IN OILSEEDS AND LEGUMES

Several deleterious constituents (Table 6) have been reported to occur in some oilseeds and these can be removed by suitable processing. Trypsin inhibitors and hemagglutinins are present in soybean and retard growth in rats. These can be inactivated by optimal heat treatment.[13] A heat-labile goitrogenic factor has been reported to be present in soybean. The goitrogenic factor of peanut is present in the red skin.[13] The pigment gossypol present in cottonseed has been found to retard the growth of rats and chicks. It is, however, not toxic to ruminants. Gossypol is inactivated when cottonseed flour is subjected to optimal heat treatment.[13] The toxic factor aflatoxin is produced by a fungus *Aspergillus flavus* growing mostly on peanut and occasionally on other oilseeds. Sreenivasa Murthy et al.[14] have developed a process for eliminating this toxin.

Selenium has been found to occur in sesame seeds grown on seleniferous soils in some countries. If selenium is present at a level higher than 300 ppb, it is toxic to mammals. No simple process for the elimination of selenium from sesame is known. A maximum level of 300 μg/kg (300 ppb) has been suggested as the safe limit in the Latin American Food Code.[15]

Table 6
DELETERIOUS CONSTITUENTS IN
SOME OIL SEEDS AND NUTS

| Oilseeds | Deleterious constituents |
| --- | --- |
| Peanut | Aflatoxin |
| | Goitrogenic factors (red skin) |
| Soybean | Trypsin inhibitor |
| | Hemagglutinins |
| | Goitrogenic factor |
| Cottonseed | Gossypol |
| Sesame | Selenium |
| | Oxalic acid (husk) |
| Rape and mustard | Glucosides and Crotonyl and allyl isothiocyanates, goitrogenic principles |

Oxalic acid is present in the form of calcium oxalate in the husk of sesame seeds. This can be eliminated by dehusking, and the dehusked sesame seed is almost free of oxalic acid.

## EFFECT OF PROCESSING ON THE NUTRITIVE VALUE

Heat processing produces both beneficial and deleterious effects on the nutritive value of proteins, depending on the severity of heat processing employed.[16] The beneficial effects are due to the inactivation by heat of inhibitors and hemagglutinins or gossypol present in them. The adverse effects are due to the decrease in the availability of certain essential amino acids such as lysine and methionine, due to reaction with reducing sugars, gossypol, and other carbonyl compounds present in food materials.

The losses of amino acids depend of the severity and duration of heat treatment and the moisture content of the sample. Moderate heat treatment (steaming at 15 lb pressure for 30 min) brings about marked improvement in the PER of soybean proteins as a result of inactivation of the growth inhibitors. Mild heat treatment as in screw pressing brings about slight improvement in the nutritive value of peanut proteins and marked improvement in the case of soybean proteins. It does not affect appreciably the PER of coconut, cottonseed, sesame, or sunflower seed proteins. Moderate heat treatment (steaming at 15 lb pressure for 60 min) brings about an appreciable decrease in the PER of cottonseed proteins due to the reaction between gossypol and the end-amino group of lysine. Severe heat treatment such as toasting, puffing, and pressure cooking for long periods causes a decrease in the PER of oilseed and nut proteins (Table 7).

## PROCESSED FOODS BASED ON OILSEEDS AND THEIR MEALS

A considerable amount of work has been carried out during recent years on the preparation of edible meals and protein isolates from oilseeds.[2,3] These have been used in the formulation of supplementary foods suitable for feeding infants and children.[3,5,6] The technological and nutritional aspects are discussed in terms of (1) preparation of edible meals and protein isolates, (2) infant foods and milk substitutes, and (3) protein foods based on oilseed meals and isolates.

**Preparation of Edible Meals**
Extensive studies have been carried out by several workers on the standardization

Table 7
EFFECT OF HEAT PROCESSING ON THE
NUTRITIVE VALUE OF OILSEED PROTEINS

| Source of protein | PER at 10% level | Ref. |
|---|---|---|
| Soybean, raw | 0.7 | 145 |
| Autoclaved at 15 lb pressure for 30 min | 2.4 | 145 |
| Cottonseed | | |
| Cooked for 20 min at 261°F | 1.7 | 146 |
| Cooked for 40 min at 261°F | 1.7 | 146 |
| Cooked for 100 min at 279°F | 0.5 | 146 |
| Peanut, raw | 1.93 | 147 |
| Roasted at 160°C for 40 min | 1.7 | 147 |
| Roasted at 180°C for 40 min | 0.2 | 147 |

of conditions for the preparation of edible meals from oilseeds and nuts.[2,3] Guidelines for the preparation of edible meals from soybean, peanut, cottonseed, and sesame have been published by the Protein Advisory Group (PAG) of the United Nations System.[17-20] Brief accounts of the steps involved in the preparation of edible meals from some oilseeds are given below:

Soybean meal

1.  Cleaning and dehulling the seed
2.  Steaming of dehulled, split seeds to inactivate trypsin, growth inhibitors, hemagglutinins, etc.
3.  Drying in a tunnel drier at low temperature (50 to 60°C)
4.  Screw-pressing or solvent extraction for removal of oil
5.  Powdering

Peanut meal

1.  Cleaning of good quality kernels
2.  Light roasting and decuticling
3.  Removal of germ- and fungus-affected kernels
4.  Screw-pressing or solvent extraction for removal of oil
5.  Powdering

Cottonseed meal

1.  Cleaning, delinting, and dehulling
2.  Steaming of the kernels to fix free gossypol in the bound form
3.  Screw-pressing or solvent extraction
4.  Powdering

Sesame meal

1.  Cleaning and dehulling of the seeds
2.  Screw-pressing or solvent extraction to remove oil
3.  Powdering

Table 8
SPECIFICATIONS FOR EDIBLE PEANUT, SESAME, COTTONSEED, AND
SOYA FLOURS SUGGESTED BY THE PROTEIN ADVISORY GROUP[17-20]

|  | Peanut flour | Cottonseed flour | Soya flour (defatted) | Soya flour (full-fat) | Sesame flour (defatted) |
|---|---|---|---|---|---|
| Moisture (% range or max.) | 7.0-11.0 | 10.0 | 12.0 | 10 | 9 |
| Crude fat (% max) | 8.0 | 6.0 | 0.5—3.0 | 18—22 | 1.5 |
| Protein (N × 6.25, % min) | 48.0 | 50.0 | 45.0—52.0 | 38—44 | 50.0 |
| Crude fiber (% max) | 3.5 | — | 3.5 | 3.5 | 6.0 |
| Ash (% max.) | 4.5 | — | 6.0 | 6.0 | 6.2 |
| FFA (% of oil, max.) | 1.0 | 1.8 | — | — | 4.0 |
| Available lysine (G/16 g N, min) | 2.5 | 3.6 | 5.0 | 5.0 | 2.4 |
| Acid insoluble ash (% max) | 0.1 | 0.1 | 0.1 | 0 | — |
| Aflatoxin (μg/kg, max) | 30.0 | 30.0 | 30.0 | 30.0 | — |
| Total bacterial (count/g) | 20,000 | 20,000 | 20,000 | 20,000 | — |
| *Salmonella* | Nil | Nil | Nil | Nil | — |
| *Escherichia coli* | Nil | Nil | Nil | Nil | — |
| Other pathogens | Nil | Nil | Nil | Nil | — |
| Total gossypol (% max) | — | 1.2 | — | — | — |
| Free gossypol (% max) | — | 0.06 | — | — | — |
| Oxalic acid (% of weight, max) | — | — | — | — | 0.5 |

Coconut meal

1.    Drying of coconut meat in a tunnel drier to obtain copra
2.    Removal of oil from copra by screw-pressing or by solvent extraction
3.    Powdering

Specifications for edible-quality flours from peanut, soybean, cottonseed, and sesame suggested by PAG are given in Table 8.

### Protein Isolates from Oilseeds and Nuts

A large amount of work has been carried out by several workers in developing methods for the preparation of protein isolates from oilseeds and nuts.[2,3] The steps involved
in the preparation of protein isolates from soybean or peanut are as follows:

1.    Solvent-extraction of edible soybean or peanut meal to remove oil
2.    Extraction of proteins with dilute sodium hydroxide
3.    Precipitation of the proteins from the extract by the addition of hydrochloric
      acid
4.    Filtration of proteins and washing with water
5.    Solubilizing the wet proteins in water by the addition of sodium hydroxide to
      pH 7.0
6.    Spray-drying

Protein isolates thus obtained have been used in the preparation of food formulations suitable for feeding infants and preschool children.[2,3]

## INFANT FOODS AND MILK SUBSTITUTES FROM OILSEEDS AND NUTS

The per capita production of milk in the developing countries is low.[7] To overcome the milk shortage, attempts have been made from very early times in China and other Asian countries to use milk substitutes based on soybean as a supplement to the diets of infants and children.[21-23] During recent years, a considerable amount of work has been carried out in different countries on the production and nutritional evaluation of milk substitutes based on soybean, peanut, coconut, and other oilseeds.[21-23] In view of the fact that oilseeds and nuts are being produced in large amounts in the developing countries (Table 1), there is the potential for manufacturing milk substitutes on a large scale to make up for the milk shortage. A brief account of the results thus far obtained on the processing and nutritive value of milk substitutes is given below.

### Infant Foods and Milk Substitutes from Soybeans
*Methods of Preparation*

Soy milk — A number of patents and processes for the preparation of soybean milk have been described.[21-23] The principle of the earlier methods is as follows: dehusked soybean is soaked in water and mashed with water or soybean flour is mixed with water. The suspension is filtered and the resulting soybean milk is boiled or steamed. Several improvements in the process have been suggested, such as removal of beany flavor and the bitter principle and modifying the flavor by treatment with enzymes, incorporating bacterial cultures, or incorporating of flavoring substances.[22]

The improved hot-water process minimizes the development of beany flavor.[23,24] The process consists of the following steps:

1.   The decuticled soybeans are soaked in water at 40 to 45°C for 1 hr.
2.   The soaked beans are mashed in boiling water in the proportion of 9 parts water to 1 part soybeans.
3.   The mash is filtered and carbohydrates (sucrose, liquid glucose) at 4% level, buffer salts (sodium and potassium phosphate), and minerals (calcium and iron salts) are added.
4.   The milk is boiled for 1 hr to destroy trypsin inhibitors, hemagglutinins, and bacteria present, and is fortified with vitamins.

The product can be used as such for feeding infants.

Dried soybean milk — A considerable amount of work has been carried out by various workers on the preparation of dried soy milk. The chemical composition of some of these products is given in Table 9. These products are being marketed in the U.S. under various trade names such as Soyalac®, Mullsoy®, etc.[25] Dean[21] developed a process for the preparation of a dried malted soy milk. A method for the preparation of dried soy milk from decuticled soybean using a hot-water extraction step has been developed by Hand et al.[23] A process for the preparation of spray-dried infant food based on soybean has been developed by Shurpalekar et al.[26] Specifications for the composition of milk substitutes and toned milk suggested by the PAG[27] are given in Tables 10 and 11.

Large-scale production — De[28] has given an account of the large-scale production of soybean milk (as fluid or dried milk) in some countries. Two Hong Kong plants have been reported to produce 12,000 cases (each case containing 24 bottles of 7 oz) of sterilized liquid soy milk daily. A plant in Indonesia has been reported to produce daily nearly 3t of dried food based on a blend of soybeans and sesame. In Manila a soybean milk plant is producing about 10,000 bottles per day. Bottled soybean milk is also sold in Bangkok and Singapore. The government of Thailand has established units for the production of soybean milk. Several units for the production of sterilized soy milk have been established at Taiwan. Dried soy milk products are being manufactured and marketed in Japan (Proton®) and in the U.S. (Soybee®, Mull Soy® and Soy-alac®).

Table 9

CHEMICAL COMPOSITION OF INFANT FOODS BASED ON CERTAIN OILSEEDS AND NUTS

| | Protein (N ×6.25, g) | Fat (g) | Carbohydrates (g) | Calcium (g) | Phosphorus (g) | Iron (mg) | Thiamine (mg) | Riboflavin (mg) | Niacin (mg) | Vitamin A (IU) | Vitamin D (IU) | Ref. |
|---|---|---|---|---|---|---|---|---|---|---|---|---|
| Infant food based on peanut protein isolate and skim milk powder | 26.2 | 18.4 | 47.3 | 0.95 | 0.73 | — | 0.9 | 1.5 | 6.0 | 1500 | 400 | 46 |
| Infant food based on peanut flour and skim milk powder | 26.1 | 18.2 | 48.2 | 0.94 | 0.60 | 5.2 | 0.6 | 1.0 | 6.0 | 1500 | 400 | 49 |
| Infant food based on soybean | 26.8 | 17.8 | 46.8 | 0.92 | 0.82 | 5.8 | 0.9 | 1.4 | 5.7 | 1450 | 380 | 26 |
| Infant food based on coconut honey, peanut protein isolate, and skim milk powder | 26.5 | 18.2 | 47.0 | 0.59 | 0.73 | — | 0.8 | 1.5 | 6.2 | 1500 | — | 62 |
| Infant food based on soy and peanut protein isolate | 26.4 | 18.2 | 47.2 | 0.95 | 0.75 | 6.0 | 0.9 | 1.5 | 6.0 | 1480 | 390 | 48 |
| Protein food based on peanut protein isolate and skim milk powder | 35.2 | 1.8 | 53.7 | 1.42 | 0.98 | — | 0.94 | 1.53 | 6.2 | 1500 | 400 | 47 |
| Full-fat milk powder | 26.4 | 27.5 | 38.2 | 0.91 | 0.71 | 0.5 | 0.29 | 1.46 | 0.7 | 1130 | — | 62 |

Note:  Values per 100 g.

Table 10
RECOMMENDED CHEMICAL COMPOSITION OF MILK
SUBSTITUTE[27]

|  | Fluid, sterilized | Dry |
|---|---|---|
| Moisture (%, max) | 89.0 | 3.5 |
| Fat (%, min) | 2.0 | 18.0 |
| Nonfat solids (%, min) | 9.0 | 78.5 |
| Protein (N × 6.25) (%, min) | 3.5 | 28.0 |
| Essential fatty acid content, expressed as linoleic acid as percent of weight of fat (min) | 2.0 | 2.0 |
| Carbohydrates (sucrose or malt sugar-dextrin, %) | 4.0 min | 51.5 max |
| Calcium (mg/100 m*l* or 100 g, min) | 100 | 800 |
| Vitamin A (μg/100 m*l* or 100 g, min) | 50 | 450 |
| Vitamin D (IU/100 m*l* or 100 g, min) | 40 | 360 |
| Iron (mg/100 m*l* or 100 g, min) | 0.4 | 4.0 |
| Thiamine (mg/100 m*l* or 100 g, min) | 0.15 | 1.0 |
| Riboflavin (mg/100 m*l* or 100 g, min) | 0.15 | 1.3 |
| Niacin (mg/100 m*l* or 100 g, min) | 1.0 | 8.0 |
| Folic acid (μg/100 m*l* or 100 g, min) | 5 | 50.0 |
| Pathothenic acid (μg/100 m*l* or 100 g, min) | 200 | 1600 |
| Vitamin $B_{12}$ (μg/100 m*l* or 100 g, min) | 0.5 | 5.0 |
| Pyridoxin (μg/100m *l* or 100 g, min) | 200 | 1600 |
| Ascorbic acid (mg/100 m*l* or 100 g, min) | 3.0 | 25.0 |
| Total ash (max) | — | 7.0 |
| Acid-insoluble ash (max) | — | 0.05 |

Table 11
RECOMMENDED CHEMICAL COMPOSITION OF TONED MILK
CONTAINING VEGETABLE PROTEIN[27]

|  | Fluid, sterilized | Dry |
|---|---|---|
| Moisture (%, max) | 89 | 3.5 |
| Fat (%, min) | 2 | 18.0 |
| Nonfat solids (%, min) | 9 | 78.5 |
| Carbohydrates (lactose/sucrose and malt sugar-dextrin, %) | 4.0 min | 35.0 min |
|  | 8.0 max | (lactose 12.0 in) |
| Protein (N × 6.25) (%, min) | 3.5 | 20.0 |
| Essential fatty acid content, expressed as linoleic aid per cent of fat (min) | 2.0 | 2.0 |
| Total ash (max) | — | 7.0 |
| Acid-insoluble (max) | — | 0.05 |

## Nutritive Value of Soybean Milk and Soybean Milk Proteins

Animal experiments — Desikachar et al.[29] reported a digestibility coefficient of 91 and biological value of 79 for the proteins of soybean milk. Chang and Murray[30] found PER values of 1.9 and 1.7 for the proteins of soy milk and curd, respectively. Shurpalekar et al.[26] reported a PER of 2.47 for soy milk proteins and 2.92 for soy milk fortified with DL-methionine as compared with 3.00 for cow's milk. Howard et al.[31] found that a soybean infant food supplemented with iron and vitamins promoted good growth, reproduction, and lactation over three generations of albino rats, comparing well with the performance of rats on a milk food fortified with iron and copper. They also found that dried infant foods based on soybean promoted good growth in rats over a period of 8 weeks comparing well with a milk food of similar composition.

**Treatment of protein malnutrition in children** — Dean[32] found that soybean milk was highly effective in the treatment of protein malnutrition in children. Bhagavan et al.[33] treated cases of protein malnutrition with milk reconstituted from spray dried infant foods based on soybean and a mixture of soybean and peanut protein isolates. They found the above foods to be almost as effective as milk in the treatment of protein malnutrition in children.

### Feeding Experiments with Infants and Children

Tso[34] fed infants successfully with soybean milk and found that they grew well and put on weight, just like breast-fed infants. Rittinger and Dembo[35] fed 50 infants for a period of 1 year on soybean milk with the addition of sugar and various salts, and they concluded that soybean milk is an adequate food for infants. Guy and Yeh[36] supplemented soybean milk with calcium, vitamin C, and cod liver oil and used it successfully for infant feeding.

Desikachar and Subrahmanyan[37] conducted feeding experiments with soybean milk on infants and toddlers. The results showed that toddlers grew somewhat better on cow's milk than on soybean milk, though the difference was not considerable. The infants, however, responded much better to soybean milk than cow's milk. They also conducted feeding trials with 30 infants in another institution. The results showed that all the infants digested the soybean milk easily and they all put on weight. No digestive disorders were observed.

Dean[21] conducted a feeding trial in infants and preschool children with malted soybean milk powder. The results showed that half the cow's milk in the diet of infants (up to 12 months old) could be replaced by malted soybean milk without affecting their growth. He also found that there was scarcely any difference between the growth rate of preschool children receiving a supplement of cow's milk and those receiving malted soybean milk containing 10% skim milk solids. Glaser and Johnstone[38] reported that infants fed a soybean formula (Mull Soy®) from the first month until 5 to 9 months of age showed satisfactory growth. Collins-Williams[39] found that infants fed a soybean formula (Soybee®) showed satisfactory weight gains. Fomon[40] reported that infants grew well when fed soybean milk providing 1.7 g protein per kilogram body weight, and the nitrogen retention was satisfactory, comparing well with infants receiving human milk. Omans et al.[41] found that out of three commercial soybean milk preparations tested, one promoted nearly as good growth as a cow's milk food while two proved inferior when fed as the sole food to premature infants.

### Milk Substitutes and Infant Foods from Peanut
*Methods of Preparation*

**Peanut milk** — Moorjani and Subrahmanyan[42] described a method for the preparation of peanut milk fortified with vitamins and minerals, consisting of the following steps:

1.    Grinding to a paste of the decuticled peanut kernels
2.    Addition of six times the weight of water and mechanical mixing for the formation of milk
3.    Filtration and addition of calcium hydroxide and buffer salts to adjust the pH to 6.8
4.    Fortification with calcium salts and vitamins
5.    Steaming for 30 min

The resulting product sweetened with cane sugar was highly acceptable to the consumers.

Mitchell and Birmingham[43] prepared a milk-like product from peanuts by grinding the nuts with water and passing the mixture through a colloid mill. They recommended the addition of $Na_2HPO_4$ and small quantities of sodium alginate, vegetable gum, or gelatin to improve the stability of the emulsions.

Moorjani[44] described a process for the preparation of peanut milk free from nutty odor by emulsifying a suspension of finely powdered, solvent-extracted peanut cake in water with refined peanut oil and lecithin in a colloid mill.

**Toned vegetable milk** — A process for the preparation of a toned vegetable milk (Miltone) based on a blend of peanut protein isolate, liquid glucose, and buffalo milk has been developed at the Central Food Technological Research Institute (CFTRI), Mysore.[45] Guidelines for the preparation of toned milk containing vegetable proteins are given by the PAG[27] and the specifications suggested by the PAG for its chemical composition are given in Table 11. Large-scale production of Miltone in developing countries may help to overcome the present acute shortage of milk.

**Infant foods** — A process for the preparation of a spray-dried infant food based on peanut protein isolate, hydrogenated vegetable fat, malto-dextrin, and skim milk powder, fortified with essential vitamins and minerals, has been described by Subrahmanyan et al.[46] The same workers[47] have described a similar process for the preparation of spray-dried protein food having a low-fat content based on peanut protein isolate, malto-dextrin, and skim milk powder. Shurpalekar et al.[48] described a process for the preparation of spray-dried infant food based on peanut protein isolate and soybeans.

A process for the preparation of an infant food based on a blend of low-fat peanut flour, gelatinized wheat flour, skim milk powder, hydrogenated peanut oil, and cane sugar also has been developed.[49] In this process, the starch present in peanut and wheat is converted into dextrin and maltose by the action of barley malt diastase. The product has been fortified with essential vitamins and minerals. The data regarding the chemical composition of the above infant foods are given in Table 9.

## Nutritive Value of Peanut Milk and its Proteins

The PER of peanut milk proteins has been found to be 1.8. Peanut milk fortified with calcium salts and vitamins promoted good growth in albino rats, comparing well with cow's milk.[50] An infant food based on peanut protein isolate and skim milk powder had a PER of 2.35. This food also promoted good growth in albino rats.[51] The PER of an infant food based on peanut protein isolate and soybean was found to be 2.19, and the value increased to 2.68 on fortification with DL-methionine, as compared with 3.00 for cow's milk. A mixture of infant food and cane sugar in the 3:1 ratio promoted good growth in albino rats, comparing well with a milk food of similar composition.[52]

## Feeding Trials with Infants and Children

Subrahmanyan et al.[53] found that a daily supplement of 12 oz of peanut milk curds (lactic fermented milk) to undernourished school children brought about a highly significant increase in their growth and nutritional status over a period of 6 months. Hanafy et al.[54] found that infants below 4 months of age did not grow well, while those of the age group of 4 to 8 months showed moderate growth and those over 8 months of age showed good growth when fed on peanut milk (not fortified with vitamins and minerals). Doraiswamy et al.[55] reported that there was no significant difference in the growth rates of two groups of infants aged 3 to 12 months, one fed on infant food based on cow's milk and the other on a mixture of peanut protein isolate and skim milk powder. A feeding trial with weaned infants and preschool children

Table 12

MEAN INCREASES IN HEIGHT AND WEIGHT
OF INFANTS ON PEANUT INFANT FOOD AND
MILK FOOD[58]

| Subjects | Initial | Final | Increase ± SE |
|---|---|---|---|
| **Height (cm)** | | | |
| Children on peanut infant food | 64.39 | 74.75 | 10.36 ± 0.384[a] |
| Children on milk food | 63.47 | 73.56 | 10.09 ± 0.483[a] |
| **Weight (kg)** | | | |
| Children on peanut infant food | 6.41 | 8.39 | 1.98 ± 0.176[a] |
| Children on milk food | 6.06 | 7.88 | 1.82 + 0.213[a] |

*Note:* Duration of experiment was 10 months, 12 infants 6 months of age per group.

[a]   Differences not significant (*t* test).

extending over a period of 4½ months showed that supplementation of their daily diet with 30 g of spray-dried protein food based on peanut protein isolate and skim milk powder brought about significant increases in height, weight, and hemoglobin content of the blood as compared with the control group.[56] This food has been found to be highly effective in the treatment of protein malnutrition in children.[57] Pereira et al.[58] found that there were no significant differences in the height and weight increases of two groups of infants (aged 6 months) fed on an infant food based on peanut flour and a milk food for a period of 10 months (Table 12).

### Coconut Milk and Products Based on Coconut Milk

Coconut has a low-protein content (on dry basis) as compared with other oilseeds. It is, nevertheless, an important additional source of protein in certain countries, e.g., the Philippines, Indonesia, Ceylon, and the West Indies where protein malnutrition is widely prevalent. The term "coconut milk" is used below to describe a milk-like emulsion obtained by pressing a suspension of grated, fresh coconut kernel in water — not to mean "coconut water" contained in fresh coconut.

De and Subrahmanyan[59] and Varadarajan[60] found that coconut milk obtained from the fresh kernel had low-protein and high-fat contents. Moorjani[61] prepared milk from coconuts of varying degrees of maturity, i.e., tender, moderately mature, and dry (copra). Tender and moderately mature coconuts yielded milk of agreeable flavor and taste, while the milk from copra had an oily taste. They found that a blend of coconut milk and peanut milk had a satisfactory protein content and was more stable than coconut milk.

Chandrasekhara et al.[62] have described a process for the preparation of an infant food based on evaporated skimmed coconut milk (known as "coconut honey"), peanut protein isolate, skim milk powder, malto-dextrin, and hydrogenated fat. Rama Rao et al.[63] found a 3:1 blend of the infant food and cane sugar promoted good growth in rats, and incorporation of the food at 20% level in a low-protein, maize-tapioca diet made up the protein deficiency in the diet and promoted good growth in rats.

## MILK SUBSTITUTES BASED ON OTHER NUTS AND OILSEEDS

Comparatively less work has been carried out on milk substitutes from other oilseeds and nuts. The available data are summarized below.

**Almond milk** — Stockert and Grunsterdt[64] described a process for the preparation of milk from sweet almonds. Ujesaghy[65] found that the retention of nitrogen and sulfur from almond milk in healthy infants was of the same order as that from cow's milk. Chapin[6] used successfully almond milk for feeding infants. Hesse[67] reported that almond milk was effective in the treatment of infantile eczema.

**Cashewnut milk** — Desikachar[68] described a process for the preparation of cashewnut milk. The stability of the milk was poor. He found a mixture of equal amounts of cashewnut milk and cow's milk was stable. Moorjani[61] succeeded in stabilizing cashewnut milk by the addition of 0.5 to 1% casein and adjusting the pH to 6.8 to 7.0 or by blending with 25 to 50% peanut flour or whole peanut followed by the hydrolysis of the starch by diastase. The milk thus obtained contained 3.3% protein and 5.4% fat.

## PROTEIN FOODS BASED ON OILSEED MEALS AND ISOLATES

A considerable amount of work has been carried out in many countries during recent years on the utilization of specially processed, low-fat oilseed flours to supplement the diets of and to treat protein malnutrition in children.[5,6] Among the oilseed meals, the most important are those derived from soybean, peanut, cottonseed, sesame, sunflower seed, and coconut. Oilseed meals are rich sources of proteins and certain B vitamins but are deficient in calcium and riboflavin. They do not contain vitamins A, D, and $B_{12}$. Data regarding the composition and protein contents of some processed protein foods based on different oilseed meals are given in Table 13.

### Supplements Based on Soybean Meal

Procssed low-fat soybean meals suitable for human consumption are being manufactured in large quantities in the U.S. for use as supplements to human diets.[2] A protein food consisting of toasted soy grits fortified with essential vitamins and minerals was developed in the U.S. This was known as multipurpose food and was distributed in several developing countries for the treatment of malnutrition in children.[69] Cooper and Bryan[70] reported that daily supplementation of the diets of school children with 1 oz of a protein food for a period of 5 months produced a marked increase in the weight of the experimental subjects.

Krishnamurthy et al.[71] have developed processed protein foods based on blends of soybean, peanut, sesame, and chickpea flours. Sure[72] prepared a low-cost composite protein food containing soybean. Gomez et al.[73] successfully treated protein malnutrition in children with a soy preparation. Doraiswamy et al.[74] reported that a daily supplement of 40 g of a protein food based on 1:1 blend of soybean and peanut flours for a period of 6 months brought about highly significant increases in the height and weight of children aged 5 to 11 years' as compared with the control group receiving an isocaloric rice supplement. Other food supplements containing soybean flour developed in the U.S. and some countries include Cerealina, Fortifex, Ceplapro, C.S.M., W.S.B., and Pronutro.[75-78] Their composition and protein contents are given in Table 13. These foods have been found to be effective in overcoming protein-calorie malnutrition in children.

### Supplements Based on Peanut Meal

In recent years a considerable amount of work has been carried out in several coun-

Table 13
## SUPPLEMENTARY FOODS FOR WEANED INFANTS AND PRESCHOOL CHILDREN

| Product | Country | Composition | Protein content (%) | Ref. |
|---|---|---|---|---|
| Multipurpose food | India | Peanut and chickpea flours with calcium carbonate and vitamins | 42.5 | 81 |
| Protein food I | India | Peanut and soy flours (1:1) fortified with calcium carbonate and vitamins | 47.8 | 74 |
| Protein food II | India | Soya, peanut and coconut flours fortified with calcium carbonate and vitamins | 31.9 | 102 |
| Balanced malt food | India | Cereal malt, peanut and chickpea flours, skim milk powder, calcium carbonate, and vitamins | 31.9 | 79 |
| Enriched macaroni | India | Wheat, cassava, peanut and chickpea flours, calcium carbonate, and vitamins | 18.0 | 118 |
| Nutro biscuits | India | Wheat flour, peanut flour, and peanut protein isolate, calcium carbonate, and vitamins | 16.5 | 113 |
| Balahar | India | Cereal flour, peanut and chickpea flours, calcium carbonate, and vitamins | 22.5 | 88 |
| Incaparina | Guatemala | Maize, cottonseed flour, vitamin A, lysine, and calcium carbonate | 27.5 | 91 |
| Fortifex | Brazil | Maize, defatted soya flour, vitamins A, $B_1$, and $B_2$, DL-methionine, and calcium carbonate | 30.0 | 76 |
| Cerealina | Brazil | Full-fat soybean flour, corn starch, skim milk powder, vitamins, and minerals | 20.0 | 75 |
| Argentirina | Argentina | Sorghum, wheat, peanut, and white bean flour fortified with minerals and vitamins | 27.8 | 76 |
| Peruvita | Peru | Quinua and cottonseed flour, skim milk powder, sugar, spices, calcium carbonate, vitamins A, $B_1$, and $B_2$ | 30.0 | 92 |
| Multipurpose Food | U.S. | Soya grits fortified with vitamins and minerals | 48.2 | 69 |
| Ceplapro | U.S. | Degerminated maize flour, wheat, defatted soya, skim milk powder, calcium carbonate, and vitamins | 20.0 | 77 |
| CSM | U.S. | Maize (precooked), defatted soya flour, skim milk powder, calcium carbonate, and vitamins | 20.0 | 78 |
| WSB | U.S. | Wheat, soybean flour and calcium slats and vitamins | 20.0 | 78 |
| Pronutro | South Africa | Maize, skim milk powder, peanut, soya, FPC, Yeast, wheat germ, vitamins A, $B_1$, and $B_2$ niacin, and sugar iodized salt | 22.0 | 76 |
| Aliment de Sevrage | Senegal | Millet flour, peanut flour, skim milk powder, sugar, vitamin A, and calcium salts | 20.0 | 76 |
| Protein-rich biscuits | Uganda | Wheat, peanut and skim milk powder, and vitamins | 20.0 | 112 |
| Arlac | Nigeria | Peanut flour and skim milk powder | 40.2 | 84 |

tries on the utilization of low-fat peanut flour as a supplement to the diets of children.[5,6] Low-fat peanut flour has been used in the preparation of soup powder, balanced food, nutro biscuits, low-cost malt foods, Indian multipurpose food, and Balahar.[79] Harris et al.[80] developed a dehydrated soup powder containing peanut flour, soy flour, precooked pea flour, and skim milk powder, together with added flavor and condiments and fortified with essential minerals and vitamins. Supplementation of the

Table 14
INCREASES IN HEIGHT, WEIGHT,
HEMOGLOBIN, AND RED BLOOD CELL
(RBC) COUNT OF CHILDREN FED RICE
DIET AND RICE-MPF DIET[82]

|  | Mean increase | |
|---|---|---|
|  | Rice diet (control) | Rice-MPF[a] diet (experimental) |
| Height (cm) | 0.07 | 2.44 |
| Weight (kg) | 0.45 | 1.19 |
| Hemoglobin (g/100 m$l$) | 0.13 | 1.00 |
| RBC ($10^6$/mm$^3$) | 0.17 | 0.33 |

*Note:* Duration of experiment was 5 months. Each group comprised of 23 girls, age 4—12 years.

[a]   Each child received daily 56 g of MPF.

diets of school children with 30 g of soup powder daily brought about a considerable improvement in their nutritional status. Parpia et al.[81] standardized a method for the large-scale production of Indian multipurpose food (Indian MPF), consisting of a blend of 75 parts of processed peanut flour and 25 parts of chickpea flour fortified with vitamins and minerals. The product was found to be an effective supplement to the diets of children bringing about marked improvement in their growth rate and nutritional status (Table 14).[82]

Purushothama Rao[83] successfully treated cases of kwashiorkor in children with Indian multipurpse food. A 3:1 blend of peanut flour and skim milk powder (known as Arlac) has been found effective in the treatment of protein malnutrition in children.[84] Senecal[85] reported that supplementation of the diets of children suffering from mild kwashiorkor with a 1:1 blend of millet and peanut flour with or without small amounts of fish flour brought about improvement in their growth and clinical symptoms. De Mayer and Vanderborght,[86] as a result of investigations on the supplementation of the basal diet with skim milk or mixtures of peanut flour with beans or soybean flour to children convalescing from kwashiorkor, concluded that a mixture of beans and peanuts produced a slightly better nitrogen retention in children than a mixture of soybean and peanut flours. Both the blends, however, were inferior to skim milk powder in the above respects.

Peanut flour fortified with vitamins and minerals markedly supplemented the diets of children, bringing about significant improvements in their growth rate and nutritional status.[87] Low-cost protein foods (Balahar) based on blends of cereal, oilseed, and legume flours and fortified with essential vitamins and minerals have been developed by Daniel et al.[88] A daily supplement of 50 g of Balahar based on a blend of sorghum, peanut, and chickpea flours brought about highly significant improvements in the growth rate and nutritional status of children over a period of 6 months.[89] These foods will be suitable for use as supplements to the diets of preschool children in the developing countries.

## Supplements Based on Cottonseed Flour

Low-fat cottonseed flour obtained by expressing dehulled cottonseed kernels in a screw press followed by solvent extraction of the meal, is rich in proteins (40 to 45%)

and can be used in the preparation of processed protein foods.[90] Cottonseed flour suffers from the defect that it contains gossypol which is toxic to animals. Technological developments, however, have resulted in the production of edible cottonseed flour containing proteins of high nutritive value and with low free and total gossypol contents. Scrimshaw and Bressani[91] developed a vegetable mixture known as INCAP mixture 9B containing specially prepared cottonseed flour. The mixture contained corn (29 parts), sorghum (29 parts) cottonseed flour (38 parts), dry torula yeast (3 parts), calcium carbonate (1 part), and vitamin A (4500 IU). This food was found to be very effective in the treatment of kwashiorkor in children. The product under the name of Incaparina is at present being produced on a large scale and distributed for feeding preschool children in Guatemala. Two protein-food formulations based on cottonseed flour, wheat flour, quina flour, alfalfa leaf meal, and torula yeast have been developed for use in Peru by Bradfield.[92] Graham et al.[93] reported that a blend of cottonseed flour and wheat flour was quite effective in curing kwashiokor and marasmus in preschool children.

### Supplements Based on Sesame Flour

The use of sesame meal as a protein source in human diets has been hampered to a considerable extent for want of efficient equipment for the large-scale dehulling of the seed before crushing it for oil.[20] The hull, which forms about 12% of the seed, is rich in fiber and oxalates and contains bitter principles. Hence, it must be removed for preparing edible meal. Processes for the removal of the hull have been described.[94-96]

Behar et al.[97] have used whole sesame flour for the preparation of vegetable protein mixture for the treatment of protein malnutrition. INCAP mixture 8 developed by the above workers consisted of a blend of corn masa (50 parts), sesame flour (35 parts), cottonseed flour (9 parts), torula yeast (3 parts), and kikuyu leaf (3 parts). The food was found to be quite effective in the treatment of kwashiorkor.

Protein-food formulations based on blends of sesame, soybean, chickpea, and peanut flours and fortified with essential vitamins and minerals have been developed in India.[98] Doraiswamy et al.[99] reported that a daily supplement of 50 g of a protein food based on a blend of sesame, chickpea, and peanut flours over a period of 6 months brought about highly significant increases in height and weight of children aged 5 to 11 years as compared with an isocaloric control group.

### Supplements Based on Conconut Meal

Edible coconut meal contains about 20 to 25% proteins. As it contains excessive amounts of fiber, it can be used only in small amounts (10 to 20%) as a supplement to human diets.[2,100] Edible coconut meal fortified with vitamins and minerals has been found to be an excellent supplement to poor Indian diets when incorporated at 15 to 18% levels to provide about 2% extra proteins.[101] Krishnamurthy et al.[100] standardized the conditions for the preparation of a protein food from a blend of coconut meal (25 parts), peanut flour (50 parts), and chick pea flour (25 parts) fortified with vitamins and minerals. Animal experiments and feeding trials on children have shown that this food has significant supplementary value to poor Indian diets.

A protein-food formulation based on blends of coconut, soybean, and peanut meals and fortified with essential vitamins and minerals has been developed in India.[102] Doraiswamy et al.[103] found that a daily supplement of 50 g of such protein food over a period of 6 months brought about a highly significant improvement in the growth and nutritional status of children aged 5 to 11 years subsisting on poor-quality diets as compared with an isocaloric control group.

**Sunflower Seed Meal**

Processes for the preparation of sunflower seed meal were standardized by some workers.[104,105] The PER of the proteins of the sunflower seed meal has been reported to be 2.57. A weaning food formulation based on blends of sunflower seed meal, rice flour, malt extract, and sugar fortified with calcium carbonate was reported to promote good growth in weaned infants.[106] Weaning food formulations based on blends of sunflower seed meal, chickpea, and wheat flours were developed in Algeria.[107]

## OTHER PROCESSED PRODUCTS BASED ON OILSEEDS AND NUTS AND THEIR MEALS

Several other processed products based on oilseeds and nuts are consumed in different parts of the world. Studies have also been carried out on the development of enriched biscuits, bread, and macaroni products and on the use of peanut flour for enriching tapioca flour. The nutritive vaues of some of these products are summarized below.

### Products Based on Peanut and Peanut Flour

**Roasted decuticled peanuts** — Roasted decuticled peanuts are consumed widely all over the world. They have the disadvantage that they cannot be easily consumed by weaned infants and preschool children.[108]

**Peanut butter** — Peanut butter is manufactured on a large scale in the U.S. and is used as a supplement to human diets. Peanut butter has been reported to be quite effective in the treatment of protein malnutrition in children.[109]

**Peanut candies** — Candies based on peanut kernel and sugars are rich sources of protein and calories.[110] The traditional candy preparations based on roasted peanut and jaggery (crude cane sugar) are prepared on home or cottage scale in India and consumed quite extensively. Peanut candies prepared from broken peanut kernel and sugar have been successfully used in the treatment of protein malnutrition in children.[111]

**Peanut biscuits** — Peanut biscuits based on peanut, wheat flour, and skim milk powder and containing 20% proteins have been effective in the treatment of protein malnutrition in children.[112] Nutro biscuits containing 16 to 17% proteins have been prepared from blends of peanut flour and wheat flour fortified with vitamins and minerals.[113] These biscuits have been found to be effective in curing mild cases of protein malnutrition.[114]

### Enriched Tapioca Flour and Macaroni Products

Peanut flour can be used for enriching tapioca flour, which is very low in protein content. These blends can also be processed into macaroni-type products. In addition to contributing protein to the diet, such foods provide extra calories. In several developing areas where tapioca is grown and consumed in large quantities these blends have helped to overcome protein malnutrition among preschool children in Africa, Latin America, Mexico, Indonesia, and Kerala State in India.[115]

A mixture of 25 parts of peanut flour and 75 parts of tapioca (cassava) flour known as Mysore flour, having a protein content of 12% has been used as a partial substitute for cereals in large scale feeding in famine-affected areas of South India. Feeding trials carried out for 6 months on girls aged 6 to 10 years showed that 50% of cereals in their diets could be replaced by an equal quantity of Mysore flour without significantly affecting the growth, general health, and nutritional status.[116]

Tapioca macaroni has been prepared from a blend of 60 parts tapioca flour, 15 parts peanut flour, and 25 parts wheat semolina. The product cooks readily in 5 to 6 min.

Feeding trials with children (6 to 10 years of age) have shown that rice in their diets could be replaced completely by tapioca macaroni without significantly affecting their growth, general health, and nutritional status.[117] Enriched macaroni products containing about 18 to 19% proteins and fortified with calcium salts and essential vitamins have been prepared from: (1) blends of peanut flour, tapioca flour, chickpea flour, and wheat semolina and (2) wheat semolina (4 parts) and peanut flour (1 part).[118] A daily supplement of 2 oz of enriched tapioca macaroni to diets of weaned infants over a period of 6 months gave a significant increase in their growth and nutritional status as compared with the control group receiving ordinary tapioca macaroni.[119] In another experiment the substitution of enriched wheat macaroni for 50% rice in the basal diet of school children over an equal period resulted in a significant increase in growth and nutritional status.[120]

### Products Based on Soybean and Soybean Meal

**Baked products** — Adding soybean flour to bread at 3 to 5% levels brought about an increased protein content and improved nutritive value of the proteins.[4,121,122] Mizrahi et al.[123] investigated the functional and nutritional properties of bread enriched with soybean protein isolate and calcium-precipitated soy protein. They found that the protein isolate could be incorporated at a level of 6% without impairing loaf volume, taste color, or odor. They also found the PER of the proteins of the enriched bread was higher than that of the control bread.

Soybean flour has also been used to enhance the nutritive value of other baked foods. Reynolds and Hall[124] reported that cakes and pastries supplemented with soybean flour were nutritionally superior to unsupplemented products as judged by increase in growth rate and PER in albino rats. Addition of soybean grits to cookies and crackers markedly improved the nutritive value of their proteins.[125]

**Macaroni products** — Paulsen[126] reported that addition of soy flour at levels varying from 12.5 to 25.0% markedly improved the nutritive value and cooking quality of different macaroni products.

**Tofu** — Tofu is an important processed product prepared from soybean and consumed extensively in Japan. It is available in different forms, e.g., fresh, dried, and fried tofu. Fresh tofu contains about 6% proteins and 88% water while dried tofu contains about 56% proteins and 8% water.

To prepare tofu, soybean milk is first treated with coagulating agents like calcium sulfate, and the mixture is warmed to about 65°C. The proteins are precipitated in the form of curd. This curd is filtered and pressed to remove adhering water.

Fresh tofu thus obtained is consumed as such or converted into dried or fried tofu.[127] Feeding experiments with weaned infants have shown that diets containing tofu as the sole protein source promoted good growth in infants who maintained positive N balance and good health.[128]

**Natto** — This product, which resembles cheese, is prepared by cooking soybeans in boiling water for about 5 hr. The cooked beans are inoculated with *Bacillus natto* culture at 60°C, wrapped in paddy straw, and allowed to undergo fermentation at 40 to 45°C for about 24 hr. The fresh, fermented product is consumed as such and has also been dried and consumed in powder form.[4]

Fresh natto contains about 18% proteins and 56% water. Studies with young albino rats have shown that a diet containing 10% proteins (6% from natto and 4% from rice) promoted good growth over a period of 80 days.[129] Muto et al.[128] reported that natto could replace part of the milk in infant diets without affecting the growth rate and N retention. Biscuits containing natto were well accepted by children.[130]

**Tempeh** — This product, consumed extensively in Indonesia, is prepared by inoculating cooked soybeans with *Aspergillus oryzae*. The mycelium is allowed to grow for

24 to 48 hr, after which the product is roasted, fried in oil, or sliced and dried.[4] Studies with albino rats have shown that the PER of tempeh proteins is similar to that of processed soybean flour.[131]

## Foods Based on Protein Isolates from Peanut and Soybean

Protein isolates have some advantage over the parent raw materials insofar as they are free from: (1) insoluble and indigestible carbohydrates, which may swell and interfere with protein digestion, especially in young children, and (2) natural odoriferous and bitter principles, growth inhibitors, and other interfering materials normally present in the seed meals, which may affect palatability, digestibility, and nutritive value. Further, isolated proteins are two to four times as concentrated as seed meals, and they possess bland taste and can be easily blended to increase the protein content of other foodstuffs without imparting any flavor of their own.[2,3] Recent investigations have shown that protein isolates from peanut and soybean can be used in the preparation of protein foods suitable for feeding infants and children and for treating protein malnutrition in children.[2,3,5]

### Products Based on Peanut Protein Isolate

**High-protein food** — This food is a blend of 85 parts peanut protein isolate and 15 parts chickpea flour, fortified with essential vitamins and minerals. The product has been prepared in unseasoned form flavored with vanillin and in seasoned form with 3% seasoning premix and 3% common salt. High-protein food contains about 80% protein and adequate amounts of other essential nutrients.[132] Studies on albino rats showed that high-protein food incorporated in poor rice and maize-tapioca diets provided 5 and 15% extra proteins, respectively, and brought about highly significant increases in the growth rates. This food's fairly high protein and nutritive values were evidenced by respective PER values of 1.92 and 2.11 in a 4-week period at 10 and 15% protein levels.[133] A 6-month feeding trial with preschool children showed that a daily supplement of 1 oz of high-protein food brought about a highly significant improvement in their weight, height, and nutritional status as compared to a control group.[134]

**Infant foods and toned milk** — Peanut protein isolate has been used in the preparation of infant foods and toned vegetable milk,[45] as described in the section above.

### Products Based on Soy Protein Isolate

During recent years processes for the preparation of edible soybean protein isolate have been developed by several workers.[2,3] This protein isolate has been used for the preparation of infant foods and textured food products.[135]

**Infant foods** — An infant food containing soy protein isolate has been prepared and tested in infants by Cherry et al.[136] The food promoted good growth, but it was somewhat inferior to an infant food based on cow's milk. There were, however, no significant differences in the levels of serum protein, free amino acids, cholesterol, hemoglobin, and red blood cells between the two groups of infants. Cowan[137] reported a lower incidence of anal irritation in infants receiving formula containing soy protein isolate than that observed in infants receiving formula based on soybean flour.

**Textured food products** — Extensive studies have been carried out in recent years on the development of textured foods from soy protein isolates simulating ground beef, ham, fish, etc. Bressani et al.[138] reported that the PER of a textured food based on soy protein and supplemented with egg albumin, wheat gluten, flavoring, and coloring was 2.30 as compared with 2.34 for natural, dehydrated beef. Studies with children showed that the protein quality of the textured product was about 80% that of milk. In another study Hodges and Koury[139] found that adult human subjects receiving diets containing textured soy protein products maintained good health and positive nitrogen balance over a period of 24 weeks.

Kies and Fox[140] conducted a controlled nitrogen-balance study with adults in order to compare the protein quality of a textured soy protein food (TSP) with the natural beef. Mean nitrogen balances of subjects receiving 8 g nitrogen per head per day on the TSP and beef diets were 0.74 and 0.78 g/day, respectively.

## CONCLUSION

It is evident from the foregoing account that large-scale production and distribution of processed supplementary foods based on oilseeds, nuts, and their meals will help to overcome malnutrition and improve the health of weaned infants and preschool children in the developing countries. The present author, while discussing the critical food problem facing the world, has suggested that the shortage in the supply of protein-rich and protective foods in the developing countries could be made up by the use of processed protein foods based on oilseeds and nuts and low-fat meals derived from them.[141] The need for the utilization of oilseed meals in the production of supplementary foods for the vulnerable sections of the populations has also been stressed in a United Nations report, "International Action to Avert the Impending Protein Crisis".[1]

## REFERENCES

1. **Protein Advisory Group, United Nations,** International Action to Avert the Impending Protein Crisis, E.1443/Rev. I, United Nations, New York, 1968.
2. **Altschul, A. M., Ed.,** *Processed Plant Protein Foodstuffs,* Academic Press, New York, 1958.
3. **Smith, A. K and Circle, S. J., Ed.,** *Soybeans: Chemistry and Technology,* Vol. 1 AVI Publishing, Westport, Conn., 1972.
4. **Abott, J. C.,** in *World Protein Resources,* Gould, R. F., Ed., American Chemical Society, Washington, D.C., 1966, 1.
5. **Food and Nutrition Board, National Research Council-National Academy of Sciences,** in *Progress in Meeting Protein Needs of Infants and Pre-School Children,* Publ. 843, National Academy of Sciences, Washington, D.C., 1961.
6. **Food and Nutrition Board, National Research Council-National Academy of Sciences,** in *Pre-School Child Malnutrition — Primary Deterrent to Human Progress,* Publ. 1282, National Academy of Sciences, Washington, D.C., 1964.
7. **Anon.,** *FAO Production Year Book,* Vol. 28.1, Food and Agricultural Organization of the United Nations, Rome, 1974.
8. **Watt, B. K. and Merrill, A. L.,** Composition of foods—Raw, Processed and Prepared, Agriculture Handbook No. 8, U.S. Department of Agriculture, Washington, D.C., 1963.
9. **Jolliffe, N.,** *Metabolism,* 10, 497, 1961.
10. **Orr, M. L. andd Watt, B K.,** Amino Acid Content of Foods, Home Economics Res. Rep. No. 4, U.S. Department of Agriculture, Washington, D.C., 1957.
11. **Howe, E. E., Jansen, G. R., and Gilfillan, E. W.,** *Am. J. Clin. Nutr.,* 16, 315, 1965.
12. **Venkatrao, S., Joseph, A. A., Swaminathan, M., and Parpia, H. A. B.,** *J. Nutr. Diet.,* 1, 192, 1964.
13. **Liener, E., Ed.,** *Toxic Constituents of Foodstuffs,* Academic Press, New York. 1968.
14. **Sreenivasa Murthy, V., Srikantia, S., and Parpia, H. A. B.,** Indian Patent No. 12057, 1971.
15. **Jaffe, W. G.,** in *The Safety of Foods: Proc. Int. Symp. Safety and Importance of Foods in the Western Hemisphere,* AVI Publishing Westport, Conn., 1968, 38.
16. **Liener, I. E.,** in *Processed Plant Protein Foods* Altschul, A. M., Ed., Academic Press, New York, 1958, 72.
17. **Protein Advisory Group United Nations,** Guideline for preparation of food quality groundnut flour, *PAG Compendium,* C2, 1519, 1975.
18. **Protein Advisory Group, United Nations,** Guideline for edible soy grits and flour, *PAG Compendium,* C2, 1945, 1975.

19. Protein Advisory Group, United Nations, Guideline for preparation of edible cottonseed protein concentrate, *PAG Compendium,* C1, 1137, 1975.
20. Protein Advisory Group, United Nations, Guideline for the preparation of defatted edible sesame flour, *PAG Bull.,* 3(1), 10, 1973.
21. Dean, R. F. A., Plant Proteins in Child Feeding, *Med. Res. Coun. (G.B.) Spec. Rep. Ser.,* No. 279, 1953.
22. Anon., Milk Substitutes of Vegetable Origin, Special Rep. Ser., No. 31, Indian Council of Medical Research, New Delhi, 1955.
23. Hand, D. B., Steinkraus, K. H., Van Buren, J. P., Hackler, L. R., El Rawi, I., and Pallesen, H. R., *Food Technol. (Chicago),* 18, 139, 1964.
24. Wilkins, W. F., Mallick, L. R., and Hand, D. B., *Food Technol. (Chicago),* 21, 1630, 1967.
25. Meyer, H. F., *Infant Foods and Feeding Practice,* Charles C Thomas, Springfield, Ill., 1960, 161.
26. Shurpalekar, S. R., Korula, S., Chandrasekhara, M. R., and Swaminathan, M., *J. Sci. Food Agric.,* 16, 90, 1965.
27. Protein Advisory Group United Nations, Guideline for the preparation of milk substitutes of vegetable origin and toned milk containing vegetable protein, *PAG Bull.,* 3(1), 14, 1973.
28. De, S. S., *J. Nutr. Diet.,* 2, 166, 1965.
29. Desikachar, H. S. R., De, S. S., and Subrahmanyan, V., *Ann. Biochem. Exp. Med.,* 6, 61, 1964.
30. Chang, I. C. L. and Murray, H. C., *Cereal Chem.,* 26, 297, 1949.
31. Howard, H. W., Block, R. J., Anderson, D. W., and Bauer, C. D., *Ann. Allergy,* 14, 166, 1956.
32. Dean, R. F. A., *Br. Med. J.,* 2, 791, 1952.
33. Bhagavan, R. K., Prasanna, H. A., Shurpalekar, S. R., Chandrasekhara, M. R., Acharya, U. S. V., Swaminathan, M., Krupanidhi, I., and Ankegowda, T., *Indian J. Pediatr.,* 1, 211, 1964.
34. Tso, E., *Chin. J. Physiol.,* 3, 353, 1929.
35. Rittinger, F. R. and Dembo, L. H., *Am. J. Dis. Child.,* 44, 1221, 1932.
36. Guy, R. A. and Yeh, K. S., *Clin. Med. J.,* 54, 1, 1938.
37. Desikachar, H. S. R. and Subrahmanyan, V., *Indian J. Med. Res.,* 37, 77, 1949.
38. Glaser, J. and Johnstone, D. E., *Ann. Allergy,* 10, 433, 1952.
39. Collins-Williams, C., *Can. Med. Assoc. J.,* 75, 934, 1956.
40. Fomon, S. J., *Pediatrics,* 24, 577, 1959.
41. Omans, W. B., Leuterer, W., and Gyorgy, P., *J. Pediatr.,* 62, 98, 1963.
42. Moorjani, M. N. and Subrahmanyan, V., *Indian J. Med. Res.,* 38, 59, 1950.
43. Mitchell, J. H., Jr. and Birmingham, A., U.S. Patent, 2, 511, 1950.
44. Moorjani, M. N., *Bull. Cent. Food Technol. Res. Inst. (Mysore),* 3, 27, 1953.
45. Chandrasekhara, M. R. and Ramanna, B. R., *Voeding,* 30, 297, 1969.
46. Subrahmanyan, V., Chandrasekhara, M. R., Subramanian, N., Korula, S., Bhatia, D. S., Sreenivasan, A., and Swaminathan, M., *Food Sci.,* 11, 9, 1962.
47. Subrahmanyan, V., Chandrasekhara, M R., Korula, S., Subramanian, N., Bhatia, D. S., Sreenivasan, A., and Swaminathan, M., *Food Sci.,* 11, 16, 1962.
48. Shurpalekar, S. R., Chandrasekhara, M. R., Korula, S., Swaminathan, M., Sreenivasan, A., and Subrahmanyan, V., *Food Technol. (Chicago),* 18, 898, 1964.
49. Chandrasekhara, M. R., Aswathanarayana, S., Shurpalekar, S. R., and Subba Rao, B. H., *J. Food Sci. Technol.,* 6, 267, 1969.
50. Shurpalekar, S. R., Chandrasekhara, M. R., Lahiry, N. L., Swaminathan, M., Indiramma, K., and Subrahmanyan, V., *Ann. Biochem. Exp. Med.,* 20, 145, 1960.
51. Korula, S., Chandrasekhara, M. R., Sankaran, A. N., Bhatia, D. S., Swaminathan, M., Sreenivasan, A., and Subrahmanyan, V., *Food Sci.,* 11, 12, 1962.
52. Shurpalekar, S. R., Korula, S., Chandrasekhara, M. R., Swaminathan, M., Chandrasekhara, B. S., Sreenivasan, A., and Subrahmanyan, V., *Food Technol (Chicago),* 18, 900, 1964.
53. Subrahmanyan, V., Reddi, S. K., Moorjani, M. N., Doraiswamy, T. R., Sankaran, A. N., Swaminathan, M., and Bhatia, D. S., *Br J. Nutr.,* 8, 348, 1954.
54. Hanafy, M. M., Ibrahim, A. H., Ek-Khateeb, S., and Seddik, Y., *Alexandria Med. J.,* 9, 477, 1963.
55. Doraiswamy, T. R., Chandrasekara, M. R., Subbarau, B. H., Sankaran, A. N., Swaminathan, M., Sreenivasan, A., and Subrahmanyan, V., *Indian J. Pediatr.,* 30, 365, 1963.
56. Doraiswamy, T. R., Chandrasekhara, M. R., Subbarau, B. H., Sankaran, A. N., and Swaminathan, M., *J. Nutr. Diet.,* 1, 98, 1964.
57. Subrahmanyan, V., Bhagavan, R. K., Doraiswamy, T. R., Chandrasekhara, M R., Joseph, K., Subramanian, N., Bhatia, D. S., Streenivasan, A., and Swaminathan, M., *Food Sci.,* 11, 22, 1962.
58. Pereira, S., Jesudian, G, Sambamurthy, R., and Benjamin, V., *J. Food Sci. Technol.,* 5, 133, 1968.
59. De, S. S. and Subrahmanyan, V., *Sci. Cult.,* 11, 692, 1946.
60. Varadarajan, S. A., *Madras Agric. J.,* 41, 35, 1954.
61. Moorjani, M. N., *Bull. Cent. Food Technol. Res. Inst. (Mysore),* 4, 60, 1954.

62. Chandrasekhara, M. R., Ramanatham, G., Rama Rao, G., Bhatia, D. S., Swaminathan, M., Sreenivasan, A., and Subrahmanyan, V., *J. Sci. Food Agric.*, 15, 839, 1964.
63. Rama Rao, G., Indira, K., Ramanatham, G., and Chandrasekhara, M. R., *J. Sci. Food Agric.*, 15, 841, 1964.
64. Stockert, K. and Grunsterdtt, E., *Z. Unters. Lebensm.*, 57, 320, 1929.
65. Ujesaghy, P., *Kinderheilk*, 81, 214, 1940.
66. Chapin, H. D., *Arch. Pediatr.*, 35, 365, 1918.
67. Hesse, R., *Dtsch. Med. Wochenschr.*, 58, 52, 1932.
68. Desikachar, H. S. R., Studies on the Nutritive Value of Soybean Milk and Other Vegetable Milks, Ph.D thesis, Bombay University, India, 1949.
69. Hafner, F. H., *Soybean Dig.*, 21(8), 20, 1961.
70. Cooper, L. G. and Bryan, M. D. G., *J. Home Econ.*, 43, 355, 1951.
71. Krishnamurthy, K., Ramakrishnan, T. N., Ganapathy, S. N., Rajagopalan, R., Swaminathan, M., Sankaran, A. N., and Subrahmanyan, V., *Ann. Biochem. Exp. Med.*, 19, 139, 1959.
72. Sure, B., *Am. J. Clin. Nutr.*, 1, 534, 1953.
73. Gomez, F., Galvan, R. R., Bienvenu, B., and Craviato, M., Jr., *Bol. Med. Hosp. Infant. Mex. Engl. Ed.*, 9, 399, 1952.
74. Doraiswamy, T. R., Narayana Rao, M., Sankaran, A. N., Rajagopalan, R., and Swaminathan, M., *J. Nutr. Diet.*, 1, 87, 1964.
75. Frost, H. C., *PAG Bull.*, No. 9, 8, 1970.
76. Kapsiotis, G. D., *PAG Bull.*, No. 7, 71, 1967.
77. Senti, F. R., in *Protein Enriched Cereal Foods for World Needs*, Milner, M., Ed., The American Association of Cereal Chemists, St. Paul, Minn., 1969, 246.
78. Odendaal, W. A., *PAG Bull.*, No. 5, 13, 1965.
79. Parpia, H. A. B., in *Pre-School Child Malnutrition — Primary Deterrent to Human Progress*, Publ. 1282, National Academy of Sciences, Washington D.C., 1966, 181.
80. Harris, R. S., Weeks, E., and Kinda, M., *J. Am. Diet. Assoc.*, 19, 182, 1943.
81. Parpia, H. A. B., Swaminathan, M., and Subrahmanyan, V., *Food Sci.*, 6, 96, 1957.
82. Subrahmanyan, V., Doraiswamy, T. R., Joseph, K., Narayana Rao, M., and Swaminathan, M., *Br. J. Nutr.*, 11, 382, 1957.
83. Purushothama Rao, G., *Indian J. Child Health*, 9, 207, 1960.
84. Brock, J. F., in *Progress in Meeting Protein Needs of Infants and Pre-School Children*, Publ. 843, National Academy of Sciences, Washington, D.C., 1961, 103.
85. Senecal, J., *Ann. N. Y. Acad. Sci.*, 69, 916, 1957-58.
86. De Mayer, E. M. and Vanderborght, H., *J. Nutr.*, 65, 335, 1958.
87. Doraiswamy, T. R., Parthasarathy, H. N., Tasker, P. K., Sankaran, A. N., Rajagopalan, R., Swaminathan, M., Sreenivasan, A., and Subrahmanyan, V., *Food Sci.*, 11, 186, 1962.
88. Daniel, V. A., Subrahmanya Raj Urs, T. S., Desai, B. L. M., Venkat Rao, S., Rajalakshmi, D., Swaminathan, M., and Parpia, H. A. B., *J. Nutr. Diet.*, 4, 183, 1967.
89. Doraiswamy, T. R., Daniel, V. A., Rajalakshmi, D., Swaminathan, M., and Parpia, H. A. B., *Nutr. Rep. Int.*, 3, 67, 1971.
90. Bressani, R., Braham, J. E., Elias, L. G., and Jarquin, R., in Cottonseed Protein Concentrates, U.S. Dept. Agric. Res. Ser., U.S. Government Printing Office, Washington, D.C., 1965, 112.
91. Scrimshaw, N. S. and Bressani, R., *Fed. Proc., Fed. Am. Soc. Exp. Biol.*, 20(Suppl.7), 80, 1961.
92. Bradfield, R. B., in Cottonseed Protein for Animal and Man U.S. Dept. Agric. Res. Ser., U.S. Government Printing Office, Washington, D.C., 1960, 29.
93. Graham, G. G., Cordano, A., and Baertl, J. M., *J. Nutr.*, 84, 71, 1964.
94. Shamanthaka Shastry, M. C., Subramanian, N., and Rajagopalan, R., *J. Am. Oil Chem. Soc.*, 46, 592(Abstr.), 1969.
95. Deschampo, I., Calderon, R., and Gonzales, A., *PAG Compendium*, C2, 1603, 1975.
96. Carter, F. L., Cirino, V. O., and Allen, L. E., *J. Am. Oil Chem. Soc.*, 38, 148, 1961.
97. Behar, M., Viteri, F, Bressani, R., Arroyave, G., Squibb, R. L., and Scrimshaw, N. S., *Ann. N.Y. Aca Sci.*, 69, 954, 1958.
98. Guttikar, M. N, Panemangalore, M., Narayana Rao, M., Rajagopalan, R., and Swaminathan, M., *J. Nutr. Diet.*, 2, 21, 1965.
99. Doraiswamy, T. R., Guttikar, M. N., Panemangalore, M., Rajalakshmi, D., and Swaminathan, M., *J. Nutr. Diet.*, 2, 71, 1965.
100. Krishnamurthy, K., Tasker, P. K., Indira K., Rajagopalan, R., Swaminathan, M., and Subrahmanyan, V., *Ann. Biochem. Exp. Med.*, 18, 195, 1958.
101. Daniel, V. A., Subrahmanya Raj Urs, T. S., Desai, B. L. M., Venkat Rao, S., and Swaminathan, M. *J. Nutr. Diet.*, 5, 104, 1968.
102. Tasker, P. K., Narayana Rao, M., Swaminathan, M., Sreenivassan, A., and Subrahmanyan, V., *Food Sci.*, 12, 173, 1963.

103. Doraiswamy, T. R., Tasker, P. K., Narayana Rao, M., Sankaran, A. N., and Swaminathan, M., *J. Nutr. Diet.,* 1, 281, 1964.
104. Wamble, A. C., *Oil Mill Gaset.,* 73, 10, 1969.
105. Jones, O. J., *Oil Mill Gazet.,* 73, 20, 1969.
106. Riberdean-Dumas, L. and Andre, E., *Chem. Abstr.,* 24, 3041, 1930.
107. Kapsiotis, G. D., *PAG Compendium,* C2, 1973, 1975.
108. Woodroof, J. G., *Peanuts — Production Processing and Products,* AVI Publishing, Westport, Conn., 1966, 165.
109. Bailey, K. V., *J. Trop. Pediatr.,* 9, 35, 1963.
110. Iyengar, J. R., Jagtiani, J. K., and Bhatia, D. S., *Food Sci.,* 9, 43, 1960.
111. Jayalakshmi, V. T. and Mukundan, R., *Indian J. Med. Res.,* 49, 1130, 1961.
112. Dean, R. F. A., *J. Pediat.,* 56, 575, 1960.
113. Subrahmanyan, V., Bains, G. S., Bhatia, D. S., and Swaminathan, M., *Res. Ind.,* 3, 178, 1958.
114. Karnad, R., in *Symposium on Proteins,* Central Food Technological Research Institute, Mysore, India, 1961, 415.
115. Murthy, H. B. N., Swaminathan, M., and Subrahmanyan, V., *J. Sci. Ind. Res. B,* 9, 173, 1950.
116. Subrahmanyan, V., Doraiswamy, T. R., Swaminathan, M., and Sankaran, A. N., *Bull. Cent. Food Technol. Res. Inst. (Mysore),* 3, 267, 1954.
117. Subrahmanyan, V., Doraiswamy, T. R., Bhagavan, R. K., Rajagopalan, R., Kurien, P. P., Sankaran, A. N., Bhatia, D. S., and Swaminathan, M., *Br. J. Nutr.,* 12, 353, 1958.
118. Bains, G. S., Bhatia, D. S., and Subrahmanyan, V., in *Symposium on Proteins,* Central Food Technological Research Institute, Mysore, India, 1961, 270.
119. Doraiswamy, T. R., Bhagavan, R. K., Bains, G. S., Sankaran, A. N., Bhatia, D. S., Swaminathan, M., Sreenivasan, A., and Subrahmanyan, V., *Food Sci.,* 10, 389, 1961.
120. Subrahmanyan, V., Bhagavan, R. K., Doraiswamy, T. R., Bains, G. S., Bhatia, D. S., Sankaran, A. N., and Swaminathan, M., *Food Sci.,* 7, 143, 1958.
121. Hoover, W. J. and Tsen, C. C. *Southwestern Miller,* 8, 26, 1970.
122. Wilding, M. D, Alden, D. E., and Rice, E. E., *Cereal Chem.,* 45, 254, 1968.
123. Mizrahi, S., Zimmermann, G., Bark, Z., and Cogan, V., *Cereal Chem.,* 44, 193, 1967.
124. Reynolds, M. S. and Hall, C., *J. Am. Diet. Assoc.,* 26, 584, 1950.
125. Hayward, J. W. and Diser, G. M., *Soybean Dig.,* 21(10), 14, 1961.
126. Paulsen, T. M., *Food Technol. (Chicago),* -15, 118, 961.
127. Smith, A. K., Watanabe, T., and Nash, A. M. C., *Food Technol. (Chicago),* 14, 332, 1960.
128. Muto, S., Taka Hashi, E., Hara, M., and Konuma, Y., *J. Am. Diet. Assoc.,* 43, 451, 1963.
129. Sano, T., in *Progress in Meeting Protein Needs of Infants and Pre-School Children,* Publ. 843, National Academy of Sciences, Washington, D.C., 1961, 257.
130. Arimoto, K., in *Progress in Meeting Protein Needs of Infants and Pre-School Children,* Publ. 843, National Academy of Sciences, Washington, D.C., 1961, 269.
131. Gyorgy, P., in *Progress in Meeting Protein Needs of Infants and Pre-School Children,* Publ. 843, National Academy of Sciences, Washington, D.C., 1961, 281.
132. Subrahmanyan, V., Chandrasekhara, M. R., Korula, S., Subramanian, N., Bhatia, D. S., Sreenivasan, A., and Swaminathan, M., *Food Sci.,* 11, 16, 1962.
133. Panemangalore, M., Joseph, K., Narayana Rao, M., Subramanian, N., Indiramma, K., Bhatia, D. S., Swaminathan, M., Sreenivasan, A., and Subrahmanyan, V., *Food Sci.,* 11, 199, 1962.
134. Dumm, M. E., Rao, B. R. H., Jesudian, G., and Benjamin, V, *J. Nutr. Diet.,* 3, 25, 1966.
135. Meyer, E. W., in Proc. Int. Conf. Soyabean Protein Foods, ARS-71-35, Agricultural Research Services, U.S. Department of Agriculture, Washington, D.C., 1966, 142.
136. Cherry, F. F., Cooper, M. D., Stewart, R. A., and Platon, R. V., *Am. J. Dis. Child.,* 115, 677, 1968.
137. Cowan, C. C., *South. Med. J.,* 61, 389, 1969.
138. Bressani, R., Viteri, F., Elias, L. G., Zaghi, S., Alvarado, J., and Odell, A. D., *J. Nutr.,* 93, 349, 1967.
139. Hodges, R. E. and Koury, S. D., *J. Am. Diet. Assoc.,* 52, 480, 1968.
140. Kies, C. and Fox, W. M., *J. Food Sci.,* 36, 841, 1971.
141. Swaminathan, M., *Borden's Rev. Nutr. Res.,* 28, 1, 1967.
142. Howe, E. E., Gillfilan, E. W., and Milner, M., *Am. J. Clin. Nutr.,* 16, 321, 1965.
143. Joseph, K., Narayana Rao, M., Swaminathan, M., Indiramma, K., and Subrahmanyan, V., *Ann. Biochem Exp.Med.,* 20, 243, 1960.
144. Joseph, A. A., Tasker, P. K., Joseph K., Narayana Rao, M., Swaminathan, M., Sankaran, A. N., Sreenivasan, A., and Subrahmanyan, V., *Ann. Biochem. Exp. Med.,* 22, 113, 1962.
145. Parthasarathy, H. N., Joseph, K., Narayana Rao, M., Swaminathan, M., Sankaran, A. N., Sreenivasan, A., and Subrahmanyan, V., *J. Nutr. Diet.,* 1, 14, 1964.
146. Horn, M. J., Blum, A. E., Womack, M., and Gresdorff, C. E. F., *J. Nutr.* 48, 231, 1952.
147. Buss, L. W. and Goddard, V. R., *Food Res.,* 13, 506, 158.

# LEAF PROTEIN

## N. W. Pirie

## INTRODUCTION

The history of academic and practical research on leaf protein (LP) is given else-where[1,2] and need not be repeated here. The main reasons for thinking that it would sometimes be advantageous to fractionate a leafy crop instead of using the crop as fodder or using the land to grow a conventional food crop are

1.  In many climates leaf crops give a greater yield of both protein and dry matter (DM) than other types of crops. They are, therefore, potentially the most abundant sources of food. This is a strong argument for growing more leafy vegetables, but some inedible leaves give larger yields than do the vegetables.
2.  When a crop is used as fodder, 10 to 30% of the protein is converted to human food, whereas 40 to 60% can be extracted. There is thus more incentive to fertilize, irrigate, and harvest a leaf crop optimally when it will be extracted rather than used as fodder.
3.  By frequent cutting rather than harvesting and resowing, continuous photosynthetic ground cover is maintained. This protects the soil from erosion — especially when perennial crops are used.
4.  The unextracted protein and most of the DM of the leaf can be used as ruminant fodder. This residue can be used fresh, as silage, or as dry winter feed. The last use is particularly important because, depending on processing conditions, its content of DM can be two to five times that of the original crop; drying is therefore economical.

## LEAF SOURCES

The process of extracting juice removes the leaf fiber, and the process of separating protein curd from the 'whey' removes toxic or strongly flavored leaf components. Leaf protein can therefore be made from the leaves of many species that are not normally eaten or even thought suitable for use by animals.

Several principles have to be borne in mind in selecting species for study. Protein extracts more readily from soft, lush leaves than from those that are fibrous and dry. Even when pulped with added alkali, acid leaves do not extract so well as those that are neutral; leaves that give glutinous or slimy extracts are difficult to handle. It is obviously advantageous to use leaves that can be harvested mechanically from a species that will regrow after cutting; this probably excludes tree leaves, though coppiced trees have potentialities.[3] Equally obvious, mixed weeds from untended ground are useless; if the growth could be harvested mechanically and is being manured to ensure an adequate yield, it would be better to use the ground to grow a desirable species. Water weeds are an exception to that generalization[2] — they often grow luxuriantly, but little is known about the extractability of protein from them. Good yields of protein have come from leaves that are by-products, e.g., bean (*Phaseolus* spp. and *Vicia faba*), jute (*Corchorus* spp., pea (*Pisum sativum*), ramie (*Boehmeria nivea*), potato (*Solanum tuberosum*), and sugar beet (*Beta vulgaris*). Surplus vegetables and the discarded outer leaves of vegetables are a potential intermittent source, but nothing would be gained by making LP from edible vegetable leaves. Few communities eat leafy vegetables on the scale that is possible and desirable, and there is little prospect of popularizing LP as food in a community that does not already make ample use of leafy vegetables.

## EXTRACTION PROCESS

Part of any dust and mud on the leaf surface will contaminate the LP. The crop should therefore be washed; the simplest method is to pass the crop through a tank of water on the way to the extraction unit.

The essential process in liberating protein-containing juices from leaves is rubbing and bruising — fine subdivision is an inessential (or even detrimental) concomitant. About 4/5 of the amount of juice that can be pressed out at extreme pressure comes out at 1 to 2 kg/cm² (0.1 to 0.2 MPa), and the gentler the pressure, the greater its protein content and the smaller the amount of fiber carried out in it. Ideally, extraction would take place in one operation, and the process should not waste power in friction or creating wind. Most of the protein used in human feeding trials[2] was made in a high-speed pulper coupled to a press. This wastes power by creating wind, but is a little more effective in extracting protein than the screw expellers that have been used. Progress is being made in designing a unit in which there is less frictional waste of power than in conventional screw expellers.[2a,2b]

Traces of fiber contaminate extracts made in any of these arrangements and must be removed by straining. LP can be coagulated by acidification or heating. Heating is preferable because it partly sterilizes the curd and gives it a hard texture that makes filtration easy. The suddener the heating, the better the texture and the less risk from enzymic changes. If extracts from leaves rich in chlorophyllase are heated slowly, a hazardous amount of pheophorbide may be formed.

Heating to 70°C suffices for coagulation, and heating to 90°C is preferable. The various proteins in a leaf extract coagulate at different temperatures. Those associated with the chlorophylls coagulate at 45 to 55°C (depending on species and pH). If this green fraction is removed, a pale preparation can be made by further heating. This well-known procedure is sometimes advocated, although it is technically difficult and only a third or less of the extracted protein appears in the pale fraction. Furthermore, delay in separating curd from 'whey' facilitates the conjugation of protein with tannins and other substances in the extract. These points are discussed more fully elsewhere.[4]

Coagulum containing 40% DM is easily made by pressing. If the residual water contains the amount of soluble material usually found in leaf extracts, about 7.5% of the DM of the LP will be this extraneous, soluble material. A less adequately pressed coagulum may contain 80% water; soluble material will then account for about 20% of the DM. Similarly, when a well-pressed coagulum is resuspended in so much water that there is only 1 g or less of soluble material per liter and pressed again until it contains only 60% water, only 0.15% of the final cake will be soluble. The recommended standard is <1% soluble material.[2] As already mentioned, the coagulum from a suddenly heated extract filters off easily; when resuspended in water at leaf pH, filtration is difficult. Filtration is easy if salt is added to the water or if the suspension is acidified to about pH 4. A cake made at pH 4 is more reliably free from alkaloids than one at about pH 6. On the other hand, the chlorophylls are completely converted to pheophytins through loss of Mg. The dull green is less attractive than the bright color of neutral LP, and the risk of pheophorbide formation is increased. There is more loss of carotene from acid LP, and the unsaturated fatty acids in it are more rapidly oxidized. If LP is regarded as something to be made on the farm, these defects of acid washing must probably be accepted. If it is regarded as an industrial product, it could be washed by centrifugation or, if washed by acidification and filtration, the washed, pressed, and crumbled coagulum could be neutralized again by exposure to NH³ vapor.

## PRESERVATION AND DRYING

Whenever possible, LP should be used as fresh press-cake containing about 60% water. If made by the method outlined it will be at pH 4 and so will have the keeping quality of cheese or sauerkraut. If longer preservation is needed, it can be salted, pickled, or canned. Drying, if that should be considered essential, must be circumspect or the product will be dark and gritty. A more attractive product, which is also more digestible in vitro, can be made by evaporating water from crumbled press-cake in warm air in a tumble-drier until it contains 70 to 80% DM. It is then ground finely and dried in a current of warm air.

By using water-miscible solvents, drying can conveniently be combined with solvent extraction. This is often advocated by those who think the color of chlorophyll breakdown products unappealing. The disadvantage is that it complicates what could be a process simple enough to be managed by unskilled people on a farm, and it removes carotene and unsaturated lipids, to which many authorities assign great nutritional importance.

## QUALITY

Table 1 shows the recommended standard for a food-grade preparation. The presence of fiber is evidence of inadequate straining; the presence of soluble material, of inadequate washing and pressing, and the presence of acid insoluble ash is usually evidence of inadequate removal of dirt from the leaves, but some leaves contain hydrated silica which extracts along with the protein. The β-carotene is a particularly valuable component in the many regions with a vitamin A shortage. The lipids are not fully extracted unless a polar solvent is used. This explains some anomalously small percentages of lipid that have been published.

Table 2 is compiled from all the credible amino acid analyses that have been published. At this stage of development of research of LP, there is little point in differentiating between the species from which the LP was made because there is no reason to think that differences between species are larger than differences between preparations made from the same species taken at different stages of maturity or manured in different ways. The many individual proteins that make up what is loosely called LP probably have different amino acid compositions and are probably affected to different extents by physiological differences between samples of leaf. Nevertheless, different preparations of LP have similar compositions. The greatest apparent differences in amino acid composition are shown by the three amino acids (cysteine, methionine, and tryptophan) for which analytical methods are least satisfactory. This suggests that the ranges would have been smaller if it were not for analytical error. When preparations are made from species in hitherto-untested families, they should be analyzed, but on present evidence, it would be surprising if the results differ much from those in Table 2.

## NUTRITIONAL VALUE

The results of feeding experiments on chickens, mice, pigs, and rats showed that LP was both safe and nutritionally useful. A mixture of equal parts of LP and milk gave nearly as great a nitrogen retention in malnourished infants as the same amount of protein wholly in the form of milk.[5] As a supplement to the diet of children 6 to 11 years old, LP caused greater increases in both height and weight than lysine or sesame seed.[6] In Nigeria, a group of 2- to 6-year-old children recovered from kwashiorkor

Table 1
COMPOSITION OF LEAF
PROTEIN AS USUALLY
PREPARED

| | |
|---|---|
| True protein | 60—70% |
| Lipid | 20—30% |
| Starch | 5—10% |
| β-carotene | 1—2 mg/g |
| Fiber | < 2% |
| Water-soluble components | < 1% |
| Ash | < 3% |
| Acid insoluble ash | < 1% |

Table 2
THE ESSENTIAL AMINO
ACIDS IN 56
UNFRACTIONATED
PREPARATIONS OF LEAF
PROTEIN MADE FROM 21
SPECIES

| | |
|---|---|
| Isoleucine | 4.5—5.5 |
| Leucine | 8.8—10.2 |
| Lysine | 5.6—7.3 |
| Methionine | 1.6—2.6 |
| Phenylalanine | 5.5—6.8 |
| Threonine | 4.7—5.8 |
| Tryptophan | 1.2—2.3 |
| Tyrosine | 3.7—4.9 |
| Valine | 5.9—6.9 |
| Cystine and cysteine on fewer preparations | 1.5—2.1 |

*Note:* Values expressed as grams of amino acid per 100 g of recovered amino acids.

when 10 g of LP was added to the daily diet. The report on that trial laid particular stress on the children's improved appetite and mental alertness. It seems to be established that leaves, though not as good as milk or egg as protein sources, are better than any of the seeds that are available in bulk. There is no basis for the common opinion that plant proteins are uniformly second class.

Only a summary[2] has as yet been published of a more elaborate trial in the neighborhood of Coimbatore, India. Five groups, with 60 children 2 to 4 years old in each group, get a daily energy supplement of 1.3 MJ. The supplement for one group contains no extra protein; for four of the groups it contains 10 g of protein in the form of milk, LP, a legume seed, or a legume/cereal mixture. Not unexpectedly, milk was the best supplement, but LP was better than the other two. The LP used in this experiment is all made from lucerne with careful attention to technique and hygiene. This probably explains the absence of the 'allergic' reactions that had been noticed with a few participants in the earlier trials.[5]

## ACCEPTANCE

The form in which a foodstuff is presented depends on the types of food that are familiar in a region, and on the need that the foodstuff is meant to satisfy. The methods of presentation on the dinner table that have been suggested[2] were designed to increase the percentage of protein in the diet. Consequently, no method seemed suitable unless the final product contained 20% protein (on the DM) and more than half that protein was LP. In the feeding trial described in the preceding paragraph, there is no such restraint; the 1.3 MJ in the supplement allows large amounts of jaggery (crude sugar) to be included in it. There have been no problems with acceptance.

Young children do not have firmly established food prejudices because, in the years just after weaning, their diets are changing in any event. Although adults are more conservative, their conservatism is usually grossly exaggerated.[8] All those who make food-grade LP regularly find it palatable. When properly prepared, it is as acceptable on first contact as any other really novel food component. These points, which have been a matter of general experience, were recently confirmed experimentally by some trials with tasting panels in Pakistan which also demonstrated that LP and milk had equal nutritional value.[10]

Like flour and many other starting materials, it has no intrinsic appeal. Traditional foods are used by most people with little regard for their nutritional merits or demerits. Consequently, it is unlikely that a nontraditional food will be accepted for wholly logical reasons. People do not arrange their meals with the help of food tables.

The main factor that should ultimately lead to LP being accepted as a dietary component will be familiarity gained in "Mother and Child Welfare Clinics" and in canteens. Use in such places will depend on small-scale industrial production. But the real advantage that LP has over some other novel foodstuffs is that it could easily be made on small farms or in villages where, in the less-developed countries, the need for improved nutrition is greatest. Fortunately, this point is gradually being recognized by those concerned with planning.[9] LP will not be used widely until more administrators realize that it is a good protein and potentially the most abundant protein in wet, tropical regions. Acceptance will obviously be hastened if LP is known to be used by people with local prestige.

## REFERENCES

1. Pirie, N. W., Leaf protein as a human food, *Science,* 152, 1701-1705, 1966.
2. Devadas, R. P., Appropriate technology with reference to infant weaning foods, *Proc. 1st Household Nutr. Appropriate Technol. Conf.,* Colombo, July 1981, 199.
2a. Butler, J. B. and Pirie, N. W., An improved small scale unit for extracting leaf juice, *Exp. Agric.,* 17, 39-47, 1981.
2b. Nelson, F. W., Bruhn, H. D., Koegel, R. G., and Straub, R. J., Rotary extrusion devices, *Trans. Am. Soc. Agric. Eng.,* 23, 1596, 1980.
3. Pirie, N. W., Food from the forests, *New Sci.,* 40, 420-422, 1968.
4. Pirie, N. W., The effect of processing conditions on the quality of leaf protein, in *Protein Nutritional Quality of Foods and Feeds,* Friedman, M., Ed., Marcel Dekker, New York, 1975, 341-354.
5. Waterlow, J. C., The absorption and retention of nitrogen from leaf protein by infants recovering from malnutrition, *Br. J. Nutr.,* 16, 531, 1962.
6. Doraiswamy, T. R., Singh, N., and Daniel, V. A., Effects of supplementing ragi *(Eleusine coracana)* diets with lysine or leaf protein on the growth and nitrogen metabolism of children in India, *Br. J. Nutr.,* 23, 737-743, 1969.
7. Olatunbosun, D. A., Adadevoh, B. K., and Oke, O. L., Leaf protein: a new protein source for the management of protein calorie malnutrition in Nigeria, *Niger. Med. J.,* 2, 195, 1972.

8. **Pirie, N. W.**, The direction of beneficial nutritional change, *Ecol. Food Nutr.*, 1, 279-294, 1972.
9. **Joy, J. L.**, Nutrition and national development planning. III. Planning to reduce nutritional deprivation, *Food Nutr.*, 1, 10, 1976.
10. **Shah, F. H., Sheikh, A. S., Farrukh, N., and Rasool, A.**, A comparison of leaf protein concentrate fortified dishes and milk as supplements for children with nutritionally inadequate diets, *Plant Foods Hum. Nutr.*, 30, 245-258, 1981.

# PROTEIN TEXTURIZATION FABRICATION AND FLAVORING*

## John E. Kinsella

## INTRODUCTION

### World Food Situation

The world food supply, particularly that of protein is presently precarious, and massive localized shortages are anticipated if the population continues to increase as predicted.[25] More food protein will be needed from both conventional and nonconventional sources, particularly the latter because of the limitations on land and energy. The current and prospective problems in protein nutrition have been extensively and repeatedly addressed.[4,5,12,25,42,76,86,129,181,193] Data have been compiled on the overall protein supply and consumption.[12,25] Some controversy exists as to the extent of the shortage.[76,95,236,257] Nevertheless, too many humans are suffering from protein malnutrition because they are not getting enough dietary protein, though averaged statistics may not reveal this situation.

People in many of the densely populated regions of the world suffer from protein-calorie malnutrition, and as the world population continues to expand at an increasing rate toward 7 to 8 billion by the 21st century, the need for more protein will become accentuated. It has been estimated that by that time the world demand for protein will range from 130 to 150 million metric ton/annum. Statistically the average world protein supply exceeds requirements by approximately 70%.[12] However, marked inequities in distribution and in the capacity to redistribute this protein prevail. Many approaches for increasing protein supply and nutritive value have been proposed and research is in progress on several novel sources. Thus proteins from oilseeds, grains, legumes, fish, microbes, algae, and leaves are being investigated.[4,5] In recognition of the magnitude of world needs, it is expedient to examine all potential sources.

### Resources

Excluding energy, the two major factors in determining the adequacy of the world's food supply are population and availability of arable land. At the present level of food production and with a world population of 3.5 billion, approximately 0.4 ha of land per person is in use. Malnutrition is rampant, i.e., estimates indicate that 50% of world's population is undernourished. If the world population continues to grow from 3 billion in 1970 to 7 billion by 2000, with a possible 12 billion by 2025, it is anticipated that three times the area of cultivated land (i.e., 5 billion ha) will be needed. This far exceeds available arable land.[202] Though crop productivity can be expanded somewhat and waste reduced, the overall need for food cannot be met using conventional approaches. Population growth must diminish or local famine(s) appear inevitable.

The current rates of food production are attributed to several scientific or technological advances, i.e., the green revolution, improved fertilizers, irrigation, etc. Sustaining present production, however, will require the expenditure of the most important nonrenewable resource in crop food production, — energy. Because of the very limited area of new arable land available, expanded food production will depend increasingly on increasing energy inputs. But because energy is a very finite resource, the most efficient methods for food production and utilization must be adopted. Thus the use of green leaves directly would be most efficient, e.g., alfalfa produces 1 kcal

* Supported in part by the National Science Foundation Grant 7519123.

of protein per kcal of fossil fuel used in its cultivation while soybean requires about 2.1 kcal of energy per kcal protein produced.[211] Protein production by intensive animal husbandry methods is most energy consuming, requiring about 47 kc/kcal of protein. Thus it seems that to further postpone the Malthusian prophecy, more direct consumption of plant foods is inevitable. In the U.S. over 90% of the plant protein produced is inefficiently processed into high-quality protein via animals. In India the corresponding figure is less than 1%. Approximately 10 kg of plant protein is required to produce 1 kg of animal meat protein. This means that if only 1% of vegetable protein was used for human consumption instead of being used for animal feed, the available protein supply would be increased almost 10%, though its biological value would be somewhat less.

With the rising costs of energy, and the limited availability of land, greater emphasis on crop agriculture seems inevitable. In the future, plant proteins must provide an even greater proportion of our food protein. Cereals, as they have traditionally, may supply most of this. However, soybean and, to an increasing extent, sunflower, peanuts, cottonseed, and other seeds will become significant sources of food proteins for the human population.

### Protein Properties

Because of the high cost of crop production and the inefficiency of food protein conversion by animals, an increased emphasis and reliance on the direct consumption of plant proteins seems certain. Proteins may be produced from numerous sources. Unless these proteins are converted to acceptable foods or food ingredients, however, they will have limited value.

As real demand expands with a burgeoning population and as the emphasis changes from animal agriculture to the direct consumption of plant and microbial proteins, the necessity for new processes and new products will increase and thereby accentuate the requirement for critical physicochemical properties in new proteins. Such properties, generally referred to as functional properties, are important in determining the potential uses of new proteins for the development of food products. The principal functional properties required vary with markets, geographic location, and ethnic traditions. When considering and developing proteins for worldwide use, all the quality, technical, and functional attributes of proteins need to be evaluated. The world demand for functional protein ingredients from plant sources has been estimated at 10 million metric tons.[42,86]

There are several criteria that a protein intended for food use must fulfill, and of these, functional properties are very important in determining the uses of such proteins in the development of simulated or novel foods. Functional properties refer to the composite physical behavior of proteins in foods and reflect interactions that are influenced by: (1) composition of protein, (2) its structure and conformation, (3) intra- and intermolecular associations of the protein with other food components, and (4) the nature of the medium in which these reactions may occur.[129] Typical functional properties include solubility under a variety of conditions, thermal stability, gelation, and emulsifying capacity (Table 1). Solubility is perhaps the most critical property because many of the common functional attributes of food proteins depend on initial solubility, e.g., foam formation, emulsifying power, and gelation.[129]

Therefore, novel proteins should have satisfactory intrinsic properties, i.e., nutritional value and acceptable flavor, color, and texture, ideally, however, they should also possess the additional functional properties of solubility, gelling, emulsifying, and foaming- and fiber-forming properties that make them compatible with and possibly able to enhance the food to which they are added.[96] These criteria are frequently overlooked in discussing new protein sources for which quantity of protein and its biolog-

Table 1
TYPICAL FUNCTIONAL PROPERTIES OF
PROTEINS IMPORTANT IN FOOD APPLICATIONS

| Property | Examples[a] |
| --- | --- |
| Organoleptic } Kinesthetic | Color, flavor, odor, texture, mouthfeel |
| Hydration | Solubility, dispersibility, wettability, water absorption, swelling, thickening, gelling, water-holding capacity, syneresis, viscosity |
| Surface | Emulsification, foaming, aeration, whipping, protein/lipid film formation, lipid binding, flavor binding |
| Structural } Rheological | Elasticity, grittiness, cohesiveness, chewiness, viscosity, adhesion, network cross-binding, aggregation, stickiness, gelation, dough formation, texturizability, fiber formation, extrudability, etc. |

[a]   These properties vary with pH, temperature, protein concentration, protein species or source, prior treatment, ionic strength, and dielectric constant of the medium. They are also affected by other treatments, macromolecules in the medium, processing treatments, and modification.

ical value are normally the only ones considered. The successful supplementation of existing foods, the replacement or simulation of traditional proteinaceous foods, and the fabrication of new foods will depend on the availability of new proteins with the critical functional characteristics that enable them to be successfully used and be acceptable to people of both affluent and developing countries.[129]

Foods fabricated to compete in contemporary markets must possess functional characteristics, aesthetic appeal, and cost advantage when compared to conventional products. Better functionality provides greater flexibility in choice of proteins and should ensure reliable ingredient uniformity, both of which should facilitate modern manufacturing processes.

## TEXTURIZATION

Though plant proteins are relatively plentiful in many parts of the world, little innovation in their preparation as food products has been accomplished. In the past quarter century numerous efforts to increase the consumption of plant proteins in nutritionally balanced formulated foods have failed. Several problems emanate from the fact that the formulated foods did not resemble some traditional food commodity in their quality attributes, i.e., flavor, color, odor, and texture.

In the fabrication of new foods, the raw materials should have properties to facilitate their manipulation and transformation into desirable food items. At present food scientists are restricted and limited in the modifications that they can employ to facilitate fabrication and to improve physical properties of raw materials. The chemical modification of food proteins for improving physicochemical properties requires exhaustive safety testing to satisfy current regulatory standards. Thus the food technologist is largely restricted to manipulation or alteration of secondary bonds and tertiary structures (hydrogen bonding, hydrophilic associations, and electrostatic interactions) for restructuring of proteins in food fabrication.[74,247] However, in limited cases, e.g., gluten development, fiber spinning, extrusion, and rupture and reformation of disulfide bonds (thiol/disulfide interchange reactions) may have some importance.

The ability to alter the tertiary structure of many novel plant proteins and thereby impart texture to otherwise amorphous powders has expanded the potential uses of plan proteins. Textured protein products are those protein-rich items that have been modified in structure, shape, texture, flavor, and appearance to simulate conventional food items, especially meat products.

Meats are universally accepted and desirable foods, and the recently developed technology for simulating meats has provided the flexibility in product design necessary to meet the widely diverse textural and taste qualities required if plant proteins are to be successfully used in providing a significant quantity of food protein in the future.

### Historical

The practice of texturizing plant and animal proteins to improve their mouthfeel or kinesthetic properties is long established, as many traditional foods depend on textured proteins for their unique physical structure, e.g., muscle in meat, gluten in bread, coagulated casein in cheese, and coagulated soy protein in tofu. In the present paper, however, the recent innovative technological developments for texturizing proteins will be reviewed. In the present context the first recorded purposeful endeavors to fabricate textured foods exclusively from plant proteins were those of John Harvey Kellogg (around 1880), who was a vegetarian.[91]

Much of the impetus for fabricated foods emanated from the early pioneering work of Kellogg and the Seventh-Day Adventists. In 1866 a sanitarium was established in Battle Creek, Mich., and Dr. Kellogg experimented to develop palatable diets devoid of meat. This led to the development of textured vegetable cereals (flakes and granola), coffee substitutes, and peanut butter. Kellogg also developed meat analogs termed "nut meats". Nuts were ground into a paste, and with the addition of water an emulsion was formed. Following the addition of flour, cereals, and other ingredients, and upon retorting or cooking, this blend set into a solid mass. This coagulated or textured food could be diced and fried or used directly with condiments.[91] Wheat gluten obtained by elution of starch and sugars from wetted flour has been the basis for many textured proteins. By boiling gluten pieces, expansion and denaturation of the protein yielded expanded chewy products. These were used in bouillon type broths, minced, and used as imitation meats. Larger pieces were cooked to produce solid textured loaf-type products.[91]

These were the forerunners of today's textured proteins. Textured protein foods obtained by fermentation techniques, e.g., fermented soya, tofu, and soy cheeses, precede those cited above by thousands of years. These traditional processes are briefly reviewed later in this chapter.

The initial attempts at texturization were impelled by a desire to make meat-like products from other proteins, and this has been the principal motivating factor in the development of present-day texturized proteins or meat analogs. In 1907, Kellogg[122] patented a process for the fabrication of a comminuted meat-like product from mixtures of wheat, gluten, and casein.[91] Using nonfat milk powder and various starchy materials, as texturizing agents, Wrenshall[268] later prepared various sausage-type products. Simulated sausage- and bologna-type comminuted meats were prepared from soy proteins by Circle and Frank.[55]

Stimulated by Boyer's patent,[36] methods for fabricaton of textured vegetable proteins have developed very rapidly, and the topic of vegetable proteins has received much publicity. In the present context texturized proteins generally refer to vegetable proteins that have been processed so that they are composed of bits or pieces larger than soy grits.

Several methods have been devised for texturizing food proteins, e.g., steam texturization, fiber spinning, thermal extrusion, chewy gel formation, extrusion fiber formation, and the meophase process. The product types, the precursor raw materials, and the methods of texturization are discussed.

Meat extenders are, or technical and economic reasons, presently the most widely used texturized form. Pyke[183] has written that "the problem of presenting synthetic protein as a food stuff or food ingredient with some sort of recognizable and acceptable structure and appearance may be difficult. Meat and many protein foods have a recognizable structural anatomy of 'grain.' The structure of meat which gives it one of the culinary qualities for which it is esteemed is due to the orderly arrangement of muscle fibers. In order for synthetic or isolated proteins to compete with and complement meat, they will need to be fabricated into something not entirely dissimilar to meat." It is now possible to produce numerous types of simulated meats, i.e., simulated in texture, color, flavor, taste, mouthfeel, though the validity of these characteristics, being subjective, is open to some criticism.

## Terminology

Numerous terms have been and are in use for textured commodities, e.g., textured vegetable protein, protein food analogs, vegetable protein foods, protein extenders, and meat analogs. Textured vegetable proteins are food products made from edible proteins. They are characterized by possessing structural integrity and discrete, identifiable texture, as the ability to withstand hydration during cooking and other procedures used for preparing the food for consumption.[10,11]

Simulated meats are called meat analogs not because they are meat because they perform the functions of meat in possessing or providing similar functional characteristics, i.e., texture, color, appearance, taste, and sometimes aroma.

Meat extenders denote small-particle, textured items intended for use in combination with comminuted or chopped meats. These are preponderantly made of extruded soy flour and, according to trade experts, may be used up to 50% of the meat. However, a content above 20% of extruded extenders may exert undesirable effects on flavor and texture.

The food industry has expended great amounts of effort and money toward developing meat substitutes from vegetable proteins. This new category of food has been designated by the Food and Drug Administration (FDA) as "textured protein products."[11] In order to be acceptable to the consumer, these sources of protein must simulate the texture, flavor, and appearance of a natural meat product. They must also retain their texture after cooking, so that the masticatory properties of the cooked product approximate those of cooked meat.

## PROTEIN SOURCES

Statistical trends, economic developments, and circumstances have indicated that the importance of plant proteins will increase rapidly in industrialized countries while demand for meat and fish protein will increase more slowly. Holmes[104] concluded that the probability of protein from vegetable protein becoming commercially available as simulated meat products via texturization is very high. While it is conceivable that numerous materials may be used as sources of protein for textured food products, from a practical, contemporary viewpoint, oilseed protein are expected to be the primary sources in the foreseeable future. Soybean will undoubtedly be the major commodity protein for some time although the present technoloy should easily be adapted to other sources such as cottonseed, sunflower, peanut, microbial, or leaf proteins.

## Soy Proteins

Soy protein preparations are the preponderant sources of plant protein for texturization. A brief summary of their preparation and composition is therefore warranted to aid the subsequent discussions.

Though soybeans were grown in the U.S. as early as 1804, they were an agricultural curiosity for over a century. In 1925 production was around 5 million bushels; in 1970 it was 1.1 billion bushels.[105] Production is rapidly increasing worldwide. Initially soybeans were grown for edible oil. In the 1940s production increased rapidly and the domestic oil extraction industry developed, particularly with the improvement in solvent extraction techniques. Further expansion accompanied the increased use of soybean oil following the successful exploitation of selective hydrogenation. Soybean oil is presently the preponderant source of edible oil in the U.S. With the increased use of oil, the by-product meal gradually became a major source of livestock feed. With the increased demand and price, soybean meal, i.e., soy protein, has currently become more valuable than the oil.[105]

The objective of soybean processing is to remove maximum oil from the bean while preserving maximum nutritional value of the meal. Approximately 70% of the domestic crop is processed by solvent extraction. Currently, however, only 3 to 5% of the 17 million tons of soybean meal thus produced is used in human foods.

The soybean contains approximately 40, 22, 32, and 5% protein, fat, carbohydrate, and ash, respectively. The processing of soybeans has been described in detail by Smith and Circle.[218] Basically the cleaned beans are cracked, dehulled, milled, flaked, and the lipids in the flakes are extracted with hexane. The hexane/oil miscella is further processed to produce oil and lecithin. The defatted flakes are mildly heated to remove residual solvent. These flakes are then steam treated (temperature 85°C) to deodorize them. After desolventization and heat treatment soy flakes are milled and classified according particle size. Soy grits (coarse to medium) are retained by −5 to +40 mesh (U.S. standard sieve size). Soy flour or meal is finely ground soy grits. The extent of heating during these processes can be carefully controlled to minimize denaturation of protein, which is undesirable where proteins are intended for uses requiring specific functional proerties (Figure 1).

The composition and nutrient content of soy grits or flour is summarized in Table 2. The soluble carbohydrates are composed of 4.5% sucrose, 1.1% raffinose and 3.7% stachyrose, with small quantities of arbinose and glucose.[105-108] These are important in relation to the flatulence problem associated with the consumption of soy flours. To circumvent this problem, to increase protein content and to improve nutritional value, the flour is converted to soy protein concentrate by leaching out the soluble carbohydrates, and minerals using successive washes with aqueous alcohol, dilute acid, and water.[105] Commercial yields are about 60% (80% of the protein). These treatments markedly improve protein content (Table 3). Soy protein isolates are made by acid (isoelectric) precipitation of the protein from an alkali dispersion of soy flour. Good-quality isolates contain 95% protein (Table 3). Information concerning the protein fractions and their physicochemical properties has been compiled by Smith and Circle.[218] The average essential amino acid composition is shown in Table 4. The use of these untextured soy protein preparations in meats has been discussed by Rakosky.[191,192]

## FIBER SPINNING

The numerous patents pertaining to protein processing, including texturizing, have been compiled by Hanson,[87] and Gutcho[84] has devoted a complete volume to details of texturizing processes described in the patent literature up to 1973. Duda[65] has collated information on protein meat extenders and analogs.

The major problem with fabricating meat-like products has always been the difficulty of reproducing the appearance and texture of the natural product. Texturizing is

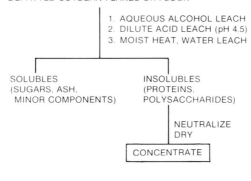

DEFATTED SOYBEAN FLAKES OR FLOUR

1. AQUEOUS ALCOHOL LEACH
2. DILUTE ACID LEACH (pH 4.5)
3. MOIST HEAT, WATER LEACH

SOLUBLES
(SUGARS, ASH,
MINOR COMPONENTS)

INSOLUBLES
(PROTEINS,
POLYSACCHARIDES)

NEUTRALIZE
DRY

CONCENTRATE

A

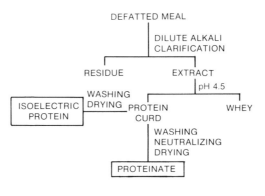

COMMERCIAL ISOLATION OF SOYBEAN PROTEINS

DEFATTED MEAL

DILUTE ALKALI
CLARIFICATION

RESIDUE          EXTRACT
                     pH 4.5
          WASHING
ISOELECTRIC  DRYING   PROTEIN          WHEY
PROTEIN               CURD
                 WASHING
                 NEUTRALIZING
                 DRYING

PROTEINATE

B

FIGURE 1. An outline of the processes involved in the preparation of (A) soy protein concentrates and (B) isolates. (From Horan, F. E., *J. Am. Oil Chem. Soc.*, 51, 67A, 1974. With permission.)

the critical process in the simulation of meat structure from plant proteins. Most proteins, being polymers, can be processed to form filaments or fibers which can be fabricated into meat-like items. Fiber spinning using classical textile fiber spinning techniques pioneered the way for the reasonable initial acceptance of these new products.

## Basic Process

The pioneering work on the experimental production of protein fibers directed at textile applications was performed by Boyer.[35] In 1954, however, Boyer[36] applied the spinning technique to the preparation of meat-like structures. The original basic patent has expired, but companies now engaged in this business hold numerous patents on improved versions of the original invention and on methods for assembling the fibers into meat analogs.[77,78,84,90,106,138,243,245,260]

The first stage in the manufacture of meat analogs is the production of filaments or "fibers." The term filaments is best since most, though not all, possess the structural characteristics of fibers.[246] The principal steps in the typical process are outlined in Table 5.

## Table 2
## AVERAGED COMPOSITIONAL DATA OF SOY FLOUR OR GRITS

| Component | Quantity (g/100 g) | Vitamin | Quantity |
|---|---|---|---|
| | | **Vitamin content of defatted soy flour** | |
| Protein (N × 6.25) | 51.5 | | |
| Nitrogen | 8.2 | Vitamin A | 0.7—4.0 IU |
| Moisture | 7.0 | Thiamin | 1.10—1.50 mg/100 g |
| Fat (ether extract) | 1.0 | Riboflavin | 0.24—0.44 mg/100 g |
| Fat (acid hydrolysis) | 3.5 | Niacin | 4.09—6.70 mg/100 g |
| Fiber | 3.0 | Vitamin D | 0 |
| Ash | 5.8 | Vitamin E | 1.5 IU |
| Carbohydrates | 30.0 | Vitamin $B_6$ | 0.48—1.20 mg/100 g |
| Hexose | Trace | Folic acid | 0.03—0.09 mg100 g |
| Sucrose | 5.7 | Vitamin $B_{12}$ | 0.06—0.20 mg/100 g |
| Stachyose | 4.6 | Biotin | 0.17—0.66 mg/100 g |
| Raffinose | 4.1 | Pantothenic acid | 1.3—5.1 mg/100 g |
| Neutral arabinogalactan | 8—10 | Choline | 2.2—3.8 mg/100 g |
| Acidic polysaccharide | 5—7 | | |
| Arabinan | 1 | | |

| Amino acid | Quantity (mg/16 g N) | Quantity (g/100 g flour) | Mineral | Quantity (mg/100 g) |
|---|---|---|---|---|
| | **Amino acid content** | | **Mineral Content** | |
| Essential amino acid | | | Aluminum | 2.33 |
| Cystine | 1.22 | 0.62 | Arsenic | 0.01 |
| Isoleucine | 4.69 | 2.39 | Calcium | 220.00 |
| Leucine | 7.90 | 4.03 | Clorine | 132.0 |
| Lysine | 6.25 | 3.19 | Cobalt | 0.05 |
| Methionine | 1.27 | 0.65 | Copper | 2.3 |
| Phenylalanine | 5.27 | 2.69 | Fluorine | 0.14 |
| Threonine | 3.86 | 1.97 | Iodine | 0.001 |
| Tryptophan | 1.27 | 0.65 | Iron | 11.0 |
| Valine | 5.08 | 2.59 | Lead | 0.02 |
| | | | Magnesium | 309.0 |
| Nonessential amino acid | | | Manganese | 2.8 |
| Alanine | 4.39 | 2.24 | Phosphorus | 680.0 |
| Arginine | 7.06 | 3.60 | Potassium | 2360.0 |
| Aspartic acid | 11.78 | 6.01 | Selenium | 0.06 |
| Glutamic acid | 19.61 | 10.00 | Sodium | 25.4 |
| Glycine | 4.33 | 2.21 | Sulfur | 250.0 |
| Histidine | 2.84 | 1.45 | Zinc | 6.1 |
| Proline | 5.22 | 2.66 | | |
| Serine | 4.92 | 2.51 | | |
| Tyrosine | 3.78 | 1.93 | | |

Data adapted from Kellor, R. L., *J. Am. Oil Chem. Soc.*, 51, 77A, 1974.

The protein preparation containing above 90% protein, e.g., soy isolate, is dispersed in water, and then the pH is adjusted above 10 to give a spinning dope containing approximately 20% solids. This colloidal solution has a translucent appearance and upon standing (with agitation) its viscosity increases (100 to 1000 P) because the protein

Table 3

## AVERAGE PERCENT COMPOSITION OF SOY FLOURS, CONCENTRATES, AND ISOLATES

| Component | Soy flours | Concentrates | Isolates |
|---|---|---|---|
| Protein | 56.0 | 72.0 | 96.0 |
| Fat | 1.0 | 1.0 | 0.1 |
| Fiber | 3.5 | 4.5 | 0.1 |
| Ash | 6.0 | 5.0 | 3.5 |
| Carbohydrates | | | |
| Soluble | 14.0 | 2.5 | 0 |
| Insoluble | 19.5 | 15.0 | 0.3 |

Table 4

## AVERAGE AMINO ACID CONTENT OF SOY PROTEINS (G/16 G N)

| Amino acid | Flour | Concentrates | Isolates |
|---|---|---|---|
| Lysine | 6.2 | 5.6 | 5.5 |
| Threonine | 3.8 | 3.7 | 3.3 |
| Valine | 5.1 | 4.7 | 4.6 |
| Methionine | 1.3 | 1.2 | 1.1 |
| Isoleucine | 4.7 | 4.5 | 4.4 |
| Leucine | 7.9 | 7.9 | 7.6 |
| Phenylalanine | 5.3 | 5.1 | 5.1 |

Table 5

## GENERAL OUTLINE OF A CONVENTIONAL SPINNING PROCESS

1. Raw material, i.e., protein isolate with >90% protein, prepared from soybean or other source
2. Dope preparation: protein dispersed and dissolved at 20% concentration, adjustment to pH ∼11
3. Color, some flavors, gums, other proteins (gluten, casein) may be added to the dope
4. Dope is aged to allow viscosity to increase to approximately 300 P, with unfolding of polypeptide chains
5. Dope is pumped and forced through spinnerets, possessing numerous orifices (15,000 with diameters of 0.01—0.04 mm) into an acidic (acetic, phosphoric, lactic) saline (sodium chloride, ∼10%) bath at pH 2 to yield coagulated filaments
6. Filaments collected on godets and pulled through the acid bath
7. The fibers or tows are squeezed between rollers to remove coagulating fluid and then passed through a neutralization tank (dilute sodium bicarbonate) around pH 5.5—6 to neutralize the acid (sourness)
8. The coagulated individual fibrils or filaments are stretched up to fourfold their original length by the revolving pick-up reels; the fibrils from each spinneret are collected into bundles ∼6.5 mm in diameter, and these in turn are assembled into tows ∼10 cm in diameter
9. The fibers or tows are drawn through a bath containing binders, flavors, lipids, etc; the tows may then be heated to coagulate binding materials and to set the tows; the tows are sliced as desired into various pieces and stored in saline (4%) or dilute acetic acid before use

unfolds from its aggregate or globular conformation into coiled polypeptides. This facilitates realignment and association between chains during extrusion flow through the spinneret. This viscous dope is then filtered to remove insoluble particles and is pumped via a metering pump through a battery of thin, membranous platinum or glass spinnerets into an acidic coagulating bath. Each spinneret contains 5,000 to 15,000 tiny holes with an average diameter at 0.025 mm.

As the protein stream emerges from the spinneret it is almost instantaneously coagulated by the acid at pH 2 to 4. Several food-grade acids are used, e.g., phosphoric, lactic, acetic, citric, and hydrochloric. The acid bath contains 7 to 12% sodium chloride to minimize solubilization of the protein.

The dynamics of wet spinning may be summarized as follows:[275] when the stream of protein dope emerging from the spinneret contacts the coagulating medium (e.g., acid saline solution) immediate coagulation of the outer layer of protein occurs along with countercurrent diffusion of the alkaline dope solution from the coagulating fibers and infusion of the fibers with coagulating solution. As the latter solution diffuses inward, progressive structural rearrangement and coagulation of the protein polymer occurs. Thus, as the filaments are drawn through the coagulating bath, coagulation occurs until the entire filament is insoluble. The rate of drawing and the tensile force applied (which progressively decrease filament diameter) affects the rate of coagulation. A fine filament of protein about 20 $\mu$ in diameter proceeds from each orifice in the spinneret. The filaments emerging from each spinneret are collected into bundles or fibers of about 0.5 cm in diameter picked up on drawing or take-away reels. These reels rotate more rapidly than the rate of emergence of the filaments from the spinneret. This causes stretching of fibers, which causes the alignment and cohesion of the protein polypeptide chains, improves elasticity with concomitant strengthening of the fibers, whose diameters decrease. If the filaments are not stretched they are weak, kinky, tender, and inelastic. Synthetic products made from kinky or unstretched fibers lack chewiness and resilience, whereas those from stretched oriental fibers have better meat-like chewiness and resilience. Bundles of fibers from several spinnerets are collected into tows (about 7.5 cm in diameter) and further stretched. The fibers or tows are pulled via a series of reels through a hardening bath containing salt solution that may be heated. Then the tows are drawn through a neutralizing bath containing sodium bicarbonate and salt at a pH of 5 to 6. This solution infuses the fibers thereby eliminating the sourness by neturalizing the free acid and bringing the pH of the fibers up to 5 to 6.

Then the tows are washed, passed between squeeze rollers to eliminate excess water. The tows are then sliced or cut several ways depending upon their intended use. These cut pieces are stored in dilute acetic acid or sodium chloride. Numerous modifications and variations have been made in this basic process, particularly in the order and methods of adding binders, lipids, and flavors. The engineering, technology, and practical aspects of fiber spinning has been covered in detail in the textile literature.[149,165,242,267,275,162]

The basic spinnng process used in the food industry is based on Boyer's work.[36] Subsequently, numerous patents have been granted on variations of the original process, i.e., different proteins used, variatons in dope preparation, composition of coagulating bath, and a variety of fiber treatments.[84,87] These are discussed below.

### Protein Sources

Numerous proteins have been converted to fibers by spinning.[84] Soy protein is by far the most common. Casein and wheat gluten are frequently used, usually in combination with other plant proteins. The language of the patent claims indicates that most common plant proteins have been used for fiber spinning but most available information is concerned with soy protein.[84,87] For best results refined protein isolates containing in excess of 90% protein is required, and while most proteins can be manipulated to form fibers, not all can be converted to fibers suitable for edible products. Most common oilseed protein isolates have been converted to protein fibers, e.g., soy. cottonseed, peanut, sesame, sunflower, and safflower.[84] Boyer[36] spun fibers from soybean, corn, peanuts, casein, and keratin. Zein, the alcohol-soluble protein of corn, is a useful fiber-forming protein because of its composition and molecular dimensions.[26,149] Elmquist[69] has described a successful method for spinning fibers from safflower seed meal dope containing 25% solids and 10% oil. Huang and Rha[111] have reported the formation of fibers from Torula yeast protein via extrusion. The protein isolated from Cellulomonas forms very weak fibers, but the addition of casein improved their mechanical properties.[57] Young and Lawrie[269,270] have described the process of successfully spinning fibers from proteins of blood plasma and lung and stomach tissue. Hayakawa et al.[93] compared the spinnability and fiber characteristics of yeast protein with soy and casein. Fabre[70] described the optimum conditions for fiber spinning from sunflower seed protein.

Schmandke et al.[205-208] have reported in detail the spinning of rapeseed proteins, sunflower proteins, and horse bean protein and mixtures of these with casein. Hidalgo et al.[99] patented the fabrication of a nutritional fiber from blends of soybean protein with lactalbumin. Jaynes and Asan[117] spun fibers from whey proteins. However, fibers made from whey protein alone were brittle and weak, and the inclusion of detergent in the dope solution was essential for the spinning of fibers with satisfactory physical characteristics. Lundgren[148] had earlier shown that detergents improves the spinnability of egg albumin.

## Dope Solution

Protein isolates are usually hydrated and dispersed in water or slightly alkaline solution. After thorough dispersion concentrated alkali is added to raise the pH to 11 to 12. The final protein concentration is usually between 15 and 20% by weight, depending upon viscosity of the dope. Other alkali-stable ingredients may also be added to the dope, i.e., colorants, some flavors binders, fiber strengtheners, and lipid compounds. Care should be exercized, however, since certain additives weaken the resultant fibers. Fabre[70] reported that the addition of 5 to 20% gluten, starch, and casein, respectively, to a sunflower dope (containing 20% dry matter) improved elasticity, water absorption, and color of the resultant fibers. Schmandke et al.[208] claimed that the addition of sulfated starch, containing about 7.4% sulfur at a level of 2% to protein dopes, significantly increased the heat stability of the spun fibers and reduced their tendency to disintegrate. Deaeration of the dope is advocated to minimize air bubble formation during extrusion at the spinneret with subsequent weakening of the fibers.

Within the dope vat the alkaline conditions causes unfolding of the globular proteins from their tightly and naturally folded conformation into loose, long polypeptides with a concomitant increase in viscosity of the dispersion. The pH of the dope must not be so drastic as to cause hydrolysis, and both storage time and temperature must be controlled to avoid or minimize hydrolysis, racemization of amino acids, or formation of new interpeptide cross-links.[59,60,182] Upon mixing of the protein with the alkali, a gradual increase in viscosity occurs. This viscosity should stabilize between 50 and 350 P to be suitable for spinning. If viscosity becomes too high (i.e., gelation occurs) reduction of protein concentration and/or pH reduction should be tested although these may only delay the onset of gelation.[269,270]

Rheological characteristics of dope solution are critical factors in spinning. Viscosity is related to degree of polymerization and also polypeptide chain length and configuration. Thompson[242] reported that the highest viscosity preceding gel formation was best for spinning. Viscosity, reflecting mutual attraction between component molecules, is essential for fiber formation; otherwise dispersion resolubilization or disintegration may occur upon emergence of the protein from the spinneret. The flow characteristics of spinning dope depends mostly upon the solute:solvent ratio, however temperature, pH, and molecular properties (physical and chemical) of the protein also influence the liquidity of the dispersion.

The viscosity of an alkaline dope made with about 15% soy protein markedly increases with a concomitant change in ultracentrifugal components to a preponderantly 3S component. The viscoscity increase is time- and temperature-dependent and also is affected by thiol reagents.[122] Native soy protein particles unfold in the alkaline dope to produce long polypeptide chains that cause the dramatic increase in viscosity. In alkaline solution, thiol disulfide exchange is favored so that new intermolecular disulfide cross-links between unfolded polypeptides can occur.

Some proteins, i.e., peanut, blood serum, whey, and yeast proteins tend to become too viscous and form gels when dispersed in alkali. This tendency creates serious problems in spinning because of the difficulty of pumping such solutions throug the spinnerets. Blood serum proteins demonstrated marked tendency to form a gel above pH 10, so that when these are dispersed at a 10% concentration in an alkali dope (approximately 1% NaOH), the viscosity increases very rapidly from 25 to 500 P within 15 to 20 min. Gel formation ensues.[269] Peanut proteins demonstrate a similar tendency. Young and Lawrie[269,270] reported that reduction in pH to 10.5 with acetic acid after dispersion at pH 12 yielded a dope with a stable viscosity of 250 P suitable for spinning. Blood serum proteins dispersed at a concentration of 10 to 12% (g/100 m$\ell$) in dilute alkali took 15 min to attain a suitable spinning viscosity. The tendency of blood plasma dope to gel rapidly was controlled by reducing the pH to 10.5 to 11 with acetic acid after viscosity exceeded 50 P within 15 min. However, the quantity of acid required was closely related to the protein concentration, being optimum at acid-to-protein ratio of 0.075.

The viscosity of dope made from alkaline  dispersions of protein from lung or stomach increased with protein concentrations, and at high concentration, i.e., over 15%, gelation occurred.[269,270] These dopes were of a relatively stable viscosity with time, and they yielded acceptable fibers.

Schmandke et al.[205,207] reported that the viscosity of dope solutions containing sunflower protein isolate, horse bean protein, casein, or mixtures of casein with horse bean or sunflower proteins were mainly affected by protein concentration and, to a lesser extent, by alkali, sodium chloride concentration, and temperature.

Huang and Rha[112] showed that dope containing 20% protein from Torula yeast behaved in a pseudoplastic manner as the apparent viscosity decreased with the rate of shear. Apparent viscosities increased with protein concentration. Dopes containing 15, 20, and 25% protein showed increased viscosities up to pH 9.0, probably caused by unfolding of the protein. Between pH 9 and 10 viscosity decreased, possibly because of depolymerization, and gelation occurred above pH 10.

Reasonable stability of dope at optimum viscosity over time is necessary to provide enough time for batch processing. This varies with protein source, concentration, temperature, pH, and other dope ingredients. These parameters, which must be determined for each protein, can be manipulated to control and stabilize the viscosity.

Stability of the protein in the dope solution may also be problematical especially in the event of delays in spinning. Holding proteins at pH 11 to 12 results in degradation, racemization, hydrolysis, and loss in viscosity. Systems for the initial dispersion of protein in aqueous solutions at pH 7.0 until spinning have been patented.[260] Measured amounts of concentrated alkali are added when the whole spinning operation is ready.

### Coagulation and Drawing

Upon attaining optimum viscosity, the viscous dope solution is pumped under pressure through the orifices in the spinneret heads. These are 0.075 mm in diameter and may number from 5,000 to 15,000 per spinneret. Hence numerous, very fine and discrete streams of dope emerge into the coagulation bath in which the spinnerets are submerged. This bath contains acid (pH 2 to 3) and usually around 10% sodium chloride. Thus, as the dope streamlets emerge their outer surface is immediately coagulated to form a filament. The interior coagulates and solidifies slower as the acid penetrates the filament and reduces pH to the isoelectric point. Initially, as the dope emerges from the spinneret, it coagulates into a glob. This has to be picked up and slowly drawn and attached to the pick-up or drawing rollers (godets), which pull the filaments through the acid bath. Then the pick-up velocity can be slowly increased to optimum rate. Upon emergence from the spinneret orifice, the coagulating dope stream dilates, i.e., the die-swell phenomenon. However, the tensile force, determined by the drawing velocity, progressively reduces the diameter of the filament as it traverses the bath.

One spinneret produces several thousand filaments (20 ≫) that can be put into one fiber bundle having a diameter of 1 to 2 cm. Bundles from different spinnerets can be assembled into tows of 7 to 10 cm in diameter.

The coagulating bath is usually maintained around pH 2. A number of food-grade acids have been used, i.e., acetic, lactic, citric, hydrochloric, or phosphoric acid.[84] Salt, usually sodium chloride at a concentration of 10% is included to enhance fiber formation by a salting out phenomenon and to toughen the fibers. The composition of the coagulating solution affected the fibers obtained from blood serum proteins. Acetic acid (1 N) in a 20% sodium chloride or 11% sodium sulfate solution yielded finer, stronger, and more elastic fibers than those obtained with sulfuric acid (1 N). The latter fibers were coarse and brittle.[270]

The components of the coagulating bath may be altered to affect the properties of the resultant fibers. Frequently carbohydrate materials, i.e., compounds which form thermostable gels, e.g., alginates, pectins may be included in the proteinaceous dope solution to improve fiber properties. Coagulation of these compounds is aided by the inclusion of alkaline metals, like aluminum. The bound aluminum undergoes ion exchange very slowly thereby stabilizing the fibers against softening.[84]

The inclusion of sulfur dioxide in the coagulating bath reportedly improves the flavor of fibers for simulated meats.[138]

The toughness or tenderness, i.e., mouthfeel characteristics in synthetic meats made from spun fibers is affected by orientation of the proteins in the fibrils. This is controlled during the flow of protein through the orifice (rate of flow) and by the alignment of these molecules in the coagulating fibrils caused by stetching of the fibrils during take-up. If filaments are not continually pulled onto rollers (godets) and stretched they will be kinky, weak, and inelastic.[84] When stretched, fibrils are stronger because protein molecules can form more intermolecular associations via improved orientation. Stretching of fibers increases their tensile strength but reduces their extensibility.[117,162]

As fibers are forced through the spinneret they are taken up on the godet wheel. If the peripheral speed of the wheel is equal to the extrusion rate, zero stretching occurs. If the peripheral speed is greater than the extrusion rate, stretching of the fibrils occurs; i.e., if the peripheral speed is twice the extrusion rate then 100% stretching occurs. Thus the take-away speed controls stretching and orientation of the protein fibrils. This may be varied, and there is an optimum speed for different preparations to attain the required strength and elasticity for various meats. Excessive tension in coagulating bath will break some fibers so that the tension on energing fibers should be sufficient only to prevent kinking. Upon leaving this bath, however, stretching forces can be increased by passing the tows over a series of rollers revolving at increasing speeds. In this manner progressively increasing tensions are applied continuously as the strength of the fibers increases. In practice stretching tensions from 50 to 400% have been used for soybean fibers.[84]

Toughness (hardness, chewiness) can also be controlled by exposing the fibers to chemical agents. Concentrated sodium chloride toughens the fibers. Tannic acid, formaldehyde, or aluminum sulfate will insolubilize or fix filaments by cross-linking. These agents are not desirable in foods.

While the degree of toughness and chewiness can be controlled to some extent by the stretching protocol, further desired improvements can be obtained by immersing the stretched, loosened fibrils to a saline solution, pH 5 to 7, at 25 to 40°C and gently agitating them. This procedure toughens each fibril and increases the internal pH of the fibrils to near neutrality.

In the testing of a new protein or mixture of proteins for fiber spinning its coagulation characteristics, i.e., coagulation time and diffusion rate of the coagulant through a protein fiber or protein film, should be determined. This will indicate the time required in the coagulating bath and the drawing velocity or linear speed of the first take-up roller. The tensile strength of the fiber should also be measured to estimate its stretchability and elasticity. These parameters were measured for zein by Balmaceda and Rha.[26] Castaigne et al.[45] have developed mathematical models for analyzing diffusion rates and coagulation times during extrusion of plant protein fibers varying in diameter.

### Binders

After drawing the filaments/tows through the coagulation bath the fibers are pulled through a neutralizing bath containing dilute sodium bicarbonate (pH 5 to 6) and sodium chloride (1%). This neutralizes most of the absorbed acid and eliminate the sourness.

The next sequence of treatments are variable depending upon the intended end use of the fibers. When spun into fibers and assembled into meat-like products, casein cannot withstand cooking temperatures, and the fibers partially dissolve and disintegrate. Soy protein forms fibers that lack the tensile strength of casein fibers and they have inferior textural properties. The use of appropriate thermally stable binding agents, however, markedly improves the fiber properties. Szcznesiak and Engel[237] showed that combinations of casein and soy protein form fibers with excellent properties, which are stabilized by the addition of starch and gums.

Binders are used to hold filaments together by adhesion, gelation, chemical cross-linking, or by using casing such as edible sausage casing. After washing, filaments are treated with binders to ensure adhesion and continuity as in meat. The filaments are mostly produced in aligned bundles, and the main technical consideration is whether this alignment should be maintained through to the final product or not. There is no consensus on this point; some products appear to be highly aligned while others are not. Thus no single description can be given of this part of the overall process, and although product texture depends at least as much on this as on filament production, it has received much less attention. Binders are added to glue fibers or pieces together. Albuminoid proteins from various sources (mostly egg) are popular. Gelatin, casein, whey proteins, processed starches, and gums are also used. Frequently, blends of these materials are employed. Heat-coagulable proteins, like egg white, are excellent because they retain their strength during cooking treatments.

An essential step in the Boyer[36] process is the incorporation of an edible binder that serves to heat-set the fibers or groups of fibers to provide specific textural characteristics. Dundman,[66] fused the protein fibers together by application of heat and pressure. Anson and Pader[15-17] proposed that the binder consist of a protein gel precursor which is converted into a chewy gel upon application of sufficient heat. They found that by raising the pH of the fibers between 6.5 to 7.0, an inherent gel precursor is built directly into the fibers. Another system employed a binder composed of protein and a polysaccharide such as carrageenin.[78] Usually the fibers are coated or impregnated with binders, flavors, fat, and, in some cases, colorings or food dyes. This may be accomplished by drawing the fibers through baths containing these ingredients; they may be applied as a fine powder or the filaments may be soaked in these solutions so that they become infused with these additives. Improved neutralization, washing and impregnation of filaments with binding agents, flavors, or nutrients can be achieved by loosening the bundles of fibers by vibration of the fibrous mass as it passes through the appropriate baths.[58]

In one patented procedure[175] the fibers or tows are immersed in a fluid dispersion of various ingredients. The fibers are kneaded by passing between rollers moving at relatively different rates. This exerts mechanical pressure on the tow, facilitating impregnation of the fibers with the ingredients that flow counter to the direction of the fiber. A typical example of the ingredients used in treating fibers to be used in simulated beef is 51% water, 15% egg albumin, 10% wheat gluten, 8% soy flour, 7% onion powder, 5% sugar, 2% hydrolyzed protein, 1% salt, 0.15% monosodium glutamate, and 0.5% artificial color. The impregnated tows were treated by pulling them through a bath containing coconut oil at 34°C.

Using a combination of soy protein and casein Szczesniak and Engel[237] formed a tacky dope at pH 9 from which fibers with excellent textural and hydration characteristics were spun. These fibers were successfully dried to a moisture content as low as 3% and they facilely rehydrated. When included in compounded meat-like products they inparted masticatory properties reminiscent of meat. When formulated with modifiers, i.e., starch, gums, and fats, they displayed good heat stability and did not disintegrate upon cooking or frying at temperatures 450°C.

Schmandke and Kormann[208] studied the swelling capacity of fibers made from casein and casein/plant protein mixtures in water and sodium bicarbonate solutions as an index of their structural stability to further processing. Rehydration in 0.1% sodium bicarbonate where swelling (i.e., increased fiber diameter) was less than threefold ensured adequate structural stability.

Carbohydrates, starches, gums, dextrins, and carboxymethylcellulose, when incorporated within fibers may affect chewability, elasticity, cohesiveness, adhesiveness, moisture retention, hydration, freeze-thaw stability of hydrated textured products, and water activity.[79] These compounds may be added to spun fibers to enhance binding and cohesiveness between fibers.

After treatment with binders the fibers or tows may be heated to accomplish the final setting in a continuous gel matrix. Heating may involve baking, frying, or boiling. It is possible by appropriate heat treatments to cause binding of fibrils into tows without the application of any binding material.[66]

## Other Additives

As indicated previously the incorporation of flavoring materials, texture modifiers, or coloring agents to achieve the flavor, color, and textural characteristics of meat can be done at several stages. The inclusion of the appropriate additives in the dope solution is desirable for uniform distribution of materials within fibers. Boyer[37] reported the successful inclusion of various fats, spices, sugar, starches, protein hydrolyzates, dyes, pigments, and flavoring agents in the spinning dope. The soluble or easily miscible compounds were incorporated with satisfactory results. The inclusion of nonmiscible compounds such as lipids and lipophilic substances may result in weak points in the fibers, especially where lipid droplets occur. The amounts included will depend on "carry-through" and desired characteristics of the final product. Fibers containing relatively high proportions, above 30% of additive material show significant reduction in tensile strength and toughness.

The protein filaments or tows emerging from the acid bath are generally similar in color to the starting material. Alkaline- and acid-stable dyes may be added to the starting alkaline solution to achieve proper color. Freshly spun protein fibers are usually stored as chunks in dilute acetic acid of pH 4.5 to 6.0 or in aqueous sodium chloride of 4% concentration.

## Composition

The finished, spun, textured plant proteins may contain from 20 to 40% protein depending on the amount of moisture removed before analysis. Most foods made with spun fibers contain less than 50% of the actual fiber, the remainder consisting of other plant proteins, binders (albumin, gluten, whey proteins), emulsifiers, lipids, etc. Such product may be used as meat extenders or as complete replacements for meat in canned and frozen products.

The composition of products with spun protein, from the process of Thulin and Kuramoto[243], was 40% spun fiber, 10% binder protein, 20% fat, and 30% flavors, colors, and other ingredients. The composition of meat analogs, i.e., commercial Bontrae® was 60% protein, 20% fat, 17% carbohydrate, and 3% ash dry weight; of "beef", 40% protein, 58% fat, and 2% ash dry weight; of "pork" 36% protein, 61% fat and 3% ash dry weight; of "chicken" 50% protein, 48% fat and 2% ash dry weight.[261] Freshly spun commercial soy fibers contained 60% moisture and 30% protein.[49] The metal content was 200 ppm calcium, 54 ppm magnesium, 33 ppm iron, 14 ppm zinc, 6 ppm copper, and 2 ppm manganese.

The nutritive value of spun products (vide infra) can easily be manipulated by addition of nutrients. Proteins of high biological value, e.g., egg albumin, whey proteins, amino acids, vitamins, and minerals may be added as desired. These can be incorporated into the dope dispersion and extruded with the protein or used in the binder materials. Some losses in nutritive proteins may occur during coagulation and washing.

## PHYSICOCHEMICAL ASPECTS OF FIBER FORMATION

Theoretically, most proteins should be capable of forming fibers when subjected to the spinning process. However, the ability of various proteins to unfold into long polypeptide chains at alkaline pH values varies. Furthermore, the uncoiled polypeptides from some proteins in alkaline solution associate rapidly and become excessively viscous or form gels thereby impairing the spinning operations.

With regard to proteins, differences in amino acid composition and their arrangement and sequence affect protein conformation. This in turn governs secondary and tertiary structures that affect the ease and extent of intermolecular interactions which are important in the intermolecular binding of fibers. For example, polypeptides with relatively high concentrations of serine threonine, glutamine, and asparagine have a marked propensity to form hydrogen bonds.

The conformation of proteins must be critical in many mechanisms governing their functionality in food systems. The native conformation of globular proteins, in which the polar amino acids are exposed to the aqueous phase, favors solubility, while an unfolded, elongated conformation is more desirable in proteins for gelation, stabilizing foams, and fiber spinning. The flexibility of proteins, their ability to change conformation under certain conditions, is important in functional applications.

Some investigators have attempted to predict the conformation of proteins from their amino acid sequence on the rationale that the covalent structure of protein possesses the information for initiating and directing the folding process to attain the favored conformation. By estimating the type and magnitude of all forces and constraints acting upon a polypeptide chain of a given amino acid sequence in solution, the secondary and tertiary structure of protein molecules should be predictable. Nagano[169] has reviewed this approach and summarized the problems encountered.

With respect to the physical chemistry involved, Lundgren[149] summarized the extant information on protein fibers. He reviewed the phenomena of solubilzation, unfolding of the protein molecules, molecular orientation, and recrystalization as related to the formation and properties of the final fibers. Wormell[267] reviewed the early research on fiber spinning. Since then a large volume of information on the wet spinning of casein, soybean, zein, and peanut proteins for textile fiber production has been published.[117,162,165,178] and Huang and Rha[112] reviewed the chemical aspects of protein fibers.

Senti et al.[214] demonstrated that several proteins, casein, lactoglobulin, hemoglobin, ovalbumin, zein, edestin, peanut, and soybean proteins can be changed from globular conformations to oriented, fibrous structures by mechanical stretching of their heated solutions. This observation indicated the feasibility of fiber formation. Lundgren[149] ennumerated the molecular criteria for optimum fiber formation. The molecules should be linear (1000Å) and of molecular weight around 20,000 to 30,000 daltons. The molecules should possess a high degree of linear symmetry and be devoid of bulky side chain groups that would sterically interfere with chain apposition, lessen intermolecular association and bonding, and weaken crystalline forces thereby weakening the fiber. The component molecules should have a high content of polar amino groups to enhance intermolecular cohesive forces. The presence of cysteine residues that engage in disulfide bond formation also enhance the strength of the fibers.

Generally an average molecular weight in the range 10,000 to 50,000 daltons is required. Below 10,000 daltons only very weak fibers can be formed, if any at all, while above 50,000 daltons high viscosity and gelation become problems. Each protein, depending upon length of uncoiled polypeptides show an optimum molecular size within the above range.[149]

The exact configuration of polypeptides, i.e., the relative contents of $\alpha$ helix, $\beta$-pleated sheet and random coil in spun fibers is unknown. However, in spinning fibers from globular proteins (soy, peanut, zein, and casein) the globular proteins are unfolded (denatured) to random coils and changed into the extended $\beta$-configuration by forces prevailing during the extrusion and stretching involved in spinning.

Ziabicki[275] proposed that polypeptides become oriented longitudinally by streaming orientation in the shear flow within the spinneret and in elongational flow, as well as deformation orientation of the elastic fibril during drawing. This is affected by output rate, length and diameter of orifice, viscosity of dope, rate of coagulation and drawing force. The extent of longitudinal alignment (depending upon component amino acids) determines the degree of intermolecular bonding and therefore affects fiber strength.

Crystalline and amorphous regions exist in protein fibers. Amorphous regions occur where bulky side chains occur. Goodman[80] in discussing the crystalline regions stated that there are three major configurational structures in fibers. These are a linear configuration in which polypeptides are mostly extended, helical configuration with the long axes of the helices lying parallel to one another and probably associated via secondary bonds, and sheet-like aggregates of molecules joined by hydrogen bonds or ionic forces, these sheets being parallel. Considerable variation in these occurs in the case where molecules with bulky side chains are present. A stable fiber requires a sufficient amount of similar crystalline structure that is not disrupted by changing environmental conditions.

The secondary forces prevailing between neighboring polypeptides are electrostatic interactions and electrokinetic (dispersion, vander Waals) forces. The latter forces are supplemented by inductive forces. Hydrogen bonding is also important in stabilizing the structure of fibers.[80] The importance of hydrophobic associations has not been quantified though these are functioning in some manner.[49] Hydrophobic forces help stabilize polypeptides in the folded configuration. These forces become stronger with increasing temperatures, reaching maximum around 60°C. They may be of some significance in the thermal stabilization of protein fibers. The marked capacity of urea of dissociate and solubilize protein from soy fibers[49] demonstrated the importance of hydrophobic associations in holding protein fibers together.

Primary covalent disulfide bonds are also of significance in protein fibers[49,122] because thiol reducing agents can dissociate proteins from spun fibers.

In addition, crystalline configurational forces are functional in stabilizing fibers.[80] Thus, during drawing, localized adjustments in molecular packing and mutual alignment of molecules in certain segments occur. A staggered conformation in chains usually is preferred. Thus the chains adopt preferred conformations, and there is internal resistance to change.

During spinning, pressure, shear forces, and drawing enhance the alignment of the uncoiled chains thereby facilitating formation of crystalline regions in the filaments.[112] The shear forces disentagle the polypeptides and the flow through the spinneret causes parallel alignment and stretching, which further accentuate parallel associations and the resultant formation of essentially crystalline regions as discussed above.

Further basic research is needed to determine and measure the significant stabilizing forces in edible protein fibers and the relationship between amino acid composition, sequence, peptide conformation, and spinnability, and to develop modifications that might enhance the spinning properties of inexpensive proteins.

There are few basic studies on the dynamics of spinning protein fibers. Balmaceda and Rha[26] ennumerated some of the physical parameters influencing the spinning of zein fibers. These include composition and properties of dope (protein, other ingredients, alkali concentration, age, etc.), composition and temperature of the spinning bath (i.e., acid type and concentration, salt type and concentration), spinneret size and orifice dimensions, spinneret velocity; drawing velocity, and spinning length (i.e., length of coagulating fiber in coagulating bath from spinneret to first take-up reel). These latter parameters affect rate and extent of coagulation.

Balmaceda and Rha[26] reported that the drawing velocity increased linearly with spinning length except when high concentrations (45%) of proteins were used. The linearity was attributed to the decrease in longitudinal strain and tension along the fiber as it increased in length. Therefore, the velocity could be increased before breaking tension is reached. The relationship between drawing velocity and spinning length was denoted by the term "spinnability curve". The drawing velocity also increased with rate of extrusion from the spinneret, but this was affected by the diameter of the orifice. Thus at similar extrusion velocities the highest drawing velocity was obtained wth spinneret orifice of 0.041 cm and lowest with an orifice of 0.025 cm in diameter.

The protein concentration in the dope (and presumably its viscosity) affected the extrusion velocity. As the protein concentration was increased, the drawing velocity decreased because the viscosity increased and the rate of coagulation decreased.[26] When the coagulation rate is rapid, a skin or pellicle forms immediately as the filament emerges. This minimizes swelling of the filament, so that the dope jet velocity is not retarded. When initial surface coagulation is slow, the swelling tends to slow the dope jet velocity, and this in turn retards drawing rate.

Increasing bath temperatures from 25.6 ot 32°C markedly improved spinnabiity curves.[26] Spinnability is quite sensitive to small changes in coagulating bath temperature. The temperature effect may be twofold, i.e., increased temperature increases coagulation rate which allows increased drawing velocity. It also decreases viscosity of the filament as it emerges from the orifice allowing increased drawing rate.[26]

## Structure and Physical Properties

Aguilera[2] found that diameters of spun commercial soy fibers were very variable, ranging from 55 to 95 $\mu$m even though spinneret apertures were 100 $\mu$m. Stretching following spinning caused a reduction in diameter. The fibrils appeared as being surrounded by a thin, continuous, membranous layer or skin, which was aparently composed of a film of denatured protein formed as the protein stream from the spinneret contacted the acid precipitant in the coagulating bath. The interior of the fibrils had an uneven, grainy structure with occasional vesicles or air pockets. Microcavities in the fibrils result in fibers with weak tensile strength.

Scanning electron micrographs of rehydrated soy fibers revealed longitudinal fissures and fibrils or plates.[230] No globular protein was observed.

Limited information has been published on the properties of fibers. Stanley et al.[230] studied physical, structural, and tensile properties of spun soy protein. Dehydrated spun soy proteins, rehydrated by boiling in distilled water absorb approximately 142% water and have a density of 1.015 g/cm.[3]

Rehydrated soy fibers demonstrated load extension characteristics similar to those of wool but different from those of meat. The biphasic stress-strain curve curve shown by soy fibers was composed of an initial linear portion in which elastic recovery was nearly complete, a curvilinear portion in which recovery was incomplete, and finally, breakage of the fibers. An average elastic modulus (gram force divided by the product of cross-sectional area and change in length) of 12,700 g/cm$^2$ was calculated for the initial elastic region of the soy fiber stress — strain curves. This compared with a value of 12,500 g/cm$^2$ for muscle in rigor and 2,500 g/cm$^2$ for fresh muscle.[229]

The breaking strength, i.e., the load required to break a sample (grams load per gram sample) is a useful textural parameter. Spun fibers had an average value of 2.12 kg/g compared to 241 g and 400 g for raw and cooked pork tenderloin muscle, respectively. These breaking strengths are correlated with relative toughness and indicate that pure fibers would be judged tough. Normally, however, meat-like products contain only about 40% spun fiber material; hence they should not be as tough as fibers alone.

Spun soy fibers demonstrated a marked ability to elongate before breaking, e.g., over 300% compared to 27% observed for pork muscle fibers. Work weakening is another important physical attribute, i.e., do spun fibers become weaker upon continued chewing? Using instrumental techniques, Stanley et al.[230] showed that while stress-elongation was noticeably reduced, break strength was not significantly affected by simulated chewing. The data indicated that during the initial period of mastication spun soy protein demonstrated a greater loss of structural integrity than meat.

The elasticity, i.e., the extent to which a fiber becomes permanently deformed when it is extended and its restoration upon removal of the stress of spun soy fibers, was less than that of cooked meat. Thus soy fibers do not have the same capacity to return to their original structure upon removal of stress. This may be a significant factor in chewiness and mouthfeel characteristics.

These objective measurements reflect the differences in structure between meat and soy fibrils. The latter do not possess the tensile characteristics associated with meat tenderness. Stanley et al.[230] mentioned the difficulties in measuring these properties objectively and noted that methods and conditions used could influence the measurements. The need to investigate methods for tenderizing spun fibers was suggested.

Using a composite material approach, Miller and Morrow[161] determined the effects of fiber concentration and fiber orientation on the mechanical properties of spun-fiber meal analogs. They used dynamic compressive and parallel-creep shear tests to determine time-dependent elastic and shear moduli. The respective maximum and minimum compressive moduli occurred with the fiber parallel and perpendicular to the loading direction while the shear modulus was greatest with the fibers at a 45° orientation.

Table 6

SOME CONTROLLABLE FACTORS AFFECTING THE TEXTURE OF SPUN
PROTEIN FIBERS

| Factor | Variables |
| --- | --- |
| Protein | Source, purity, compositon, molecular weight, conformation |
| Dope | Viscosity, degree of unfolding of polypeptides; accessibility of hydrogen bonding and sulfhydryl groups, age of dope, presence of nonprotein ingredients |
| Flow rate | Rate of pumping or extrusion of dope through spinneret orifices |
| Spinneret | Diameter, dimensions, and configuration of orifices |
| Coagulating bath | Acidity, circulation rate; temperature; presence of salts and tanning agents; length of bath |
| Drawing | Rate of drawing, i.e., tensile force applied, extent of fiber stretching |
| Collection | Number of filaments collated into fiber; number of fibers included in a tow; pressure applied in assembly of fibers |
| Treatment | Nature of binders used; binders applied to filaments, fibers, or tows; quantity and type of fat applied heat treatment |
| Fabrication | Manner in which fibers are aligned — parallel, irregular, or crossed |
| Cutting | Manner in which tows are cut or sliced |
| Aging | Duration and conditions of storage |

Higher compressive and shear moduli were obtained as fiber concentration was increased.

The texture of fiber is influenced by composition and purity of protein, modification (if any), extrusion pressure, acidity of coagulating solution, diameter of fiber, degree of stretching of the fiber and tow, nature of binders and fat, extent of heating, etc. (Table 6).

*Storage Characteristics*

Unless they are used in products, fibers are placed in saline solution (pH 5 to 6) to prevent them from redissolving. Before further processing the salt solution is removed by centrifugation or gently squeezing. Schmandke and Korman[208] reported that fibers made from equal mixtures of casein and horse bean protein were stabilized to temperatures of 100°C following treatment with concentrated sodium chloride.

Freshly spun protein tows are creamy white, soft in texture, and quite elastic. During storage, fibers deteriorate in color, flavor, and texture. The inclusion of small amounts of alkaline earth metals (aluminum, calcium) with sodium, potassium, or ammonium, plus some polybasic acid (phosphoric) during the preparation of casein fibers, improve storage characteristics. Fibers containing these improve heat resistance and retain their resiliency following prolonged storage.[142] Upon prolonged storage, before utilization in end products, the fibers deteriorate. They turn a dull, greyish color, gradually become tough, and lose their resilience and elasticity. This is a serious practical problem when processing fibers into food products is delayed.

Chiang and Sternberg[49] studied some of the changes occurring and demonstrated that disulfide bonds were involved. The importance of disulfide bonds and thiol groups in fiber structure and quality was shown by Kelley and Pressy[122] and Chiang and Sternberg.[49] The latter researchers reported that of the total 72 μmol of half cystine per gram of protein, 47 μmol of free thiol (SH) groups were titratable, i.e., available for bonding. During storage at 22°C, the SH groups decreased from 47 to 25 μmol/g protein in 60 days while the number of disulfide bonds increased. At 38°C these changes were accelerated. Storage at −20°C resulted in negligible changes. The addition of ascorbic acid (0.1%) retarded the rate of thiol (−SH) oxidation during storage at 20°C. The presence of copper and iron enhanced the oxidation rate, and the inclusion of a metal chelating agent retarded oxidation.

The loss of SH groups was accompanied by a decrease in solubility of the protein, a loss of elasticity, and an increased toughening of the fibers. This was ascribed to the increased aggregation caused by disulfide cross-linking. A loss in water absorption also occurred during storage. In the case of an analogous product, Saio et al.[203] reported that tofu became harder and tougher during storage due to increased cross-linking and aggregation of the proteins. These phenomena require further research.

With regard to microbial deterioration, spun fibers are relatively stable. The initial product is sterile if aseptic conditions prevail during manufacture. This is unlikely, but storage in the acidic saline medium assures minimum microbial deterioration. Atkinson[21] described a procedure for manufacturing protein fibers that were resistant to bacterial degradation by including soluble alginate in the dope; treating the mixture with hydrogen peroxide (1%), and then heating to 160°F before storage.

### Utilization

After fabrication and binding the spun product may be sliced, ground, or dried and either consumed or further processed into frozen, canned, or dried products. Spun fibers provide great versatility for fabrication of simulated meats, though the reproduction of unique texture of specific meats has been difficult. Nevertheless the bulk of extruded and spun soy materials is used in meat analogs where texture is the more important characteristic.

After the binder is applied, the filaments may be drawn through a bath containing fat (liquid) and desirable lipophilic flavors. Then the groups of filaments are assembled into a tow by pressing them together. This may be heated to enhance binding. The pressure applied can be controlled to adjust final density and toughness of the product. Thus lengths of tow from 24 to 30 cm with diameters of 7 to 10 cm are usual. These pieces can be cut along, across, or at any angle to the fiber grain to give the desired grain appearance for the final product.[84] This product may be layered, wound, chopped, or sliced for use in fabricated, simulated meats.

In the simulation of different types of meat, different practices are followed. The spun fibers may be dispersed, layered, cross-hatched, or arranged in parallel orientation; in a variety of patterns to give different texture and chew characteristics. For pork chops the filaments emerging from each spinneret may be assembled into a group or fiber (0.5 cm). Each fiber is coated with lard (15 mm thick, binders, flavors, colors, and vitamins may also be added), and then the groups are bound into tows 7 to 10 cm in diameter. For filet mignon approximately four groups of filaments are assembled before application of tallow and are then assembled into tows following the addition of binders, flavors, color etc.[105,107,276] In simulating poultry meat, groups are assembled following the application of binder, and then fat layer is added to the outside. Fibers made from casein and soy protein are coated with binder and fat by drawing them through a bath containing oil, flavors, etc. emulsified with albumin. The ratio of wet fiber to binder is 1.2:1. The coated fiber is heated at 90°C for 45 min. The resulting product has the cohesiveness, texture, and mouthfeel of chicken. This product could be successfully included in dehydratable sauces, gravies, and soups because of its rehydratable properties, or deep fat fried to simulate fried chicken.[237]

Numerous patents describe variations of the standard methods used in the fabrication of simulated meats with spun fibers. Many involve thermosetting of chunks of tows in heat coagulable proteins to simulate a variety of meats, depending on flavorings and colorings employed.[38] These can be sold as dehydrated products and are facilely rehydratable.

By rolling tows of filaments that had already been impregnated with binders, flavoring agents, colorants, lipids, and emulsifiers, through heated rollers at 95 to 180°C, Kjelson and Page[132] produced a product with characteristics of a chopped beef prod-

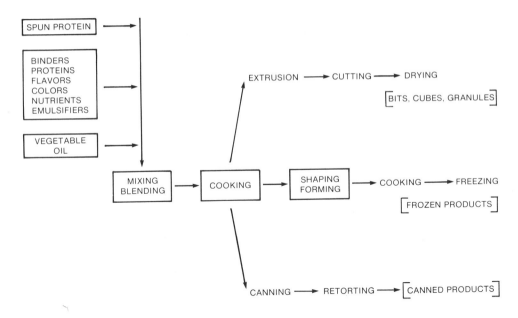

FIGURE 2.  Outline of processes for fabrication of textured products from spun protein fibers.

uct. The addition of chopped spun fibers to extend comminuted meats and sausages has also been done.

Products consisting of combined lean and fatty components simulating bacon slices, pastrami, corned beef, etc. have been made from spun fibers.[90] These products can be essentially fat free, the light and dark areas being obtained with adroit use of coloring dyes, or fat may be used for the fatty portions. This is achieved by building up a multilayered bacon-like slab product consisting of spun fibers bound together and flavored, with some layers being colored while others remain lightly colored. This slab is then sliced to give bacon-like strips.

A large number of simulated meats (e.g., beef, chicken, ham, pork, bacon, and seafood analogs) have been commercially marketed in a prepared ready-to-eat form. They contain approximately 50% water.[106,199,200] Spun fibers are used in many dried, canned products, and as frozen prepared foods. Rosenfeld and Hartman[200] have summarized the principal steps in the three major lines of fabricated foods (Figure 2). The principal advantage claimed for the use of spun fiber analogs in meat-type foods is that relatively high amounts can be included without altering the mouthfeel characteristics, because they are similar to meat in texture.

*Problems and Prospects*

Fiber spinning of edible protein is a highly sophisticated technology requiring modern equipment and highly skilled technicians. It is an expensive process, and the products are principally restricted to affluent markets. Several technical and engineering problems can be encountered in spinning, as one might expect from the intricacy of the process. The quality of protein isolates are quite variable. Insoluble particles can be problematical and clog spinnerets. Some batches of proteins occasionally fail to spin.[246] The alkaline dopes are unstable and may gel spontaneously or, if there is a delay or breakdown of the viscosity, may decrease because of alkaline hydrolysis. Weak filaments are occasionally formed. The fibers need extensive washing to remove acid. This may dissolve some protein and weaken the fibers.

The high pH of the alkaline dope causes some degradation of protein, especially if the dope is stored. Thus deamination and cross-linking may occur. The high pH also prevents the addition of alkalilabile colors, flavors, vitamins, etc. The major problems of obtaining a bland-tasting fiber from soy protein and of adequately flavoring meat analogs have not been overcome.

Nevertheless, several products being commercialized in the U.S. are evidence of significant technical success with this process. The versatility of this technique clearly points out that the spinning technology makes it possible to manufacture engineered foods. Depending on the choice of ingredients, there is literally a limitless number of ways in which a protein food can be fabricated for a specific use. New proteins from algae, oilseeds, microbes, leaf, or fish may be included with the soy protein fibers as a vehicle to impart textural characteristics into these other sources of protein.

The basic principles of the process described by Boyer in 1954 have since been subjected to several chemical engineering embellishments and have progressed through semi-works installation to a full-scale, modern plant with a capacity of 20 to 30 million pounds per year.[107]

## EXTRUSION

A uniform terminology in the area of textured food proteins has not been agreed upon. This must await the promulgation and establishment of official standards of identity and composition. "Texturized vegetable proteins" is a generic term that includes a wide range of protein made by different processes. They include spun protein fibers, extruded protein foods, various types of heat-coagulated protein pieces, and, in some cases, soy grits. Generally, however, it is assumed that texturized proteins refers to structured proteins produced by a number of extrusion-cooking processes. These are by far the more popular texturized products. Textured proteins, especially extruded products, are generally classified as meat extenders while spun products are viewed as meat replacements and have been called meat analogs.

The concept of texturizing plant proteins was advanced by the spun-fiber process, which represented the first generation of texturized plant proteins. Because of the technical requirements and overall cost, however, the simple technique of extrusion has been rapidly adopted. With regard to quantitative importance it is estimated that about 95% of textured plant proteins currently are made by the extrusion process.

Initially developed as an economical method of gelatinizing starches, extrusion cookers have been modified during the intervening years to process an ever-widening group of foods. Currently, many fabricated foods are cooked and are given desired textures, shapes, densities, and rehydration characteristics by an extrusion-cooking process. This relatively new process is used in the preparation of engineered foods, textured vegetable proteins, breakfast cereals, snacks, infant foods, breadings, croutons, and pasta products.

In 1935 extrusion processing became important to the food industry when it was used to extrude pasta products, i.e., pressure extrusion without cooking. Cooking extruders were introduced more recently, initially to expell oil from oilseeds, gelatinize starch, or mix additives.[89] The initial work of Anson and Pader[15-17] the increased anticipated demand for plant proteins, and principally the patent of Atkinson[23] have resulted in the rapid development of extrusion cooking as a means of texturizing plant proteins. This has stimulated the design and development of extruders specifically for the texturization of proteins.

A myriad of snack-type foods are produced by extrusion cooking in the U.S. These include farinaceous- and proteinaceous-type items. Their method of manufacture involves the extrusion under pressure of moist blends or slurries of a variety of raw materials. These may be cooked during the extrusion process, or the extruded, shaped item may be subsequently set by cooking (baking, deep frying). This technology has been described in detail.[156]

Numerous processes for texturing plant proteins have been described in the patent literature.[84,87] Much information on the process is proprietary and much is still secret. The major technique for fabricating textured vegetable proteins is by extrusion of protein under heat and pressure. This is a simple process compared with spinning and requires less equipment and less sophisticated technology. It does not produce well-defined fibers, but gives fibrous particulates with good mouthfeel and chewiness similar to meat. Extrusion basically involves plasticizing moistened proteinaceous material by applying shear forces at transient high temperatures and forcing the proteinaceous lava through a restricted aperture under high pressure into a cooling zone. The shearing within the extruder tube results in elevated product temperatures within the tube, gelatinization of starchy components present, denaturation of proteins, stretching or restructuring of tractile components, shaping of the end product, and expansion of the extrudate upon emergence. Within the tube, mechanical agitation by the screw causes partial orientation of the protein molecules and aligns the molecules prior to expansion. The structure of the plastic, proteinaceous mass changes, and it acquires a fibrous texture. Pressures up to 100 psi and temperatures of 115 to 175°C are attained within the extruder cone.

Upon emergence from the nozzle, the plastic mass expands to give a continuous, ropy stream of puffed, fibrous, textured protein that is either cut into strips or chunks or ground into powder or granules. Depending upon the type and condition of the starting material and other factors, the extruded particles may be compacted or expanded. The expanded form is generally preferred. These particles, usually bite size, can be made in a wide array of sizes and shapes to resemble a variety of products from beef granules to nut meats. The particles are light tan in color and have a bland, nutty flavor. About 60% of the protein-texturizing capacity in the U.S. is licensed under the patent of Atkinson.[40] This process yields a spongy, plexilamellar product with relatively large, branched plates or flat fibers.

### Materials

A significant advantage of extrusion is that a wide range of raw materials can be effectively texturized. Thus proteinaceous flours, grits, and concentrates ranging in protein content from 30 to 75% protein can be facilely transformed into textured products. Products have been made from soy, cottonseed, peanut, corn, wheat gluten, sesame protein, and yeast proteins.[22-24,40,84,87] Most commercial texturized-plant protein is made from soy flour and/or soy grits, though the use of soy protein concentrate is increasing because of its superior flavor characteristics. Occasionally, depending upon product specifications, wheat gluten may be included. This forms a continuous gluten network during the extrusion process and sets well upon cooling to yield a strong, nonfriable product.

Extrusion of full-fat vegetable oil flours (soybean, cottonseed, peanut) has been successfully developed. In this process, the oil apparently minimizes the extent of protein denaturation during the cooking/extrusion process. Lorenz et al.[146] and Spadaro et al.[228] have successfully applied this process to triticale and rice.

Many of the factors affecting the properties of extruded products are still unknown. Close control of the composition and properties of the raw materials is recommended, however, to ensure consistent products.

### Extrusion Process

Atkinson[23] stimulated the application of the thermal extrusion process with the de-

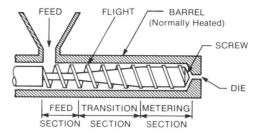

FIGURE 3. Functional sections of a typical cooking extruder. (Reprinted with permission from *J. Food Sci.*, 39, 1099, 1974. Copyright © by Institute of Food Technologists, Chicago, Ill.)

velopment of the simple process whereby moistened protein in the form of plastic mass is extruded through an orifice at elevated temperatures into a medium of low pressure. This produces porous protein product with plexilammellar structure containing longitudinal vacuoles. "The extrudate is a tough, resilient semi-dry, open-celled, funicular structure composed of interlaced interconnected funicali of varying widths and thickness."[24] The real significance is that this product does not disintegrate upon contact with boiling water, could be rehydrated by steaming or boiling, and demonstrated the coherence, texture, and appearance of cooked meat.

The typical essential steps in the extrusion process are outlined below (refer to Figure 3). Soy flour from defatted soy flakes and containing approximately 50% protein is placed in a preconditioning chamber where it is moistened with water or steam to a moisture content of 15 to 40%, depending upon the product characteristics needed. Additives such as salt, alkali, pH controllers, colorants, and flavors can be added as desired. The ingredients are mixed to obtain a homogeneous blend and are fed through a feeder/hopper into the extruder. The basic extruder consists of a hollow barrel or tube (which can be temperature controlled segmentally), inside of which is a tapered screw with whorled flights or ridges whose heights decrease toward the exit end. This, together with the decreasing clearance between the flights and inner barrel surface towards the exit orifice, causes high shearing and concurrent temperature increases as the material is moved along.[88,89] As the preconditioned raw material is fed into this extruder, the screw is rotating at high speed. The speed can be regulated as desired. The deep flights, with pronounced pitch, convey this material down the extruder tube and by continuous shearing action rapidly work it into a continuous, moist matrix. As the clearance diminishes, the temperature and internal pressure rises rapidly from 120 to 175°C and 400 to 600 psi, respectively, changing the material into a plastic, viscous state in the metering section of the extruder. In the transition section of the extruder, both solid material (in aqueous slurry or dough) and melted fluid protein exist. Melting occurs at the barrel surface in a thin film, and it flows to a melt pool at the rear of the flight.[88,89] This phenomenon is influenced by the screw speed and geometry; the thermal conductivity, viscosity, and latent heat of fusion of the material in the barrel, and the temperature control. Because of the high pressures (back pressure from the restrictor orifice or die), the moisture remains trapped in the molten material, and cooking of the ingredients occurs at the high temperatures. The shearing action of the rotating flights tends to align the unfolding, denaturing proteins into parallel sheaths. After a total residence time of 30 to 60 sec in the extruder (variable as desired), the molten mass squirts out through the die orifice. As the material passes through the die, the protein fibers are further aligned. With the instantaneous release of the high pressure the superheated moisture entrapped in the structured, denatured protein, flashes off and leaves vacuoles in the interstices between branching protein strands, and there is concurrent puffing of the extrudate resulting in a porous structure. The evaporation causes rapid dissipation of heat with concurrent cooling of the product. This cooling results in thermosetting of the product. The product, which may contain 20% moisture is usually passed through a drier and the moisture content is reduced to 8% before packaging.[84,87,88,89,276]

### Extruder Types

Most systems designed to create structural and textural properties in foods utilize extruders, which impart these characteristics by mixing, molecular shearing, cooking, forming, and puffing. The extrusion process is a combination of one or more of these functions. Extruder types may range from the pasta extruders that operate at low temperatures to the high-shear cooking extruders that produce the thermoplastic-extruded textured vegetable protein products. Thermoplastic extruders are used in the plastics industry and have been used in the cereals industry for gelatinizing starch and extruding various shaped breakfast cereals. Numerous extruder types have been developed for the texturization of protein rich foods and modifications and improvements in design and applications continue to be patented.

There are several types of extrusion cookers. There is the basic pressure-cooking unit fitted with a rotary steam-lock feeder, i.e. an enlarged cooking chamber, feeding into a shaping extruder. There is the popular, more traditional, tubular extruder with the attached feeding device described in the preceding section. The tube is fitted with steam and water injectors for moistening the proteinaceous material. During extrusion the internal temperatures may be kept relatively low by circulating water or steam.[219,220]

Most cookers include a method of steam preconditioning at controlled temperatures (65 to 100°C) and at atmospheric pressures; a method of uniform application of moisture; an extruder assembly designed to work the moisturized oilseed or cereal into a dough at moderate temperatures (85 to 110°C); a means of elevating the temperature of the dough in the coned nose section of extruder to a desired higher temperature (115 to 175°C) during a very short period of time (12 to 20 sec); a method of forming the dough into the desired shape by use of a die; and a mechanism for cutting the expanding dough into segments of desired length.[219-222]

The popular modern type is the high-temperature, short-time (HTST) extrusion cooker. It has a continuous feeding device for dry materials, an optional steam preconditioner, a high-speed mixer, and an extruder assembly built in several sections, the last section of which is conical and progressively reduced in a cross-sectional area. Hence process temperatures are raised above 100 to 121°C only in the last 12 to 20 sec to the higher temperatures (121 to 186°C) required in the cone section. A tunnel-type dryer, designed for sanitary operation and continuous removal of fines, is a specialized system component.

The high-temperature, short-time extrusion cooking system has become the most popular method for fabrication of textured foods of varying shapes, densities, textures, and rehydration characteristics.[219-222] This system is versatile and energy efficient. It is able to successfully texturize a variety of materials of different protein contents, and to effectively inactivate antinutritive factors and provide a pasteurized product. High-pressure cooker extruders possess a feeder, a compression screw enclosed in a hollow-walled barrel of progressively decreasing diameter.

The feeder may simply be a hopper, vibratory feeder, or screw feeder to conduct the feed meal into the extruder barrel. It may also possess blending units for ingredient mixing and valves for the addition of set quantities of steam or water to precondition the feed stock for specific objectives.

The extruder barrel may be smooth, rifled or grooved and may possess pins that coincide with interruptions in the screw flite. The size (diameter and length) of barrels vary. Different designs and configurations affect mixing and extent of shearing within the barrel when the screw is rotating. The speed of the screw may also be varied.

The heating system usually consists of sectional steam jackets that are modular components of the extruder barrel. Occasionally electric strip heaters are used. Appreciable heat is generated within the extruder barrel by friction and shear as the rotating screw moves the materials under increasing pressure.

Outlet dies or orifices control the back pressure that can be manipulated to regulate the exposure time to high temperatures, and of course it affects the extent or degree of pressure drop experienced by the extruded material as it emerges from the barrel and thereby influences porosity of the extrudate. The die also controls the shape of the emerging material, and the size of the pieces are determined by the location of the cutter knife. The die may be a simple orifice or more complicated, consisting of a two-piece arrangement that forces the flowing material to change directions and thereby increases shearing and aligning of the proteinaceous material as it emerges from the die.[219-222]

The technique of extrusion and the versatility of extruders provide several benefits. Smith[219-222] has enumerated the advantages of extrusion cooking in relation to the manufacture of textured foods. The inactivation of antinutritive factors and the volatilization of off-flavors and off-odors is achieved in conjunction with the fabrication process. The facile control of temperature and dwell time allows antinutrients, allergens, and antitryptic factors to be destroyed, while potential deleterious interactions between lysine and sugars and degradation of sulfur-containing amino acids are minimal. The precise sectional temperature control means that high temperatures are attained for short times, effective pasteurization is achieved, and the shelf life of extruded products is excellent.

The versatility in processing parameters enables a wide range of raw materials to be successfully handled. Extrusion can be manipulated to control product texture and mouthfeel through a wide range of product densities. It successfully forms expanded, plexilamellar, fibrous extrudates with desired thermosetting properties and stability upon rehydration.[220]

**Physical and Chemical Changes**

While the technology of thermoplastic extrusion of protein materials has developed rapidly, basic information concerning the chemical and physical changes occurring to the protein is limited. Within the extruder barrel the globular proteins (glycinins) in the aleurone granules become hydrated, gradually unravelled, and stretched by the shearing action of the rotating screw flites. The protein becomes aligned in sheaths in the direction of flow. The moisture becomes entrapped within these proteinaceous sheaths. In passing through the die, the proteins become further compressed and laminated longitudinally, and denaturation occurs at the high temperature. At the instant of emergence from the die, the pressure drops and the moisture vaporizes and flashes off. This leaves vacuoles within the laminated extrudate. The cooling accompanying vaporization allows the rapid thermosetting or solidification of the stretched protein fibers and a porous structure with parallel arrays or lamellae of protein fibers result.

**Factors Affecting Texture**

The physical characteristics (i.e., texture, density, chewiness, rehydratability, and color) of extruded products can be altered by manipulating several processing parameters. Variables that can influence product quality include ingredients, moisture content, pH, temperature gradients, pressure, shear rates (screw speed), residence time in extruder, extruder type, configuration of extruder, shape, size, and geometry of the die, presence (or absence) of a post-die restricted cooling zone, and post-extrusion treatments. Several of these factors are interrelated.

Though title information has been published the composition of ingredients has a marked impact on the characteristics of extruded products. Proteins from different sources, varying in composition and structure, are expected to significantly affect texture. For example, the inclusion of gluten prepared from hard wheat in the proteinaceous mix yields a tougher, chewier product, while the use of gluten prepared from soft wheat yields a more tender, friable product.[220] The presence of lipids tends to weaken the extrudate. Starches (amylose, amylopectin) and reducing sugars exert marked effects on product texture, depending upon their gelatinizing characteristics and interactions with proteins, respectively.

The moisture concentration in the mix markedly affects product texture. Normally, feed material contains 7 to 10% moisture, and then moisture is added in the mixer or preconditioner. The amount of water added affects the degree of expansion of the product upon extrusion. For maximum expansion soy flour should have around 35% moisture. This facilitates maximum expansion upon emergence from the die. When the proteinaceous material is too dry the temperature increase in the extruder rises excessively, and there is limited expansion of the extruded product. Desirable product qualities of maximum expansion and crisp texture are obtained when the fluid plastic mass emerging from the die can expand, releasing sufficient moisture by vaporization for the product to set with acceptable structure. If moisture is too high the product does not expand, insufficient water vaporizes, and the product remains moist, soft, and occasionally collapses and becomes tough and hard.[51,52]

The effects of moisture concentration largely depend upon the prevailing[23,24] temperatures and pressure especially during the actual extrusion. Atkinson stated the physical structure and characteristics of the extruded product are primarily affected by the concentration of water in the protein mix, the temperature during extrusion, and the pressure developed in the extruder. These are interrelated factors. Thus water facilitates the mixing of the proteinaceous material to form the necessary plastic mass, it causes expansion of the extrudate upon emergence, and by vaporization it forms the vacuoles in the extrudate. Higher levels of water generally result in greater plasticization and expansion. However, the intrinsic water bound by the proteinaceous material cannot accomplish these effects; hence water must be added in varying amounts depending on the composition of the material being extruded. The concentration of this "nonreleasable" water tends to increase with protein concentration in the feed material and with decreasing temperatures. Water should be added to at least 15% more than this nonreleasable water.[23,24,84,87]

Temperatures at extrusion must be above the vaporization temperature of water, i.e., 100°C, to permit expansion and flash evaporation. Temperatures of 120 to 150°C are recommended. In order to produce a textured, rehydratable, structurally stable product, both temperatures and pressure must critically exceed minima, e.g., 120°C and 300 psi, respectively. If extruded at lower temperatures the particles become unstable and disintegrate in boiling water. Approximately 0.8 m$\ell$ of water are added for each gram of protein.

Using response surface analyses, Aguilera[2] attempted to optimize initial moisture content, processing temperature, and screw speed to obtain textured protein pieces with good rehydration characteristics. He found that high processing temperature (above 140°C) and moisture levels, especially below 30%, resulted in extruded pieces with superior rehydration characteristics. However, extrudates made from soy flour with less than 33% moisture exhibited excessive toughness and hardness.

Moisture is also significant in relation to nutritional quality of the extrudate. The heat required for the inactivation of the trypsin inhibitor varies inversely with moisture levels in the protein, i.e., higher temperatures are required for meals with lower moisture contents.[188] Aguilera[2] showed that this relationship also applied to the destruction of trypsin inhibitor during extrusion of soy flour.

Operating temperatures and conditions should be such as to destroy anti-tryptic factors and inactivate antinutrient components without damaging the nutritional value of the protein and, of course, should induce the appropriate physical changes in the ingredients. Trypsin inhibitors are most heat resistant of the undesirable components in soy protein,[27] so that extrusion temperature and times should be sufficient to destroy these but not to degrade protein or cause interactions between the proteins and carbohydrates. In the short-time, high-temperature extruders most of the heat required for product fabrication is generated from the viscous dissipation of the mechanical energy applied through the screw, i.e., friction and from viscous shear within the product itself. Further temperature control is achieved by heating and cooling (with steam or water) at specific segments of the sectional extruder. The ability to precisely control temperature at each point in the extruder system and to adjust it rapidly is critical for the control of product quality.[219,220]

Manipulation of the pH of the proteinaceous materials is a useful approach for varying the textural characteristics of extruded plant proteins. The pH of the material affects fluidity of the dough in the extruder, as well as the shaping, density, chewiness, and rehydration propensities of the product. acidic pH values (pH 5 to 6.5) result in extruded products that are dense and chewy, shape easily, harden (thermoset) slowly, and show poor rehydration properties. These effects may be partly caused by the lower solubility of the protein at acidic pH values and their increased susceptibility to thermal denaturation. Thus the proteins may aggregate sooner in the extruder and form a denser network, thereby decreasing the size of entrapped moisture droplets. This makes it more difficult for this moisture to evaporate upon extrusion, and it results in smaller vacuoles. These in turn retard thermosetting, increase the density, and prolong rehydration of the finished product. In contrast, alkaline pH values result in a softer, looser, more hydratable textured soy protein that is less chewy and less plastic.

Most textured soy proteins are not pH modified and have fairly light density, 10 to 15 lb/ft³.[221] Extruded products with bulk densities ranging from 9 to 37 lb/ft³ can be produced. Denser products of 16 to 24 lb/ft³ are produced at lower temperatures because there is less volatilization of vapor and less expansion upon emergence from the die. This can also be controlled by manipulating the pH.

Much research needs to be done in determining the various factors that affect texture and other properties of extruded products. Studies to establish quantitative interrelationships between operating parameters are needed. Aguilera[2] concluded that statistical approaches such as response surface analyses were very useful in determining optimum operational parameters for the extrusion process.

## New Developments

Recent innovations in extrusion technology have resulted in the fabrication of highly structured extruded products with meat-like texture and improved flavors. These products represent marked improvements over the first generation of extruded texturized proteins because they resemble meat in physical appearance and texture more faithfully than do the previous products. Two recent developments have resulted in significant improvements in the texture and flavor quality of extruded products.

### Tempering Die

In a novel process,[56] the extruded material emerging from the die under pressure and at high temperatures enters a tempering die, a hollow cylinder attached to the die with a diameter greater than that of the extruder die. In the tempering die the hot molten protein does not explode due to flash evaporation of the entrapped moisture, as occurs in the conventional extruder. Instead, the moisture remains entrapped within the molten protein, and some of the entrained droplets may coalesce. Because the pressure is least in the direction of flow, the water droplets tend to be longitudinal in shape as they move toward the exit, where pressure is lowest. This forms channels in the longitudinally aligned laminar flowing protein. As the molten protein approaches the exit port of the tempering die the temperature drops and the protein thermosets or coagulates. At the exit port of the tempering die the temperature (100°C) results in controlled vaporization of the moisture. There is no explosive-type evaporation and hence no puffing of the extrudate. The moisture evaporates and leaves longitudinal vacuoles where the droplets originally were. This results in a fibrolamellar protein matrix in which the protein strands are arranged parallel, with limited cross-branching.

The key factors in this new process are careful control of the initial moisture level and of the temperature and pressure to minimize vaporization within the extruder and tempering barrel. The product has superior texture to the previous generation of extruded products, can be shaped to simulate a variety of meat types, and rehydrates very well. The pieces made by this process lack the interconnecting fibers and spongy structure of products made by conventional extrusion processes; hence they simulate meat fibers better and they are stable to retorting treatments.

*Double Extrusion*

Another innovation resulting in significant improvements in the texture of products involves double extrusion, i.e., the Uni-Tex process.[221,259]Two specialized extrusion cookers are used, one feeding directly into another to produce meat-like, fibrous-to-lamellar chunks of fabricated proteins.[259] The first cooking extruder discharges a moistened, heat-denatured protein into a long-barrel extrusion cooker from which bite size chunks are extruded then dried, flavored, and cooled. The first extruder (fitted with special screws, steamlocks, and dies) is used to: (1) feed, moisten, and heat process the materials, (2) denature the protein, (3) destroy growth inhibitors, and (4) volatilize and remove phenolic acids from process materials. The purposes of the second long-barrel extruder are (1) to reheat the materials fed into it by the first extruder, (2) to stretch, layer, and subsequently cool the process materials, (3) to form them into uniform layers of parallel orientation, and (4) to cut the extrudate into bites of desired size.[219,220,259]

The double extrusion process employs relatively low pressure in both extruders and produces texturized pieces with even, parallel layers of flat, untwisted ribbons or fibers of protein. These pieces have parallel, untwisted, rectilinear fibers devoid of the sponginess associated with pieces produced by high-pressure, single-extrusion cooking.

The product is dense, approximately 25 lb/ft³ (or 400 g /ℓ) at 7% moisture. The pieces are very stable to retorting and upon rehydration retain their layered lamellar structure. This process can produce meat analogs from soy flour, soy concentrates, wheat gluten, peanut, protein, rapeseed protein, and cottonseed.[259] The products made by this latter process show superior properties when compared to the traditional textured products. They lack the undesirable sponginess following rehydration, and they are stable to rehydration at 100°C and above. The high temperatures of the water used in rehydration more effectively leach out stachyose and raffinose, thereby reducing the flatulence-causing agents. There is greater removal of off-flavors during the double-extrusion process to produce a bland product.[222,259]

The extruded product is dense and contains around 30% moisture. This is dried to a moisture content of approximately 7% at which level it is stable and may be safely stored without refrigeration for over 6 months without bacteriological deterioration. The dry product is dense (approximately 2 lb/ft³). After 20 to 30 min in water at

100°C, it rehydrates to about 65% moisture. When the product is appropriately colored and flavored it simulates meat in appearance, mouthfeel, and textural properties. Texture can be modified to resemble different meat types. The rehydrated pieces can be used in a variety of ways in numerous products.

## Structure and Properties

There is little published information available on the macrostructure and microstructure of extruded proteins or on their classical physical or mechanical properties. Cumming et al.[54] observed fiberization of the proteins of soy flour following extrusion. Many irregular holes and fissures were observed in and around the fibers. Aguilera[2] examined the progressive changes in structure of soy flour grits in the barrel of an extruder using scanning electron microscopy. Close to the exit die an increasing degree of strand formation was evident, indicating flow and plasticity in this region. Elongated fibers were very obvious at the die. Outside the die "explosion" effects broke the fibrils, and new surfaces and conjoining networks of irregular branching fibers were apparent. Globular proteins were not observed.

### Physical Properties

Some basic physical properties related to textural characteristics have been examined using soy flour extruded under experimental conditions.[54,61,158] For instance, the density of extruded products decreased as extrusion temperature was increased above 130°C, i.e., from 1.5 to 1.1 g/cm³ at temperatures of 130 and 190°C, respectively.[54] The density had a significant impact on physical characteristics of the extruded product. Rehydration was closely related to density being markedly more rapid with more porous extrudates of low density.[54]

A high positive correlation ($r^2 = 0.926$) was observed between shear force as measured with a Kramer shear press and an increase in process temperature from 110 to 200°C. This was attributed to the large amount of compression required by the spongy pieces before actual shearing began. As the temperature of extrusion was increased from 130 to 180°C, the extruded product became more resistant to shear and compression. This indicated a greater cohesiveness and structural integrity.[158]

When measured using a Warner-Bratzler shear, a sigmoid relationship between processing temperature and shear force was observed. This reflected a rapid change in product characteristic between 140 and 170°C when shear force increased from 1.7 to 2.9 kg. The product extruded at 170°C had a much more distinctive fibrous or laminated structure.

The tensile properties, i.e., breaking strength of pieces extruded at different temperatures progressively increased with the temperature from 120 to 150°C but decreased rapidly above 160°C. This reflected the structure of the pieces where increased orientation and fiberization was obtained at extrusion temperatures between 120 and 150°C, whereas at the higher temperature excess fissuring occurred and thereby weakened the cohesive strength of the pieces.[54,61]

Harper and Harmann[89] have emphasized the need for research to develop quantitative data concerning the interrelationships between operating parameters, extruder design, materials composition and their physical properties, and final product quality. These workers point out that the available knowledge of extrusion theory has been developed in the plastics industry. Research is needed to determine material flow and predict output as a function of barrel dimension, screw design, and rotating speed. Little is known about fusion of the food materials within the extruder barrel, and the effects of extruder design, screw speed, etc. on melting, and how these are related to physical characteristics of the final product. Research on die design is warranted. Design criteria for shape control, flow uniformity and pressure distribution through the breaker plates behind the die have evolved through empirical experience. If the physical properties of these were known, the effect of pressure drop across the die could be determined.[89] Reliable information is needed concerning the physical properties of viscosity, thermal conductivity, heats of reaction, fusion, friction factors, and extrudable raw materials. Other needed research includes measuring nutrient stability (vitamins, proteins, lipids, etc.); and determining fate of antinutrients, extent of Maillard reactions and Strecker-type degradations, and of reduction (if any) of the biological value of proteins during extrusion under the range of conditions that might be encountered in commercial production.

*Composition and Uses*

Textured soy protein pieces are dried, cooled, and screened prior to packaging. Drying is normally in a tunnel-type dryer with air at 115°C. Flavoring and vitamin supplements are usually added to the final dry product to avoid heat destruction and vaporization during extrusion and drying. Hydrogenated fat may be used as a flavor carrier.

The composition of extruded products are essentially identical to the raw materials from which they are manufactured. Extruded products vary in moisture content. An unflavored dried product made from soy flour has a composition of 52, 8, 3, 5, and 1% protein moisture, fiber, ash, and fat, respectively. In the hydrated state this product contains about 70% moisture.[191,192] It may be infused with from 6 to 30% fat.

The advantages of textured soy products include ease of manufacture, low cost, and long storage life. The bacterial count for these products is low, and under normal storage conditions they can keep for at least a year. They are, however, limited in their applications because they do not have the high degree of meat-like texture characteristic of spun-fiber products, though the products developed by newer extrusion processes can be used as meat analogs.

The largest market for textured plant proteins is in their use as meat extenders. Textured plant protein has gained utilization as a meat extender, expecially in school lunch programs, which permit a 30% addition of plant protein products to meat items.[10] Extrusion cooked products in rehydrated state are used as extenders in the formulation of comminuted and other meat items (e.g., spaghetti sauce, chili) and in meat patties, meat loaves, salisbury steak, etc.

In addition to conforming to special health, religious or economic needs, textured protein products should find wide application in convenience foods such as dry-mix entrees, seasoning, sauces and gravy products. There is an ever increasing interest in easily prepared packaged entrees containing all necessary ingredients in one mix. Adolphson and Horan,[1] Horan,[105,108] and Rakosky[191,192] reviewed the technical aspects, cost, and consumer impact of textured soy proteins, particularly in reference to meat extenders.

Functional properties and palatability characteristics associated with the use of textured soy protein in ground beef formulations are well documented.[62,120,223] Although the advantages of using textured soy proteins in ground beef formulations are numerous, some problems still exist. Robinson[198] reported a survey in which 71% of consumers were prejudiced against meat analogs even before trying them. Seidman et al.[213] showed that the addition of textured soy protein above 10% changed the appearance of raw beef patties and decreased the flavor desirability of the cooked product. The problem of the mealy flavor has been a major drawback to the more widespread acceptability of textured products. However, much improved products are available in the 1980's in terms of color, texture, and especially flavor. This will greatly accelerate consumer acceptance of texturized products.

## OTHER METHODS FOR TEXTURIZING PROTEINS

Because of the desire to produce textured proteins with fibrous structure that simulate meats, several other methods for producing texturized products have been developed. Thus in addition to the current, major, commercially practiced methods for texturizing protein, i.e., fiber spinning and extrusion, numerous other modifications of these and several uniquely novel procedures have been developed on experimental, pilot-plant, or commercial scale.[84,87,107] These processes, which are arbitrarily divided into fiber type and textured pieces, are briefly summarized below.

### Fiber Type

Giddey[78] described a process for spinning fibers from a mixture of protein and polysaccharide. The properties and reactions of the polysaccharides having acidic side groups vary with the nature of the side groups. For carrageenin, the sulfate groups are strongly acidic, whereas the alginate polysaccharide contains the weakly acidic carboxyl groups. A combination of polysaccaharide and protein in aqueous solution developed a viscosity suitable for spinning. To coagulate the filamentous streamlets, a pH range of 1 to 3 is required for carrageenin, but it is necessary to supplement this with 10% solution of calcium chloride to insolubilize the alginate.

Ishler and MacAllister[116] used a combination of polysaccharides and proteins. The polysaccharides sodium alginate or pectin were the principal structural components of the fiber, which was coagulated by extruding the dope into a bath containing alkaline earth metals.

A simplified process for converting proteinaceous slurries (soy, peanut, casein, or yeast protein isolates) into edible fibers consists of pumping a protein slurry (up to 35% solids) at high pressure through a heat exchanger and then expelling it through a small nozzle. The protein emerges as fibers (4 to 6 cm long) that are cooled by dropping 20 ft through ambient air into a collecting vessel. Excess water is removed by centrifuging.[102]

Lange[140] described a simple process that yields a protein monofilament. Soy isolate mixed with water, sodium sulfite, glycerine, plus an acid or base was heated until it became plastic (95 to 120°C) and then it was extruded through tiny orifices into air. The resulting fiber can be combined with binders, flavors, and color to form simulated meats. These "dry" spinning processes eliminate the preliminary spinning dope step, thereby avoiding alkali-induced alterations of the protein and the acid-salt coagulating bath employed in the usual fiber-spinning operation.

Casein fibers that are stable to boiling are made by extruding into a gaseous environment a homogenous mixture of calcium casinate, calcium and orthophosphate at 80°C around pH 5.5 to 6.0. When bonded with a proteinaceous binder, these fibers are particularly suitable for reconstituted fish products.

The mesophase process, although it produces filaments and uses a spinneret, is different from the Boyer process. In this process the protein is produced in the form of a mesophase, i.e., under conditions where they would be expected to form a precipitate, some proteins instead produce a homogeneous liquid phase that can coexist with the solution. Soy proteins, and many other vegetable proteins form these liquid protein-rich phases providing they have retained their native structure.[245,247] Thus soy proteins that are scarcely soluble in water at their isoelectric pH remain in a liquid, crystalling mesophase state when sodium chloride concentration is above 0.45 $M$. Exploiting this behavior has led to a variation of the classical fiber-spinning process and has eliminated the need for alkaline treatment. Thus soy protein isolate prepared in the customary way is dispersed in water ($\sim$pH 5) by adding solid salt to a final molarity of 0.4 to

0.5 *M* instead of dissolving it with alkali. The curd does not dissolve completely, but the soluble portion or mesophase is separated by centrifuging and then extruded through spinnerets into a hot-water (80°C or higher) bath. The elution of the salt, the acidic pH, and particularly the high temperature cause coagulation of the protein into fibers. The remaining salt is removed by leaching into the water.[245,246] The filaments are weak unless heated. The process is most conveniently done at the isoelectric point ($\sim$pH 5).

In this mesophase process there is no need to stretch the filaments to give them mechanical strength. In order to avoid the mechanical limitations of collecting on a drum they are simply collected on a conveyor belt and washed and stored frozen or dehydrated. Flavors, colors and other materials may be incorporated in the spinning dope, and the problems of high pH are avoided. The filament can be made in any required size and, within limits, of any required cross section. No binder is necessary.

Although this process avoids many of the problems of the Boyer method, it has some limitations. It requires an essentially undenatured protein isolate as well as a low level of particulate matter. This requires great care in the protein isolation process, and protein isolates meeting these criteria are not normally commercially available. With soy protein, sulfite is needed to control the disulfide interchain linking in the protein, and although the sulfite is removed during spinning, regulations in some countries may preclude its use in fabrication of edible fibers.[246]

### Textured Pieces

The pioneering research of Anson[13] and Pader[14] in developing texturized, chewy proteins stimulated much creativity and changed general attitudes toward the potential of plant protein foods. In a series of patents,[13,17] Anson and Pader described several methods for making thermal setting-structured gels (simulating meats in texture) from aqueous slurries of soy protein by the application of heat. Other proteins, were also used i.e., casein. Oils, flavors, and colors could be included as desired. Anson and Pader[16] described a method by which enmeshed protein filaments in a thermal gelling protein (e.g., peanut protein) formed an irreversible chewy protein gel following heating. Thus peanut protein was made into a plastic paste containing 28% protein. This was extruded and the protein cylinders were layered in parallel arrays and then thermally set by autoclaving. The product supposedly possessed the texture and chewiness of meat.[17]

Anson and Pader[15,17] described a simple process for the manufacture of a "chewy protein gel" by thermal gelation of an aqueous dispersion of protein. They claimed that this product had the chewiness, moisture, and texture of cooked meat, i.e., when pieces were chewed they had the physical properties of resilience, elasticity, and resistance to shear that are typical of meat. In addition, they had the property of heat stability, retaining their firmness when subjected to heat, particularly in products subjected to heat processing or normal cooking conditions prior to eating. The gels were clear and smooth. Appropriate ingredients, i.e., carbohydrates, flavors, colors, etc., could be included to obtain the desired meat-type impression, and the gel could easily be molded into a variety of shapes.

A variety of products could be made from this, i.e., it could be shaped into cylinders or large fibers or small pieces and used as simulated pot roast or in chopped meats. These gels are heat stable and retain their properties following cooking. To obtain a variety of textures and nonuniform appearance, other proteins like gluten may be incorporated. This does not form a chewy gel but improves the handling of the gel.[84] These blends are very useful in hamburger and laminated-type luncheon meats.

Texture and mouthfeel of these gels can be modified by incorporating hydrocolloids into the gel or by coating them on the gel particles. The incorporation of carbohydrate additives makes the gels weaker and less gelatinous. The addition of gums, such as locust bean gum, reduces the rubberiness of the gel and makes it softer. Alginates, seaweed extracts, and locust bean gum facilitate extrusion and provide products with smoother textural characteristics. Because of their water absorption characteristics, gums may also be used to modify and control the rehydration properties of a dehydrated gel.[79] Small particles of the gelable protein may be coated with flavorings, colorants, etc. and then thermally gelled, the resultant particles being useful in chopped meats, chili, soups, meat pies, etc.

Anson and Pader[14] described a simple extrusion device (a spaghetti-type extruder die) whereby multiple parallel cylinders (0.007-in. diameter) of chewy gel-forming proteins were extruded on to a reciprocating platform. As the protein cylinders emerged from the apertures in the extrusion apparatus they were individually coated with an edible additive or heated with steam, which caused the formation of coagulated film and prevented adhesion of the fibers. The cylinders of protein were thus layered to form a mass of cylinders arranged in parallel layers. Each layer was pressed lightly as it is deposited on top of the previous layer. The mass was then heat treated with steam and a chewy mass resembling meat in appearance and texture was obtained. This could be cooked as desired and retained its texture.

Robbins et al.[197] prepared an isoelectric (pH 4.5), precipitable soy protein devoid of water-soluble albumins and globulins and it formed a continuous elastic gel when heated to 100°C. This protein could also be spun into fibers using a dope at pH 6.5.

Coleman and Creswick[50] patented a method for preparing texturized "meats" for soup mixes. Portions of meats (chicken, pork, beef) are shredded into small fibers and recombined with soy sodium proteinate, egg albumen as binder, and fat. This combination is mixed, extruded and cut into small particles, heat coagulated, and dried to a moisture level of 2%. These can be flavored and colored as desired.

Subjecting soybean meal to temperatures above 100°C and pressures up to 5000 psi for short periods debitters and coagulates the soybean into tough, chewable particles that can be used as meat extenders because they expand without disintegration upon rehydration.[103]

A technique that does not require fiber spinning or extrusion equipment for the manufacture of chewy protein fibers was patented by Arima and Harada.[20] This involves the formation of a coagulum of mixtures of vegetable, cereal, egg, or milk proteins and alginate and calcium salts. This curd is cut with rotating blades to form soft, flat fibers or ribbons of random lengths. These are immersed in an acid bath of pH 2.5 and then boiled, drained, and thoroughly washed. These are boiled again to remove contaminants, washed, and dried. The fibers are 1 to 4 mm wide and 8 to 20 mm in length, exhibiting superior elasticity and strength compared to spun fibers. Various combinations of proteins may be used to simulate different meat types in texture and when appropriate fat and flavors are added, color.

Okumura and Wilkinson[172] described a method for freezing soymilk curd so that the entrapped water forms ice crystals that coalesce and expand. This compacts and toughens protein sponge structure ensuring stability during subsequent processing. By heating this mass the water is drained from the protein sponge together with undesirable carbohydrates. Defatted sesame, cottonseed, or alfalfa protein may also be used. Lugay and Kim[277] reviewed the freeze alignment process for protein texturization.

Cabot[43] developed a process whereby soy protein curd (pH 7) was modified by extrusion at 100 to 130°C and pressure of 75 to 200 psi to yield a product with textural properties resembling seafood (shrimp, scallops) amenable to breading and deep frying.

## Steam Texturization

Another commercial process for preparing expanded textured proteins without extrusion is the steam texturization process.[67,233-235] The process consists of adding water to a blend of defatted soy flour or soy concentrate or isolate to raise the moisture to 20%. The mixture is then fed into a rotating multichambered valve device. As the valve turns the mixture is subjected to high-pressure steam, which results in volatilization of much of the undesirable flavors of the soy. The pressurized material is expelled through a nozzle into a zone of low pressure. The sudden pressure release causes puffing, texturizing, and flash evaporation of the undesirable volatilized flavor compounds. Residence time in the apparatus may be less than a second; hence, the product does not turn dark but is light in color and has a bland flavor. A variation of this process has also been developed in which a slurry of the protein material is sprayed into a stream of high-pressure steam. The excess moisture is flashed off and a textured product is obtained.[234]

Press Texturization

McAnelly[159] patented a method for the texturization of soy flour by making a dough and cooking it under pressure. This dough assumes a cellular or spongy structure when the pressure is released.

Calvert and Atkinson[44] reported that the inclusion of cysteine or ammonium hypophosphite in an oilseed protein dispersion followed by application of high pressure at 65 to 90°C (i.e., passage between heated rollers revolving at different speeds, which causes plastic flow) yielded a dry, dense mechanically strong protein structure. This could be rehydrated into a firm, flexible, spongy structure that retained its shape without any evidence of disintegration. Any device that can induce plastic flow may be used, e.g., extruders and drum rollers. The cysteine, apparently by reducing disulfide cross-links between proteins, facilitates plastic flow of the proteins under pressure. The protein molecules slide, realign, and reorient with the pressure, forming strong intermolecular bonds which stabilize the protein against disintegration upon rehydration and cooking. The protein sheets from the rolls can be cut and shaped as desired. The pieces rehydrate and swell facilely absorbing three to five times their weight in water. Jenkins[118] used sulfides (0.1%) and a cooker-extruder to prepare expanded fibrous protein products from soybean meal containing 5% oil. Apparently the sulfides, via sulfhydryl/disulfide exchange reactions by disrupting intra- and intermolecular disulfide bonds, allow the proteins to unravel and realign when subjected to the shear forces during extrusion through the die. This causes the longitudinal orientation of the proteins and improves the fibrous nature of the finished product.

Waggle[253] subjected an aqueous protein dispersion or dough to a high temperature (100°C) under pressure and mechanically rolled, stretched, or worked it with mechanical beaters. This mechanical working imparted a high degree of orientation to the protein structure prior to the final thermal setting. This reputedly yielded a resilient, chewy, and meat-like product that was stable to heating. The inclusion of humectants such as glycerol improved the mechanical tempering and orientation.

Other

A process for making synthetic caviar was patented by Nesmeyanov et al.[168] The "caviar" is composed of an encapsulated protein solution or suspension. The capsule is a membrane composed of gelatin and vegetable tanning agents. The process consists of making an aqueous alkaline solution or suspension of the protein, to which a gel-forming agent such as gelatin is added. Other texture-modifying ingredients are also added, such as glycerol, vegetable oil, and starch. The mixture is then formed into granules by adding it in a drop-wise stream to an immiscible-medium bath, such as oil, which has an upper layer heated above the gelling temperature of the mix (15 to 40°C) and a lower layer cooled to temperatures below gel melting (0 to 20°C). The granules are washed and tanned by immersion in a solution containing tannins such as tea extract. They can be colored by soaking them in appropriate food dye.

## Gluten

Wheat gluten has traditionally served as a basis for textured vegetable proteins for vegetarian diets.[90,91] Upon being placed in boiling water, gluten expands, the protein denatures, and a spongy, chewy product is obtained. This can be used in broths, chopped to simulate meats, or made into meat loaves.

Gluten is made by the elution of starch from dough. When this gluten is dried carefully and milled to a flour it is commercialized as vital gluten. Generally freshly prepared gluten is far superior to vital gluten for the preparation of texturized protein foods. Problems of rehydrating vital gluten for use in vegetarian products have been solved by the uniform rehydration process.[91]

Finucane and McAllister[71] described various formulations of wheat gluten, soy flour, protein binders, flavors, etc. which, when thoroughly blended and extruded through a macaroni press, yielded chewy particles that were usable in meat dishes and pies when cooked. Blends of wheat gluten and oilseed flour can be thermally set to give a meat-like gel when properly flavored and colored.[176]

## Oriental Textured Food

The traditional oriental textured products, both the nonfermented type (i.e., kori-tofu and yuba) and fermented types (sufu and tempeh) will not be described in great detail in this article.

Tofu is soybean curd made by coagulating soybean milk with a calcium salt. It is a white, soft, gelatinous mass containing 88% moisture, 6% protein, and 3% lipid. It is a soybean protein concentrate because soluble and insoluble carbohydrates are at least partly removed during the processing, and thus the protein content on a dry basis in tofu is higher than in the original soybean. Kori-tofu is tofu dried into a porous, spongy matrix without case hardening, by the process of freezing, aging, pressing, and thawing. It has 53.4% protein and 9% water. This is essentially a freeze-texturing process that is practiced in Japan.[255]

Sufu is a traditional Chinese cheese made from calcium-precipitated soybean curd by pressing it into molds to eliminate water. The pressed curd is cut into small cubes, sprayed with an acidic saline solution and exposed to hot-air sterilization at 100°C for 10 min. This minimizes bacterial contamination. These pieces are then inoculated with *Actinomucor elegans*, and the mycelium forms a mat around the particles.[98]

Tempeh is made from dehulled soybeans that are soaked, cooked briefly, and then inoculated with *Rhizopus oligosporms*. Within 24 to 48 hr a continuous mat of mycelium has overgrown the beans to form a firm cake. This can be sliced, dipped in salt brine, and deep-fat fried or used as chunks of protein.[231,232] Soybean curd or cheese has been traditionally made in China. The process was reviewed by Yang and Jackson.[273]

## SENSORY CHARACTERISTICS

With regard to development of completely new products, i.e., analogs and/or modified conventional foods, it must be remembered that most people select food primarily for the enjoyment they derive from its consumption. Thus the quality attributes or sensory properties of new foods are critical factors in determining their acceptability and commercial success. However, nutritional value and dietary and perhaps therapeutic properties will play an increasingly important role as the consumer becomes more knowledgeable about nutrition and optimum nutrient combinations.

Sensory properties connote those characteristics of a food whose evaluation is based on the integrated input from five senses: sight, taste, smell, touch, and hearing. The evaluation is subjective and complex, involving physical and psychological phenomena. The important sensory properties are broadly classified under the terms appearance (shape, color, size), texture, and flavor.[136] All of these are important criteria in food selection and acceptance. The color, shape, and size of a food item are critical traits in the initial selection, testing, and acceptance of a food. Food analogs should faithfully reproduce or closely simulate a familiar original food item. Otherwise, the first impression (based on unfamiliarity) will tend to be negative unless motivated subjects are involved. This is a challenging area in food development and Sidel et al.[216] have noted the lack of specific methods for the comprehensive sensory testing of fabricated foods.

## Texture

Texture, which is a composite of several properties, is one of the three primary sensory properties of food that relates to the sense of touch or feel and is capable of objective measurement. The analogous psychological and physical terms are kinesthesis and rheology, respectively.[136] Bourne[34] has stated that there is no satisfactory definition for texture, and he proposed using the term "textural properties" to reflect the numerous physical property components underlying texture. A food may have up to 30 different discrete textural properties.[33,34] Bourne defined the textural properties of food as those physical characteristics that are sensed by touch or feel, are related to the deformation, disintegration, and flow of food under force, and can be measured objectively by functions of force, time, and distance.[34] Therefore, texture represents a plurality of sensory impulses that reflect physical characteristics, i.e., the rheological properties of deformation and the manner in which food disintegrates in the mouth. Textural properties include: (1) mechanical characteristics like hardness, cohesiveness (brittleness, chewiness, gumminess), viscosity, elasticity and adhesiveness, (2) geometrical characteristics like particle size, shape, and orientation (grainy, coarse, fibrous, etc.), and (3) miscellaneous characteristics like moist, fatty, greasy, and other textures.[238]

Textural properties are often compositely referred to as "mouthfeel", i.e., the sensations perceived during entry, biting, mastication, and swallowing of food. Mouthfeel connotes the nonchemical tactile stimuli sensed in the mouth during mastication, savoring, and swallowing of food. Textural characteristics include chewiness (meat), crispness (chips), smoothness (whole milk), flakiness (fish), crumbliness (cookie), shortness (ginger cookie), gumminess, stickiness, plasticity, stringiness, etc. These are attractive properties in foods and determine consumer acceptance in many cases. Textured protein foods like meat analogs must possess the textural characteristics that duplicate those found acceptable in the original food or provide a new texture. Szczesniak[238-240] has extensively categorized descriptive terms for textural properties of foods, and her studies demonstrate the importance of these characteristics in food acceptability.

The various objective methods for evaluating textural characteristics of foods, the specific physical properties/components measured, and their reliabilities and limitations have been described and discussed by Kramer and Szczesniak[135] and Bourne.[33,34] Corey[53] has addressed, to a limited extent, the problems in testing the textural properties of meat analogs. The difficulties involved in measuring these textural properties and problems of terminology and lack of standard definitions have also been discussed by Sherman.[215]

Oral impressions of relative hardness, shape, and moisture or dryness can form the basis of specific subjective procedures to assess the textural properties of textured foods.[238] Trained sensory panels provided with appropriate reference standards can provide precise and reproducible results.

Textural properties and their importance vary from food to food. In beverages they are of minor significance; in numerous foods they are equally as important as flavor (fruits, vegetables), and in certain foods they constitute the principal sensory attribute (e.g., celery, potato chips and several meats). Thus in meats, toughness, tenderness, juiceness, dryness, and chewiness are prime quality traits. Hence texturized protein products intended for use as meat analogs or extenders should possess these attributes. In foods where flavor is not the primary sensory impact or response, texture is a preeminent requisite.[240] However, only when the genuine textural properties or mouthfeel diverge from the normal or anticipated texture are consumers aware of their importance. If the texture is not as expected, it becomes a focal point for criticism and rejection of food.[239,240]

In most meats both textural and flavor properties are very important, and both of these composite qualities must be effectively simulated in meat analogs. To simulate meats, protein analogs should be highly deformable (compressable), possess a measurable shear strength (toughness), show a lack of brittleness, require an intermediate amount of work for mastication (not too tough, nor too tender), require some grinding or tearing in addition to compression for proper mastication, and impart a sensation of juiceness when first compressed during mastication and subsequent chewing.[33] Tenderness is a critical palatability factor in determining the acceptance of meats. In this specific case, mouthfeel is composed of the impression of the initial ease of penetration and shearing of the meat by the teeth, the ease with which meat breaks into chewable fragments, and the texture of the residue upon chewing. The physical basis of these traits in meats needs to be quantified to facilitate their duplication in meat analogs.[33,34,277]

In Bourne's summary of textural characteristics of fabricated foods, meat analogs are categorized as chewy foods, that is, they are deformable, nonrigid, not subject to brittle fracture, but they possess shear strength as shown by toughness and work required to masticate. Chewy foods require compression, grinding, and shear-tearing for proper mastication. These should not be excessive or the food will be considered too tough. Using force/compression plots, Bourne[34] showed extensive differences within beef cuts that were greater than those between beef cuts and meat analogs. The meat analog had initial bite characteristics intermediate between cooked tenderloin and chuck steak. Chewability, as reflected in the ratios of initial and second compressability curves, were approximately the same for all three products. The initial deformation curve was much larger for the meat analog than for the meat, however. In addition, the analog demonstrated much greater recovery from the initial compression, i.e., greater springiness than the meat. Furthermore, the meats gave a sensation of juiciness throughout mastication, whereas the protein analog felt dry and the sensation of dryness became more pronounced as mastication progressed.[33] These are only two aspects of meat texture that have not yet been replicated in meat analogs. In the analogs made from soy fibers, toughness and chewiness were matched quite well.[33] Several other properties were not duplicated, however, and these are among the most challenging problems confronting the fabrication of meat analogs from textured plant foods.

Bourne[34] has cogently stated that new technology, particularly in the area of fabricated foods, will require a full understanding of the physical and chemical bases of texture. This is necessary to obtain the desired textural characteristics and to design texturized foods that are acceptable.

## Flavor

Several physical, chemical, psychological, and possibly nutritional factors both consciously and subconsciously affect food selection and consumer acceptance. While no single factor is predominant, flavor, which represents a composite sensory impact including odor, taste, and mouthfeel, is usually a primary criterion of quality. The importance of flavor in governing the acceptance of foods has been well emphasized both from the point of view of desirable and undesirable flavors in food, particularly off-flavor problems. Because flavor is a major and decisive factor in the selection, acceptance, and ingestion (or rejection) of a food item, an understanding of flavor attributes must be an integral objective in the development of new or specially formulated foods for various target groups. Ignorance, neglect, or minimization of the critical role of flavor (and texture) has been a common cause of failure in the history of fabricated, formulated, and commerciogenic foods.[180]

Flavor has two connotations; viz. it refers to the psychosomatic impression preceived following stimulation of appropriate nerve (taste, smell) receptors by odoriferous and taste-producing chemicals, and it also may refer to a group of chemicals responsible for the overall flavor sensation produced by a food.

Except for water and odorless gases, most volatile components have traditionally been considered the basis of food flavors. It is now known, however, that many nonvolatile substances found in foods affect flavor and its perception. Flavor chemistry is a complex area of significant practical importance in food fabrication. Knowledge of the nature of flavor chemicals, their origin and synthesis, their physical and chemical properties, their interactions with each other and with food components, their partitioning and adsorption characteristics, and their chemical alteration during processing, storage and cooking are important aspects that have been reviewed.[29,73,75,81-83,129,130,150,155,173,209,224-227] The perceived flavor of food is affected by several parameters: interactions, such as additive, synergistic and masking, differential adsorption on food components and the physical structure of the food, particle size, succulence, emulsion etc.

In formulating flavor blends for various foods, a knowledge is needed of the major flavor precursors and mechanisms by which flavors are generated via thermal reactions during cooking. Thus in meat analogs, appropriate thermolabile precursors might be included. More information concerning flavors is needed to improve the acceptability of food analogs, to make formulated nutritious foods attractive to a variety of ethnic or regional taste preferences, to facilitate development of superior flavor ingredients, and, importantly, to devise flavors that mask or modify undesirable flavors that currently cannot be eliminated by practical processing methods.

Food flavors (taste, aroma) usually are composed of a broad array of chemical compounds including volatile and nonvolatile compounds.[173,209] Solms[226] broadly divided flavors into the volatile compounds affecting odor, nonvolatile compounds affecting taste and mouthfeel, and compounds possessing potentiating and synergistic effects. Natural flavors may be direct metabolites of exogenous or endogenous biogenesis (enzymatic) the products of chemical reactions (e.g., autoxidation, hydrolysis), or of thermally induced reactions. Lipids, proteins, amino acids, carbohydrates, vitamins, and salts are the principal sources of food flavors. The relative importance of each varies from commodity to commodity.

Carbohydrates, particularly the reducing sugars, through nonenzymatic browning or the Maillard reaction, are the sources of numerous flavors, especially in foods subjected to cooking like meats. The chemistry of sugars with emphasis on changes that can occur in food systems has been summarized by Hodge and Osman.[101] Hodge[100] has reviewed the significance of sugars in the synthesis of numerous important flavor compounds during the heat treatment of foods.

Lipids, including hydrocarbons, are sources of flavors in foods of plant, animal, fish, and avian origin. Lipids also act as flavor solvents and carriers, and their physical state in foods affects the partitioning of flavors and their perception by the consumer. The functions of lipids in flavors have been reviewed extensively.[73,130,209]

In addition to the lipids and sugars, the nitrogenous components like amino acids, peptides, and nucleotides can also impart flavors to foods, especially meats. The importance of these compounds to flavor has been reviewed by Solms,[224-227] Kirimura et al.,[131] Yamaguchi et al.,[271] and Ney.[170]

Because of the increased demand for meat flavors and the incorporation of hydrolyzed vegetable and yeast proteins into imitation meat flavors, much interest has been focused on the composition of these flavors.[153-154] Amino acids constitute a major class of components of these hydrolyzed flavors, hence the flavor of amino acids have been studied in detail. Solms[225] and Kirimura et al.[131] reviewed the information on the taste of amino acids, peptides, and proteins. Only certain amino acids impart flavor. Solms[225] divided amino acids into those possessing little taste, those with complex taste (cysteine, methionine, and glutamic acid), and those in which the L an D enantiomorphs taste bitter and sweet. Ranking in decreasing order of sweetness are D-tryptophan, D-histidine, D-phenylalanine, D-tyrosine, D-leucine, L-alanine, and glycine, with D-tryptophan 35 times as sweet as sucrose. In order of decreasing bitterness, there are L-tryptophan, L-phenylalanine, L-tyrsine, and L-leucine, with L-trypophan half as bitter as caffeine. Sulfur-containing amino acids may possess a sulfurous taste believed attributable to some decomposition; alanine and glycine taste sweet while leucine, tryptophan, tyrosine, and phenylalanine and glycine taste sweet while leucine, tryptophan, tyrosine, and phenylalanine taste bitter at low concentrations and sweet at higher concentrations.[225] Glutamic acid, especially the Na salt, imparts a brothy flavor and may act as flavor enhancer in foods.

Thus while amino acids can impart flavors directly (e.g., glycine is an important flavorant in lobster and crab[131] and glutamic acid — especially its sodium salt-imparts "brothy" flavors to meat dishes and soups), they also function as important precursors of many volatile flavors generated via Strecker degradation reactions. Furthermore, mixtures of amino acids are very important in the flavor of many foods. They provide an essential background flavor note to many foods upon which the more perceptible and characteristic flavors are superimposed .[225,226] This is particularly true for cheese, fish, meats, sauces, and broths where amino acids and peptides provide taste and tactile impressions. They may also act as flavor potentiators and flavor synergists.

In 1909 Ikeda[115] demonstrated that monosodium glutamate (MSG) was the major compound for imparting a meaty, brothy sensation to foods and soups. Produce by microbial synthesis, MSG is presently a major ingredient of meat-type and soup flavors.[92,170] It markedly intensifies the taste of food and significantly reduces flavor threshold concentration (i.e., minimum concentration at which flavors are perceptible in a particular food system) of other flavor components. Ney[170] showed that several chemical compounds with two negative charges located four to six carbons from one another like MSG, act as flavor enhancers. The presence of an alpha amino group further accentuates this effect.

Depending on their composition, peptides can exert bitter, brothy, pleasant, and sweet tastes.[131,225,226] Most attention has been given to bitter-tasting peptides, though the dipeptide L-aspartyl-methylphenylalanine (aspartame) is a successful sweetener. Many peptides exert bitter tastes that can be related to their net hydrophobicity.[170] Bitterness is usually associated with peptides containing a high proportion of valine, leucine, isoleucine, phenylalanine, and tyrosine. Kirimura et al.[131] reported that peptides which taste sour possess two acidic amino acids or an acidic and an aromatic amino acid. They attributed sourness to hydrogen bonding. Some peptides taste sweet. Mazur et al.[157] discovered that L-aspartyl-L-phenylalanine methyl ester was at least 100 times sweeter than sucrose.

Thus the flavor potential of amino acids and peptides is slowly being elucidated, and this will inevitably result in the formulation of improved meat and cheese-like flavors. The ability of glutamyl peptides to mask bitter flavors is particularly significant for fabricating novel foods.[171]

The contribution of proteins to food flavors must also be recognized. While proteins per se have no intrinsic flavor, they may modify flavor by their differing capacities to bind flavors, to act as off-flavor carriers, to generate flavors on cooking, and to release reactants that may produce falvors — especially following hydrolysis or proteolysis. These are important factors to be considered in fabricating foods from different proteins. In the fabrication of foods, the same formulas may not apply for all proteins because texture, colors, and flavor binding of the processed protein will vary with its composition and structure. This is particularly true when various oilseed meals are used, e.g., in cooking extrusion.

Several flavors are generated from proteins by heating. Manley and Fagerson[153,154] identified numerous compounds following heating of vegetable proteins, demonstrating that proteins per se can serve as sources of many flavors, especially during thermal processing. The production of various volatile sulfur and carbonyl compounds following the heating of $\beta$-lactoglobulin was reported by Nakanishi and Wada.[166] Maga[151] reported on the sensory evaluation and flavor quality of a number of food proteins. The capacity of proteins to impart desirable and undesirable flavors to foods must always be evaluated.

Quist and Von Sydow[184,185] isolated over 150 volatile flavor compounds (hydrocarbons, alcohols, aldehydes, ketones, furans, and sulfur-containing compounds) following the heating of casein, soy, or fish proteins. The amount of each class varied with each protein, but in all cases concentrations increased with intensity of heating. These studies showed that flavors generated by heating proteins may be significant in the flavor of the final food products, especially if they become entrapped or adsorbed, e.g., in lipids associated with the proteinaceous food.

In addition to acting as sources of flavors per se, protein also bind flavors.[29,75,227] Thus when used as ingredients in foods or when exclusively used in the manufacture of simulated foods, the capacity to bind added flavors (i.e., flavor adsorption, binding, and retention) is a critical attribute of new proteins. A important criterion in the successful utilization of meat extenders is their ability to adsorb and retain added flavors, and the most important limitation to consumer acceptance is undesirable product flavor. Flavor loss during commercial processing, storage, and home preparation, as well as undesirable protein ingredient flavor are significant problems in extended-meat products and in meat analogs.

## Meat Flavors

The success or failure of fabricated textured foods will depend to a significant extent on whether they can be flavored to faithfully and consistently simulate the imitated products or establish themselves as bona fide foods. Because the initial use of texturized proteins has been mostly in meats and simulated meat products, there is currently intensive research activity concerned with the elucidation of meat flavors and the formulation of good imitation meat flavors.

Bird[30] predicted that vegetable proteins would displace around 2 billion pounds of meat and other proteins in the U.S. by the 1980s. This has not been realized yet. The successful formulation of a meat flavor with good aroma, taste, and mouthfeel (full, brothy, and without undesirable residual notes) is a major challenge in the successful expansion of the analog market.

The complexity of meat flavor is dramatized by the identification of over 500 components to date. Many of the compounds have been quantified and tabulated.[47,63,97,109,110,155,256]

Kuramoto and Katz[139] briefly reviewed the evolution of information on the chemistry of meat flavors. Hornstein[109-110] showed that the flavors of red meats are mostly attributable to low molecular weight; water-soluble extracts of muscle though the aqueous extracts of adipose tissue apparently contain precursors of the compounds responsible for species characteristics.[177,254] The adipose tissue serves as a reservoir for the precursors of aroma compounds, mostly aldehydes, which might be termed the "bouquet" of meat, and they contribute to mouthfeel aroma even when present in low concentration.[263]

Reducing sugars (ribose, deoxyribose, glucose, mannose, and galactose), several amino acids (methionine, cysteine, and glutamine), and thiamine are the important common precursors of the thermally generated flavors in meat. While recognizing that the lipid components give rise to varying amounts of several carbonyl compounds, Chang[47] concluded that these are of minor importance to meat flavor because meat flavor can be generated from lean muscle alone. However, the addition of lipids or adipose of the appropriate species is helpful in the generation of flavor reminiscent of meat from a particular species. Aliphatic lactones can be generated from lipids, and these contribute important flavor notes.

Various sulfur compounds (mercaptans, thiophenes) and various heterocyclic compounds (pyrazines and various alkyl derivatives thereof) are important components of the flavor of cooked beef. Chang[49] has isolated over 160 flavor compounds from boiled beef but could identify no particular compound that was genuinely reminiscent of beef, indicating that subtle combinations of flavorants at low concentrations are essential for true meat flavor.

Meat flavor is generally characterized by the high concentration of inosine-monophosphate (IMP) present. This is derived by the sequential hydrolysis and deamination of adenosine triphosphate.[119] Nonvolatile compounds identified as being important in meat flavor are alanine, glycine, glutamate, hydroxyproline, lysine, methionine, phenylalanine, tyrosine, creatine, creatinine, taurine, hypoxanthine, purine nucleotides, purine nucleosides, inosine-5-monophosphate, lactic acid, and inorganic potassium salts.[226]

In foods — and especially in meats — amino acids, peptides and mononucleotides interact in a complex manner involving synergism and potentiation.[119,131,170,225,226] Kuninaka[137] has reviewed in detail the role of 5'-mononucleotides and sodium glutamate as flavorants and flavor potentiators in meat-type flavors. Flavor potentiators are compounds that may possess no flavor impact themselves but significantly accentuate the effects or impact of other flavorants in the mixture. Sodium glutamate (MSG) improves the flavor impact, "the fulless" of mixtures of amino acids and peptides especially in the presence of mononucleotides [inosine 5'-nucleotide (IMP) and guanosine-5'-nucleotide (GMP)]. These mutually reduce flavor threshold levels by an order of magnitude or more. In model systems the flavor threshold values of IMP and GMP are reduced over 100-fold to approximately 6.0 and 0.3 ppm in the presence of 0.1% MSG. IMP and GMP at concentrations of approximately 100 and 2 mg/100 g have been found.[92] The addition of a methyl or ethyl thiol group to IMP causes a fivefold enhancement of its synergistic effect with MSG.[272]

In meat condiments or seasonings, MSG should be added at approximately 20% of the sodium chloride concentration, and nucleotides at around 5% of the MSG concentration.[92] The levels of IMP and GMP used vary with food; in meat seasonings, the use of meat flavor to about 0.1% by weight of final product is advocated.

Mason and Katz[155] reviewed the various factors affecting the development of meat flavors and the respective roles of lipids, mono- and oligosaccharides, and nitrogenous substances in the final flavor. They concluded that there was little doubt that the lipid material of adipose cells contributes some of the most characteristic and potent flavor chemicals in the overall mixture of flavor constituents formed during cooking.Reducing sugars and phosphosphorylated sugars are the precursors of many important, thermally produced flavors in meat. These interact with amino acids or products of amino acids to generate unique and important products. For example, 4-hydroxy-5-methyl-3(2H) furanone, an important flavorant in beef broth, is formed from ribose-5-phosphate and glutamine or glutamic acid.[248] Furthermore, the carbonyl compounds derived from the thermal alteration of sugars interact with amino acids, resulting in Strecher degradation and release of aldehyde, ammonia, and hydrogen sulfide. These volatile products may in turn interact to produce a range of novel flavor compounds. For example, thiol groups, cysteine, or hydrogen sulfide may interact with furan compounds to yield analogous thiophenes via displacement of the hydroxyl function with a thiol group.[248] Sulfur-containg amino acids like cysteine, methionine, and thiamine are key compounds in the generation of authentic and simulated meat flavors.[264]

Much of the flavor of meat results from the kind and amounts of primary precursors present, i.e., free amino acids, sugars, lipids, vitamins, and nucleotide precursors; the physical state of the medium, the prevailing pH, and pressure; and the intensity and duration of heating. These precursors and environmental conditions affect the initial products, which in turn influence the subsequent reactions and products.[63,155,264]

## Meat Flavor Formulations

The increasing consumption of textured proteins has been closely paralleled by a dramatic increase in production and use of formulated meat flavors. Intensive research concerned with the synthesis of improved meat flavor ingredients is in progress, as evidenced by the patent literature. Marked improvement in meat flavoring substances has been made in recent years.

The original imitation meat flavors produced depended heavily on species and onion as the dominant flavor notes. These are still useful for masking undesirable flavors. Then, with the discovery of their importance, mononucleotides (MSG, IMP, and GMP) were combined with the spices to enhance perceived flavor and impart brothiness. Further improvements were obtained by including hydrolyzed vegetable and yeast proteins (combinations of mixed amino acids and peptides) which provided an improved meaty flavor upon cooking. In some cases meat extracts are used.[264]

Oriental cultures have traditionally and successfully used hydrolyzed soy protein, i.e., soy sauce or shoyu, as a meat-type flavoring. Hydrolyzed vegetable proteins prepared by acid hydrolysis have a wide array of amino acids and some sugars, which undergo many reactions during heating. These reactions, i.e., Strecker degradation, Maillard reactions, deaminations, dehydrations, cyclizations — result in the generation of broad categories of acidic, basic, and neutral fractions.

Hydrolyzed vegetable or yeast proteins are usually salty as a result of neutralization of the acid used in their preparation. They are quite variable in quality due to compositional differences, i.e., varying amounts of reducing sugars, glutamates, and nucleotides are used. The extent of cooking also varies.[264] These hydrolyzed blends while imparting meat-like flavors also serve as a rich reservoir of precursors of meat-flavor compounds.

Manley and Fagerson[153,154] reviewed the nature of flavor precursors in acid hydrolyzed vegetable proteins. The acid treatment at elevated temperatures (110°C for 24 hr) produces amino acids, peptides, sugars, hydroxy furfurals, and lignin hydrolysates. Numerous acids are producd (formic,acetic, propanoic, butyric, isovaleric, valeric, crotonic, 2-butenoic, levulinic, 2-furoic, and phenylacetic) from amino acids via a combination of Maillard reaction, Strecker degradation, and oxidation. Some acids are generated from carmelization reactions. Some gamma lactones are also produced. These acids are considered integral components of meat flavors.

Several aldehydes (acetaldehyde, furfural, benzaldehyde, 5-methylfurfural, and phenylacetaldehyde) are produced by Maillard-type reactions and by Strecker degradation. These aldehydes have low flavor thresholds and may be important in aroma. Furans, degradation products of carbohydrates, are also produced, though their flavor significance is unknown.

Numerous methyl- and ethyl-substituted pyrazines are synthesized during hydrolysis. These are essential for cooked flavor. Several phenolic compounds, cresol, caffeic acid, guaiacol, ferulic acid, phenol, and derivatives thereof have been identified. The ethyl guaiacol may be a significant flavor component contributed by hydrolyzed vegetable protein. Dipeptides undoubtedly are present, but these have not been identified. The hydrolyzed vegetable proteins do not possess a meat aroma, but in combination with salt or MSG, they do possess a meat-like taste. Acid-hydrolyzed vegetable protein is used as a flavor enhancer in meat analogs at 0.2 to 2% levels.

Flavors for meat analogs must be far superior to the traditional blend of flavors used for imparting meat flavors to soups, gravies, etc.[139] In the case of extenders in comminuted meats, when the addition of textured protein (soy) exceeds 25%, the flavor generated by the meat cannot mask the natural, undesirable flavors of the extender/analog. Thus there is a real demand for flavor precursor systems whose potency is thermally generated during cooking. Complete flavors that truly simulate meat flavors are needed if analogs are to be successfully marketed.

Thermally produced imitation or processed meat flavors represent a blend of chemicals that provide flavors suggestive of cooked meats.[264] Because of the complexity of meat flavors and incomplete knowledge, a genuine facsimile has not yet been produced.

Cooking is an essential step for the generation of meat flavors from the various water-soluble, low-molecular precursors.[49,63,264] The cooking step obviously enhances

1.  Maillard-type reactions between the precursor reducing sugars and amines
2.  Strecker-type degradation of amino acids
3.  Deamination of mononucleotides
4.  Fission of methyl sulfide from methionine
5.  Dehydration of sugars and hydroxy fatty acids ($\delta,\gamma$)
6.  Carbonyl-induced browning reactions
7.  Oxidative decarboxylations

These reactions involve amino acids, peptides, sugars and their derivatives, lipids, nucleotides, and vitamins.

### Synthetic Meat Flavors

Extensive research has been carried out, and many important reactions have been patented concerned with the development of meat flavors.[264] The classical nonenzymatic browning or Maillard reaction is undoubtedly an essential step because it produces several flavors (furfurals) and generates important intermediate reactants and catalytic compounds, e.g., dicarbonyls. Numerous recent patents for meat flavorants have concentrated on the products obtained by reacting sulfur-containing organic compounds (e.g., mercaptans, methionine, cysteine, thiamine, glutathione, and thiols) with various sugars and/or protein hydrolysates (yeast or vegetable) at elevated temperatures.[264] Several patents have described methods for producing meat flavors from a variety of chemical precursors. Thus various mixtures including cysteine, taurine, methionine, cystine, hydrogen sulfide, glyceraldehyde, $\alpha$-ketobutyric acid, inosine, monosodium glutamate, glucose, lipids, and hydrolyzed animal, vegetable or yeast protein, and furanones have been used in model systems as precursors of meat flavors. These blends, however, do not generate a true meat flavor, and flavor experts are assiduously synthesizing and testing new flavors, many of which have not been found naturally.

The hydroxymethylfuranones react with hydrogen sulfide to yield thiophenes that possess meaty flavors. The compound dimethyldehydroxydithiane has a roasted-chicken flavor.[139] The thermal reaction of cysteine and cystine with reducing sugar produces a meat-like flavor attributable to mixtures of sulfides, aldehydes, furfurals, thiophenes, amines, and various cyclic compounds containing sulfur.[83,264] These findings have emphasized the significance of sulfur-containing compounds in meat flavor, and numerous patents have listed a wide variety of sulfur compounds derived from thermal reactions of methionine, cystine, cysteine, and thiamine. Many of these are heterocyclic ring compounds (thiazolines, thiazoles, and dithiazines) of limited volatility. The chemistry of these compounds are being intensively studied in private industrial laboratories.[83,155] Thiamine degradation may be another source of meaty flavors.[64] The heterogeneity of chemical products generated during cooking of various precursors (amino acids, sugars, and nucleotides) and hydrolyzed proteins were shown by Wilson,[264] but none of the products alone imparted a full meat flavor.

Van den Ouweland and Peer[250] isolated over 17 compounds following the thermal reaction of hydroxymethylfuranone with hydrogen sulfide. Several compounds were obtained by the substitution of sulfur for oxygen to yield a variety of thio analogs with strong, roasted-meat flavors. Hydroxymethylfuranone was selected because it could be derived from ribose-5-phosphate via a dephosphorylation-dehydration reaction, and when heated with sulfides, it formed meaty flavors by reactions not involving the Maillard reaction.

Grevall[83] cited the ongoing research involved in the synthesis of an array of furans and thiophenes following the thermal reactions of furanones with cysteine. These compounds were effective in making textured vegetable proteins smell like beef.

### Flavoring Problems
*Off-Flavors*

Acceptable flavoring is extremely important in the production of fabricated texturized protein foods such as meat analogs. Flavoring is the principal intractable problem surrounding the more widespread use of food analogs.[246] This problem is multifaceted, being caused by off-flavors adsorbed to the proteins, undesirable flavors generated during processing and cooking, and by the uneven adsorption and desorption of added flavors in final products.[278]

The use of novel proteins in the manufacture of textured pieces challenges the flavor chemist and technologist alike because these proteins may be a source of unusual and undesirable flavors (derived from amino acids, peptides, lipids, and lipoproteins). These off-flavors may be contaminants of the protein per se, or they may be generated during subsequent processing and storage of the formulated food. The beany flavor in soybean products is a pertinent example of the importance of flavor in limiting practical use of new proteins in traditional products. However, off-flavors may constitute problems with many food proteins, e.g., soy, casein, peanut, fish, single-cell, and leaf proteins. These usually result from the presence of small amounts of lipids in these preparations. Many of the off-flavor compounds in novel proteins (carbonyls, alcohols) originate via oxidation of the lipid components. Deterioration caused by lipids is a general problem with protein concentrates.[278] Though present at a few parts per million, these off-flavors adhere to proteins and may persist in products through processing.

Quist and Von Sydow[184,185] have characterized some of the flavor/off-flavor compounds associated with proteins. Walker and Manning[252] identified several groups of compounds as causes of the musty off-flavor of caseins. Acetophenone (derived from tryptophan under alkaline conditions) imparts a musty/stale flavor that remains adsorbed to the protein. This may be common in alkali-treated proteins.

The capacity of soy proteins to bind and retain "beany" off-flavors — especially hexanal, hexanol, and ethyl vinylketone — presents a major problem in fabricating acceptable foods from soy because these off-flavors carry through processing and cause a high rate of rejection of soy-based foods.[278] The undesirable flavor associated with soy has been a major problem retarding its expanded use in foods. When soy meal is prepared it has a bitter, beany flavor.[19,81] When the solvent-extracted meal is desolventized with steam most of the more obvious off-flavors are eliminated, but some of the desirable functional properties of the protein may be destroyed.[46,68,218] The off-flavor problem has been difficult to solve because of the low concentration of the compounds responsible for off-flavors, the mechanism of their synthesis during seed crushing and processing and the tenacity with which these compounds are bound to the protein, which renders their removal most difficult.[218] Over 35 volatile organic compounds have been identified in soy products.[46,218] These include aldehydes (alkanals, alkenals, and alkdienals), alkanones, alcohols, fatty acids, phenolic acids, amines, and aliphatic esters. The alcohols were major flavor components of beans, soy flour, and soy protein. Pentanol, hexanol and heptanol, which apparently are generated by lipoxygenase, become tightly bound to the protein and are very difficult to remove.[278] These possess a distinct, green bean-like taste. Hexanal, which is derived from the oxidation of fatty acids, is tightly bound to soy protein and has a grassy flavor.[19] Ethyl vinyl ketone has a strong, beany flavor. The formation of these off-flavors can be minimized by processing soybeans under conditions that inactivate the lipoxygenase, i.e., at high temperatures.[19,218]

The phenolic acids (syringic, vanillic, ferulic, gentisic, chlorogenic) possess flavors that are astringent, bitter and sour. In conjunction with the aliphatic alcohols and carbonyls, these may be significant components of the beany flavor[81,83]

When soy flour is heated, a cooked off-flavor develops that can become quite repulsive.[83] Two compounds that have been identified as the main contributors to this off-flavor are 4-vinyl phenol and 4-vinyl guaiacol, which are derived from the corresponding cinnamic acids by thermal decarboxylation. These acids can be extracted from soy flour with polar solvents with the resultant flour not developing these cooked off-flavors.

Much of the off-flavor associated with soy protein can be removed by extraction with polar solvents or by vacuum steam distillation techniques. These treatments increase the cost of production, however, and may impair functional properties of protein. Rackis et al.[186] reviewed the problems of off-flavors in soy products and described a solvent-extraction procedure for minimizing this problem. Improvements in processing have resulted in better products especially in the textured product lines.[279]

Proteolysis facilitates the distillation of these off-flavors,[18,19] but this reduces the potential uses of the soy protein. In fermented soy products the off-flavors are eliminated or masked. Several treatments have been advocated for minimizing off-flavors in soybean products, i.e., heat treatment to inactivate lipoxygenase and minimize lipid oxidation,[19] presoaking of beans in weak alkali, and distillation or steaming to eliminate the flavors from starting materials. Treatment of the soy protein with sulfur-containing compounds (cysteine, cystine) followed by cooking extrusion improves the flavor, as does treatment of defatted soybean with reducing thiol reagents.[92]

Another approach in the use of soy proteins has involved the addition of desirable flavors that mask the impact of undesirable flavors. In addition, blends of flavorants are added to impart the desired product flavor. The addition of flavor may not have the desired effect, however, because of interactions between flavors and the soy proteins. The specific sorption properties of soy proteins for many flavorful organic compounds influence the perceived flavor.[82]

*Physical Effects*

In addition to the challenges of eliminating the off-flavors associated with the protein source and formulating a bonafide meat flavor, there are practical problems involving the actual flavoring of the textured product. The ability to mask undesirable flavor(s) and simulate the desired meat flavor is significantly influenced by the flavor-binding capacity of the protein used. The porous nature of texturized vegetable proteins markedly enhances their capacity to absorb added flavors. In several applications this proves quite expensive because large amounts of flavor chemicals must be added to obtain the desired flavor impact. Therefore, techniques for reducing adsorption of specific flavors must be sought and exploited in fabricated foods. The binding of flavors by plant proteins, the uneven retention of flavors during processing treatments and storage, and the preferential release (or retention) of some components of a flavor blend during mastication are problems confronting the manufacture of fabricated foods from plant proteins. Thus typical problems are selective adsorption of particular components, disproportionate volatilization, masking of essential flavor notes, chemical decomposition of flavors, and generation of off-flavors.

For the flavorist creating a specific food flavor, it is important to know how the added flavor chemicals will interact with the components of the textured product, particularly the proteins. It is necessary to know if there is selective adsorption or entrapment of specific components, if some of the essential flavor notes are masked, and if, during subsequent storage, processing or cooking, a disproportionate amount of a particular flavor chemical is chemically altered or dissipated. These questions constitute aspects of texturizing protein foods that warrant systematic study because their elucidation or solution is essential for the ultimate acceptability of these fabricated foods.

The problem of binding of flavors to proteins has received limited attention.[29,75,152,224,227] Much basic information is needed concerning protein flavor interactions in terms of the thermodynamics of adsorption and description of chemical, physical, compositional, and environmental factors affecting this.

Arai et al.[18] showed that hexanal binding increases as soy protein is denatured. This binding was extremely tight and was not removable by distillation.

Solms et al.[227] showed that binding increases with ligand concentration and that soybean protein has a high affinity for apolar ligands. The quantity of flavor bound depended upon the nature of the flavor (ligand), the tertiary conformation of the protein, the content of apolar residues and their disposition, and other components in the system. Hydrophobic interactions are very important in the adsorption of flavors and in determining the facility of desorption of unwanted flavors.[280]

Maier[152] showed that binding varies with protein source and increases with hydrophobicity, and that moisture facilitates desorption. Some hydrogen bonding may be involved in flavor binding.

Using headspace analyses, Gremli[82] studied the interaction or binding of several aliphatic alcohols, aldehydes, and ketones with soy protein. The aldehydes, particularly the unsaturated species and ketones, showed considerable interaction with the protein, whereas alcohols were much less reactive. There was a gradual increase in retention of flavor molecules by the protein with molecular weight of the flavor compounds. The retention or binding was the same whether each volatile substance was tested individually or in the presence of a mixture. The protein facilely bound heptanal and nonanone, respectively. The binding of ketones by the protein was reversible, whereas a significant proportion of the aldehydes were irreversibly bound. The degree of irreversible binding increased with molecular weight of the aldehydes, e.g., 10 and 50% of the octanal and 2-dodecanal were irreversibly bound, respectively.

The binding of these flavors suppresses their primary flavoring impact.[82] In textured foods, however, the flavors may be released during mastication, though this may not be a desirable situation in many cases because of the uneven distribution of the component classes of volatile substances.

*Practical Problems*

Currently, an array of meat flavors (beef, chicken, bacon, ham, and pork) based on hydrolyzed proteins and including the appropriate precursors required for heat-generated flavors are available in liquid, paste, or spray-dried states. These flavors may be added to proteinaceous materials before or after texturization. It is more practical to add the flavor mixtures before the texturizing process. Because of alterations caused by physical and chemical changes during spinning or extrusion, however, the flavorants are usually added after texturization. In spun fibers the flavors are usually added with the binders during the binding phase of processing. Extruded proteins are usually flavored by infusion of an aqueous or emulsion dispersion into the pieces.

There are many problems associated with flavoring fabricated proteins. In the case of extruded products, flavor blends may be added to the mixture either before or after extrusion; or some before and the remainder after. Mixing flavors with proteins prior to extrusion frequently results in masking, uneven retention, and/or excessive evaporation during processing. Hence flavoring after extrusion is more practical.[72] The differential adsorption of water-soluble and lipophilic flavors is another problem. The latter flavors may be applied in emulsified form. Use of flavor suspension or emulsions can result in very uneven distribution of flavors, with pockets or excessive concentrations in some portions. In certain foods, e.g., meat patties, the textured soy absorbs water and fat and thus retains the flavors quite well. In foods cooked in aqueous media, like soups, leaching of flavors occurs, so that the flavor of the final product may be inferior. Infusion of textured or spun product with lipid or oil enhances the retention of lipid-soluble flavors.

To minimize the undesirable flavor in textured soy proteins, spices and seasonings should be added to the hydration water and allowed to permeate the protein matrix. In certain types of products, such as "sloppy joes", the lower pH tends to accentuate the perception off-flavors.

Alden[3] described a method for flavoring textured protein products. Initially, the expanded (extruded) protein was exposed to a solution of flavoring materials (salt, hydrolyzed proteins, nucleotides, sucrose, etc.) and then coated with a film of fat. This film entrapped the flavors and also absorbed lipophilic flavors when exposed to them, e.g., smoke flavors. The use of flavored-coating materials, however, frequently results in unequal distribution of flavorants. Furthermore, exposure on the surface may result in excessive volatilization and/or oxidative, hydrolytic, photoinduced flavor degradation.

Encapsulation of flavors using gum/gelatin combinations or other appropriate chemical or thermally stable encapsulating agents is a significant development. It may facilitate the successful addition of flavors to the starting proteinaceous mixture prior to extrusion texturization.[6,150]

## NUTRITIONAL ASPECTS

The nutritional value of textured plant proteins ultimately is a most important criterion of practical concern when these food items constitute a significant dietary source (more than 10%) of protein and other nutrients. Nutritional value of textured foods denotes their nutrient content, composition, and the biological availability of the nutrients. The potential of textured fabricated foods to become significant sources of nutrients has not yet been realized. Currently these are being used mostly in meat-based foods, with up to 30% textured-protein content permitted in meats served in school lunch programs. This has spurred interest in the nutritional value and particularly the protein quality of textured proteins.

It should be realized that the human requires about 50 nutrients in the diet and perhaps additional materials, e.g., fiber. Too frequently, food technologists emphasize proteins and vitamins, but all nutrients are essential. This is particularly pertinent as more refined ingredients are used in the fabrication of foods. Therefore, while nutritive value of protein is important the ability of food analogs to supply other essential nutrients in appropriate quantities must be considered — especially if the analog is replacing some other significant source of nutrients. Soybean is currently the predominant protein source for texturizing. Therefore, the nutritional properties of soybean are discussed below since these largely determine the nutritional value of the texturized product. The nutritional properties of soybean products have been reviewed in detail by Liener.[144]

Antinutritive Factors

In developing texturized protein foods from new protein sources, the manufacturer and consumer must be fully knowledgeable about their nutritional value. In addition they should be aware of possible biological or physiological factors producing antinutritive or allergenic properties. These components of soy protein have been examined in detail,[143,144,186-190] and the associated research exemplifies the systematic studies that may be required of other plant protein sources to ensure maximum nutritive value and consumer safety.

Raw, nonheat treated-, nonfermented-form soybean, soybean flours, and soy proteins contain a variety of substances that cause differing physiological responses in various species of animals. Feeding of raw, full-fat, or unroasted defatted soy flours depresses growth rates; reduces metabolizable energy and fat absorption, inhibits protein digestibility; causes pancreatic hypertrophy; results in hypersecretion of pancreatic enzymes; reduces amino acid, vitamin, and mineral availability; and may induce allergic reactions. The extent and intensity of these reactions vary in rats, chickens, pigs, calves, and dogs.[188] There are few data available on humans. Rackis[188,190] in reviewing these effects, stated that they are interrelated and they reflect the animals' inability to use essential nutrients fully because of exogenous factors rather than as responses to toxic substances. Thus the antinutritive factors in uncooked soy proteins are not toxic agents and the abnormalities caused in animals following consumption of uncooked soy meal can be redressed. Several long-term feeding trials with rats, dogs, pigs, and poultry have failed to show any toxicity following consumption of raw soy meals.[190]

Liener[143, 144] has reviewed in detail the subject of the antinutritive components in plant foods wih particular emphasis on effects of proteinase inhibitors. There are at least five proteinase inhibitors (trypsin inhibitors or TI) in soybean that inhibit trypsin and chymotrypsin activity. These account for all of the pancreatic hypertrophic effect and for up to 60% of growth-inhibiting properties of raw soybean meal in rats.[188] In one study removal of the TI eliminated 40% of the growth inhibitors. Fortunately, trypsin inhibitors are reasonably heat labile, as are other antimetabolic factors in soybean. The quantity of TI varies with soybean varieties, and the amounts occurring in soy meal and soy protein preparations vary with previous heat treatments. The nutritive values of several soybean varieties, with varying contents of trypsin inhibitors, were thus improved from 61 to 180% after heat treatment.[188] Following toasting (i.e., live steam treatment) the nutritive value of soy flours, soy concentrates, and soy isolates are significantly improved. The protein efficiency ratio (PER) value of soy flour is increased from 1.45 to 2.5 following moist-heat treatment at 100°C for 15 min at atmospheric pressure. Maximum PER is obtained by autoclaving the protein at pressures of 15 psi for 20 to 30 min.

Rackis[188-190] showed that steaming of soybean meal at 100°C reduced TI activity by 50% within 4 min and by approximately 85% after 10 min. PER values increased concurrently from an initial 1.5 to 2.3 and 3.1 after 4 and 10 min heating, respectively. Thus TI activity accounts for much of the poor growth rate observed in experimental animals receiving uncooked soy protein. In addition, however, hemagglutinin activity is destroyed and protein digestibility is improved following heating.

The particle size and moisture content of soy flour, (or soy concentrate) affect the rate of TI destruction. Thus in samples of dry meals of large particle size, the TI is more heat resistant.[144] Autoclaving is very effective for improving the nutritional value of soy protein. Trypsin inhibitor acivity is destroyed in soy flour by autoclaving at pressures of 5, 10, 15, and 20 psi for 45, 30, 20, and 10 min, respectively.

The PER values of various commercial soy protein preparations show considerable variation and reflect the extent of prior moist-heat treatment. In some instances heat treatment is minimal or is not applied, so as to avoid protein denaturation and loss of functional properties. During the heat treatment, conditions must be carefully controlled to minimize alteration of essential amino acids and the resultant loss of nutritive value. Heat treatment of soy protein under alkaline conditions accelerates destruction of TI, but alkali concentration, time, and temperatures must be controlled to minimize formation of cross-links via lysinoalanine.

Phytohemagglutinins may account for 25% of the growth inhibition of raw soybean meal in rats.[143] There are, however, no substantial data to indicate that these compounds have antinutritional properties, though the low levels in other legumes definitely inhibit growth.[188] Those present in soy proteins are destroyed by roasting.

Phytic acid occurs as a phytate-mineral-protein complex in soy flour and soy isolates, and it significantly decreases the availability of zinc, manganese, copper, molybdenum, calcium, magnesium, and iron. Moist-heat treatment reduces these effects.[188] By chelating the metal ions, the phytic acid present in the soy protein greatly accounts for much of the mineral deficiencies observed when animals are fed solely on unsupplemented soy isolate as a protein source or soy protein concentrate.[186,188] Zinc deficiency can occur in humans existing mostly on plant proteins (e.g., cereals and beans). Supplementation of diets high in soy protein with zinc may be necessary where the consumption of animal protein is limited. In the case of vegetable-protein diets where calcium is added, the zinc deficiency may be exacerbated.[188]

In addition to these antinutritive factors, others (i.e., goitrogenic, allergenic, and oestrogenic factors) may be of significance where consumption of soy protein is high. Normally these are of marginal significance, however.[144]

With appropriate heat treatment and controlled processing, the nutritive value of soy flour can be markedly improved. Properly, heat-treated soy protein has an adequate essential amino acid content except for a deficiency in methionine. Soy protein has PER values of at least 80% of that for casein.[144, 188] Defatted soy flour, soy protein concentrate, and soy protein isolate have protein efficiency ratios of 2.16 to 2.48, 2.02 to 2.48, and 1.08 to 2.1 respectively, compared to casein at 2.5. Supplementation of these with 1.0 to 1.5% methionine improves the PER of soy protein to around 3.0. Following heating, soy protein concentrates have PER values comparable to those of soy flour. There is no information available on the effect of soy concentrate diets upon vitamin and mineral requirements in animals.[188]

Soy proteinate or soy isolate have a greater deficiency of sulfur amino acids than the more heterogeneous proteins found in soy flour, and they have lower PER values as shown above. Heat treatments improve the protein efficiency values of soy concentrates and isolates.[147]

A different spectrum of nutritional and biological factors may result from ingestion of soy protein isolates. Feeding soy isolate increases the requirements for vitamins (particlarly E, K, B₂, B₃, and B₁₂) and induces deficiency symptoms typical of calcium, magnesium, manganese, molybdenum, copper, iron, and particularly zinc deficiency. Phosphorus is also utilized poorly.[188] Rachitogenic and perotic factors are also concentrated in soy isolates, while growth-promoting, antiperotic, antirachitogenic, and antithyrotoxic factors are found in meal extracts.[188] Proper heat treatments, appropriate supplementation, and addition of chelating agents can be used to correct these nutritional deficiencies of soy isolates. The above information is very relevant to the use of spun fibers made from soy isolate. However, these fibers invariably are used in products containing other proteins which help balance the nutritive value of these foods.

More definitive knowledge is needed to establish optimum conditions for removal or inactivation of antinutritional factors, particularly in relation to the new technological processes now in use.

### Effects of Heating

The presence of antinutritive compounds; i.e., proteinase inhibitors, amylase inhibitors, phytohemagglutinins, phytic acid, goitrogens, saponins, and phenolic compounds; in soy preparations imposes certain processing requirements of which heat treatment is most important. The first three factors listed above are destroyed by adequate thermal treatment, while the remainder are normally not of major nutritional importance.

It is of concern that the biological value and digestibility of soybean proteins are significantly lower than those for egg proteins. Liener[144] reported the biological value, measured with human subjects, of heat-treated, full-fat soybean flour was 64, while that of egg was 87. Supplementation of the soybean flour with methionine increased the biological value only to 75. Digestibility values, also measured on human subjects, were 84 and 97 for soybean flour and eggs, respectively, and the digestibility of soybean flour was not improved by addition of methionine.

The presence of active inhibitors and phytohemagglutinins in improperly heat-treated soybean flour undoubtedly accounts for some of the observed decreased digestibility. Rackis[188] indicates that undenatured soy protein in its tightly packed globular state is quite resistant to digestive enzymes and that this resistance to digestion may account for 40 to 60% of its poor nutritional quality. Thus the tertiary structure of soy protein, in which the molecules are compactly folded with the hydrophobic region in the interior, are somewhat resistant to proteolysis. Destruction of this structure by heat denaturation is necessary for complete digestibility. Agents that disrupt disulfide bonds enhance digestibility, e.g., heating under acidic[31] or alkaline conditions. During extrusion the globular structure of native soy is destroyed, and this is aided by disulfide bond-reducing agents. Presumably these changes also facilitate subsequent digestion of texturized protein. Thus heat application improves the nutritional value of soy proteins by destroying inhibitors and increasing susceptibility of the protein to digestion by proteolytic enzymes.

Heat treatments can also reduce biological value of proteins, however. Bender[28] and Osner[174] have reviewed information concerning the beneficial and deleterious effects of heat treatments on proteins. The beneficial effects are mostly observed when legume proteins are heated as discussed above. Thermal damage may result from destruction of amino acids via oxidation; modification of linkages ($\alpha$-elimination) between amino acids which retards their hydrolysis; and possibly formation of cross-linkages which are resistant to digestive enzymes, e.g., β-elimination reactions or Schiffs base formation with reducing sugars. These cause losses in biological availablity. The extent of these interactions depends upon temperature and duration of heating, presence of moisture, and reducing substances. Damage is usually proportional to the extent of heating, particularly at temperatures above 100°C. Damage is most severe at moisture levels between 10 and 14%. Of course, the presence of reducing sugars markedly accelerates these reactions.[101]

In evaluating heat damage to proteins, certain methods used for assessing changes are inadequate or incomplete and may result in invalid conclusions. Thus measures such as biological value, net protein utilization, and protein efficiency ratio may only reveal processing effects when they affect limiting amino acids, while changes in other amino acids present in abundance may not be noticed.[28] Furthermore, many studies of processing changes in proteins emphasize the Maillard reaction involving lysine, whereas methionine may be the critical limiting amino acid. Thus combined chemical and biological tests should be employed[113] in such evaluations.

The most commonly studied cause of thermal deterioration in proteins is the Maillard reaction involving the initial interaction between ε-amino groups of lysine and the carbonyl group of reducing sugars and other compounds.[110,101,194] The nutritional effects of this reaction have been studied.[113]

Thermally induced racemization of amino acids in peptides and protein may also occur, especially at temperatures above 110°C. Hayase et al.[94] reported that aspartic acid, glutamic acid, alanine, and lysine are facilely racemized during heating of proteins at 180°C for 20 min. Other amino acids except proline were also racemized. Free amino acids and those in oligopeptides were more susceptible to racemization. Basic, β-hydroxy and sulfur-containing amino acids are most susceptible to heat degradation at high temperatures. In most thermal processes, however, the temperature employed rarely exceeds 110°C, or if it does it is for short times; hence thermally induced racemization of amino acids is assumed to be insignificant. Racemization of amino acids is accentuated by heating under alkaline conditions, a fact relevant to fiber spinning and extrusion at alkaline pH.

With regard to biological value, alkali treatment also causes formation of dehydroalanine from cysteine and serine via β-elimination-type reactions. This may result in cross-linking of polypeptides and render proteins resistant to proteolysis, thereby reducing their nutritive value. Lanthionine and ornithinoalanine may be formed via the reaction of dehydroalanine with cysteine and ornithine, respectively.[164,182] Thus by causing racemization; destruction of some limiting amino acids (serine, arginine, threonine, lysine, isoleucine, and methionine); and cross-linking, alkali treatment may reduce the nutritional value of protein.[59, 60, 182]

Provensal et al.[182] carefully determined the conditions under which alkali caused formation of undesirable compounds. Increasing alkali concentration (pH 9.6 to 12.9), increasing temperatures up to 60°C, and duration of exposure cause a progressive destruction of the labile amino acids and formation of ornithine, lysinoalanine, and alloisoleucine. The changes caused by alkali treatment depend upon the concentration of the alkali the duration and temperature of the treatment. Increasing alkali concentration from 0.1 to 1.0 *M* while heating sunflower protein at 80°C for 16 hr caused a sixfold increase in ornithine and alloisoleucine with concurrent diminution of arginine and isoleucine. Lysinoalanine showed no significant increase, though at higher concentrations of alkali its formation was signifcant. Alkaline (0.2 *M*) treatment at 80°C for 1 hr or more results in isomerization of lysine.[48]

The biological effect of lysinoalanine is controversial. Woodward and Short[266] reported that cytomegalia of kidney tubules occurred in rats receiving alkaline treated soy protein. DeGroot and Slump[59] and DeGroot et al.[60] failed to observe this effect but reported the occurrence of nephrocalcinosis in female rats fed alkali-treated, spun soy isolate. Cheftel et al.[48] and Provensal et al.[182] concluded that alkaline treatments should be mild and brief to minimize destruction of cysteine, threonine, isoleucine, and lysine and the formation of nonhydrolyzable cross-links.

Because of the numerous interrelated factors, it is impossible to be specific and state the optimum heat treatments and conditions for plant proteins. However, it is generally held that during the normal processing of soy proteins, the heat applied during roasting and cooking extrusion result in minimal destruction of amino acids.[48]

### Flatulence Factors

Though not a nutritional problem, flatulence usually associated with the consumption of soy products has retarded their acceptance. Flatus activity, i.e., the formation of gastrointestinal gas, which may result in nausea, cramps, diarrhea, pain, and social discomfort is common following the consumption of soy flour, though the gravity of symptoms varies with the subject.[187] The flatulence-causing facors are low-molecular weight carbohydrates that are concentrated mostly in defatted soy flour and, to an decreasing extent, in full-fat soy flour, soy protein concentrate, and soy isolate. The flatulence is caused by anaerobic fermentation of oligosaccharides in the lower gut (ileum and colon) with the generation of hydrogen and carbon dioxide. Gas production is caused by the low-molecular weight oligosaccharides — mostly sucrose, raffinose, and stachyose. The latter is apparently the principal sugar causing flatulence.

Defatted soy flour has the highest content of oligosaccharides, i.e., 8% sucrose, 5% stachyose, 2% raffinose, and 1% verbacose. Soy flour and products manufactured therefrom are the major sources of flatus activity. Textured soy flour, i.e., extruded flour, causes flatulence when consumed in excess of 50 g/meal. Wide variations among humans have been observed, however.[187] Extruded soy flour products may be less active if they are extracted with water, e.g., during the rehydration process. Smith[221-222] described a method whereby soy flour may be first lightly toasted by extrusion. This minimizes protein loss during the subsequent aqueous washing to remove the oligosaccharides. Because they have been extracted with an aqueous alcohol solvent, soy concentrates are less troublesome, as most of these oligosaccharides have been removed. Soy proteinates are essentially devoid of flatus activity. Textured soy concentrates and isolates are devoid of flatus activity.[187]

### Nutritive Value of Textured Protein

While fabricated foods should provide essential nutrients at least to the extent provided by the foods they might displace, some precautions are warranted in connection with the increased use of food analogs. The average intake of protein in the American diet (100 g/day) is almost twice the basic requirement. It would seem that further fortification of protein-rich foods with proteinaceous, fabricated foods is wasteful and may be deleterious, as intimated by Visek.[251] Furthermore, the dilution of the traditional American diet with fabricated food items may conceivably result in the inadequate consumption of less "topical" but equally essential micronutrients.

The biological value of protein in textured products is, at best, as good as the protein in the raw material, other things being similar.

### *Spun Fibers*

Heat treatment of soy isolate improves its nutritional value,[39,144,147,188] indicating the presence of residual antinutritive factors. Fibers made from unheated isolates have better PER values than the original protein, indicating that the spinning process may cause elution or inactivation of antinutritive agents. In discussing nutritional value it must be remembered that spun-fiber, textured products contain proteinaceous materials other than the spun fiber. While spun protein fibers are made mostly from soy protein, the fabricated products containing these fibers usually contain proteins from several other sources, i.e., milk proteins, egg albumin, and wheat gluten which are added as binders. These are used for their functional effects, but they also improve the nutritional value of the food. Thus some spun-fiber-based products cited by Rosenfeld[199] and Rosenfeld and Hartman[200] had PER values of 2.5, i.e., equivalent to casein. Thulin and Kuramoto[243] claimed that spun fibers had PER values from 2.2 to 2.4.

In dietary studies using rats, spun soy protein fibers supplemented with egg albumin, wheat gluten, and soy flour gave PER values of 2.3, compared to 2.34 and 2.5 for casein. In young children this same textured food produced growth rates and nitrogen balance values similar to those obtained following the feeding of a dehydrated beef product. The protein quality of this textured product was about 80% that of milk.[39]

In another study a controlled feeding regime was carried out using spun soy fibers in products resembling chicken, seafoods, ham, and beef on hospitalized adults for 24 weeks. The diet was virtually devoid of animal protein. These "volunteers", who received all their protein from vegetable sources, maintained excellent health as well as normal biochemical values for hemoglobin, hematocrit, and urea nitrogen, and the nitrogen balance remained positive.[106]

Koury et al.[134] reported that textured soy isolate adequately maintained human subjects in good health, though some complained of abdominal gas pains. Turk et al.,[249] following appropriate studies with humans, concluded that products made with spun soy fibers containing egg albumin were an adequate dietary source of protein. The PER values of extruded textured soy are very similar to those of heated soy protein. Changes in digestibility and PER of soy protein are small, e.g., digestibilities of heated soy flour averages 89% while the extruded protein averages 80%.[85]

*Extruded Proteins*

Textured vegetable proteins are limiting in the sulfur-containing amino acids, both cystine and methionine (Table 7). Supplementation can correct this, though some technical problems, especially off-flavor development, can render this impractical.

Though the present discussion focuses on soy protein, it must be recognized that any blend of proteins (plant, animal, avian, fish) may be extruded and texturized to yield a product with optimum protein values. If heating is involved in texturizing, some improvement in nutritional value may result via destruction of the antinutrients and improved digestibility of the protein. If heating is excessive, however, destruction of some limiting essential amino acids may occur. Aguilera[2] reported that extruder temperatures of 120 to 150°C, with initial moisture levels of 25 to 40%, were effective in reducing TI activity below levels having measurable antinutritional effects.[189] Short-time extrusion cooking is very effective in destruction of TI and improving PER of soy proteins. Mustakas et al.[163] and Cheftel et al.[48] reported no destruction of amino acids following extrusion of soy and sunflower protein at temperatures of 210°C.

Sautier and Camus[204] reported that extrusion (at 100°C) of soy and sunflower protein improved in vitro proteolysis by about 150 and 26% when moisture levels were at 30 and 60%, respectively. These workers reported that feeding various mixtures of textured proteins up to 65% of total protein intake showed no adverse effects on nitrogen, sodium, or potassium balance in humans.

Kies and Fox[124-128] showed that nitrogen balances in human subjects fed at a level of 8 g of nitrogen (i.e., approximately 50 g protein) per day from extruded soy proteins or cooked beef were almost identical. When fed at 4 g of nitrogen per day both sources resulted in negative nitrogen balances. Beef was the superior protein source, however. Supplementation of the extruded soy proteins improved their biological value, e.g.,

Table 7

COMPARISONS OF ESSENTIAL
AMINO ACID CONTENT OF
TEXTURED SOY PROTEIN, BEEF,
AND FAO PATTERN (MG/16 G N$_2$)

| Amino acid | Textured protein | | Beef | FAO pattern |
| | A | B | | |
|---|---|---|---|---|
| Isoleucine | 4.3 | 5.24 | 4.82 | 4.8 |
| Valine | 4.1 | 5.74 | 5.00 | 4.2 |
| Leucine | 7.0 | 7.54 | 8.11 | 4.8 |
| Lysine | 6.1 | 5.88 | 8.90 | 4.2 |
| Methionine | 1.1 | 1.10 | 2.70 | 2.2 |
| Cystine | 1.2 | 1.47 | 1.28 | 2.0 |
| Threonine | 3.7 | 3.78 | 4.6 | 2.8 |
| Tryptophan | 1.2 | 1.36 | — | 1.4 |

Data adapted from Hamdy, M. M., *J. Am. Oil Chem. Soc.*, 51, 85A, 1974.

beef, textured soy, and textured soy with 1% methionine had PER values of 2.4, 2.1, and 2.8, respectively.[107,124]

Kies and Fox[124,127] showed that a negative nitrogen balanced occurred at low levels of dietary textured protein intake, i.e., supplying 4 g/day to adolescent boys. Supplementation with 1% DL-methionine made nitrogen retention values equivalent to those of subjects receiving their nitrogen exclusively from beef. In other feeding trials with textured soy protein there was no significant difference between the protein value of milk and textured protein when fed to young children at a rate of 2 g protein per kilogram body weight per day.

The respective biological value, digestibility, and net protein utilization data for humans fed beef were 43.6, 89.5, and 39.3 and 35.7, 87.7, and 30.9, respectively, for textured soy flour. The respective PER values were 2.37 and 2.1 for the two protein sources.[84] Supplementation of soy protein with 1% DL-methionine increased its PER to 2.82.[133]

Textured soy proteins are used to replace meats and/or as meat extenders. A comparison of the PER values revealed that textured soy protein, casein, beef, beef/texturized plant protein blends at ratios of 70:30 and at 55:45, and beef/texturized protein blend at a 55:45 ratio also supplemented with 0.3% DL-methionine had PER values of 2.1, 2.5, 2.99, 2.95, 2.73, and 2.82, respectively.[107] Compared to 45 g beef which supplied enough methionine, 45 g textured soy supplies only 50% of the recommended methionine intake. Wilding[262] reported that textured proteins, when included up to levels of 30% of total protein in meat or chicken patties, had PER values significantly above those of casein. Blends containing 50% meat protein and 50% extruded soy protein had PER values of 2.72.

The studies of Kies[126-128] and colleagues have shown that textured soy protein is a good source of protein for both adolescent and adults, especially when blended with beef protein. The inclusion of methionine significantly improves biological value of the protein. Supplementation of textured protein with vitamins, particularly niacin, improves nitrogen balance 15 to 23%. In addition to nitrogen balance, Kies and Fox[124,125] also monitored blood proteins, hemoglobin, and hematocrit of human subjects on textured soy protein or beef protein, and reported that they were similar in

Table 8
VITAMIN CONTENT OF TEXTURED
SOY PROTEIN

| Vitamin | Normal[a] | Enriched[a,b] |
|---|---|---|
| C | <1.0 | <1.0 |
| A | — | — |
| D | — | — |
| Thiamin (B$_1$) | 0.3 | 0.3 |
| Riboflavin (B$_2$) | 0.3 | 0.6 |
| Pyridoxin (B$_6$) | 0.4 | 1.4 |
| Cyanocobalamine (B$_{12}$) $\mu$g | <0.1 | 6.0 |
| Folic acid | 0.2 | 0.2 |
| Pantothenic acid | 2.5 | 2.5 |
| Niacin | 2.3 | 16.0 |

[a]    Content expressed in mg/100 g except where noted.
[b]    As specified by USDA.

Data adapted from Hamdy, M. M., *J. Am. Oil Chem. Soc.*, 51, 85A, 1974.

both groups. Iron as measured by hemoglobin level is also adequate, and blood calcium is also maintained on textured soy protein. No digestive disturbances were experienced by subjects being maintained on extruded soy protein.

*Vitamins and Minerals*

Soy proteins are generally not considered to be significant sources of vitamins. Though the bean has reasonable quantities, toasting destroys much of them, e.g., more than 50% of the thiamin is lost. Soy proteins are essentially devoid of vitamins C, D, E, K, and B$_{12}$.[262] Thus where soy proteins constitute a significant proportion of diets (10% of protein) precautions must be taken to provide appropriate amounts of vitamins and minerals.[84,107] The vitamin levels in textured soy protein vary from sample to sample and with processing treatment, especially heat treatments. The levels shown in Table 8 are representative. Vitamins A, C, and D are negligible, and enrichment with these may be required depending on intended use. The most stable vitamin is niacin, while riboflavin and pyridoxine are less stable. Vitamins B$_1$, cyanocobalamine (B$_{12}$), and panthothenate are most unstable.[32] It is advisable to add vitamins in a blend to the protein material and then process if the heating regime is not too rigorous. According to Borenstein,[32] the times and temperature required to texturize do not cause significant degradation of the labile vitamins. However, destruction of B$_1$ ranges from 10 to 80% during extrusion at 380 and 300°F, respectively. Riboflavin destruction is highly influenced by moisture levels. Ascorbic acid is very sensitive to thermal oxidation. Borenstein[32] cogently points out that destruction of labile vitamins is dependent not only on temperature-time factors but also on moisture levels. The pH can also markedly alter the kinetics of vitamin destruction.

The minerals associated with textured soy protein are extremely variable (cultural conditions, variety, and processing treatments). The quantities found (Table 9) are potential sources of required elements. However, the availability of these minerals varies. Thus zinc may be largely unavailable because of binding with phytic acid.[188]

## REGULATIONS

In the U.S., the use of textured plant proteins in foods is regulated by the Food and

Table 9
MINERAL CONTENT OF TEXTURED
SOY PROTEINS

| Mineral | Amount[a] | Mineral | Amount[a] |
|---|---|---|---|
| Sodium | 0.9 | Iron | 9.6 |
| Potassium | 2090.0 | Copper | 1.6 |
| Calcium | 252.0 | Manganese | 3.6 |
| Magnesium | 302.0 | Zinc | 5.6 |
| Phosphorus | 740.0 | Boron | 3.8 |
| Chloride | 0.01 | Aluminum | 0.9 |
| Iodine | 5 ng | Cobalt | 0.1 gn |

[a]    Content expressed mg/100 g protein except where noted.

Drug Administration (FDA) and the Food Quality and Safety Service (FQSS) of the U.S. Department of Agriculture (USDA). The latter agency regulates meat standards.

The major impetus for the use of textured proteins followed the sanctioning of their inclusion in the school lunch program by the Food and Nutrition Service[10] of the USDA. This also encouraged the improvement in the nutritional value of these products through fortification. With regard to blending of textured proteins with meat, the regulations stipulate that the ratio of hydrated protein product to uncooked meat (poultry or fish) must not exceed 30:70 in percent of total weight. The protein efficiency ratio (PER) of the textured protein must be at least 1.8 on a scale where casein is 2.8, i.e., the PER must be 72% of casein and the meat-textured vegetable protein mixture must have a PER of 2.5 or above. Actually, the PER of textured soy proteins is approximately 85% of the casein PER.[145] In addition, the Food and Nutrition Service[10] requires that texturized vegetable protein for use in school lunches must be fortified with minerals and vitamins.[10] The specifications for textured proteins to be permitted in school lunches are summarized (Table 10).

The specifications of textured proteins for the school lunch program proposed in 1974,[10] required nutritional information (PER), a minimum protein content of 18% in the hydrated product, a definition of physical structure or texture, and permission to use plant proteins other than soy. The name "textured meat alternates" was introduced, and all of these intended for consumer use must bear a label indicating their acceptability to USDA.

The procedural test for physical characteristics and structural integrity, i.e., measuring the amounts of textured plant protein remaining on a 20-mesh screen after cooking, was described. This essentially is a measure of particle size and their ability to remain intact upon cooking. A number of improved methods for measuring particle size and particle stability have been described.[277] All of these are somewhat arbitrary. Breen[229] developed the Minnesota texture method, which employs instrumental methods for measuring textural quality of extruded proteins, rehydrated meat extenders, and extender/ground-bean mixtures. Textural parameters could be evaluated by this test, i.e., hardness, chewiness, and packability.

At present FDA are formulating standards and guidelines governing the nomenclature, classification, and use of textured plant proteins. The criteria being used are essentially that if a fabricated food resembles, simulates, or is intended to replace a traditional food it must contain at least the same amount of the recommended daily allowance of nutrients as the traditional food. Furthermore, where used as a blend, if the hydrated protein product is more than 30% by weight of the mixture when mixed

## Table 10
### THE SPECIFICATIONS OF TEXTURED VEGETABLE PROTEINS FOR USE AS MEAT EXTENDERS IN SCHOOL LUNCH PROGRAMS

| Component | Amount (min) |
| --- | --- |
| Protein (weight %)[a,b] | 50.0 |
| Fat (weight %)[c] | 2.0 |
| Magnesium (mg/100 g) | 70.0 |
| Iron (mg/100 g) | 10.0 |
| Thiamin (mg/100 g) | 0.30 |
| Riboflavin (mg/100 g) | 0.60 |
| Niacin (mg/100 g) | 16.0 |
| Vitamin B$_6$ (mg/100 g) | 1.4 |
| Vitamin B$_{12}$ (μg/100 g) | 5.7 |
| Pantothenic acid (mg/100 g) | 2.0 |

[a] Nitrogen times 6.25 (dry weight basis).
[b] Biological value of protein: The protein efficiency ratio (PER) of the textured vegetable protein shall be not less than 1.8 on basis of PER = 2.5 for casein. PER of a meat-textured vegetable protein combination shall not be less than 2.5 PER. Moisture content of the hydrated form shall not exceed 65.0% or be less than 60.0%.
[c] Fat must not exceed 30%.

Data adapted from **Anon.**, Textured Vegetable Protein Products, Food and Nutrition Notice #219, U.S. Department of Agriculture, Washington, D.C., 1971.

with meat, seafood, poultry, eggs, or cheese; or, if the hydrated protein product is used unmixed in a way that it substitutes for and resembles meat, seafood, poultry, eggs, or cheese; the biological quality of the protein (including amino acids added thereto) is at least 108% that of casein.[11,199]

Because one can fabricate textured proteins from a variety of raw materials, PER values of 2.5 can readily be attained, and this is permitted under current regulations. For analogs not to be labeled "imitation", they must contain the same percentage of Recommended Daily Allowance (RDA) for protein and other nutrients. The RDA for protein is 45 g if the PER of the textured product is equal to or greater than that of casein (2.5) and 65 g if it is less than casein. A food shall not be deemed an imitation if it complies with the applicable requirements of a standard of identity and nutritional quality guidelines. Ingredient statements for fabricated foods must list the variety or source of proteins used.[199]

The FDA proposed ruling on common names for plant protein products required clear distinctions between soy flour, concentrates, and isolates. It stated that a product with less than 65% protein may not use the word "protein" in its name and stipulated that nutrients be expressed on a "per gram of protein" basis.[11]

Currently, the manufacturers of texturized proteinaceous foods are obliged to ensure that food analogs are equivalent to the food items they might replace in significant quantities. However, the philosophy behind this requirement imposed by regulatory agencies should not negate the potential of fabricated foods being exploited as ideal vehicles for the improvement of the nutritional status of particular consumers. Texturized protein foods, which can be fabricated in a wide variety of shapes, textures, and flavors should be useful for exploiting the idea of total nutrification, i.e., to contain all the nutrients known to be required by humans in the optimum proportions so that a serving of the food provides a uniform percentage of the daily needs.[126]

A complete, updated listing of processors and private-label distributors of textured vegetable protein products permitted in the USDA, Food and Nutriton Service, Child Nutrition Programs is available from the Food and Nutrition Service. All the suppliers listed provide nutrient analyses and per values for their product (available from USDA).

## PROSPECTS

In the early 1970s, the prospects for textured proteins seemed excellent. The general optimism was generated by the volume of literature appearing, the numerous meetings focusing on this topic, the mutual encouragement of interested groups, the rising prices of meat, and, significantly, by the Food and Nutrition Service Notice 219 permitting textured vegetable proteins in school lunch servings.[10]

The study of Hammonds and Call[86] forecasted that textured proteins would account for 10% of all domestic meat consumption, i.e., around 2 billion lb/year by 1985. In 1972 it was predicted that 2 to 4 billion lb (wet) of meat extenders would be in use by 1980.[30] In retrospect, however, this prediction was grossly overinflated, and since 1972 there has been relatively little movement in volume. Bird[30] maintains that prices will inevitably determine that the American population will consume vegetable protein products to an increasing extent. Because of the economic situation in 1972, many products of inferior quality were rushed onto the market and this may have adversely affected the consumer's image of meat extenders. Thus instead of educating the young consumer, their use may have engendered a dislike for such products. Many extenders cannot or should not be used above 5 to 10% of the meat because of their dominating beany off-flavor above that level. Estimates in 1973 indicated that 50 million lb of hydrated protein extenders were used. Few reports of the acceptance/rejection rates of extended meat products by school students are available. Such information should be very useful. The use of textured proteins in school lunch programs continues to increase and presently it has been estimated that 65% of such programs are using these products.[8]

The greatest expansion is expected to occur with meat extenders and meat analogs. The data in Table 11 projected a sixfold increase in textured proteins by the year 2000. This report predicted a large increase in spun fiber-type proteins. With the recent developments and improvements in extrusion techniques,[56,259] however, it is anticipated that extruded products will displace some of the spun-fiber products and also significantly expand the market for meat analogs.

The major determinants of growth of textured protein are availability of protein, price, manufacturer attitudes, consumer attitudes, technological progress, and government regulations.[86] These factors are not independent but obviously are highly correlated, e.g., supply, price, and manufacturer attitudes. Currently these three factors are favorable and well disposed. However, the other three are more uncertain. Technological progress in the area of texturization has been marked in the past decade. Processes that can use a wide range of basic starting materials to produce foods of desired structure and rheological properties are now available.

Table 11
MARKET PROJECTIONS FOR TEXTURED
VEGETABLE PROTEINS, SELECTED YEARS, 1975-
2000

|  | Year | | | | |
|---|---|---|---|---|---|
|  | 1975 | 1980 | 1985 | 1990 | 2000 |
|  | Million Pounds | | | | |
| School lunch | 113 | 180 | 210 | 270 | 348 |
| Public eating | 28 | 352 | 1,095 | 1,968 | 2,372 |
| Federal institutions | 12 | 27 | 40 | 58 | 79 |
| Commercial and others | 35 | 1,248 | 3,139 | 7,423 | 9,413 |
| Total | 188 | 1,807 | 4,484 | 9,719 | 12,212 |
| Extruded type | 117 | 1,066 | 2,107 | 3,888 | 4,885 |
| Spun type | 71 | 741 | 2,377 | 5,831 | 7,327 |

From Anon., Edible Soy Protein: Operational Aspects of Producing and
Marketing, Farmers Cooperative Service, Rep. #33, U.S. Department of
Agriculture, Washington, D.C., 1975, 43.

It is now possible to increase the protein value of foods by proper blending of ingredients prior to extrusion cooking. This capability is an asset for societies or particular
groups who require more options for increasing protein levels in their diets. The capacity to fabricate protein foods that do not concomitantly furnish excess fat and cholesterol should ease the burden of reducing the excessive intakes of calories and other
nutrients in affluent societies.

While the emphasis in this survey has focused on soybean protein, the technology
developed for the soybean can be easily adapted to other oilseed proteins and, with
further modification, to proteins from microbial cells and plant leaves. Thus proteinaceous foods with a variety of physical properties, nutrient compositions and specific
consumer types can be fabricated. However, the ultimate success of these fabricated
foods will depend on consumer acceptance.

Many factors such as appearance, flavor, texture, convenience, nutrition, selling
price, and cultural background, influence the consumer's decision to buy a particular
food. Acceptance depends upon complex reactions emanating from general cultural
and economic values and attitudes that reflect numerous interacting factors (geographic, familial, ethnic, peer-group, etc.). These influence the initial examination of
a new product or new concept and precede the impact that sensory properties might
have.[210] Where endogenous consumer motivation is lacking, some educational efforts
(advertising, labeling) may be required to overcome the initial aversion to testing of
new products by the potential consumer. Marketing of these products as simulated
meats equivalent to meats in flavor, texture, and nutritive value will convey an initial
advantage, especially if prices are favorable. This will only be sustained if these new
products perform as advertised. Schutz[210] stated that the more acceptable products
would be those in which textured proteins cannot be identified. This is corroborated
by the relative success of the meat extenders. As stated earlier, flavoring is perhaps
the major technical problem militating against the more facile acceptance of textured
protein foods, and this is where the next innovative developments must occur. This
problem reflects the subtle interrelationships between technological progress and consumer acceptance.

Finally, the impact of government regulations is considerable. Whether a new textured protein product is labeled as imitation or given a standard of identity classifying it as a distinct genus will have a marked impact on the success of such a product. The preliminary guidelines governing the use of textured protein products were published by FDA[11] The meat inspection service (Food Quality and Safety Service, USDA) has jurisdiction over meat inspection regulations and in situations where textured protein/ meat blends are used, this agency sets standards for usages. Regulatory guidelines are discussed elsewhere in this handbook.

The development of improved technology, while essential to expand the availability of a greater variety of foods, has been viewed as totally beneficial. However, advocation of the widespread adoption of this modern technology should be very carefully assessed in relation to its energy requirements, labor displacement, pollution, etc. Current economic circumstances and political considerations should not be the only criteria applied, but possible social and cultural impacts should also be assessed. Both the domestic and world food situations are inextricably involved with the problems of energy and cost economics. Some experts maintain that energy requirements must be the principal criterion in programs relating to long-term planning for food production in developing countries[217] and that labor-intensive systems less dependent on fossil energy should be emphasized. Others claim that the burgeoning population dictates the need for energy-intensive agriculture to ensure production of adequate food.[244] It would appear at present that a compromise between these two approaches is necessary.

This problem is quite relevant to the present topic. Thus sociologically and psychologically, meats are the most desired universal foods. However, their production is costly in terms of consumption of energy and protein. The capacity to fabricate reasonable facsimiles of meats from inexpensive vegetable proteins by modern technological procedures like extrusion and spinning may provide an acceptable alternative to meat at appreciable savings in energy and food protein. Thus Aguilera[2] computed relative total energy requirements (production and processing) for production of ground beef, spun soy protein fibers, and extruded soy pieces at 37,700, 13,900, and 5,680 kcal/kg protein, respectively. Although several assumptions were made, these values show a marked advantage for extruded soy protein. The nutritional value of these extruded products could be improved at a very modest cost. This suggests that extrusion has marked energy-saving advantages over beef production. Furthermore, considering the inefficient conversion rate of beef cattle consuming soy protein (i.e., 10%) and the greater versatility and stability of extruded products, this technique may offer great advantages to developing countries.

In discussing the prospects for textured proteins in developing countries, Weisberg[258] summarized the favorable aspects:

1.  They can be fabricated from local protein sources.
2.  They should be cheaper than animal proteins.
3.  They can be engineered for shape, size, color, texture, flavor, and nutritional value to fulfill any desired form.
4.  Because they are dehydrated, they should have a long shelf-life, which would minimize storage problems and facilitate packaging and transport needs.
5.  They are very amenable to institutional-type feeding programs, and in the case of extruded products, the technology is relatively simple, easy to learn, and cheap to operate.

The unfavorable aspects include the substantial initial capital outlay in equipment and physical plant, lack of information on marketing systems, protein availability, indigenous consumer preferences, quality control, and consumer disposition to such products.

The record of successfully introducing new foods into developing countries is a poor one when judged by any of several criteria. Numerous examples may be cited, and the failures may be attributed to several causes. The obvious conclusions are that balanced nutrition and good will, will not guarantee success. Price is very important. But perhaps the organoleptic qualities of new products, which frequently are sacrificed to nutrition or economy, are the critical factors in the determining ultimate acceptance of new foods by a target group — if they can afford to purchase it.

Meat is universally acceptable, and using the most recent, relatively simple extrusion processes it is now feasible to fabricate acceptable meat analogs. With appropriate flavoring applications, these can make a significant breakthrough in the alleviation of worldwide malnutrition. This technology gives cause for qualified optimism.

# REFERENCES

1. Adolphson, L. C. and Horan, F. E., Textured vegetable proteins as meat extenders, *Cereal Sci. Today*, 19, 441, 1974.
2. Aguilera, J. M., Texturization of Foods: Raw Materials, Processes and Products, Ph.D. thesis, Cornell University, Ithaca, N.Y., 1976.
3. Alden, D. E., Improvements in Flavoring Expanded Protein Material, U.S. Patent 3,615,656, 1971.
4. Altschul, A. M., Ed., Protein food technologies and the politics of food: an overview, in *New Protein Foods*, Vol. 1A, Academic Press, New York, 1974a, 1.
5. Altschul, A. M., Ed., *New Protein Foods,* Vol. 1A, Academic Press, New York, 1974b.
6. Andress, C., Flavors withstand extrusion heat without loss of flavor or aroma, Food Process. (Chicago), 38, 72, 1977.
7. Anon., Strategy on Action to Avert Protein Crisis in Developing Countries, U.N. Report E5018, June 1971, United Nations, New York. See also *PAG Bull.*, Vols. 1-4, 1971-1974 inclusive.
8. Anon., User acceptance spurs demand for vegetable protein analogs, *Institutional/Volume Feeding*, 79, 31, 1976.
9. Anon., Edible Soy Protein : Operational Aspects of Producing and Marketing, Farmers Cooperative Service, Report #33, U.S. Department of Agriculture, Washington, D.C., 1975, 43.
10. Anon., Textured Vegetable Protein Products, Food and Nutrition Notice #219, U.S. Department of Agriculture, Washington, D.C., 1971.
11. Anon., Food and Drug Proposals, Nutritional value of meat protein — soy protein blends, *Fed. Regist.*, 39(16), 20892, 1974.
12. Anon., A Hungry World: The Challenge to Agriculture, General Report, University of California Task Force, Berkely, 1974.
13. Anson, M. L., Method of Making Protein Food Product and the Resulting Product, U.S. Patent 2,813,025, 1954.
14. Anson, M. L. and Pader, M., *Methods for Preparing a Meat-Like Product,* U.S. Patent 2,879,163, 1959.
15. Anson, M. L. and Pader, M., Chewy Protein Gel Derived from Heat Denatured Seed Protein, U.S. Patent 2,830,902, 1958a.
16. Anson, M. L. and Pader, M., Chewy Protein Gel Binder for Protein Filaments, U.S. Patent 2,813,025, 1957.
17. Anson, M. L. and Pader, M., Method of Making Protein Food Product, U.S. Patent 2,833,651, 1958b.
18. Arai, S., Noguchi, M., and Fugimaki, M., Studies on flavor components in soybean, *Agric. Biol. Chem., (Tokyo)*, 34, 1569, 1970.
19. Arai, S., N-hexanal and some golatile alcohols: their distribution in raw soybean tissue and formation in soy concentrate by lipoxidase, *Agric. Biol. Chem. (Tokyo)*, 34, 1420, 1970.

20. Arima, T. and Harada, Y., Method of Producing Proteinaceous Fibers, U.S. Patent 3,627,536, 1971.
21. Atkinson, W. T., Bacteria Inhibited Protein Alginate Composition, U.S. Patent 3,645,746, 1972.
22. Atkinson, W. T., Aluminum-Modified Alginate Fiber, U.S. Patent 3,455,697, 1969.
23. Atkinson, W. T., Meat-Like Protein Food Products, U.S. Patent 3,488,770, 1970.
24. Atkinson, W. T., Process for Extruding Oilseed Protein Material, U.S. Patent 3,845,228, 1974.
25. Autret, M., World protein supply and needs, in *Proteins as Human Foods,* Lawrie, R. A., Ed., AVI Publishing, Westport, Conn., 1970, 3.
26. Balmaceda, E. and Rha, C., Spinning of zein, *J. Food Sci.,* 39, 226, 1974.
27. Baker, R. C. and Mustakas, G. C., Heat inactivation of trypsin inhibitor, lipoxygenase and urease in soybeans: effect of acid and base additives, *J. Am. Oil Chem. Soc.,* 50, 37, 1973.
28. Bender, A. E., Processing damage to protein food: a review, *J. Food Technol.,* 7, 239, 1972.
29. Beyeler, M. and Solms, J., Interaction of flavor model compounds with soy protein and bovine serum albumin, *Lebensm. Wiss. Technol.,* 7, 4, 1974.
30. Bird, K., Plant proteins, progress and problems, *Food Technol. (Chicago),* 28, 31, 1974.
31. Boonvisut, S. and Whitaker, J. R., Effect of meat, amylase and disulfide cleavage on the in vitro digestibility of soy protein, *J. Agric. Food Chem.,* 24, 1130, 1976.
32. Borenstein, B., Vitamin and mineral fortification, in *Fabricated Foods,* Inglett, C., Ed., AVI Publishing, Westport, Conn., 1975, 207-212.
33. Bourne, M. C., Desired textures of food analogs and methods of measuring their textural properties, paper presented at Annual Meeting of the American Institute of Chemical Engineers, Washington, D.C., 1974.
34. Bourne, M. C., Texture properties and evaluations of fabricated foods, in *Fabricated Foods,* Inglett, G. E., Ed., AVI Publishing, Westport, Conn., 1975.
35. Boyer, R. A., Soybean protein fibers: experimental production, *Ind. Eng. Chem.,* 32, 1549, 1940.
36. Boyer, R. A., High Protein Food Product and Process for its Preparation, U.S. Patent 2,682,466, 1954.
37. Boyer, R. A., Method of Manufacturing a High Protein Food product. Inclusion of Modifiers in Spinning Dope, U.S. Patent 2,730,447, 1956.
38. Boyer, R. A., Schultz, A. A., and Schultzman, E. A., Meat-Like Rehydratable Dehydrated Protein Products, U.S. Patent 3,644,121, 1972.
39. Bressani, R., Viteri, F., Elias, L., Alvardo, J., and Odell, A., Protein quality of soybean protein textured food in experimental animals and children, *J. Nutr.,* 93, 349, 1967.
40. Brian, R., Texturized protein products, *J. Am. Oil Chem. Soc.,* 53, 325, 1976.
41. Briggs, G., Nutritional aspects of fabricated foods, in *Fabricated Foods,* Inglett, G., Ed., AVI Publishing, Westport, Conn., 1975, 170-185.
42. Burrows, V., Green, A. H., Korol, A., Melnchyn, P., Pearson, G., and Sibbald, I., Food Protein from Grains and Oilseeds, Report, Canadian Wheat Board, Ottawa, Canada, 1972.
43. Cabot, J. M., Method of Producing Vegetable Protein Seafood Substitutes, U.S. Patent 3,852,484, 1974.
44. Calvert, F. E. and Atkinson, W. T., Use of Flow Inducing Salts for Expanded Proteins, U.S. Patent 3,498,794, 1970.
45. Castaigne, F., Rield, R., and Boulet, M., Mathematical model of water and soluble solids diffusion during protein fiber coagulation in meat analog fabrication, *Can. Inst. Food Sci. Technol. J.,* 9, 39, 1976.
46. Circle, S. J. and Smith, A. K., Functional properties of commercial edible soybean products, in *Symposium: Seed Proteins,* Inglett, G. E., Ed., AVI Publishing, Westport, Conn., 1972, 242-254.
47. Chang, S. S., Recent advances in meat flavor research, *Flavors,* p. 77, March 1976.
48. Cheftel, C., Cuq, J., Provensal, M., and Besancon, P., Influence de procedes technologiques sur la composition et la valeur nutritionelle D'aliments proteiques, *Rev. Fr. Corps Gras,* 23, 7, 1976.
49. Chiang, J. P. and Sternberg, M., Physical and chemical changes in spun soy protein fibers during storage, *Cereal Chem.,* 51, 465, 1974.
50. Coleman, R. J. and Creswick, N. S., Dried Meat Pieces, U.S. Patent 3,142,571, 1964.
51. Conway, H. F., Extrusion cooking of cereals and soybeans. I, *Food Prod. Dev.,* 5, 27, 1971.
52. Conway, H. F., Extrusion cooking of cereals and soybeans. II, *Food Prod. Dev.,* 5, 14, 1971.
53. Corey, H., Texture in foodstuffs, *CRC Crit. Rev. Food Technol.,* 1, 161, 1970.
54. Cumming, D. B., Stanley, D. W., and deMan, J. M., Texture-structure relationships in texturized soy protein. II. Textural properties and ultrastructure of an extruded soybean products, *Can. Inst. Food Sci. Technol. J.,* 5, 124, 1972.
55. Circle, S. and Frank, S. S., Use of isolated soybean protein for non-meat simulated sausage products, *Food Technol. (Chicago),* 13, 307, 1959.
56. Crocco, S. E., Better texture for vegetable protein foods, *Food Eng.,* 48, 15, 1976.
57. Daly, W. H. and Ruiz, L. P., Reduction of RNA in single cell protein in conjunction with fiber formation, *Biotechnol. Bioeng.,* 16, 285, 1974.

58. **Dechaine, R. C. and Callaghan, R. W.**, Vibrating Method for Impregnating Fibrous Protein Products, U.S. Patent 3,269,841, 1966.

59. **DeGroot, A. R. and Slump, P.**, Effects of severe alkali treatment of proteins on amino acid composition and nutritive value, *J. Nutr.,* 98, 45, 1967.

60. **DeGroot, A. P., van Beek, L., and Loewe, R. J.**, Feeding studies with alkali-treated proteins in rats, *Cereal Sci. Today,* 18 (Abstr.), 308, 1973.

61. **DeMan, J. M.**, Texture:structure relationships in new protein foods, *Cereal Foods World,* 21, 10, 1976.

62. **Drake, S. R., Hinnergardt, L. C., Kluter, R. H., and Prell, P. A.**, Beef patties: effect of textured soy protein and fat levels on quality and acceptability, *J. Food Sci.,* 40, 1065, 1975.

63. **Dwivedi, B. K.**, Meat flavor, *CRC Crit. Rev. Food Sci. Nutr.,* 5, 487, 1975.

64. **Dwivedi, B. K. and Arnold, R. G.**, Thiamine, *J. Agric. Food Chem.,* 21, 54, 1973.

65. **Duda, Z.**, *Vegetable Protein, Meat Extenders and Analogs,* Food and Agricultural Organization of the United Nations, New York, 1974.

66. **Dudman, R. K.**, Binding of Protein Fibers, U.S. Patent 2,785,069, 1957.

67. **Dunning, H. N., Strommer, P. K., and VanHulle, G.**, Steam Deodorization, Texturization, U.S. Patent 3,707,780, 1972.

68. **Eldridge, A. C.**, Organic solvent treatment of soybean and soybean fractions in soybeans, in *Chemistry and Technology I,* Smith, A. K. and Circle, S. J., Eds., AVI Publishing, Westport, Conn., 1973, 144.

69. **Elmquist, L. F.**, Preparation of Protein Fibers Using Safflower Seed Meal and Resulting Product, U.S. Patent 3,175,909, 1965a.

70. **Fabre, M.**, Spinning of sunflower proteins. Physical properties in relation to the organoleptic quality of spun protein, *Rev. Fr. Corps Gras,* 22, 591, 1975.

71. **Finucane, T. P. and MacAllister, R. V.**, Textured Protein Pieces, U.S. Patent 3,102,031, 1963.

72. **Fischetti, F.**, Flavoring textured soy proteins, *Food Prod. Dev.,* 9, 64, 1975.

73. **Forss, D. A.**, Odor and flavor compounds from lipids, *Progr. Chem. Fats Other Lipids* 13, 177, 1972.

74. **Franks, F.**, Physical-chemical principles of food fabrication, *in Fabricated Foods,* Inglett, G., Ed., AVI Publishing, Westport, Conn. 1975, 32.

75. **Franzen, K. and Kinsella, J. E.**, Physicochemical aspects of food flavoring, Chem. Ind., p. 505, June 1975.

76. **Gallimore, W. W.**, Synthetics and substitutes for agricultural products: projections for 1980, *U.S. Dep. Agric. Res. Serv. Mark. Rep.,* No. 947, U.S. Department of Agriculture, Washington, D.C., 1972.

77. **Giddey, C.**, Artificial edible structure from non-animal proteins, *Cereal Sci. Today,* 10, 56, 1973.

78. **Giddey, C.**, Protein Compositions and Process of Producing the Same, U.S. Patent 2,952,542, 1960.

79. **Glicksman, M.**, Carbohydrates for fabricated foods, in *Fabricated Foods,* Inglett, G., Ed., AVI Publishing, Westport, Conn., 1975, 68.

80. **Goodman, I.**, in *Fibre Structure,* Hearle, J. and Peters, R., Eds., The Textile Institute, Butterworth's, London, 1963, 111.

81. **Goossens, A. E.**, Protein foods: its flavors and off-flavors, *Flavour Ind.,* 273, 1974.

82. **Gremli, H. A.**, Interaction of flavor compounds with soy protein, *J. Am. Oil Chem. Soc.,* 51, 95A, 1974.

83. **Greuell, E. H.**, Some aspects of research in the applications of soy proteins in foods, *J. Am. Oil Chem. Soc.,* 51, 98A, 1974.

84. **Gutcho, M.**, *Textured Foods and Allied Products,* Noyes Data Corp., Park Ridge, N.J., 1973.

85. **Hamdy, M. M.**, Nutritional aspects in textured soy proteins, *J. Am. Oil Chem. Soc.,* 51, 85A, 1974.

86. **Hammonds, T. M. and Call, D. L.**, Utilization of protein ingredients in the U.S. food industry. II. The future market for protein ingredients, Department of Agricultural Economics, Cornell University, Ithaca, N.Y., 1970.

87. **Hanson, L. P.**, *Vegetable Protein Processing,* Noyes Data Corp. Park Ridge, N.J., 1974.

88. **Harman, D. V. and Harper, J. M.**, Modeling a forming foods extruder, *J. Food Sci.,* 39, 1099, 1974.

89. **Harper, J. and Harmann, D. V.**, Research needs in extrusion cooking and forming, *Am. Soc. Agric. Eng. Trans.,* 16, 941, 1973.

90. **Hartman, W. E.**, Worthington Foods, Inc., Vegetable Base High Protein Food Product, U.S. Patent 3,320,070, 1967.

91. **Hartmann, W. E.**, Plant Protein Foods: from Whence They Came to Where They are Going, paper presented at American Chemical Society Symposium, San Francisco, Calif., April 1976.

92. **Hashida, W.**, Flavor potentiation in meat analogs, *Food Trade Rev.,* p. 21, January 1974.

93. **Hayakawa, I., Kawasaki, S., and Nomura, D.**, Spinnability of yeast protein and its viscoelastic properties, *J. Agric. Soc. Jpn. (Nihon Nogei Kagakki-Shi),* 49, 641, 1975.

94. Hayase, F., Kato, H., and Fujimaki, M., Racemization of amino acid residues in proteins, *J. Agric. Food Chem.,* 23, 491, 1975.

95. Hegstead, D. M., Protein needs and possible modifications of the American diet, *J. Am. Diet. Assoc.,* 68, 317, 1976.

96. Hermansson, A. M., Determination of functional properties of protein foods, in *Problems in Human Nutrition,* Porter, J. and Rolls, B., Eds., Academic Press, New York, 407.

97. Herz, K. O. and Chang, S. S., Meat flavor, *Adv. Food Res.,* 18, 1, 1970.

98. Hesseltime, C. H., Fermented Products — Miso, Sufu and Tempeh, in Proc. Int. Conf. Soybean Proteins, Agricultural Research Service, U.S. Department of Agriculture, Peoria, Ill., 1966; *Biotechnol. Bioeng.,* 9, 275, 1967.

99. Hidalgo, J., DeRham, O., and Van De Rovaart, P., Fibers from Edible Proteins with High Nutritional Value, German Patent 2,604,234, 1 975.

100. Hodge, J., Origin of flavor in foods: nonenzymatic browing reactions, in *Chemistry and Physiology of Flavors,* Schultz, H., Day, E., and Libbey, L., Eds., AVI Publishing, Westport, Conn., 1967, 465.

101. Hodge, J. E. and Osman, E. M., Carbohydrates, in *Principles of Food Science: Food Chemistry,* Fennema, O., Ed., Marcel Dekker, New York, 1976.

102. Hoer, R. A., Protein Fiber Forming, U.S. Patent 3,662,672, 1972.

103. Hoffman, H., Soybean Meal Pieces Impregnated with Coconut Oil, U.S. Patent 3,485,636, 1969.

104. Holmes, A. W., Substitute foods: a practical alternative, *Philos. Trans. R. Soc. London Ser. B,* 267, 157, 1973.

105. Horan, F. E., Soy protein products and their production, *J. Am. Oil Chem. Soc.,* 51, 67A, 1974.

106. Horan, F. E., Meat analogs, in *New Protein Foods,* Vol. 1A, Altschul, A. M., Ed., Academic Press, New York, 1974b, 367-411.

107. Horan, F. E. and Wolff, H., Meat analogs: a supplement, in *New Protein Foods,* Altschul, A. M., Ed., Academic Press, New York 1976, 274-298.

108. Horan, F. E. and Burket, R. E., Engineered foods — the place for oilseed proteins, *Food Technol. (Chicago),* 25, 815, 1971.

109. Horenstein, I., Flavor of red meats, in *Chemistry and Physiology of Flavors,* Schultz, H., Day, E. A., and Libbey, L. M., Eds., AVI Publishing, Westport, Conn., 1967, 228-250.

110. Horenstein, I. and Crowe, P. F., Flavor studies on beef and pork, *J. Agric. Food Chem.,* 8, 494, 1960.

111. Huang, F. and Rha, C. K., Fiber formation from single cell protein, *Biotechnol. Bioeng.,* 14, 1047, 1972.

112. Huang, F. and Rha, C., Protein structures and protein fibers: a review, *Poly. Eng. Sci.,* 14, 81, 1974.

113. Hurrell, R. F. and Carpenter, K. J., Mechanism of heat damage in proteins: the reactive lysine content of heat damaged material, *Br. J. Nutr.,* 32, 589, 1974.

114. Inglett, G. E., Ed., *Fabricated Foods,* AVI Publishing, Westport, Conn., 1975.

115. Ikeda, K., On a new seasoning, *J. Tokyo Chem. Soc.,* 30, 820, 1909.

116. Ishler, N. H. and MacAllister, R. V., Textured Proteins with Polysaccharides, U.S. Patent 3,093,483, 1963.

117. Jaynes, H. O. and Asan, T., Fibrous protein from cottage cheese whey, *J. Food Sci.,* 41, 787-790, 1976.

118. Jenkins, S. L., Use of sulfides in extrusion, as cited in Gutcho, M., *Textured Foods and Allied Products,* Noyes Data Corp., Park Ridge, N.J., 1973.

119. Jones, N. R., Meat and fish flavors, significance of ribomononucleotides and their metabolites, *J. Agric. Food Chem.,* 17, 712, 1969.

120. Judge, M. D., Haugh, C. G., Zachariah, G. L., Parmalee, C. E., and Pyle, R. L., Soy additives in beef patties, *J. Food Sci.,* 39, 137, 1974.

121. Kakade, M. L., Rackis, J. J., McGhee, J. E., and Puski, G., Determination of trypsin inhibitor activity of soy products: a collaborative analysis of an improved procedure, *Cereal Chem.,* 51, 376, 1974.

122. Kelley, J. J. and Pressy, R., Studies with soy protein and fiber formation, *Cereal Chem.,* 43, 195, 1966.

122a. Kellogg, J. H., U.S. Patent 869,371,1907.

123. Kellor, R. L., Defatted soy flour and grits, *J. Am. Oil Chem. Soc.,* 51, 77A, 1974.

124. Kies, C. and Fox, H. M., Comparison of the protein nutritional value of TVP, methionine enriched TVP, and beef at two levels of intake for human adults, *J. Food Sci.,* 36, 841, 1971.

125. Kies, C. and Fox, H. M., Vitamin/protein interrelationships influencing the nutritive value of a soy TVP product for humans, *Cereal Sci. Today,* 18 (Abstr.), 298, 1973.

126. Kies, C., Nutritional implications of textured protein products, *Cereal World,* 19, 450, 1974.

127. Kies, C. and Fox, H. M., Effect of varying the ratio of beef and textured vegetable protein nitrogen on protein nutritive value for humans, *J. Food Sci.,* 38, 1211, 1973.

128. **Kies, C.,** Nutritional evaluation of fabricated foods, in *Fabricated Foods,* Inglett, G., Ed., AVI Publishing, Westport, Conn., 1975, 186-195.

129. **Kinsella, J. E.,** Junctional properties of proteins in foods. A survey, *CRC Crit. Rev. Food Sci. Nutr.,* 7(3), 219, 1976.

130. **Kinsella, J. E.,** Butter flavor, *Food Technol. (Chicago),* 29, 82, 1975.

131. **Kirimura, J., Shimizu, A., and Katsuya, N.,** The contribution of peptides and amino acids to foodstuffs, *J. Agric. Food Chem.,* 17, 689, 1969.

132. **Kjelson, N. A. and Page, J. A.,** Simulated chopped beef product, U.S., Patent 3,210,195, 1965.

133. **Korslund, M., Kies, C., and Fox, H. M.,** Comparison of the protein nutritional value of TVP, methionine enriched TVP and beef for adolescent boys, *J. Food Sci.,* 38, 637, 1973.

134. **Koury, J. J., Honig, D. H., Dessa, D. J., and Stegerda, F. R.,** Flavor and flatulence factors in soybean products, *J. Agric. Food Chem.,* 18, 977, 1970.

135. **Kramer, A. and Szczesniak, A. S.,** *Texture Measurement of Foods,* Reidel Publishing, Dordrecht, Holland, 1973.

136. **Kramer, A.,** Texture, its definition, measurement and relation to other attributes of food quality, *Food Technol. (Chicago),* 26, 34, 1972.

137. **Kuninaka, K.,** Flavor potentiators, in *Chemistry and Physiology of Flavors,* Schultz, H., Day, E. A., and Libbey, L. M., Eds., AVI Publishing, Westport, Conn., 1967, 505-535.

138. **Kuramoto, S., Westeen, R. W., and Keen, J.,** U.S. Patent 3,177,079, 1975; as cited in Gutcho, M., *Textured Foods and Allied Products,* Noyes Data Corp., Park Ridge, N.J., 1973, 31.

139. **Kuramoto, S. and Katz, I.,** Flavoring fabricated foods, in *Fabricated Foods,* Inglett, G., Ed., AVI Publishing, Westport, Conn., 1975, 159.

140. **Lange, D. H.,** Process for Preparing Protein Microfilaments, U.S. Patent 3,800,053, 1974.

141. **Lawrie, R. A., Ed.,** *Proteins as Human Food,* AVI Publishing, Westport, Conn., 1970.

142. **Lecluse, W. J.,** Edible Protein Fibers Based on Casein and a Process for Preparing Same, U.S. Patent 3,865,959, 1975.

143. **Liener, I. E.,** *Toxic Constituents of Plant Foodstuffs,* Academic Press, New York, 1969.

144. **Liener, I. E.,** Nutritional value of food protein products, in soybeans: Chemistry and Technology, Smith, A. and Circle, S., Eds., AVI Publishing, Westport, Conn., 1972, 203-224.

145. **Lockmiller, N. R.,** Textured protein products, *Food Technol. (Chicago),* 26, 57, 1972.

146. **Lorenz, K., Welsh, J., Norman, R., and Frey, A.,** Extrusion processing of triticale, *J. Food Sci.,* 39, 572, 1974.

147. **Longenecker, J. B., Martin, W. H., and Sarett, H. P.,** Improvement in the protein efficiency of soybean concentrates and isolates by heat treatment, *J. Agric. Food Chem.,* 12, 411, 1964.

148. **Lundgren, H. P.,** Synthetic protein fibers from protein detergent complexes, *Textile Res. J.,* 15, 335, 1945.

149. **Lundgren, H. P.,** Synthetic fibers made from proteins, *Adv. Protein Chem.,* 5, 305, 1949.

150. **Maarse, H. and Groenen, P. J.,** Aroma Research, Center for Agricultural Publication and Documentation, Wageningen, Netherlands, 1975.

151. **Maga, J.,** A review of flavor investigations associated with soy products, flours and isolates, *J. Agric. Food Chem.,* 21, 864, 1973.

152. **Maier, H. G.,** Binding fluchtiger aromastoffe an proteine, *Dtsch. Lebensm. Rundsch.,* 10, 349, 1974.

153. **Manley, C. H. and Fagerson, I. S.,** Major volatile compounds of hydrolyzed soy proteins, *J. Food Sci.,* 35, 286, 1970; *J. Agric. Food Chem.,* 18, 340, 1970.

154. **Manley, C. H. and Fagerson, I. S.,** Aspects of aroma and taste characteristics of hydrolyzed vegetable protein, *Flavour Ind.,* 2, 686, 1971.

155. **Mason, M. E. and Katz, I.,** Role of flavor in new protein technologies, in *New Protein Foods,* Vol. 2, Altschul, A., Ed., Academic Press, New York, 1976, 122-170.

156. **Matz, S.,** *Cereal Technology,* AVI Publishing, Westport, Conn., 1971.

157. **Mazur, R., Schlatter, J., and Goldkamp, V.,** Structure taste relationship of some dipeptides, *J. Am. Chem. Soc.,* 91, 2684, 1969.

158. **Maurice, T., Burgess, L. D., and Stanley, D. W.,** Texture evaluation of extruded products, *Can. Inst. Food Technol. J.,* 9, 173, 1976.

159. **McAnelly, J. K.,** Method for Producing a Soybean Product and the Resulting Product, U.S. Patent 3,142,571, 1964.

160. **McAnelly, J.,** Textured Products from Defatted Cooked Soybean Flour, U.S. Patent 3,142,571, 1964.

161. **Miller, W. and Morrow, C. T.,** Mechanical characterization of fibrous materials as related to meat analogs, *J. Texture Stud.,* 6, 473, 1975.

162. **Moncrieff, R. W.,** *Man-Made Fibers,* John Wiley & Sons, New York, 1963.

163. **Mustakas, G. C., Albrecht, W. F., Bookwalter, G. N., McGhee, J. E., Kwolek, W. F., and Griffin, E. L., Jr.,** Extruder processing to improve nutritional quality, flavor and keeping quality of full-fat soy flour, *Food Technol. (Chicago),* 24, 102, 1970.

164. Nashef, A. S., Osuga, D. T., Lee, H. S., Ahmed, A., Whitaker, J. R., and Feeney, R. E., Effect of alkali on proteins. Disulfides and their products, *J. Agric. Food Chem.*, 25, 245, 1977.

165. Naismith, W. W. F. and Thomson, R. H. K., Studies in the formation of fiber from groundnut protein, *J. Appl. Chem.*, 5, 192, 1955.

166. Nakanishi, T. and Wada, Y., Production of volatile sulfur anc carbonyl compounds by heat degradation of β-lactoglobulin, *Rokuno Kagaku No Kenkyu*, 24, A33, 1975.

167. NAS/NRC, *Toxicants Occurrring Naturally in Foods,* Publ. 1354, National Academy of Sciences-National Research Council, Washington, D.C., 1960.

168. Nesmeyanov, A. N., Rogozhin, S. V., Slonimsky, G. L., and Ershova, V. A., Synthetic caviar and Method of Preparing it, U.S. Patent 3,589,910, 1971.

169. Nagano, K., Logical analysis of the mechanism of protein folding. The nucleation process, *J. Mol. Biol.*, 84, 337, 1974.

170. Ney, K. H., Contribution of amino acids and peptides toward food flavor. in *Contributions to Chemical Food Supplies,* Morton, I. and Rhodes, D., Eds., Butterworth's London, 1974, 411.

171. Noguchi, M., Yamashita, M., Arai, S., and Fujimaki, M., On the bitter masking activity of a glutamic rich oligopeptide fraction, *J. Food Sci.*, 40, 367, 1975.

172. Okumura, G. K. and Wilkinson, J. E., U.S., Patent 3,490,914, as cited in Gutcho, M., *Textured Foods and Allied Products,* Noyes Data Corp., Park Ridge, N.J., 1973, 166.

173. Ohloff, G. and Thomas, A. F., *Gustation and Olfaction,* Academic Press, New York, 1971.

174. Osner, R. C., Nutritional and chemical changes in heated casein, *J. Food Technol.*, 10, 533, 1975.

175. Page, J. and Bauer, W. G., Method for Processing Protein Fibers, U.S. Patent 3,403,027, 1965.

176. Palmer, H. C., Filaments and Expanded Cellular Structure Formed by Heating Dough-Like Slurry of Wheat Gluten and Water, U.S. Patent 3,645,747, 1972.

177. Pepper, F. A. and Pearson, A. M., Possible role of adipose tissue in meat flavor. The nondialyzable aqueous extract, *J. Agric. Food Chem.*, 19, 964, 1971.

178. Peters, R. H., Production of fibers, in *Textile Chemistry,* Vol. 1, Peters, R., Ed., Elsevier, New York, 1963, 404.

179. Pirie, N. W., *Leaf Protein,* IBP Handbook No. 20, Blackwell Scientific Publications, Oxford, England, 1971.

180. Popkin, B. M. and Latham, M. C., The limitations and dangers of commerciogenic nutritious foods, *Am. J. Clin. Nutr.*, 26, 1015, 1973.

181. Porter, J. W. and Rolls, B. A., *Proteins in Human Nutrition,* Academic Press, New York, 1973.

182. Provensal, M. M. P., Cuq, J-L. A., and Cheftel, J-C., Chemical and nutritional modifications of sunflower proteins due to alkaline processing. Formation of amino acid cross-links and isomerixation lysine residues, *J. Agric. Food Chem.*, 23, 938-943, 1975.

183. Pyke, M., *Snythetic Food,* St. Martin's Press, New York, 1971.

184. Quist, I. H. and VonSydow, E., Chemical analysis of the volatile compounds in unheated and heated rapeseed protein model systems, *J. Agric. Food Chem.*, 24, 437, 1976.

185. Quist, I. H. and VonSydow, E. C., Unconventional protein as aroma precursors. Chemical analysis of the volatile compounds in heated soy, casein and fish protein model systems, *J. Agric. Food Chem.*, 22, 1077, 1974.

186. Rackis, J. J., Honig, D., Sessa, D., and Stezzerda, F. R., Flavor and flatulence factors in soybean protein products, *J. Agric. Food Chem.*, 18, 977, 1970.

187. Rackis, J. J., Sessa, F. R., Stezzerda, T., Shiizu, T., Anderson, J., and Pearl, S. L., Soybean factors relating to gas production by intestinal bacteria, *J. Food Sci.*, 35, 634, 1970.

188. Rakis, J. J., Biological and physiological factors in soybeans, *J. Am. Oil Chem. Soc.*, 51, 161A, 1974.

189. Rackis, J. J. and McGhee, J. E., Biological threshold levels of soybean trypsin inhibitors by rat bioassay, paper presented in part at 58th Annual Meeting of the American Association of Cereal Chemists, November 4-8, St. Louis, Mo., 1973.

190. Rackis, J. J., Biological active components, in *Soybeans: Chemistry and Technology,* Vol. 1, Smith, A. K. and Circle, S. J., Eds., AVI Publishing, Westport, Conn., 1972, 171.

191. Rakosky, J., Soy products in the meat industry, *J. Agric. Food Chem.*, 18, 1005, 1970.

192. Rakosky, J., Soy grits, flour, concentrates and isolates in meat products, *J. Am. Oil Chem. Soc.*, 51, 123A, 1974.

193. Rao, M. N. and Swaminathan, M., Plant proteins in the amelioration of protein deficiency states, *World Rev. Nutr. Diet.*, 11, 106, 1969.

194. Reynolds, T. M., Chemistry of nonenzymatic browning, *Adv. Food Res.* 14, 168, 1965.

195. Rechcigl, M., Ed., *World Food Problem,* CRC Press, Cleveland, Ohio, 1975.

196. Rha, C. K. and Clayton, J. T., *Synthetic and Simulated Foods* Paper No. 70-882 (Abstr.), American Society of Agricultural Engineers, Chicago, Ill., 1970.

197. **Robbins, R. M., Bonagura, A. G., and Yare, R. S.,** Preparation of a Soy Protein Having Improved Heat Gelable Properties, U.S. Patent 3,261,822, 1966.

198. **Robinson, R. F.,** What is the future of textured protein products, *Food Technol.,* 26, 59, 1972.

199. **Rosenfeld, D.,** Protein considerations for fabricated foods, in *Fabricated Foods,* Inglett, G., Ed., AVI Publishing, Westport, Conn., 1975, 196.

200. **Rosenfeld, D. and Hartman, W. E.,** Spun-fiber textured products, *J. Am. Oil Chem. Soc.,* 51, 91A, 1974.

201. **Rusoff, I. I., Ohan, W., and Long, C.,** Shred-Like Texture from Vegetable or Animal Protein, U.S. Patent 3,047,395, 1962.

202. **Sabry, Z. I.,** Coordinating food production with human needs, in *Western Hemisphere Nutrition Congress IV,* White, P. and Selvey, N., Eds., Publishing Sciences Group, Acton, Mass., 1975, 6.

203. **Saio, K., Kajikawa, M., and Watanabe, T.,** Effect of sulfhydryl groups on physical properties of tofu-gel, *Agric. Biol. Chem.,* 35, 890, 1971.

204. **Sautier, C. and Camus, M.,** Nutritive value and acceptability of textured vegetable proteins, *Rev. Fr. Corps Gras,* 23, 203, 1976.

205. **Schmandke, H., Maune, R., Webers, V., Anger, H., and Kormann, I.,** Experiments on spinning of rapeseed protein into fibers, *Nahrung,* 20, 25, 1976a.

206. **Schmandke, H., Paul, D., Friebe, R., and Webers, V.,** Rheology and spinning of alkaline solutions of sunflower seed globulin and casein, *Nahrung,* 20, 195, 1976b.

207. **Schmandke, H., Genrisch, H., Luther, H., and Maune, R.,** Rheology and spinning of alkaline solution of horse-bean protein and casein, *Nahrung,* 20, 531, 1976c.

208. **Schmandke, H. and Kormann, I.,** Swellability and stability of the structure of spun protein fibers, *Nahrung,* 20, 383, 1976.

209. **Schultz, H. W., Day, E. A., and Libbey, L.,** *Chemistry and Physiology of Flavors,* AVI Publishing, Westport, Conn., 1967.

210. **Schutz, H. G.,** Textured proteins, consumer acceptance and evaluation considerations, *Cereal Sci. Today,* 19, 453, 1974.

211. **Scrimshaw, N. S. and Hwang, D.,** Protein Resources and Technology: Status and Research Needs, NSF Rep. #NSF-RA-T-75-037, National Science Foundation, Washington, D.C., 1975.

212. **Scrimshaw, N. S. and Altschul, A. M., Eds.,** *Amino Acid Fortification of Protein Foods,* MIT Press, Cambridge, Mass., 1971.

213. **Seidman, S. C., Smith, G. C., and Carpenter, Z. L.,** Addition of textured soy protein and mechanically deboned beef to ground beef formulations, *J. Food Sci.,* 42, 197, 1977.

214. **Senti, F. R., Eddy, C. R., and Nutting, G. C.,** Conversion of globular to oriented fibrous proteins, *J. Am. Chem. Soc.,* 65, 2473, 1943.

215. **Sherman, P.,** Evaluation of textural properties of protein foods, in *Protein in Human Nutrition,* Porter, J. W. and Rolls, B., Academic Press, New York, 1973, 425.

216. **Sidel, J., Woolsey, A., and Stone, H.,** Sensory analysis: theory, methodology and evaluation, in *Fabricated Foods,* Inglett, G., Ed., AVI Publishing, Westport, Conn., 1975, 109.

217. **Slesser, M.,** Energy subsidy as a criterion in food policy planning, *J. Sci. Food Agric.,* 24, 1193, 1973.

218. **Smith, A. K. and Circle, S. J.,** *Soyabeans: Chemistry and Technology,* AVI Publishing, Wetsport, Conn., 1972.

219. **Smith, O. B.,** Textures by extrusion processing, in *Fabricated Foods,* Inglett, G. E., Ed., AVI Publishing, Westport, Mass., 1975.

220. **Smith, O. B.,** Extrusion cooking, in *New Protein Foods,* Vol. 2., Altschul, A. M., Ed., Academic Press, New York, 1976, 86.

221. **Smith, O. B.,** Extrusion and forming: creating new foods, *Food Eng.,* 47, 48, 1975.

222. **Smith, O. B.,** Textured Vegetable Proteins, paper presented at World Soybean Res. Conf., University of Illinois, Champaign, August 1975.

223. **Smith, G. C., Marshall, W. H., Carpenter, Z. L., Branson, R. E., and Meinke, W. W.,** Textured soy proteins for use in blended ground beef patties, *J. Food Sci.,* 41, 1148, 1976.

224. **Solms, J.,** Geschmackstoffe und Aromastoffe des Fleisches, *Fleischwirtschaft,* 48, 287, 1968.

225. **Solms, J.,** The taste of amino acids, peptides and proteins, *J. Agric. Food Chem.,* 17, 686, 1969.

226. **Solms, J.,** Nonvolatile compounds and the flavor of foods, in *Gustation and Olfaction,* Ohloff, G. and Thomas, A. F., Eds., Academic Press, New York, 1971, 92.

227. **Solms, J., Ismail, F. O., and Beyeler, M.,** The interaction of volatiles with food components, *Can. Inst. Food Sci. Technol. J.,* 6, A10, 1973.

228. **Spadaro, J., Mottern, M., and Gallo A.,** Extrusion of rice with cottonseed and peanut flavors, *Cereal Sci. Today,* 16, 238, 1971.

229. **Breene, W. M.,** Problems in determining textural properties of textured protein products, *Food Technol. (Chicago),* 31, 95, 1977.

230. Stanley, D. W., Cumming, D. B., and DeMan, J., Texture-structure relationships in texturized soy protein: textural properties and ultrastructure of rehydrated spun soy fibers, *Can. Inst. Food Sci. Technol. J.,* 5, 118, 1972.

231. Steinkraus, K. H., Hwa, Y. B., VanBuren, J., Providenti, M., and Hand, D., Studies on tempeh, *Food Res.,* 25, 777, 1960.

232. Steinkraus, K. H., Exotic fermented foods for Americans, *N. Y. Food Life Sci. Q.,* 8, 8, 1975.

233. Strommer, P. K., Continuously Puffing Finely Divided Particulate Food Materials Utilizing Opposing Steam Forces, U.S. Patent 3,730,729, 1972.

234. Strommer, P. K., Process for Texturizing a Protein Slurry, U.S. Patent 3,863,019, 1975.

235. Strommer, P. K. and Beck, C. I., Method for Texturizing Protein Material, U.S. Patent 3,754,926, 1973.

236. Sukhatme, P. V., India and the protein problem, *Ecol. Food Nutr.,* 1, 267, 1972.

237. Szczesniak, A. S. and Engel, E., Spinning Dope from Blend of Casein and Soy Meal, U.S. Patent 2,952,543, 1960.

238. Szczesniak, A. S., Classification of textural characteristics, *J. Food Sci.,* 28, 385, 1963.

239. Szczesniak, A., Consumer awareness of texture and other food attributes, *J. Texture Stud.,* 2, 196, 280, 1971.

240. Szczesniak, A. S., Consumer awareness of and attitudes to food texture, *J. Texture Stud.,* 3, 206, 1972.

241. Tannenbaum, S. and Wang, D. C., *Single Cell Protein II,* M.I.T. Press, Cambridge, Mass., 1975.

242. Thompson, R. H. K., *Symposium on Fibrous Proteins,* Society Dyers Col., Chorley Pickersgill, Leeds, England, 1946, 173.

243. Thulin, W. W. and Kuramoto, S., "Bontrae" — a new meat-like ingredient for convenience foods, *Food Technol. (Chicago),* 21, 168, 1967.

244. Timmer, P., Interaction of energy and food prices in less developed countries, *Am. J. Agric. Econ.,* 57, 219, 1975.

245. Tombs, M. P., Protein Products, British Patent 1,265,661, 1972.

246. Tombs, M. P., The significance of meat analogs: vegetable proteins, in *Proc. 21st Easter School Agric. Sci.,* University of Nottingham, England, 1975, 525.

247. Tombs, M. P., The significance of meat analogs, in *Proc. 21st Easter School. Agric. Sci. Univ. Nottingham on Vegetable Proteins,* Lawrie, R. A., Ed., University of Nottingham England, 1975, 27.

248. Tonsbeeck, C. H., Plancken, A. J., and vanderWeerdhof, T., Components contributing to beef flavor: isolation of 4-hydroxy-5-methyl-3(2H) furanone and its dimethyl hemolog from beef broth, *J. Agric. Food Chem.,* 16, 1016, 1968.

249. Turk, R. E., Cornwell, P., Brooks, M., and Butterworth, C., Adequacy of spun soy protein containing egg albumin for human nutrition, *J. Am. Diet. Assoc.,* 63, 519, 1973.

250. Van den Ouweland, G., and Peer, G. H., Components contributing to beef flavor, *J. Agric. Food Chem.,* 23, 501, 1975.

251. Visek, W. J., Biochemical considerations in utilization of non-specific nitrogen, *J. Agric. Food Chem.,* 22, 174, 1974.

252. Walker, N. J. and Manning, D. J., Components of the musty off-flavor of stored dried lactic casein, *N.Z. J. Dairy Technol.,* 11, 1, 1976.

253. Waggle, D. H., Method of Producing Expanded, Textured Protein Products, U.S. Patent 3,810,764, 1974.

254. Wasserman, A. and Spinelli, A. M., Effect of water soluble components on aroma of heated adipose tissue, *J. Agric. Food Chem.,* 20, 171, 1972.

255. Watanabe, T., Ebine, H., and Okada, M., New protein food technologies in Japan, in *New Protein Foods,* Altschul, A. M., Ed., Academic Press, New York, 1974, 415-454.

256. Watanabe, K. and Sato, Y., *Meat Flavor,* Rep. 45, Faculty of Agriculture, Nagoya University, Japan, 1974, 113.

257. Waterlow, J. C. and Payne, P. R., The protein gap, *Nature (London),* 258, 113, 1975.

258. Weisberg, S., Food Products intended to improve nutrition in the developing world, *Adv. Food Res.,* 22, 187, 1976.

259. Wenger, D., The Uni-Tex process, personal communication, 1977.

260. Westeen, R. W. and Kuramoto, S., General Mills, Inc. Preparation of Shaped Protein Products, U.S. Patent 3,118,959, 1964.

261. Wilding, M. D., Textured and shaped oilseed protein food products, *J. Am. Oil Chem. Soc.,* 48, 4-9, 1971.

262. Wilding, M. D., Textured proteins in meats and meat-like products, *J. Am. Oil Chem. Soc.,* 51, 129A, 1974.

263. Wilson, R. A. and Katz, I., Review of literature on chicken flavor and isolation of new flavor components from aqueous cooked chicken broth, *J. Agric. Food Chem.,* 20, 741, 1972.

264. Wilson, R. A., Review of thermally produced imitation meat flavors, *J. Agric. Food Chem.*, 23, 1032, 1975.
265. Wolf, W. J., Chemistry and technology of soybeans, *Adv. Cereal Sci. Technol.*, 1, 325, 1976.
266. Woodard, J. C. and Short, D. D., Toxicity of alkali-treated soyprotein in rats, *J. Nutr.*, 103, 569, 1973.
267. Wormell, R. L., *New Fibers from Proteins,* Butterworth's, London, 1954.
268. Wrenshall, C. L., Imitation Meat Products, U.S. Patent 2,560,621, 1951.
269. Young, R. H. and Lawrie, R. A., The spinning of blood plasma proteins, *J. Food Technol.*, 9, 171, 1974.
270. Young, R. H. and Lawrie, R., Isolation and spinning of proteins from lung and stomach, *J. Food Technol.*, 10, 453, 1975.
271. Yamaguchi, S., Yoshikawa, T., Ikeda, S., and Ninomiya, T., Measurement of the relative taste intensity of some amino acids and nucleotides, *J. Food Sci.*, 36, 846, 1971.
272. Yamazaki, A., Kumashiro, I., and Takenishi, T., Synthesis of 2-alkylthio inosine-5 phosphates, *Chem. Pharm. Bull.*, 16, 338, 1968.
273. Yang, Y. D. and Jackson, H., Preparation of soybean cheese using lactic starter organisms, *J. Food Technol.*, 21, 95, 1967.
274. Yang, J. H. and Olsen, R. A., Meat Analogs Having the Fiber Structure of Meat, U.S. Patent 3,814,823, 1974.
275. Ziabicki, A., Protein fibers, in *Man-Made Fibers: Science and Technology,* Vol. 1, Mark, H., Atlas, S., and Cernia, E., Eds., Interscience, New York, 1967.
276. Ziemba, J., Simulated meats, *Food Eng.*, 41, 72, 1969 and 43, 66, 1971.
277. Lugay, J. and Kim, M., Freeze alignment: a novel method for protein texturization, in *Utilization of Protein Resources,* Stanley, D. W., Ed., Food and Nutrition Press, Westport, Conn., 1981, 177.
278. Kinsella, J. E. and Dawsdaran, S., Flavor problems in soy proteins origin, nature, control and binding phenomena, in *Analysis and Control of Less Desirable Flavors in Foods,* Charalambous, G., Ed., Academic Press, New York, 1980, 95.
279. Anon. Proc. of World Conf. on Soya Processing and Utilization, *J. Am. Oil Chem. Soc.*, 58, 1981.
280. Dawsdaran, S. and Kinsella, J. E., Interaction of carbonyls with soy proteins, *J. Agric. Food Chem.*, 29, 1253, 1981.

# FISH PROTEIN

## Audrey L. Loomis and Virginia D. Sidwell

Throughout the ages fish has been the main source of animal protein for man living near fresh or salt water. Fish protein contains a well-balanced ratio of amino acids; in fact, they make an excellent complement to the amino acids in cereal proteins. Fish should be considered in a diet not only for its protein, but also for its nutritionally important minerals and vitamins and its low calories.

Tables 1 and 2 are a resume of the protein and amino acid values for 50 species of finfish, crustaceans, and mollusks that are landed and marketed in large quantities for human consumption. The values are obtained from 310 pieces of literature. Values for the same species, raw or processed, are grouped together and averaged. In each instance the average, the range of the values used to calculate the average, and the number of values used to calculate the average are recorded in the tables.

Generally, there is from 18 to 22% protein in raw finfish muscle. In certain species, there is a notable seasonal variation in the amount of protein in the muscle tissue. When the fat content is high, the tendency is for the amount of protein and moisture to be lower than when the percent fat is low. This seasonal variation may cause the protein content to drop 2 to 3%. Due to loss of moisture, cooked or canned finfish muscle will contain as much as 30% protein. In fish muscle that is dried, salted, or both, there is no consistent value for protein since it is associated with the degree of dryness.

In crustaceans, the amount of protein in the muscle tissue is not too different from that found in other fishery products. The mollusks contain about half the amount of protein of finfish and crustaceans. Again, there is a large seasonal, as well as sampling, variation. If mollusks are analyzed with their liquor, protein values will be lower than if the muscle is drained of liquor. The description of the sample used in the analysis is frequently unclear.

The muscle alone or the whole fish can be minced, defatted and dehydrated, and then ground to make a fine, powdered material called fish protein concentrate (FPC). FPC can be used to fortify cereal products such as bread, cookies, and tortillas. The addition of 5 to 10% FPC to wheat or corn flour improves the nutritive value of the cereal protein to a quality equal to or better than that of milk protein.[241]

All of man's protein requirements can be met by a diet with fish as the sole protein source. It has a well-balanced distribution of amino acids essential to man. There is an especially high amount of lysine in fish muscle; therefore, it is an excellent amino acid supplement to cereals.

From the scattered data found in literature, the nutritive quality of finfish, crustaceans, and mollusks is equal to or better than that of the classical reference — milk protein (casein).

## Table 1
## PROTEIN OF SOME COMMONLY CAUGHT FISH[311]

| Species | Values | Species | Values |
|---|---|---|---|
| Alewife — *Alosa* sp. | | Carp — *Cyprinus carpio* | |
| Raw | 16.5[a] | Raw[d] | 16.9 |
| | 11.7—19.4[b] | | 10.6—20.9 |
| | 4[c] | | 26 |
| Anchovy — *Engraulidae* sp. | | Boiled | 16.2 |
| Raw[d] | 19.7 | Fried[d] | 38.9 |
| | 13.2—23.5 | Catfish and Bullhead — *Ictalurus* sp. | |
| | 20 | Raw[d] | 17.8 |
| Canned | 19.9 | | 14.4—20.9 |
| Dried | 55.2 | | 9 |
| | 37.8—68.7 | Dried and seasoned[d] | |
| | 4 | Smoked[d] | |
| Paste | 20.6 | Chub — *Coregonus* sp., *Leucichthys* sp. | |
| Salted and dried[d] | 64.2 | Raw[d] | 20.8 |
| | 52.6—83.9 | | 16.8—23.6 |
| | 6 | | 7 |
| Salted and fermented | 21.6 | Canned | 16.2 |
| | 14.3—28.8 | Fried[d] | 36.9 |
| | 2 | Grilled | 22.6 |
| Unspecified cooked | 22.0 | Paste | 20.1 |
| FPC[d] | 73.4 | Clam — mixed spp. | |
| | 64.5—79.1 | Raw[d] | 11.6 |
| | 4 | | 4.4—19.0 |
| Bass (Striped) — *Morone* sp. | | | 71 |
| Raw[d] | 18.4 | Canned | 12.7 |
| | 14.0—20.0 | | 7.8—18.7 |
| | 18 | | 13 |
| Bluefish — *Pomatomus* sp. | | Salted | 9.8 |
| Raw | 20.4 | Steamed[d] | 10.1 |
| | 18.6—23.4 | Cod (Atlantic) — *Gadus morhua* | |
| | 12 | Raw[d] | 17.5 |
| Baked | 26.6 | | 15.8—19.6 |
| | 25.9—27.2 | | 13 |
| | 2 | Dried | 77.9 |
| Broiled | 25.2 | Fried | 19.3 |
| Fried | 22.7 | Salted[d] | 28.6 |
| Salted and dried[d] | 58.9 | | 19.0—42.3 |
| | 58.9—58.9 | | 4 |
| | 2 | Steamed | 22.4 |
| Steamed | 19.7 | Cod (Pacific) — *Gadus macrocephalus* | |
| Unspecified cooked | 25.9 | Raw[d] | 16.0 |
| Bonito — *Sarda* sp. | | | 14.1—17.9 |
| Raw[d] | 22.9 | | 3 |
| | 12.4—29.3 | Salted | 35.0 |
| | 13 | Unspecified cooked | 53.0 |
| Roasted | 24.0 | Crab — mixed spp. | |
| Salted and dried | 44.5 | Raw[d] | 17.4 |
| | 32.3—56.6 | | 10.8—23.4 |
| | 2 | | 56 |
| Buffalofish — *Ictiobus* sp. | | Baked | 12.8 |
| Raw[d] | 16.9 | Boiled | 19.2 |
| | 15.3—18.0 | Canned | 18.3 |
| | 3 | | 15.1—21.8 |
| Smoked | 19.0 | | 21 |

## Table 1 (continued)
## PROTEIN OF SOME COMMONLY CAUGHT FISH[311]

| Species | Values | Species | Values |
|---|---|---|---|
| Fried | 16.4 | Hake (Pacific) — *Merluccius productus* | |
| Paste | 15.6 | Raw | 15.8 |
| Salted | 14.8 | | 14.0—18.4 |
| | 11.3—18.3 | | 8 |
| | 2 | Hake (White) — *Urophycis* sp. | |
| Unspecified cooked[d] | 17.7 | Raw | 15.1 |
| | 14.3—20.8 | | 12.8—16.1 |
| | 7 | | 3 |
| Crayfish (Freshwater)— *Astacus* sp., | | FPC[d] | 88.0 |
| *Cambarus* sp. | | | 86.4—88.9 |
| Raw[d] | 16.5 | | 3 |
| | 12.0—24.1 | Halibut (Pacific) — *Hippoglossus stenolepis* | |
| | 9 | Raw | 19.3 |
| Boiled | 19.4 | | 15.4—21.5 |
| Croaker — *Micropogon undulatus* | | | 9 |
| Raw | 18.5 | Herring (Atlantic) — *Clupea harengus harengus* | |
| | 15.8—20.5 | Raw[d] | 18.3 |
| | 7 | | 17.7—18.9 |
| Flounder — mixed spp. | | | 3 |
| Raw[d] | 17.7 | Canned[d] | 21.3 |
| | 12.1—23.6 | | 17.5—23.9 |
| | 143 | | 8 |
| Baked | 30.0 | Herring (Pacific) — *Clupea harengus pallasi* | |
| Broiled | 25.2 | Raw[d] | 16.8 |
| Canned | 20.7 | | 16.0—17.7 |
| Dried | 20.5 | | 3 |
| Fried | 18.4 | Canned[d] | 20.8 |
| | 17.0—20.1 | Dried | 44.5 |
| | 5 | Salted | 18.5 |
| Smoked | 13.4 | | 17.4—19.6 |
| Steamed | 19.8 | | 2 |
| | 17.6—22.7 | Smoked | 32.8 |
| | 7 | Jack Mackerel — *Trachurus* sp. | |
| Grouper — *Epinephelus* sp., *Mycteroperca* sp. | | Raw[d] | 19.1 |
| Raw | 19.5 | | 16.1—21.3 |
| | 15.9—21.4 | | 16 |
| | 27 | Canned | 22.4 |
| Dried | 38.9 | | 21.5—23.2 |
| Haddock — *Melanogrammus aeglefinnus* | | | 2 |
| Raw[d] | 17.2 | Fried[d] | 35.2 |
| | 15.4—20.4 | Salted and dried[d] | 53.5 |
| | 23 | | 46.0—60.9 |
| Canned[d] | | | 2 |
| Fried | 18.7 | Lingcod — *Ophiodon elongatus* | |
| | 15.8—20.4 | Raw[d] | 17.6 |
| | 5 | | 14.9—20.0 |
| Salted and smoked | 23.7 | | 6 |
| Smoked | 23.3 | Lobster (American) — *Homarus* sp. | |
| Smoked and canned | 21.8 | Raw | 19.1 |
| Smoked and steamed | 22.3 | | 16.2—20.2 |
| Steamed[d] | 21.0 | | 4 |
| | 19.9—22.0 | Canned | 18.1 |
| | 2 | Lobster (Spiny) — *Panulirus* sp. | |
| FPC[d] | 83.7 | Raw[d] | 20.7 |
| | 73.6—90.3 | | 15.3—27.2 |
| | 5 | | 3 |

## Table 1 (continued)
## PROTEIN OF SOME COMMONLY CAUGHT FISH[311]

| Species | Values | Species | Values |
|---|---|---|---|
| Mackerel — *Scomber* sp. | | Raw | 19.0 |
| Raw[d] | 19.8 | | 17.9—21.7 |
| | 13.5—25.3 | | 6 |
| | 66 | Perch (Pacific Ocean) — | |
| Broiled | 21.8 | *Sebastes alutus* | |
| Canned[d] | 19.9 | Raw | 18.1 |
| | 17.3—25.4 | | 17.2—19.2 |
| | 14 | | 3 |
| Dried | 39.1 | Pollock — *Pollachius virens,* | |
| | 35.1—43.1 | *Theragra chalcogramma* | |
| | 2 | Raw[d] | 18.4 |
| Fried | 21.1 | | 16.2—20.9 |
| | 20.0—22.1 | | 19 |
| | 2 | Canned | 24.3 |
| Marinated | 20.8 | Paste | 17.8 |
| Salted | 27.0 | Steamed | 22.6 |
| Salted and dried[d] | 35.3 | Rockfish — *Sebastes* sp. | |
| | 20.9—43.1 | Raw[d] | 18.5 |
| | 3 | | 14.5—20.3 |
| Smoked | 26.0 | | 15 |
| | 21.5—30.4 | Sablefish — *Anoplopoma fimbria* | |
| | 2 | Raw | 12.1 |
| Unspecified cooked | 23.7 | | 11.0—13.6 |
| FPC | 89.9 | | 10 |
| | 89.5—90.3 | Salmon — *Oncorhynchus* sp. | |
| | 2 | Raw[d] | 20.0 |
| Mullet — *Mugil* sp. | | | 16.2—23.8 |
| Raw[d] | 19.4 | | 44 |
| | 14.0—22.6 | Baked | 26.1 |
| | 54 | Broiled | 28.0 |
| Boiled | 25.0 | Canned[d] | 20.6 |
| Canned, fried | 26.9 | | 16.3—25.9 |
| Dried | 50.7 | | 61 |
| | 32.0—69.3 | Salted | 29.8 |
| | 2 | | 23.2—36.4 |
| Salted and dried | 40.5 | | 2 |
| | 32.0—46.6 | Salted and smoked | 35.5 |
| | 4 | Slightly cured | 21.8 |
| Salted and smoked | 40.0 | Smoked | 21.4 |
| Steamed | 21.6 | Steamed | 19.1 |
| Oyster — *Ostrea* sp. | | FPC | 88.6 |
| Raw | 8.9 | Scallop (Sea) — *Patinopecten caurinus,* | |
| | 4.7—14.3 | *Placopecten magellanicus* | |
| | 61 | Raw | 17.0 |
| Canned | 9.5 | | 16.6—17.3 |
| | 7.3—12.4 | | 3 |
| | 6 | Scup (Porgy) — *Calamus* sp., | |
| Dried | 40.9 | *Stenotomus* sp. | |
| | 35.4—46.0 | Raw[d] | 18.8 |
| | 3 | | 18.4—19.1 |
| Fried | 8.6 | | 5 |
| Salted | 36.8 | Shad — *Alosa sapidissima* | |
| Salted and fermented | 3.3 | Raw[d] | 17.8 |
| Smoked and canned | 15.1 | | 15.7—19.9 |
| FPC | 62.3 | | 8 |
| Perch (Atlantic Ocean) — | | Canned[d] | |
| *Sebastes marinus* | | Sheepshead (Freshwater) — | |

## Table 1 (continued)
## PROTEIN OF SOME COMMONLY CAUGHT FISH[311]

| Species | Values | Species | Values |
|---|---|---|---|
| *Aplodinotus grunniens* | | | 5 |
| Raw | 17.4 | Salted and dried | 44.4 |
| | 15.9—18.4 | | 25.4—63.3 |
| | 11 | | 2 |
| Shrimp — mixed spp. | | Unspecified cooked | 25.6 |
| Raw[d] | 19.6 | | 20.9—27.8 |
| | 14.1—25.0 | | 5 |
| | 34 | Trout (Sea) (Gray Weakfish) — | |
| Canned[d] | 23.1 | *Cynoscion regalis* | |
| | 15.0—26.8 | Raw[d] | 17.9 |
| | 18 | | 15.7—19.6 |
| Dried[d] | 70.2 | | 4 |
| | 55.4—92.3 | Trout (Sea) (Spotted Weakfish) — | |
| | 10 | *Cynoscion nebulosus* | |
| Dried and salted | 50.0 | Raw | 16.8 |
| | 32.2—55.4 | | 15.6—18.6 |
| | 4 | | 4 |
| Fried | 11.8 | Salted and dried[d] | 48.8 |
| Paste | 24.9 | Tuna — mixed spp. | |
| | 18.4—30.0 | Raw[d] | 23.5 |
| | 4 | | 11.7—27.5 |
| Salted and fermented | 12.3 | | 67 |
| | 12.2—12.5 | Boiled | 27.0 |
| | 3 | Broiled | 33.4 |
| Unspecified cooked | 22.6 | | 31.9—34.9 |
| | 21.2—25.0 | | 2 |
| | 4 | Canned[d] | 25.6 |
| FPC | 91.0 | | 18.8—29.4 |
| Smelt — *Osmeridae* sp., *Mallotus* | | | 35 |
| *villosus* | | Dried[d] | 64.7 |
| Raw[d] | 15.2 | | 53.5—75.6 |
| | 10.7—18.9 | | 4 |
| | 17 | Fried | 31.1 |
| Canned | 21.1 | | 30.2—32.0 |
| Fried[d] | 31.3 | | 2 |
| | 25.0—37.5 | Salted and dried[d] | 55.2 |
| | 2 | | 49.5—60.9 |
| Snapper (Red) — *Etelis* sp., | | | 2 |
| *Lutjanus* sp. | | Smoked | 33.0 |
| Raw | 21.0 | FPC | 81.6 |
| | 19.8—22.4 | Whitefish (Common) — *Coregonus* | |
| | 9 | *clupeaformis* | |
| Fried | 16.4 | Raw[d] | 18.6 |
| Spot — *Leiostomus xanthurus* | | | 17.2—19.8 |
| Raw | 18.4 | | 12 |
| | 14.8—20.0 | Whiting — *Merluccius bilinearis* | |
| | 5 | Raw[d] | 17.1 |
| Squid — *Loligo* sp., *Illex* sp. | | | 15.2—20.4 |
| Raw[d] | 17.5 | | 7 |
| | 11.8—21.0 | Whiting (Kingfish) — *Menticirrhus* sp. | |
| | 38 | Raw | 17.4 |
| Dried[d] | 58.1 | | 15.5—18.9 |
| | 55.2—62.3 | | 3 |

*Note:* Values are expressed as percent of protein.

[a]  Average.
[b]  Range.
[c]  Number of figures used in computing the average.
[d]  Indicates that amino acids for this category appear in Table 2.

Table 2
AMINO ACIDS OF SOME COMMONLY CAUGHT FISH[311]

| | Lysine | Histidine | Cystine | Arginine | Tryptophan | Aspartic acid | Threonine | Serine | Glutamic acid |
|---|---|---|---|---|---|---|---|---|---|
| **Anchovy — *Engraulidae* sp.** | | | | | | | | | |
| Raw | 10.0[a] / 9.6—10.3[b] / 2[c] | 2.7 / 2.6—2.7 / 2 | 1.0 / 1.0—1.0 / 2 | 6.5 / 6.4—6.5 / 2 | 1.3 / 1.3—1.3 / 2 | 11.9 / 11.6—12.1 / 2 | 5.2 / 5.1—5.2 / 2 | 4.8 / 4.8—4.8 / 2 | 16.2 / 15.2—17.1 / 2 |
| Salted and dried | 8.7 / 7.8—9.5 / 2 | 1.9 / 1.8—2.0 / 2 | 1.4 / —[d] | 5.3 / 4.5—6.1 / 2 | 1.0 / 0.9—1.0 / 2 | 10.9 | 2.8 | 6.1 | 15.9 |
| FPC | 7.8 / 7.3—8.9 / 4 | 2.7 / 2.5—2.8 / 2 | 1.8 | 4.0 / 3.9—4.0 / 2 | 0.9 / 0.9—1.0 / 3 | 8.1 / 7.5—8.6 / 2 | 3.7 / 3.7—3.7 / 2 | 3.9 / 3.8—3.9 / 2 | 9.2 / 9.0—9.3 / 2 |
| **Bass (Striped) — *Morone* sp.** | | | | | | | | | |
| Raw | — | — | 0.9 / 0.8—1.0 / 2 | — | 1.1 / 1.0—1.1 / 2 | — | — | — | — |
| **Bluefish — *Pomatomus* sp.** | | | | | | | | | |
| Salted and dried | 11.6 | — | 1.2 | — | 1.2 | — | 6.1 | — | — |
| **Bonito — *Sarda* sp.** | | | | | | | | | |
| Raw | — | 1.0 | — | — | 1.2 | — | — | — | — |
| **Buffalofish — *Ictiobus* sp.** | | | | | | | | | |
| Raw | 7.2 | 2.9 | 1.9 | 7.1 | 1.1 | 6.6 | 4.7 | 4.4 | 13.9 |
| **Carp — *Cyprinus carpio*** | | | | | | | | | |
| Raw | 9.6 / 6.2—11.7 / 6 | 2.4 / 0.5—3.2 / 6 | 0.9 / 0.7—1.1 / 3 | 6.4 / 4.9—7.6 / 5 | 1.1 / 1.0—1.3 / 4 | 11.6 / 10.9—13.0 / 3 | 4.9 / 3.7—6.3 / 7 | 4.8 / 4.2—5.2 / 4 | 16.2 / 15.7—16.6 / 3 |
| Fried | 6.2 | — | — | — | 1.1 / 1.0—1.1 / 2 | — | 2.5 | — | — |
| **Catfish and Bullhead — *Ictalurus* sp.** | | | | | | | | | |
| Raw | 10.3 | 2.3 | — | 5.6 | — | — | 4.7 | 4.7 | — |
| Dried and seasoned | 9.8 | 2.2 | 0.6 | 6.0 | 1.0 | 10.0 | 4.5 | 5.7 | 14.7 |
| Smoked | 8.8 | 2.1 | 0.9 | 6.3 | 0.8 | 10.0 | 4.2 | 4.7 | 14.2 |
| **Chub — *Coregonus* sp., *Leucichthys* sp.** | | | | | | | | | |
| Raw | 12.6 / 6.7—19.8 / 3 | 1.8 / 1.7—1.8 / 2 | 1.5 / 0.7—2.3 / 2 | 6.2 / 5.0—7.4 / 2 | 1.1 / 1.0—1.3 / 3 | — | 5.8 / 4.6—8.1 / 3 | — | — |
| Fried | 8.1 | — | — | — | — | — | 4.0 | — | — |
| **Clam — mixed spp.** | | | | | | | | | |
| Raw | 7.5 / 5.1—9.1 / 31 | 1.7 / 1.0—2.5 / 25 | 1.7 / 1.3—2.9 / 16 | 7.0 / 4.0—10.4 / 25 | 1.2 / 0.8—1.8 / 21 | 10.3 / 7.2—12.7 / 20 | 4.4 / 3.2—5.5 / 31 | 4.5 / 3.5—5.4 / 20 | 14.3 / 11.4—17.1 / 19 |

| | | | | | | | | | |
|---|---|---|---|---|---|---|---|---|---|
| **Steamed** | 7.3 | 1.7 | — | 7.1 | 1.0 | 9.8 | 4.4 | 4.3 | 13.6 |
| **Cod (Atlantic) — *Gadus morhua*** | | | | | | | | | |
| Raw | 8.9<br>8.0—10.0<br>5 | 1.2<br>0.9—1.6<br>5 | — | 6.2<br>5.5—6.7<br>5 | — | 10.8<br>9.3—11.5<br>5 | 3.3<br>2.9—3.8<br>5 | 3.6<br>3.3—3.7<br>5 | 16.2<br>14.0—17.2<br>5 |
| Salted | 8.1 | 2.1 | 1.4 | 6.6 | 1.2 | — | 4.6 | — | 5 |
| **Cod (Pacific) — *Gadus macrocephalus*** | | | | | | | | | |
| Raw | — | — | 1.3 | — | — | — | — | — | — |
| **Crab — mixed spp.** | | | | | | | | | |
| Raw | 7.9<br>4.8—9.7<br>15 | 2.0<br>1.5—2.6<br>15 | 1.4<br>1.1—1.7<br>5 | 8.3<br>4.9—13.5<br>14 | 1.5<br>1.0—3.9<br>12 | 9.2<br>7.5—12.0<br>10 | 3.9<br>3.3—5.2<br>13 | 3.8<br>3.2—4.9<br>10 | 13.7<br>11.1—16.2<br>10 |
| Unspecified cooked | 8.1<br>7.2—9.0<br>2 | 2.1<br>1.7—2.4<br>2 | — | 9.7<br>8.2—11.2<br>2 | — | 11.6<br>11.6—11.6<br>2 | 4.4<br>3.9—4.8<br>2 | 4.0<br>3.8—4.2<br>2 | 15.3<br>13.8—16.8<br>2 |
| **Crayfish (Freshwater) — *Astacus* sp., *Cambarus* sp.** | | | | | | | | | |
| Raw | 6.4<br>5.7—7.0<br>2 | 4.4<br>3.3—5.4<br>2 | 2.3<br>2.1—2.4<br>2 | 4.9<br>3.8—5.9<br>2 | — | 8.5<br>8.0—8.9<br>2 | 5.3<br>4.6—5.9<br>2 | 5.8<br>4.3—7.3<br>2 | 15.6 |
| **Flounder — mixed spp.** | | | | | | | | | |
| Raw | 9.0<br>6.2—10.7<br>16 | 2.4<br>0.9—3.7<br>15 | 1.0<br>0.4—1.5<br>9 | 7.0<br>6.0—9.6<br>11 | 1.2<br>0.6—1.9<br>18 | 8.9<br>4.2—11.8<br>9 | 4.4<br>2.0—5.7<br>12 | 4.5<br>2.4—6.1<br>9 | 16.1<br>14.4—17.3<br>7 |
| **Haddock — *Melanogrammus aeglefinnus*** | | | | | | | | | |
| Raw | 9.6<br>6.4—11.0<br>10 | 2.5<br>1.2—3.7<br>8 | 1.2<br>1.0—1.4<br>4 | 6.6<br>5.0—9.2<br>8 | 1.2<br>0.9—1.4<br>8 | 10.7<br>9.3—11.6<br>4 | 4.7<br>4.0—5.8<br>7 | 5.3<br>3.9—6.1<br>4 | 15.7<br>13.3—17.4<br>4 |
| Canned | 8.1 | 1.5 | — | 5.2 | 1.1 | — | 4.4 | 4.3 | 13.0 |
| Steamed | 10.7 | 2.2 | — | 6.9 | 1.2 | 8.9 | 3.9 | — | — |
| FPC | 11.6 | — | 2.0 | — | 1.1 | — | 7.8 | — | — |
| **Hake (White) — *Urophycis* sp.** | | | | | | | | | |
| FPC | 7.9<br>7.7—8.2<br>3 | 1.9<br>1.8—1.9<br>3 | 1.0<br>0.9—1.1<br>2 | 6.6<br>6.2—7.1<br>3 | 1.1<br>1.0—1.2<br>2 | 10.2 | 4.3<br>4.2—4.5<br>3 | 4.7 | 15.4 |
| **Herring (Atlantic) — *Clupea harengus harengus*** | | | | | | | | | |
| Raw | 8.7<br>7.0—10.3<br>2 | 2.7<br>1.6—3.7<br>2 | — | 6.2<br>5.1—7.3<br>2 | 1.3<br>1.2—1.4<br>2 | 11.0 | 5.3 | 5.6 | 17.0 |
| Canned | 8.2<br>7.8—9.0<br>4 | 2.3<br>2.0—2.5<br>3 | — | 5.4<br>5.2—5.6<br>3 | 0.8<br>0.7—1.0<br>4 | 8.3 | 4.5<br>4.3—4.7<br>4 | — | 12.8 |

## Table 2 (continued)
## AMINO ACIDS OF SOME COMMONLY CAUGHT FISH[311]

| | Lysine | Histidine | Cystine | Arginine | Tryptophan | Aspartic acid | Threonine | Serine | Glutamic acid |
|---|---|---|---|---|---|---|---|---|---|
| **Herring (Pacific) — *Clupea harengus pallasi*** | | | | | | | | | |
| Raw | 8.4 (7.2—9.9) 3 | 2.2 (2.0—2.7) 3 | 1.1 | 5.5 (4.3—6.2) 3 | 0.9 (0.7—1.0) 3 | 12.0 (3) | 4.4 (3.6—5.1) 3 | 4.8 | 17.6 |
| Canned | 8.3 | 5.0 | — | 4.9 | 1.1 | — | 4.0 | — | — |
| **Jack Mackerel — *Trachurus* sp.** | | | | | | | | | |
| Raw | 9.2 (8.2—10.7) 6 | 3.1 (2.3—3.6) 6 | 1.2 (1.1—1.5) 3 | 6.4 (5.1—9.4) 6 | 1.0 (0.4—1.3) 6 | 9.0 (6.5—10.8) 4 | 4.6 (4.2—5.6) 5 | 3.6 (2.5—4.8) 4 | 14.6 (14.0—15.8) 3 |
| Fried | 7.3 | — | 0.9 | — | — | — | 3.6 | — | — |
| Salted and dried | 6.3 | — | — | — | — | — | 5.3 | — | — |
| **Lingcod — *Ophiodon elongatus*** | | | | | | | | | |
| Raw | — | — | 1.5 | — | 0.8 | — | — | — | — |
| **Lobster (Spiny) — *Panulirus* sp.** | | | | | | | | | |
| Raw | 9.5 | 2.2 | 2.8 | 7.4 | — | 12.3 | 4.4 | 4.9 | 17.0 |
| **Mackerel — *Scomber* sp.** | | | | | | | | | |
| Raw | 8.8 (5.1—11.5) 12 | 3.1 (1.4—5.6) 11 | 1.1 (0.8—1.4) 8 | 5.9 (5.0—7.6) 11 | 1.2 (0.6—1.5) 14 | 9.6 (8.0—11.5) 6 | 4.7 (3.9—5.7) 9 | 4.6 (3.6—5.0) 4 | 12.9 (12.0—14.3) 6 |
| Canned | 8.0 | 3.7 | — | 5.6 (5.2—5.9) 3 | 0.9 (0.7—1.0) 3 | 7.8 | 4.8 (4.7—5.0) | 4 | 11.7 |
| Salted and dried | 6.9 | 3.2 | 0.8 | 4.6 | 1.2 | 8.2 | 3.8 | 3.7 | 13.3 |
| **Mullet — *Mugil* sp.** | | | | | | | | | |
| Raw | 8.5 (6.7—10.7) 5 | 2.2 (0.6—3.7) 7 | 1.0 (0.5—1.4) 4 | 6.3 (5.4—6.8) 6 | 1.2 (0.4—1.6) 5 | 11.8 (9.1—14.1) 3 | 4.6 (3.3—7.1) 5 | 3.9 (3.4—4.2) 3 | 15.4 (13.9—16.2) 3 |
| **Perch (Atlantic Ocean) — *Sebastes marinus*** | | | | | | | | | |
| Raw | 9.2 | 2.0 | 1.1 | 6.1 | 1.0 | 10.6 | 4.8 | 5.2 | 15.4 |
| **Pollock — *Pollachius virens, Theragra chalcogramma*** | | | | | | | | | |
| Raw | 10.3 (4.1—11.0) 4 | 2.2 (2.0—2.4) 2 | 1.0 | 6.5 (6.0—7.0) 2 | 1.1 (1.0—1.2) 2 | 8.3 (6.3—10.2) 2 | 5.1 (4.4—5.8) 2 | 5.0 (4.6—5.3) 2 | 15.2 (14.5—15.9) 2 |

| | | | | | | | | | |
|---|---|---|---|---|---|---|---|---|---|
| Rockfish — *Sebastes* sp. <br>Raw | 14.4 | 1.6 | — | 4.3 | — | — | 5.1 | — | — |
| Salmon — *Oncorhynchus* sp. <br>Raw | 7.9<br>5.7—10.7<br>7 | 2.2<br>1.3—3.2<br>7 | 1.3<br>0.8—1.4<br>7 | 5.5<br>5.0—5.9<br>6 | 1.3<br>1.1—1.4<br>9 | 9.5<br>8.7—10.8<br>3 | 5.0<br>4.3—6.0<br>3 | 4.3<br>3.9—4.9<br>3 | 14.1<br>11.9—15.5<br>3 |
| Canned | 8.4<br>6.8—10.6<br>5 | 2.5<br>1.9—2.9<br>5 | — | 5.7<br>5.4—5.8<br>5 | 1.0<br>0.7—1.3<br>5 | 9.8<br>8.8—10.8<br>2 | 4.7<br>4.2—6.0<br>5 | 4.9 | 13.8<br>12.7—14.8<br>2 |
| Scup (Porgy) — *Calamus* sp., *Stenotomus* sp. <br>Raw | — | — | — | — | — | — | — | — | — |
| Shad — *Alosa sapidissima* <br>Raw | 8.2<br>6.5—9.8<br>2 | 1.7<br>1.1—2.3<br>2 | 1.2 | 5.1<br>4.5—5.7<br>2 | 1.2<br>1.1—1.2<br>2 | — | 4.1 | — | — |
| Canned | 9.0 | 1.9 | — | 5.2 | 0.8 | — | 4.1 | — | — |
| Shrimp — mixed spp. <br>Raw | 11.6<br>6.8—19.8<br>8 | 2.0<br>1.6—2.6<br>8 | 1.5<br>1.1—1.5<br>6 | 8.4<br>7.2—9.3<br>5 | 1.1<br>0.4—1.8<br>7 | 9.3 | 4.3<br>3.8—4.7<br>6 | — | 15.5 |
| Canned | 12.7<br>8.1—18.7<br>9 | 1.9<br>1.3—2.4<br>9 | 1.6<br>1.6—1.6<br>3 | 9.1<br>8.5—9.5<br>6 | 1.4<br>1.0—1.6<br>5 | 9.3 | 4.0<br>2.8—4.8<br>9 | — | 15.5 |
| Dried | 10.0<br>9.2—10.4<br>4 | 2.2<br>2.0—2.3<br>4 | 1.3<br>1.2—1.5<br>4 | 9.1 | 1.3<br>1.0—1.6<br>4 | 10.0 | 4.2<br>3.8—4.4<br>4 | 4.8 | 14.8 |
| Smelt — *Osmeridae* sp., *Mallotus villosus* <br>Raw | 11.3<br>11.1—11.4<br>2 | — | — | — | — | — | 4.3<br>4.2—4.3<br>3 | — | — |
| Fried | 6.3 | — | — | — | — | — | 4.0 | — | — |
| Squid — *Loligo* sp., *Illex* sp. <br>Raw | 8.7<br>6.6—12.1<br>13 | 2.1<br>1.0—3.8<br>13 | 1.3<br>1.1—1.8<br>3 | 7.1<br>3.6—11.6<br>13 | 1.0<br>0.3—1.8<br>8 | 9.3<br>5.6—11.6<br>11 | 4.1<br>2.1—6.6<br>13 | 3.6<br>2.2—5.6<br>10 | 14.0<br>12.4—16.5<br>9 |
| Dried | 7.2 | 1.7 | 0.9 | 7.3 | 0.8 | 8.9 | 3.6 | 4.5 | 12.8 |
| Trout (Sea)(Gray Weakfish) — *Cynoscion regalis* <br>Raw | 6.8 | 1.4 | — | 5.9 | 1.0 | — | — | — | — |
| Trout (Sea)(Spotted Weakfish) — *Cynoscion nebulosus* <br>Salted and dried | 8.8 | — | 1.1 | — | 1.1 | — | 6.3 | — | — |
| Tuna — mixed spp. <br>Raw | 9.0<br>7.8—10.8<br>8 | 4.0<br>2.5—5.5<br>8 | 1.1<br>0.8—1.3<br>3 | 5.4<br>4.3—6.1<br>6 | 1.2<br>0.4—1.7<br>12 | 10.2<br>8.3—12.0<br>6 | 3.9<br>2.7—5.9<br>8 | 3.9<br>3.1—4.7<br>5 | 13.7<br>10.0—16.8<br>7 |

## Table 2 (continued)
## AMINO ACIDS OF SOME COMMONLY CAUGHT FISH[311]

| | Lysine | Histidine | Cystine | Arginine | Tryptophan | Aspartic acid | Threonine | Serine | Glutamic acid |
|---|---|---|---|---|---|---|---|---|---|
| Canned | 8.7<br>8.2—10.1<br>8 | 5.8<br>5.7—6.0<br>6 | 0.9<br>0.9—0.9<br>2 | 5.3<br>5.2—5.4<br>6 | 1.0<br>0.8—1.2<br>8 | 8.7<br>8.7—8.7<br>2 | 4.5<br>4.1—4.7<br>6 | —<br>— | 13.0<br>12.9—13.0<br>2 |
| Dried | 7.4 | 6.6 | 1.0 | 5.1 | 1.2 | 10.1 | 4.2 | 3.4 | 12.2 |
| Salted and dried | 10.2 | — | 1.2 | — | 1.3 | — | 7.0 | — | — |
| Whitefish (Common) — *Coregonus clupeaformis* | | | | | | | | | |
| Raw | 11.7 | — | — | — | — | — | 4.9 | — | — |
| Whiting — *Merluccius bilinearis* | | | | | | | | | |
| Raw | 9.1 | 1.7 | 2.1 | 5.7 | 1.1 | 11.1 | 4.6 | 4.1 | 16.3 |

*Note:* Values are expressed as percent of protein.

a   Average.
b   Range.
c   Number of figures used in computing the average.
d   Dashes indicate data not available.

| | Proline | Glycine | Alanine | Valine | Methionine | Isoleucine | Tyrosine | Phenylalanine | Leucine |
|---|---|---|---|---|---|---|---|---|---|
| Anchovy — *Engraulidae* sp. | | | | | | | | | |
| Raw | 3.8<br>3.5—4.0<br>2 | 4.9<br>4.5—5.2<br>2 | 6.9<br>6.7—7.0<br>2 | 5.7<br>5.5—5.9<br>2 | 3.6<br>3.4—3.7<br>2 | 5.4<br>5.4—5.4<br>2 | 3.6<br>3.4—3.8<br>2 | 4.4<br>4.2—4.5<br>2 | 9.3<br>9.0—9.5<br>2 |
| Salted and dried | 4.2 | 6.1 | 7.0 | 5.4 | 3.2<br>3.1—3.2<br>2 | 5.5 | 3.5 | 4.2 | 7.8 |
| FPC | 3.1<br>3.0—3.2<br>2 | 4.0<br>3.7—4.3<br>2 | — | 4.5—6.2<br>2 | 3.0<br>2.8—3.3<br>3 | 4.3—6.6<br>2 | 3.3<br>3.2—3.4<br>2 | 3.5<br>3.4—3.6<br>2 | 6.7—8.9<br>2 |
| Bass (Striped) — *Morone* sp. | | | | | | | | | |
| Raw | — | — | — | 4.4<br>4.3—4.5<br>2 | 3.4<br>3.2—3.5<br>2 | 4.3<br>4.0—4.6<br>2 | 3.5<br>3.3—3.6<br>2 | 4.8<br>4.5—5.0<br>2 | 6.2<br>6.1—6.3<br>2 |
| Bluefish — *Pomatomus* sp. | | | | | | | | | |
| Salted and dried | — | — | — | 7.0 | 4.4 | 6.3 | — | 4.8 | 8.9 |

| Species / Preparation | Col 1 | Col 2 | Col 3 | Col 4 | Col 5 | Col 6 | Col 7 | Col 8 | Col 9 |
|---|---|---|---|---|---|---|---|---|---|
| **Bonito — *Sarda* sp.** | | | | | | | | | |
| Raw | — | — | — | — | 3.5 | — | — | — | — |
| **Buffalofish — *Ictiobus* sp.** | | | | | | | | | |
| Raw | 6.9 | 3.8 | 3.2 | 5.7 | 3.3 | 6.7 | 3.8 | 4.7 | 3.5 |
| **Carp — *Cyprinus carpio*** | | | | | | | | | |
| Raw | 8.0 / 6.7–9.2 / 6 | 4.4 / 3.6–5.1 / 6 | 3.5 / 2.4–4.0 / 5 | 5.1 / 4.5–6.2 / 6 | 3.2 / 2.7–3.7 / 7 | 5.5 / 4.5–6.6 / 6 | 6.7 / 6.2–7.0 / 4 | 4.4 / 3.7–5.1 / 3 | 3.1 / 2.3–3.8 / 4 |
| Fried | 4.0 | 2.1 | — | 3.0 | 1.4 | 2.8 | — | — | — |
| **Catfish and Bullhead — *Ictalurus* sp.** | | | | | | | | | |
| Raw | 9.6 | 5.1 | — | 7.9 | 3.1 | 6.5 | 6.8 | 5.6 | 4.1 |
| Dried and seasoned | 9.1 | 4.0 | 3.1 | 6.6 | 2.9 | 6.2 | — | — | — |
| Smoked | 8.1 | 3.8 | 3.0 | 6.5 | 2.6 | 5.2 | 6.5 | 6.6 | 4.1 |
| **Chub — *Coregonus* sp., *Leucichthys* sp.** | | | | | | | | | |
| Raw | 7.6 / 6.5–8.8 / 3 | 4.4 / 3.6–4.5 / 3 | 1.6 / 1.6–1.6 / 2 | 5.7 / 4.7–7.3 / 3 | 3.0 / 2.5–3.7 / 3 | 5.9 / 5.4–6.5 / 3 | — | — | — |
| Fried | 5.7 | 1.7 | — | 2.8 | 2.0 | 4.3 | — | — | — |
| **Clam — mixed spp.** | | | | | | | | | |
| Raw | 7.5 / 5.5–9.6 / 31 | 3.6 / 1.8–5.1 / 31 | 3.8 / 2.7–6.6 / 25 | 4.8 / 3.2–8.0 / 31 | 2.3 / 0.5–3.1 / 31 | 4.5 / 2.4–6.7 / 31 | 6.2 / 3.7–7.6 / 20 | 5.4 / 4.3–6.9 / 20 | 3.7 / 2.8–5.6 / 20 |
| Steamed | 6.6 | 3.3 | 3.3 | 4.1 | 2.3 | 4.1 | 6.4 | 7.2 | 3.7 |
| **Cod (Atlantic) — *Gadus morhua*** | | | | | | | | | |
| Raw | 7.7 / 6.2–8.3 / 5 | 3.4 / 3.2–3.6 / 5 | 3.0 / 2.8–3.3 / 5 | 4.3 / 4.1–4.7 / 5 | 3.0 / 2.7–3.2 / 5 | 5.1 / 4.4–5.4 / 5 | 6.0 / 5.1–6.4 / 5 | 5.0 / 4.0–6.4 / 5 | 4.0 / 3.4–4.8 / 5 |
| Salted | 9.4 | 4.3 | 4.7 | 4.3 | 3.2 | 5.4 | — | — | — |
| **Cod (Pacific) — *Gadus macrocephalus*** | | | | | | | | | |
| Raw | — | — | — | — | 2.2 | — | — | — | — |
| **Crab — mixed spp.** | | | | | | | | | |
| Raw | 6.5 / 3.5–9.0 / 13 | 3.7 / 3.0–4.8 / 12 | 3.6 / 2.6–4.7 / 11 | 4.4 / 3.2–9.2 / 13 | 2.7 / 1.6–5.0 / 13 | 4.5 / 3.3–5.8 / 13 | 5.7 / 4.8–6.7 / 10 | 6.2 / 4.0–8.4 / 10 | 3.9 / 3.1–4.8 / 10 |
| Unspecified cooked | 7.8 / 6.9–8.6 / 2 | 4.0 / 3.5–4.4 / 2 | 3.8 / 3.1–4.4 / 2 | 4.5 / 4.0–5.0 / 2 | 2.4 / 2.3–2.5 / 2 | 4.8 / 4.1–4.9 / 2 | 5.6 / 5.3–5.8 / 2 | 5.9 / 4.7–7.0 / 2 | 4.2 / 4.0–4.3 / 2 |
| **Crayfish (Freshwater) — *Astacus* sp., *Cambarus* sp.** | | | | | | | | | |
| Raw | — | 6.1 / 5.5–6.7 / 2 | 5.9 / 5.3–6.4 / 2 | — | 1.8 / 1.7–1.8 / 2 | 3.5 / 3.2–3.8 / 2 | 7.4 / 6.7–8.0 / 2 | 4.2 / 3.2–5.1 / 2 | 4.2 / 3.0–5.3 / 2 |
| **Flounder — mixed spp.** | | | | | | | | | |
| Raw | 7.3 / 3.6–9.0 / 11 | 3.5 / 1.7–4.9 / 13 | 3.0 / 1.2–4.2 / 11 | 4.8 / 2.6–6.2 / 11 | 2.9 / 1.3–4.5 / 15 | 5.8 / 3.4–7.0 / 11 | 6.6 / 5.6–8.1 / 7 | 4.5 / 3.9–5.4 / 9 | 3.7 / 3.0–4.7 / 9 |

## Table 2 (continued)
## AMINO ACIDS OF SOME COMMONLY CAUGHT FISH[311]

| | Proline | Glycine | Alanine | Valine | Methionine | Isoleucine | Tyrosine | Phenylalanine | Leucine |
|---|---|---|---|---|---|---|---|---|---|
| **Haddock — *Melanogrammus aeglefinnus*** | | | | | | | | | |
| Raw | 3.9<br>3.0—4.8<br>4 | 4.7<br>3.9—5.2<br>4 | 6.9<br>5.4—8.0<br>4 | 5.7<br>4.5—6.3<br>7 | 3.2<br>2.8—4.1<br>7 | 5.3<br>4.6—6.2<br>6 | 3.2<br>1.0—4.3<br>5 | 4.0<br>3.3—4.7<br>7 | 8.3<br>7.3—9.3<br>7 |
| Canned | 3.1 | — | — | 5.1 | 3.1 | 5.2 | — | 3.7 | 7.6 |
| Steamed | — | 4.0 | 5.9 | 4.5 | 3.1 | 4.7 | 2.9 | 3.8 | 7.7 |
| FPC | — | — | — | 6.1 | 4.6 | 5.7 | — | 4.3 | 7.9 |
| **Hake (White) — *Urophycis* sp.** | | | | | | | | | |
| FPC | 5.7 | 9.2 | 7.0 | 5.1<br>5.0—5.1<br>3 | 3.2<br>3.1—3.4<br>3 | 4.5<br>4.4—4.5<br>3 | 3.3 | 4.1<br>4.0—4.1<br>3 | 7.4<br>7.2—7.5<br>3 |
| **Herring (Atlantic) — *Clupea harengus harengus*** | | | | | | | | | |
| Raw | 4.4 | 5.1 | 7.4 | 6.0 | 2.0 | 5.1 | 4.1 | 4.7 | 9.6 |
| Canned | — | 5.0 | — | 5.2<br>5.0—5.6<br>4 | 2.9<br>2.7—3.2<br>4 | 4.8 | — | 3.6<br>3.3—3.8<br>4 | 7.5<br>6.9—8.6<br>4 |
| **Herring (Pacific) — *Clupea harengus pallasi*** | | | | | | | | | |
| Raw | 3.8 | 5.0 | 6.7 | 5.2<br>4.5—6.0<br>3 | 2.6<br>2.0—3.5<br>4 | 5.4<br>4.6—6.4<br>3 | 2.6<br>1.8—3.7<br>3 | 4.0<br>3.7—4.5<br>3 | 8.1<br>7.2—9.0<br>3 |
| Canned | — | — | — | 4.9 | 2.6 | 4.3 | — | 3.4 | 6.2 |
| **Jack Mackerel — *Trachurus* sp.** | | | | | | | | | |
| Raw | 3.1<br>3.0—5.0<br>4 | 4.6<br>4.2—5.0<br>4 | 6.0<br>5.4—7.2<br>3 | 5.7<br>4.9—7.4<br>6 | 2.6<br>1.5—3.6<br>7 | 4.7<br>3.2—6.1<br>3 | 3.3<br>1.7—4.6<br>5 | 3.5<br>2.1—4.9<br>6 | 7.5<br>7.1—9.1<br>5 |
| Fried | — | — | — | 3.9 | 2.1 | 3.6 | — | 2.7 | 5.1 |
| Salted and dried | — | — | — | 5.4 | 3.2 | 4.9 | — | 3.3 | 7.2 |
| **Lingcod — *Ophiodon elongatus*** | | | | | | | | | |
| Raw | — | — | — | — | 2.8<br>1.8—3.8<br>2 | — | — | — | — |
| **Lobster (Spiny) — *Panulirus* sp.** | | | | | | | | | |
| Raw | 3.4 | 4.6 | 5.9 | 4.5 | 2.8<br>2.4—3.2<br>2 | 4.1 | 4.1 | 4.7 | 8.6 |

| | (1) | (2) | (3) | (4) | (5) | (6) | (7) | (8) | (9) |
|---|---|---|---|---|---|---|---|---|---|
| **Mackerel — *Scomber* sp.** Raw | 3.6 (3.5—3.8) 4 | 4.9 (3.8—6.4) 6 | 6.2 (5.6—7.8) 4 | 5.8 (4.7—7.8) 9 | 3.0 (1.9—3.5) 13 | 5.5 (4.5—7.4) 9 | 3.5 (2.9—4.0) 4 | 3.8 (3.0—4.6) 10 | 7.6 (7.1—8.8) 9 |
| Canned | — | 7.2 | — | 5.3 (5.0—5.6) 3 | 2.8 (2.7—2.8) 3 | 4.9 (4.2—5.3) 3 | — | 3.4 (3.1—3.5) 3 | 7.2 (7.0—7.3) 3 |
| Salted and dried | 3.7 | 5.2 | 7.4 | 6.4 | 3.1 | 6.1 | 3.6 | 3.8 | 8.6 |
| **Mullet — *Mugil* sp.** Raw | 3.5 (3.3—3.8) 3 | 4.9 (4.6—5.5) 3 | 6.2 (5.5—6.6) 3 | 5.3 (4.3—6.3) 5 | 3.2 (2.3—4.4) 6 | 5.2 (3.6—6.6) 5 | 2.8 (1.6—3.9) 7 | 3.8 (3.2—4.2) 5 | 9.1 (7.1—11.2) 5 |
| **Perch (Atlantic Ocean) — *Sebastes marinus*** Raw | 3.4 | 4.6 | 8.5 | 5.9 | 3.0 | 6.3 | 3.2 | 4.0 | 8.6 |
| **Pollock — *Pollachius virens, Theragra chalcogramma*** Raw | 3.6 (3.4—3.8) 2 | 4.7 (4.3—5.0) 2 | 6.9 (5.9—7.9) 2 | 5.9 (5.7—6.1) 2 | 3.3 (3.0—3.6) 2 | 6.7 (6.2—7.2) 2 | 3.6 (3.3—3.9) 2 | 4.1 (3.8—4.3) 2 | 8.2 (8.1—8.3) 2 |
| **Rockfish — *Sebastes* sp.** Raw | — | — | — | 5.0 | 2.6 | 6.8 | 0.4 | 4.4 | 11.4 |
| **Salmon — *Oncorhynchus* sp.** Raw | 3.9 (3.7—4.3) 3 | 5.0 (3.5—6.1) 3 | 6.5 (5.8—7.2) 3 | 6.1 (4.6—7.4) 3 | 3.2 (2.9—3.6) 5 | 4.9 (4.0—5.4) 3 | 3.4 (2.8—4.1) 3 | 4.1 (3.0—4.8) 3 | 7.6 (6.6—9.1) 3 |
| Canned | 3.7 | 5.0 | 6.6 | 5.9 (5.5—7.4) 5 | 3.1 (3.0—3.4) 5 | 5.0 (4.8—5.2) 5 | 4.1 | 3.9 (3.7—4.8) 5 | 7.7 (7.1—9.1) 5 |
| **Scup (Porgy) — *Calamus* sp., *Stenotomus* sp.** Raw | — | — | — | — | 2.3 | — | — | — | — |
| **Shad — *Alosa sapidissima*** Raw | — | — | — | 6.2 | 2.8 | 5.0 | — | 3.7 | 7.7 |
| Canned | — | — | — | — | — | 4.6 | — | 3.8 | — |
| **Shrimp — mixed spp.** Raw | 3.6 | 6.8 | 4.6 | 4.6 (4.1—5.0) 6 | 3.6 (2.9—4.6) 7 | 5.4 (5.0—5.6) 6 | 2.5 (1.0—3.3) 5 | 4.7 (3.8—6.2) 8 | 11.5 (7.8—14.3) 7 |
| Canned | — | 6.3 | — | 5.0 (4.2—5.7) 9 | 3.6 (2.6—4.4) 9 | 5.4 (4.6—6.0) 9 | 3.6 (3.6—3.6) 3 | 4.5 (3.8—5.0) 9 | 10.1 (8.0—11.6) 9 |
| Dried | 3.2 | 7.3 | 5.8 | 5.0 (4.8—5.1) 4 | 3.0 (2.9—3.1) 4 | 5.5 (5.3—5.6) 4 | 3.5 (3.5—3.6) 4 | 4.3 (4.2—4.6) 4 | 8.1 (7.6—8.7) 4 |

Table 2 (continued)
## AMINO ACIDS OF SOME COMMONLY CAUGHT FISH[311]

| | Proline | Glycine | Alanine | Valine | Methionine | Isoleucine | Tyrosine | Phenylalanine | Leucine |
|---|---|---|---|---|---|---|---|---|---|
| **Smelt — *Osmeridae* sp., *Mallotus villosus*** | | | | | | | | | |
| Raw | — | — | — | 5.3 | 2.6 | 4.8 | — | 4.0 | 7.7 |
| | | | | 5.2—5.4 | 2.4—2.8 | 4.8—4.8 | | 3.9—4.0 | 7.6—7.8 |
| | | | | 2 | 2 | 2 | | 2 | 2 |
| Fried | — | — | — | 3.3 | — | 2.1 | — | 2.1 | 4.4 |
| **Squid — *Loligo* sp., *Illex* sp.** | | | | | | | | | |
| Raw | 4.8 | 4.9 | 5.6 | 4.6 | 2.3 | 4.3 | 2.8 | 3.7 | 6.9 |
| | 3.8—5.6 | 4.5—6.0 | 5.1—6.2 | 2.9—7.0 | 1.0—3.6 | 3.3—8.1 | 1.4—5.5 | 1.9—6.2 | 4.8—9.1 |
| | 9 | 10 | 9 | 13 | 14 | 11 | 11 | 13 | 11 |
| Dried | 4.1 | 6.8 | 5.9 | 4.2 | 2.7 | 4.8 | 2.8 | 3.5 | 7.3 |
| **Trout (Sea)(Gray Weakfish) — *Cynoscion regalis*** | | | | | | | | | |
| Raw | — | — | — | — | — | — | — | — | — |
| **Trout (Sea)(Spotted Weakfish) — *Cynoscion nebulosus*** | | | | | | | | | |
| Salted and dried | — | — | — | 6.2 | 4.4 | 6.6 | — | 4.1 | 9.7 |
| **Tuna — mixed spp.** | | | | | | | | | |
| Raw | 3.5 | 3.6 | 4.6 | 7.9 | 2.9 | 4.9 | 4.3 | 3.5 | 6.6 |
| | 2.5—5.7 | 2.3—4.6 | 2.8—6.8 | 5.7—9.8 | 2.4—3.7 | 3.5—8.5 | 3.8—5.3 | 2.3—4.5 | 4.5—9.1 |
| | 7 | 8 | 6 | 8 | 9 | 8 | 4 | 8 | 8 |
| Canned | — | 4.6 | — | 5.2 | 2.9 | 4.7 | — | 3.6 | 7.2 |
| | | | | 5.0—5.6 | 2.8—3.4 | 4.4—5.0 | | 3.4—3.8 | 6.9—7.3 |
| | | | | 6 | 8 | 6 | | 6 | 6 |
| Dried | 3.4 | — | 5.9 | 5.1 | 2.6 | 4.6 | 3.7 | 3.5 | 8.2 |
| Salted and dried | — | 4.5 | — | 8.5 | 3.6 | 7.8 | — | 5.1 | 11.3 |
| **Whitefish (Common) — *Coregonus clupeaformis*** | | | | | | | | | |
| Raw | — | — | — | 5.9 | 3.1 | 5.3 | — | 4.2 | 8.3 |
| **Whiting — *Merluccius bilinearis*** | | | | | | | | | |
| Raw | 3.6 | 4.7 | 6.4 | 5.4 | 3.3 | 5.0 | 3.5 | 4.3 | 8.5 |

# REFERENCES

1. Adrian, J. and Jacquot, R., Comparison between dried fish of the Portuguese province of Angola and industrial fish flours: global composition, amino acids and B-complex vitamins, in Inter-Afr. Nutr. Conf., Session III, Luanda, Angola, 1956, 99—111.

2. Adrian, J., Composition and nutritive value of fish preserved under different conditions: African samples, salted and dried, commercial meals and nuoc mam, *Ann. Nutr. Aliment.*, 11, 27—44, 1957.

3. Adriano, F. T. and De Guzman, M. S., The proximate chemical analyses of some Philippine food products, *Philipp. Agric.*, 20, 580—592, 1932.

4. Albrecht, M. and Wunsche, J., Der Gehalt an aminosauren im protein niederer Wassertiere und dessen Bedeutung fur die Fischernahrung, *Arch. Tierernaehr.*, 22(1—2), 423—430, 1972.

5. Albrecht, P. G., Chemical study of several marine mollusks of the Pacific coast, *J. Biol. Chem.*, 57, 395—405, 1920.

6. Alcarez-Bayan, A. and Leverton, R. M., The composition of dilis fish flour, *Philipp. J. Sci.*, 86(3), 247—258, 1957.

7. Alvarez-Seoane, G., Seasonal variations in chemical composition of clam, *Invest. Pesq.*, 17, 3—32, 1960.

8. Analytical Methods Committee (England), Nitrogen contents of raw fish, *Analyst*, 98, 456—457, 1973.

9. Ang, C. Y. W., unpublished data, Food Science Associates, Inc., Dobbs Ferry, New York, 1974.

10. Anon., unpublished data, Pacific Utilization Research Center, Seattle, 1965.

11. Anon., The chemical composition and food value of British Columbia marine products, *Prog. Rep. Pac. Biol. Stn. Fish. Exp. Stn.*, 19, 20—23, 1934.

12. Anon., Note: nutrition and composition, *Commer. Fish. Rev.*, 12(6), 9—10, 1950.

13. Anon., Strained tuna baby food introduced by Van Camp, *Pac. Fisherman*, 43(4), 30, 1950.

14. Anon., Note: composition and cold-storage life of fresh-water fish, *Commer. Fish. Rev.*, 14(1), 17, 1952.

15. Anon., Cold-storage life and composition of fresh-water fish, *Commer. Fish. Rev.*, 14(5), 13, 1952.

16. Anon., Composition and cold-storage life of fresh-water fish, *Commer. Fish. Rev.*, 14(6), 21—23, 1952.

17. Anon., Composition and cold-storage life of fresh-water fish, *Commer. Fish. Rev.*, 14(8), 13, 1952.

18. Anon., Composition and cold-storage life of fresh-water fish, *Commer. Fish. Rev.*, 14(10), 26—27, 1952

19. Anon., Analysis and composition: composition and cold-storage life of fresh-water fish, *Commer. Fish. Rev.*, 14(11), 10—11, 1952.

20. Anon., Composition and cold-storage life of fresh-water fish, *Commer. Fish. Rev.*, 14(2), 13—15, 1952.

21. Anon., Composition of fish, *Commer. Fish. Rev.*, 15(10), 17, 1953.

22. Anon., Composition of fish, *Commer. Fish. Rev.*, 15(12), 14—15, 1953.

23. Anon., Food composition tables for international use, in *FAO Nutritional Studies*, No. 3, Food and Agricultural Organization of the United Nations, Rome, 1949.

23a. Anon., FAO composition tables. Minerals and vitamins, in *FAO Nutritional Studies*, No. 11, Food and Agricultural Organization of the United Nations, Rome, 1954.

24. Anon., unpublished data, Booth Fisheries, Chicago, 1970.

25. Appanna, T. C. and Devadatta, S. C., Comparative studies on the nutritive value of fish and prawn muscle, *Curr. Sci.*, 11, 333—335, 1942.

26. Arakaki, J. and Suyama, M., Amino acid composition of the protein of anchovy, *Bull. Jpn. Soc. Sci. Fish.*, 32(1), 70—73, 1966.

27. Arevalo, A., Estudio de la variación en la composición quimica del jurel, *Trachurus trachurus* L., *Bol. Inst. Esp. Oceanogr.*, 8, 1—13, 1948.

28. Arnesen, G., Total and free amino acids in fishmeals and vacuum-dried codfish organs, flesh, bones, skin, and stomach contents, *J. Sci. Food Agric.*, 20(4), 218—220, 1969.

29. Atwater, W. O., The chemical composition of American food materials, *U.S. Dep. Agric. Exp. Stn. Bull.*, 28, 7—53, 1906.

30. Baba, H., The components of short neck clams, *Annu Rep. Nat. Inst. Nutr. Tokyo*, 45, 46, 1954.

31. Baba, H., On the available lysine in protein of fish and algae, *Bull. Jpn. Soc. Sci. Fish.*, 26(3), 330—333, 1960.

32. Bailey, B. E., The nutritive value of the flesh of red and white spring salmon, *Prog. Rep. Pac. Biol. Stn. Fish. Exp. Stn.*, 41, 8—9, 1939.

33. Bailey, B. E., "Chalky" halibut. II, *Prog. Rep. Pac. Biol. Stn. Fish. Exp. Stn.*, 88, 61, 1951.

34. Bailey, B. E., Chart of the nutritive values of British Columbia fishery products, *Prog. Rep. Pac. Biol. Stn. Fish. Exp. Stn.*, 53, 9, 1952.

35. **Balagtas, A. N.**, Chemical composition of Philippine fish, *Philipp. Agric. Rev.*, 17, 253—260, 1928.
36. **Balland, M.**, Sur la composition des poissons, des crustaces et des mollusques, *C. R. Acad. Sci.*, 126, 1728—1731, 1898.
37. **Barker, R. and Idler, D. R.**, Transport and storage of fish in refrigerated sea water, *Prog. Rep. Pac. Biol. Stn. Fish. Exp. Stn.*, 104, 16, 1955.
38. **Beach, E. F., Munks, B., and Robinson, A.**, The amino acid composition of animal tissue protein, *J. Biol. Chem.*, 148, 431—439, 1943.
39. **Berezin, N. T.**, Use of fish and sea products in nutrition, *Pishch. Prom. (Moscow)*, 1967.
40. **Bergeret, B. and Masseyeff, R.**, Tables de composition de quelques aliments tropicaux, *Ann. Nutr. Aliment.*, 11(5), 47—69, 1957.
41. **Bergeret, B.**, Note sur la valeur alimentaire des poissons du wouri, *Med. Trop. (Madrid)*, 18(1), 131—136, 1958.
42. **Beveridge, J. M. R.**, Sulfur distribution in fish flesh proteins, *J. Fish. Res. Board Can.*, 7(2), 51—54, 1947.
43. **Block, R. J.**, *The Amino Acid Composition of Proteins and Foods*, Charles C Thomas, Springfield, Ill., 1945, 270—271.
44. **Braekkan, O. R. and Boge, G.**, Vitaminer i norsk fisk. IV. Vitamin B⁶ og biotin i forskjellige organer fra torskefisker (Gadidae) fanget langs norskekysten, *Fiskeridir. (Norw.) Skr. Ser. Teknol. Unders.*, 4(12), 1—11, 1965.
45. **Brooke, R. O., Ravesi, E. M., and Steinberg, M. A.**, The composition of commercially important fish taken from New England waters. II. Proximate analyses of butterfish, flounder, pollock, and hake, and their seasonal variation, *Food Res.*, 27, 73—76, 1962.
46. **Brooke, R. O., Ravesi, E. M., Gadbois, D. F., and Steinberg, M. A.**, Preservation of fresh unfrozen fishery products by low-level radiation, *Food Technol. (Chicago)*, 18, 116—120, 1964.
47. **Brooke, R. O., Ravesi, E. M., Gadbois, D. F., and Steinberg, M. A.**, Preservation of fresh unfrozen fishery products by low-level radiation, *Food Technol. (Chicago)*, 20, 1479—1482, 1966.
48. **Busson, F. and Postel, E.**, Nutritional value of the fish caught off the coasts of the Cape Verde Peninsula, *Med. Trop. (Madrid)*, 13, 534—537, 1953.
49. **Butler, C.**, Nutritional value of fish in reference to atherosclerosis and current dietary research, *Commrer. Fish. Rev.*, 20(7), 7—16, 1958.
50. **Cabbat, F. S. and Standal, B. R.**, The composition of essential and certain nonessential amino acids in selected Hawaii fish, *J. Food Sci.*, 30, 172—177, 1965.
51. **Carlson, C. J., Thurston, C. E., and Stansby, M. E.**, Chemical composition of raw, precooked, and canned tuna. I. Core sampling methods, *Food Technol. (Chicago)*, 14, 477—479, 1960.
52. **Carteni, A. and Aloj, G.**, Zime chimica di animali marini del golfo di napoli, *Quad. Nutr.*, 1, 49—63, 1934—1935.
53. **Carteni, A. and Aloj, G.**, Composizione chimica di animali marini del golfo di napoli. II. Selaci, mollusci, crostacei, *Quad. Nutr.*, 2, 219—235, 1935.
54. **Carter, N. M.**, The nutritive value of marine products. VIII. Proximate analysis of canned British Columbia sockeye and pink salmon, *J. Biol. Board Can.*, 2(5), 439—455, 1936.
55. **Causeret, J.**, La valeur alimentaire des produits de la peche. III. Composition chimique et valeur alimentaire des produits de la peche, *Bull. Soc. Sci. Hyg. Aliment.*, 38, 20—34, 1950.
56. **Chari, S. T.**, Nutritive value of some of the west coast marine food fishes of the Madras Province, *Indian J. Med. Res.*, 36, 253—259, 1948.
57. **Chari, S. T. and Venkataraman, R.**, Semi-drying of prawns and its effect on amino acid composition, *Indian J. Med. Res.*, 45(1), 81—84, 1957.
58. **Cheftel, H.**, *La Valeur Alimentaire des Conserves Appertisees*, Bull. No. 11, J. J. Carnoud, Paris, 1951, 74—105.
59. **Chong, Y. H. and Soh, C. C.**, The protein nutritive quality of Ikan Bilis (*Stolephorus* spp.), *Med. J. Malaya*, 20(3), 230—233, 1966.
60. **Clark, B. S. and Berglund, R. M.**, Canning of Maine sardines, in *Fish as Food — IV*, Borgstrom, G., Ed. Academic Press, New York, 1965, 291—297.
61. **Clark, E. D. and Almy, L. H.**, A chemical study of food fishes, *J. Biol. Chem.*, 33, 483—498, 1918.
62. **Clark, E. D. and Almy, L. H.**, A chemical study of frozen fish in storage for short and long periods, *J. Ind. Eng. Chem.*, 12(7), 656—663, 1920.
63. **Clark, E. D., Clough, R. W., Fellers, L. R., and Shostrom, O. E.**, Examination of canned salmon, *Pac. Fisherman*, 21(9), 8—10, 1923.
64. **Cohen, E. H. and Peters, J. A.**, Effect of storage in refrigerated sea water on amino acids and other components of whiting (*Merluccius bilinearis*), *Fish. Ind. Res.*, 2(2), 5—11, 1963.
65. **Collazos Chiriboga, C., White, P. L., White, H. S., Vinas, T. E., Alvistur, J. E., Quiroz, M. A., Roca, N. A., Hagsted, D. M., and Bradfield, R. B.**, La composicion de los alimentos peruanos, *Arch. Venez. Nutr.*, 8(1), 129—166, 1956.

66. Connell, J. J. and Howgate, P. F., The amino-acid composition of some British food fishes, *J. Sci. Food Agric.*, 10(4), 241—243, 1959.

67. Coppini, R., Determination and comparison of the nutritive and commercial value of edible mollusk species of the Adriatic Sea, *Ateneo Parmense Sez. 2 Acta Biomed.*, 8(1), 51—65, 1972.

68. Cox, H. E., The composition of fish pastes, *Analyst*, 60, 71—77, 1935.

69. Creach, Y. and Serfaty, A., Proteolysis in the common carp (*Cyprinus carpio*) in the course of starvation: importance and localization, *C. R. Soc. Biol.*, 159, 482—486, 1965.

70. Crooks, G. C. and Ritchie, W. S., Seasonal variation in chemical composition of common haddock, *Food Res.*, 4, 159—171, 1939.

71. Dabrowski, T., Kolakowski, E., Wawreszwk, H., and Choroszucha, C., Studies on chemical composition of American crayfish (*Orconectes limosus*) meat as related to its nutritive value, *J. Fish. Res. Board Can.*, 23(11), 1653—1662, 1966.

72. Dabrowski, T., Kolakowski, E., and Sikolowski, E., Composition and nutritional value of crayfish meat from *Astacus leptodactylus*, *Z. Lebensm Unters. Forsch.*, 129(6), 337—344, 1965.

73. Dambergs, N., Extractives of fish muscle. III. Amounts, sectional distributon, and variations of fat, water-solubles, protein and moisture in cod (*Gadus morhua* L.) fillets, *J. Fish. Res. Board Can.*, 20(4), 909—919, 1963.

74. De Giacomi, R., Fish and meat pastes and other savoury spreads as food, *J. Chem. Ind.*, 43, 902—903, 1951.

75. De Ibarra, C., Tabla de composicion de alimentos para uso practico, *Inst. Nac. Nutr. Venez.*, 17, 3—24, 1954.

76. De la Torre A., M. C., Valuacion de metionina, Cistina y cisteina en algunos crustaceous consumidos en el Peru, *An. Fac. Farm. Bioquim. Univ. Nac. Mayor San Marcos* (1950—57), 3, 141—149, 1952.

77. Deas, C. P. and Tarr, H. L. A., Amino acid composition of fishery products, *J. Fish. Res. Board Can.*, 7(9), 513—521, 1949.

78. Del Monte Corporation, unpublished data, Walnut Creek, Cal., undated.

79. Deuel, H. J., Hrubetz, M. C., Johnston, C. H., Winzler, R. J., Geiger, E., and Schnakenberg, G., Studies on the nutritive value of fish proteins. I. Evaluation by the rat growth method and by the McCannon method, *J. Nutr.*, 31, 175—185 (Abstr.), 1946.

80. Dill, D. B., A chemical study of certain Pacific coast fishes, *J. Biol. Chem.*, 48, 73—82, 1921.

81. Dubrow, D. L. and Stillings, B. R., Chemical and nutritional characteristics of fish protein concentrate processed from heated whole red hake, *Urophycis chuss*, *Fish. Bull.*, 69(1), 141—144, 1971.

82. Dubrow, D. L., Brown, N. L., Pariser, E. R., Miller, H., Sidwell, V. D., and Ambrose, M. G., Effect of ice on the chemical and nutritive properties of solvent-extracted whole fish — red hake, *Urophycis chuss*, *Fish. Bull.*, 69(1), 145—150, 1971.

83. Dugal, L. C., Proximates of some freshwater fish, *Biol. Stn. Technol. Unit Fish. Rec. Board Can.*, Circ. 5, 1—6, 1962.

84. Dunn, M. S., Camien, M. N., Eiduson, S., and Malin, R. B., The nutritive value of canned foods, *J. Nutr.*, 39, 177—185, 1949.

85. Dupont, A., Amino acid content of Indonesian fresh water fish, *Biochem. Z.*, 330, 174—176, 1958.

86. Dyer, J. A., Nelson, R. W., and Barnett, H. J., Pacific hake (*Merluccius productus*) as raw material for a fish reduction industry, *Commer. Fish. Rev.*, 28(5), 12—17, 1966.

87. Edwards, L. E, Sealock, R. R., O'Donnell, W. W., Bartlett, G. R., Barclay, M. B., Tully, R., Tybout, R. H., Box, I., and Murlin, J. R., Biological value of proteins in relation to the essential amino acids which they contain. IV. The analysis of fifteen protein foods for the ten essentials, *J. Nutr.*, 32, 597—612, 1946.

88. El Rawi, I. and Geiger, E., The growth-promoting effect of commercial strained meat and fish products investigated with infantile rats, *J. Nutr.*, 47, 119—132, 1952.

89. Endo, K., Hujita, M., and Simidu, W., Studies on muscle of aquatic animals. XXXIII. Seasonal variation of nitrogenous extractives in squid muscle, *Bull. Jpn. Soc. Sci. Fish.*, 28(11), 1099—1103, 1962.

90. Establier, R., Variación estacionál de la composición quimica de la chirla (*Venus gallina* L.), *Invest. Pesqu.*, 33(1), 7—13, 1969.

91. Establier, R. and Gutierrez, M., Aspectos bioquimicos de la maduracion enzimatica del boqueron (*Engraulis encrasicholus*), *Invest. Pesq.*, 36(2), 327—340, 1972.

92. Food and Agriculture Organization of the United Nations, The use of fish flours as human food, *Proc. Nutr. Soc.*, 17(2), 153—160, 1958.

93. Farragut, R. N., Proximate composition of Chesapeake Bay blue crab (Callinctes sapidus), *J. Food Sci.*, 30, 538—544, 1965.

94. Farragut, R. N. and Thompson, M. H., Proximate composition of the Pacific coast dungeness crab (*Cancer magister*), *Fish. Ind. Res.*, 3(3), 1—4, 1965.

95. Fallers, C. R. and Parks, C. T., Biochemical study and proximate composition of Pacific coast crabs, *Univ. Wash. Publ. Fish.*, 1(7), 143—156, 1926.

96. **Fellers, C. R. and Harris, S. G.,** Canned Atlantic crab meat, *Ind. Eng. Chem.,* 32(4), 592—594, 1940.
97. **Ferreira Goncalves, F. A.,** Composicao e valor alimentor de algunas especies de peixe, *Bol. Pesca (Lisbon),* 8, 89—102, 1951.
98. **Finch, R.,** Fish protein for human foods, *Crit. Rev. Food Technol.,* 1(4), 519—580, 1970.
99. **Flores Castanon, C.,** Valoración de los amino-acidos azufrados, metionina, cistina y cisteina en algunos moluscos, *An. Fac. Farm. Bioquim. Univ. Nac. Mayor San Marcos* (1950—57), 4, 89—98, 1953.
100. **Fox, F. W. and Goldberg, L.,** South African food tables, *S. Afr. J. Med. Sci.,* 125—218, 1944.
101. **Fraga, F.,** Variación estacional de la composicion quimica de la anchoa (*Engraulis encrasicholus*), *Invest. Pesq.,* 2, 21—31, 1955.
102. **Fraser, D. I., Mannion, A., and Dyer, W. J.,** Proximate composition of Canadian Atlantic fish. III. Sectional differences in the flesh of a species of Chondrostei, one of Chimaerae, and of some miscellaneous teleosts, *J. Fish. Res. Board Can.,* 18, 893—905, 1961.
103. **Gangal, S. V. and Magar, N. G.,** Chemical composition of crabmeat, *Indian J. Appl. Chem.,* 25(4—6), 133—136, 1962.
104. **Gangal, S. V. and Magar, N. G.,** Biological evaluation of crab meat (*Scylla serrata*) in the rat, *Br. J. Nutr.,* 21, 1—6, 1967.
105. **Gatti, M. L. F.,** Contenido de aminoacidos en algunos mariscos Chilena, *An. Fac. Far. Bioquim. Univ. Nac. Mayor San Marcos,* 21, 27—30, 1969.
106. **Gilpin, G. L., Murphy, E. W., Marsh, A. C., Dawson, E. H., Bowman, F., Kerr, R. G., and Snyder, D. G.,** Meat, fish, poultry, and cheese home preparation time, yield, and composition of various market forms, *U.S. Dep. Agric. Home Econ. Res. Rep.,* 30, 1—67, 1965.
107. **Gimenez, J. C. and Rodriguez de las Heras, A.,** Chemical studies upon Spanish fishes, *Inst. Esp. Oceanogr. Trabajos,* 17, 5—58, 1943.
108. **Gonzalez-Diaz, C., Fernandez, V. O., and Cravioto, R. O.,** Valor nutritive del pescado fresco que se consume en la ciudad de Mexico, *An. Esc. Nac. Cienc. Bio. Mexico City,* 5, 283—290, 1948.
109. **Gormosova, S. A.,** Seasonal variations in the chemical composition of Black Sea oysters (*Ostrea turica*), *Gidrobiol. Zh.,* 4(3), 72—76, 1968.
110. **Gowri, V., Vasantha, M. S., Srinisasan, K. S., and Moorjani, M. N.,** Methionine content of some of the important species of Indian Fishes, *Fish. Technol. (India),* 9(2), 180—181, 1972.
111. **Greene, C. W.,** Biochemical changes in the muscle tissue of king salmon during the fast of spawning migration, *J. Biol. Chem.,* 39, 435—456, 1919.
112. **Greshoff, M.,** Zusammensetzung indischer Nahrungsmittel, *Chemekes Z.,* 27, 499, 1903.
113. **Grigsby, H. D.,** Report on fish and other marine products, *J. Assoc. Off. Anal. Chem.,* 25(3), 709—710, 1942.
114. **Hanover, L. M., Webb, N. B., Howell, A. J., and Thomas, F. B.,** Effects of cooking and rinsing on the protein losses from blue crabs, *J. Milk Food Technol.,* 36(8), 409—413, 1973.
115. **Harry, R. G.,** The composition of certain cooked fish, *J. Soc. Chem. Ind. (London),* 14, 150—151, 1936.
116. **Harvey, D.,** Tables of the amino acids in food and feedingstuffs, *Common. Bur. Anim. Nutr. Tech. Commun.,* 119, 1—52, 1970.
117. **Hatakoshi, Y.,** Composition of canned meat of the crab, *J. Chem. Soc. (Japan),* 53, 1026—1027, 1932
118. **Hatakoshi, Y.,** The contents of methionine and threonine in meat-proteins of various fishes, *J. Agric. Chem. Soc. Japan,* 27(11), 795—798, 1953.
119. **Hayes, O. B. and Rose, G.,** Supplementary food composition table, *J. Am. Diet. Assoc.,* 33, 26—29, 1957.
120. **H. J. Heinz Company Research Center,** *Heinz Nutritional Data,* 6th ed., H.J. Heinz, Pittsburgh, 1972, 106—121.
121. **Herrera, J. and Munoz, F.,** Chemical composition of the red mullet (*Mullus barbatus* L.) of castellon and biological consideration concerning the same, *Invest. Pesq.,* 23, 91—113, 1963.
122. **Herzberg, A.,** Preliminary data on proximate composition of some Mediterranean Sea and Red Sea fishes, *Extrait Rapp. Proces-Verb. Reunions C.I.E.S.M.M.,* 18(2), 253—255, 1965.
123. **Herzberg, A. and Pasteur, R.,** Proximate composition of commercial fishes from the Mediterranean Sea and the Red Sea, *Fish Ind. Res.,* 5(2), 39—65, 1969.
124. **Higashi, S.,** Seasonal variations in the chemical components of the principal mollusks in Lake Biwa-Ko, *Bull. Jpn. Soc. Sci. Fish.,* 31(8), 610—617, 1955.
125. **Anon.,** unpublished data, Icelandic Fisheries, Reykjavik, Iceland, 1973.
126. **Idler, D. R. and Bitners, I.,** Biochemical studies on sockeye salmon during spawning migration. II. Cholesterol, fat, protein, and water in the flesh of standard fish, *Can. J. Biochem. Physiol.,* 36, 793—798, 1958.

127. **Idler, D. R. and Bitners, I.**, Biochemical studies on sockeye salmon during spawning migration. V. Cholesterol, fat, protein, and water in the body of standard fish, *J. Fish. Res. Board Can.*, 16(2), 235—241, 1959.
128. **Igarashi, H. and Zama, K.**, Biochemical studies of the salmon *Oncorhynchus keta*. I. The changes in the chemical components of the body tissues during the spawning migration, *Bull. Jpn. Soc. Sci. Fish.*, 18(11), 618—622, 1953.
129. **Ingalls, R. L., Klocke, J. F., Rafferty, J. P., Greensmith, R. E., Chang, M. L., Tack, P. I., and Ohlson, M. A.**, Nutritive value of fish from Michigan waters, *Mich. Agric. Exp. Stn. Bull.*, 219, 1—24, 1950.
130. **Intengan, C. L., Alejo, L. G., Concepcion, I., Corpus, V. A., Salud, R. D., del Rosario, I., Gomez, R., and Henson, J.**, Composition of Philippine foods. V., *Philipp. J. Sci.*, 85, 203—213, 1956.
131. **Ito, K.**, Amino acid composition of the muscle extracts of aquatic animals. II. The amounts of free amino acid in the muscle of shellfishes and their variation during spoilage, *Bull. Jpn. Soc. Sci. Fish.*, 25(10—12), 658—660, 1959.
132. **Iverson, J. L.**, Technical note no. 48 — Pacific Ocean perch — proximate composition, *Commer. Fish. Rev.*, 20(12), 22—25, 1958.
133. **Jaffe, W. G., Nolberga, B., Embdens, C., Garcia, S., Olivares, H., and Gross, M.**, Composition of Venezuelan fishes, *Arch. Venez. Nutr.*, 7, 163—166, 1956.
134. **Jafri, A. K., Khawaja, D. K., and Qasim S. Z.**, Studies on the biochemical composition of some freshwater fishes, *Fish. Technol. (India)*, 1(2), 148—157, 1964.
135. **Johnstone, J.**, The cod as a food fish, *Fish. Invest. Minist. Agric. Fish. Food(G.B.) Ser. II Salmon Freshwater Fish.*, 6(7), 11—14, 1923.
136. **Jowett, W. G. and Davies, W.**, A Chemical Study of Some Australian Fish, Pamphlet 85, Commonwealth of Australia Council for Scientific and Industrial Research, Melbourne, 1938.
137. **Karrick, N. L. and Thurston, C. E.**, Proximate composition of silver salmon, *Agric. Food Chem.*, 12(3), 282—284, 1964.
138. **Karrick, N. L. and Thurston, C. E.**, Proximate composition and sodium and potassium contents of four species of tuna, *Fish. Ind. Res.*, 4(2), 73—78, 1968.
139. **Kawata, H. and Takahashi, T.**, Studies on the utilization of cuttlefish. I. The seasonal variations of the weight and constituents in the various parts of fish body, *Bull. Jpn. Soc. Sci. Fish.*, 20(10), 888—890, 1955.
140. **Khorana, M. L., Sarma, M. L., Seshagiri Rao, P., and Giri, K. V.**, Investigations of the food value of fish and other marine products. II. The protein and mineral contents, *Indian J. Med. Res.*, 31, 25—27, 1943.
141. **Kik, M. C.**, Nutritive value of buffalofish, *J. Am. Diet. Assoc.*, 41, 119—123, 1962.
142. **Kochi, M. and Era, S.**, Studies on the canned tuna. I. Determining of various components in canned tuna, *J. Shimonasiki Coll. Fish.*, 7(1), 33—36, 1957.
143. **Koga, Y.**, Studies on cholesterol in foods. III. On cholesterol crude protein index C.C.P.I.): studies on Japanese foods, report 46, *J. Jpn. Soc. Food Nutr.*, 23(6), 46—55, 1970.
144. **Konosu, S., Katori, S., Ota, R., Eguchi, S., and Mori, T.**, Amino acid composition of fish muscle protein, *Bull. Jpn. Soc. Sci. Fish.*, 29(11), 1163—1166, 1956.
145. **Konosu, S. and Mori, T.**, Amino acid composition of shellfish proteins, *Bull. Jpn. Soc. Sci. Fish.*, 25(2), 153—155, 1959.
146. **Konosu, S. and Matsuura, F.**, Tryptophan content of fish meat, *Bull. Jpn. Soc. Sci. Fish.*, 26(10), 1040—1049, 1960.
147. **Konosu, S., Fujimoto, K., Takashima, Y., Matsushita, T., and Hashimoto, Y.**, Constituents of the extracts and amino acid composition of the protein of short-necked clam, *Bull. Jpn. Soc. Sci. Fish.*, 31(9), 680—686, 1965.
148. **Konosu, S., Katori, S., Akiyama, T., and Mori, T.**, Amino acid composition of crustacean muscle proteins, *Bull. Jpn. Soc. Sci. Fish.*, 24(4), 300—304, 1968.
149. **Koval'chuk, G. K. and Niro, A.**, Technological properties of yellowfin tunny from the Indian Ocean, *Rybn. Khoz. (Moscow)*, 65—69, 1970.
150. **Kramer, A.**, Nutritive value of canned foods. XVI. Proximate and mineral composition, *Food Res.*, 11, 391—398, 1946.
151. **Krzeczkowski, R. A., Tenny, B., and Hayer, M. L.**, Fatty acid content and proximate analysis of bay, calico, sea, and weathervane scallop adductor muscle, *J. Food Sci.*, 37, 300—301, 1972.
152. **Krzeczkowski, R. A. and Stone, F. E.**, Fatty acid content and proximate analysis of tanner crab, *J. Food. Sci.*, 37(2), 300—301, 1972.
153. **Krzeczkowski, R. A.**, personal communication, 1972.
154. **Lahiry, N. L. and Proctor, B. E.**, The microbiological determination of the essential amino acid fish protein, *Food Res.*, 21, 87—90, 1956.
155. **Landgraf, R. G., Jr.**, Technical note no. 27 — Alaska pollock: proximate composition; amino acid, thiamine, and riboflavin content; use as mink feed, *Commer. Fish. Res.*, 15(7), 20—22, 1953.

156. Langworthy, C. F., Fish as food, *U.S. Dep. Agric. Farmers Bull.*, 85, 7—29, 1898.

157. Lanham, W. B. and Lemon, J. M., Nutritive value for growth of some proteins of fishery products, *Food Res.*, 3, 549, 1938.

158. Lauer, B. H., Murray, M. C., Anderson, W. E., and Guptill, E. B., Atlantic queen crab (*Chionoectes opilio*), Jonah crab (*Cancer borealis*), and red crab (*Geryon quinquedens*). Proximate composition of crabmeat from edible tissues and concentrations of some major mineral constituents in the ash, *J. Food Sci.*, 39, 383—385, 1974.

159. Le Cornu, R. R., High food value of fish *Fish. Newsl.*, 8(6), 10—11, 1949.

160. Lee, C. F., Composition of cooked food dishes, *U.S. Dep. Inter. Circ.*, 29, 1—31, 1961.

161. Lee, C. F. and Clegg, W., Technical note No. 31 — weight range, proximate composition and thiaminase content of fish taken in shallow-water trawling in northern Gulf of Mexico, *Commer. Fish. Rev.*, 17(3), 21—23, 1955.

162. Lee, C. F. and Pepper, L., Composition of southern oysters, *Commer. Fish. Rev.*, 18(7), 1—6, 1956.

163. Lee, C. F., Pepper, L., and Kurtzman, C. H., Proximate composition of southern oysters — factors affecting variability, *Commer. Fish. Rev.*, 22(7), 1—8, 1960.

164. Lee, C. M., Toledo, R. T., Nakayama, T. O. M., and Chichester, C. D., Process requirements and properties of spray-dried squid protein, *J. Food Sci.*, 39(4), 735—738, 1974.

165. Leung, W. T. W., Nutrient values suggested for Far Eastern countries, in *Nutrient Values suggested for Far Eastern Countries,* National Academy of Sciences, Washington, D. C., 1945.

166. Leung, W. T. W., Pecot, R. K., and Watt, B. K., *Composition of Foods Used in Far Eastern Countries,* U.S. Department of Agriculture Handbook #34, U.S. Government Printing Office, Washington, D.C., 1952, 35—38.

167. Leung, W. T. W., Butrum, R. R., and Chang, F. H., *Food Composition Table for Use in East Asia,* U.S. Department of Health, Education, and Welfare, Bethesda, Maryland, 1961.

168. Leung, W. T. W. and Flores, M., *Food Composition Table for Use in Latin America,* U.S. Department of Health, Education, and Welfare, Bethesda, Maryland, 1961.

169. Leung, W. T. W., *Food Composition Table for Use in Africa,* U.S. Department of Health, Education, and Welfare, Bethesda, Maryland, 1966, 178—208.

170. Lopez-Benito, M., Composición quimica de algunos moluscos y crustaceas de la ria de vigo, *Invest. Pesq.*, 5, 127—132, 1952.

171. Lyman, C. M., Kuiken, K. A., and Hale, F., Essential amino acid content of farm foods, *Agric. Food Chem.*, 4(12), 1008—1013, 1956.

172. MacCallum, W. A., Adams, D. R., Ackman, R. G., Ke, P. J., Dyer, W. J., Fraser, D. I., and Punjamapriom, S., Newfoundland capelin: proximate composition, *J. Fish. Res. Board Can.*, 26(8), 2027—2035, 1969.

173. MacLeod, R. A., Jonas, R. E. E., and McBride, J. R., Variations in the sodium and potassium content of the muscle tissue of Pacific salmon with particular reference to migration, *Can. J. Biochem. Physiol.*, 36, 1257—1258, 1958.

174. Mankikar, S. R. and Sohonie, K., Essential amino acids, tyrosine and cystine content of purified proteins of Bombay fish, *J. Univ. Bombay*, 29(3 and 5), 82—85, 1960.

175. Mannan, A., Fraser, D. I., and Dyer, W. J., Proximate composition of Canadian Atlantic fish. I. Variation in composition of different sections of the flesh of Atlantic halibut (*Hippoglossus hippoglossus*), *J. Fish. Res Bord. Can.*, 18(4), 483, 1961.

176. Mannan, A., Fraser, D. I., and Dyer, W. J., Proximate composition of Canadian Atlantic fish. II. Mackerel, tuna, and swordfish, *J. Fish. Res. Board Can.*, 18(4), 495—499, 1961.

177. Marotta, D., Fish in the human diet, *Rend. Ist. Super. Sanita*, 1, 369—387, 1938.

178. Master, F. and Magar, N. G., Studies in the nutritive value of Bombay fish. II. Amino-acid composition, *Indian J. Med. Res.*, 42, 509—513, 1954.

179. Matsumoto, J. J., Some aspects on the water-soluble proteins of squid muscle, *Bull. Tokai Reg. Fish. Res. Lab.*, 20, 65—76, 1958.

180. Matsuura, F., Kogure, T., and Fukui, G., Methionine contents of muscle proteins of various aquatic animals, *Bull. Jpn. Soc. Sci. Fish.*, 17(11), 23—26, 1952.

181. Matsuura, F., Konosu, S., Ota, R., Katori, S., and Tanaka, K., Chemical studies on the red muscle (''Chiai'') of fishes. III. Comparative studies of amino-acid contents in the protein of the ordinary and the red muscle of fishes by microbiological assay, *Bull. Jpn. Soc. Sci. Fish.*, 20(10), 941—945, 1955.

182. McCance, R. A. and Widdowson, E. M., The chemical composition of foods, *Her Majesty's Statistical Office Med. Res. Counc. Spec. Rep. Ser.*, 297, 48—72, 1960.

183. Miller, C. D., and Branthoover B., Nutritive values of some Hawaii foods in household units and common measures, *Hawaii Agric. Exp. Stn. Circ.*, 52, 3—20, 1957.

184. Milone, N. U., Composizione, valare nutritivo ed assimilabilita della carne muscolare dei pesci, *Bull. Soc. Nat. Napoli,* 10, 311—394, 1896.

185. Mitra, K. and Mittra, H. C., The determination by chemical methods of the food values of yet another batch of edibles, *Indian J. Med. Res.*, 31, 41—43, 1943.

186. Murata, K., Yoshida, M., and Miyamoto, T., Studies on the Microbiological assay of the essential amino acids in shellfish in Japan, *Rep. Sci. Living*, 7, 7—13, 1959.

187. Anon., unpublished data, National Canners Association, Washington, D.C., 1975.

188. Consumer Services Division, National Canners Association, Canned Food Tables, National Canners Association, Washington, D.C., undated.

189. Neilands, J. B., Sirny, R. J., Sohljell, I., Strong, F. M., and Elvehjem, C. A., The nutritive value of canned foods, *J. Nutr.*, 39, 187—202, 1949.

190. Nelson, R. W. and Thurston, C. E., Proximate composition, sodium, and potassium of dungeness crab, *J. Am. Diet. Assoc.*, 45, 41—43, 1964.

191. Nguyen, T. L. and Richard, C., Le poisson dans l'alimentation du Vietnamien, *Rev. Elev. Med. Vet.*, 12, 313—324, 1959.

192. Nikolaeva, N. T., Amino acid composition in the protein of squid, *Morsk, Ryb.*, 63, 158—160, 1967.

193. Niyogi, S. P., Patwardhan, V. N., Archarya, B. N, and Chitre, R. G., Balanced diets. II. Studies on the nutritive value of fish, *Indian J. Med. Res.*, 29(2), 279—285, 1941.

194. Njaa, L. R., Uthe, F., and Braekkan, O. R., Protein value of cod and coalfish and some products for the young rat, *Fiskeridir. Skr. Ser. Teknol. Unders*, 5(4), 3—13, 1968.

195. Oishi, K., Quality of flatfish from hakodate, *Bull. Fac. Fish. Hokkaido Univ.*, 9, 131—146, 1958—59.

196. Oke, O. L., Nutritive value of some Nigerian foods from animal origin, *W. Afr. Pharm.*, 9(3), 52—53, 1967.

197. Okuda, Y., On the chemistry of "Chiai" flesh, *J. Coll. Agric. Tokyo Imp. Univ.*, 7(1), 1—28, 1919.

198. Oliveiro, C. J., The nutritive value of foods, *Proc. Alumni Assoc. Malaya*, 8(2), 105—129, 1955.

199. Orton, J. H., An account of investigations into the cause or causes of the unusual mortality among oysters in English oyster beds during 1920 and 1921, *Minst. Agric. Fish. Food (G.B.) Ser. II Salmon Freshwater Fish.*, 6(3), 146—187, 1923.

200. Ousterhout, L. E., Technical note number 56 — chemical composition and laboratory fillet yield of 13 species of middle and south Atlantic fish, *Commer. Fish. Rev.*, 22(7), 15—16, 1960.

201. Palad, J. C., Abdon, J. C., Lontoc, A. V., Dimaunahan, L. B., Eusebio, E. C., and Santiago, N., Nutritive value of some foodstuffs processed in the Philippines, *Philipp. J. Sci.*, 93(4), 355—384, 1964.

202. Pallardel Peralta, T. H., Hidrolisis y valoración de amino-acidos indispensables, histidina y metionina, en la proteina de pesces de la costa Peruana, *An. Fac. Farm. Bioquim, Univ. Nac. Mayor San Marcos*, (1950—57), 2, 248—256, 1951.

203. Pandit, A. R., and Magar, N. G., Chemical composition of *Sepia orientalis* and *Loligo vulgaris*, *Fish. Technol. (India)*, 9(2), 122—125, 1972.

204. Patashnik, M., Barnett, H. J., and Nelson, R. W., Proximate chemical composition of Pacific hake, *U.S. Fish. Wildl. Serv. Circ.*, 332, 121—125, 1970.

205. Payva Carbajal, C. A., Analysis of sixty-nine articles of food consumed in Peru, *Acta. Trabajos Congr. Peruano Quim.*, 2, 530—537, 1949.

206. Perlzweig, W. A. and Gies, W. J., A further study of the chemical composition and nutritive value of fish subjected to prolonged periods of cold storage, *Biochem. Bull. (N. Y)*, 3, 69—71, 1913.

207. Petkevich, T. A., Kandyuk, R. P., Stepanyuk, I. A., Kostylev, E. F., Lisovskaya, V. I., Antsupova, L. V., and Poludina, V. P., On the food value of flesh of some Atlantic Fish, *Rybn. Khoz.*, 1, 59—62, 1974.

208. Polansky, M. F. and Toepfer, E. W., Vitamin B$_6$ components in some meats, fish, dairy products, and commercial infant formulas, *J. Agric. Food Chem.*, 17(6), 1394—1397, 1969.

209. Popa, G., Popescu, N., Brinac, V., and Feeanu, S., Study and sanitary and veterinary survey of ocean fish, *Rev. Zool. Med. Vet.*, 6, 87—90, 1968.

210. Pottinger, S. R. and Baldwin, W. H., The content of certain amino acids in the edible portions of fishery products, *Proc. 6th Pacific Sci. Congr.*, Vol. 3, University of California Press, Berkeley and Los Angeles, 1940, 453—459.

211. Prieto Herrero, J. R., Factory methods in the United States for canning tuna, salmon, and sardines; chemical composition and nutritive value, *Rev. Sanid. Hig. Publica.*, 34, 101—151, 1960.

212. Proctor, B. E., Evaluation of amino acids in fish processed by various methods, *Food Res.*, 2, 91—92, 1956.

213. Proctor, B. E., Miller, S. A., Goldblith, S. A., Wick, E. L., Pariser, E. R., Sapors, G. M., and Solberg, M., The nutritive value of Maine sardines. I. Chemical composition, *J. Food Sci.*, 26(3), 283—287, 1961.

214. Prudhomme, M., Les Escargots, *Rev. Med. Vet.*, 23, 456—461, 1960.

215. Pugsley, L. I., The nutritive value of marine products. XV. Proximate analyses of canned British Columbia crabs, shrimps and clams, *J. Fish. Res. Board Can.*, 5(4), 344—346, 1941.

216. Qudrat-I-Khuda, M., De, N. N., and Sharif, M. A. H., Biochemical and nutritional studies on East Pakistan fish. IV. Evaluation of the mechanism of fish spoilage by measurement of tyrosine values, *Pak. J. Sci. Ind. Res.*, 3(4), 187—190, 1960.

217. Qudrat-I-Khuda, M., De, N. N., Khan, N. M., and Debnath, J. C., Biochemical and nutritional studies on East Pakistan Fish. VII. Chemical composition and quality of the traditionally processed fish, *Pak. J. Sci. Ind. Res.*, 5, 70—73, 1962.

218. Ranganathan, S., Sundaravajan, A. R., and Swaminathan, M., Survey of the nutritive value of Indian foodstuffs. I. The chemical composition of 200 common foods, *Indian J. Med. Res.*, 24(3), 689—706, 1937.

219. Reber, E. F. Burt, M. H., Rust, E. M., and Kuo, E., Biological evaluation of protein quality of radiation-pasteurized haddock, flounder, and crab, *J. Food Sci.*, 33, 335—337, 1968.

220. Riddell, W. A., The nutritive value of marine products. XI. Proximate analysis of canned British Columbia coho (Blueback) salmon, *J. Biol. Board Can.*, 2(5), 463—468, 1936.

221. Rodriguez, H. A. and Mendez Isla, M. C., Chemical studies on Spanish fishes, *An. Bromatol.*, 4, 403—410, 1952.

222. Rodriguez-Rebollo, M., Estudio del valor nutritivo y estimacion del contenido en aminoacidos aromaticos y sulfarados de pescados Espagnoles del orden perciformes, *Arch. Zool.*, 8(3), 130—184, 1959.

223. Roy, A. and Sen, P. B., The estimation of cystine, tyrosine, and tryptophan in some common fishes in Bengal, *Ann. Biochem. Exp. Med.*, 1, 321—324, 1941.

224. Russell, E. S., Report on seasonal variations in the chemical composition of oysters, *Fish. Invest. Minist. Agric. Fish. Food (G.B.) Ser. II Salmon Freshwater Fish.*, 6(1), 1—24, 1923.

225. Saha, K. C. and Guha, B. C., Nutritional investigations on Bengal fish, *Ind. J. Med. Res.*, 26(4), 921—927, 1939.

226. Saha, K. C. and Ghosh, N. C., Nutritional investigations on fish, *Ann. Biochem. Exp. Med.*, 1(2), 159—162, 1941.

227. Sambucetti, M. E. and Sanahuja, J. C., El valor nutritivo de las harinas de pescado y su relacion con el contenido en lisina y metionina disponibles, *Arch. Latinoam. Nutr.*, 20(2), 119—133, 1970.

228. Sanchez Moreno, E., Valoración de triptofano y tirosina en la proteina de peces de la Costa Peruana, *An. Fac. Farm. Bioquim. Univ. Nac. Mayor San Marcos* (1950—57), 1, 135—148, 1950.

229. Santos, F. O. and Adriano, F. T., *The Chemical Composition of Philippine Food Materials*, Office of Public Welfare, Manila, 1928.

230. Santos, F. O. and Ascalon, S. J., Amount of nutrients in philippine food materials *Philipp. Agric.*, 20(1), 402—409, 1931.

231. Savagaon, K. A., Venugopal, V., Kamat, S. V., Kumta, U. S., and Sreenivasan, A., Radiation preservation of tropical shrimp for ambient temperature storage. II. Storage studies, *J. Food Sci.*, 37, 151—153, 1972.

232. Sawant, P. L. and Magar, N. G., Studies on frozen fish. II. Some chemical changes occurring during frozen storage, *Food Technol. (India)*, 15, 347—350, 1961.

233. Sawant, P. L. and Magar, N. G., Nutritive value of canned fish: effect of canning, storage and antioxidants, *J. Sci. Ind. Res.*, 20D, 313—316, 1961.

234. Schmidt, P. J., Analyses of freshwater fishes from Canadian interior provinces, *J. Fish. Res. Board Can.*, 75, 48—51, 1948.

235. Schmidt-Hebbel, H., Investigaciones bromatologicos in pescados Chilenos, *An. Bromatol.*, 2(5), 5—11, 1950.

236. Seagran, H. L., Contribution to the chemistry of the king crab (*Paralithodes camtschatica*), *Commer. Fish. Rev.*, 20(11), 15—22, 1958.

237. Sekine, S., Tatsuno, S., and Imamura, F., On the seasonal variation in the chemical composition of oysters, in *Proc., 4th Pac. Sci. Congr.*, 3, 349—351, 1929.

238. Setna, S. R., Sarangdhar, P. N., and Ganpule, N. V., Nutritive value of some marine fishes of Bombay, *Indian J. Med. Res.*, 32, 171—176, 1944.

239. Shimizu, Y. and Simidu, W., Studies on muscle of aquatic animals. XXVIII. Protein composition of fish muscle, *Bull. Jpn. Soc. Sci. Fish.*, 26(8), 806—809, 1960.

240. Shostrom, O. E., Clough, R. W., and Clark, E. D., A chemical study canned salmon. Variations in composition of the Pacific coast salmons and steelhead trout as influenced by species and locality where caught, *Ind. Eng. Chem.*, 16(3), 283—289, 1924.

241. Sidwell, V. D., Utilization of FPC and acceptability, in *Economics, Marketing and Technology of Fish Protein Concentrate*, Tennebaum, S. R., Stillings, B. R., and Scrimshaw, N. S., Eds., MIT Press, Cambridge, 1972, 255.

242. Sidwell, V. D., Bonnet, J. C., and Zook, E. G., Chemical and nutritive values of fresh and canned finfish, crustaceans, and mollusks. I. proximate composition, calcium and phosphorus, *Mar. Fish. Rev.*, 35(12), 19—21, 1973.

243. Sidwell, V.D. and Ambrose, M. E., Nutritional and chemical evaluation of the protein of various finfish and shellfish, in *Protein Nutritional Quality of Foods and Feeds,* Part. 2, Friedman, M., Ed., Marcel Dekker, New York, 1975, 197—209.

244. Sinnhuber, R. O., Yu, T. C., Yu, T. C., and Karrick, N. L., Variation in proximate composition of right and left fillets of rockfish (*Sebastodes pinniger* ) and Dover sole (*Microstomus pacificus* ) *Commer. Fish. Rev.,* 18(2), 24—27, 1956.

245. Slutskaya, T. N., Chemical composition and structure of the meat of invertebrates, *Proc. Pac. Sci. Res. Inst. Mar. Fish. Oceanogr.,* 75, 204—208, 1971.

246. Smith, C. S., A study of the influence of cold-storage temperatures upon the chemical and nutritive value of fish, *Biochem. Bull. (N.Y.),* 3, 54—68, 1913.

247. Sohn, B. I., Carver, J. H., and Mangan, G. F., Jr., Composition of commercially important fish from New England waters. I. Proximate analyses of cod, haddock, Atlantic Ocean perch, butterfish, and mackerel, *Commer. Fish. Rev.,* 23, 7—10, 1961.

248. Sorasuchart, T., The nutritive value of Thai fish products. III. Amino acid composition, *Fiskerid, Norw. Skr. Ser. Teknol. Unders.,* 5(9), 1—13, 1972.

249. Anon., unpublished data, Southeast Utilization Research Center, College Park, Maryland, 1975.

250. Standal, B. R., Bassett, D. R., Policar, P. B., Thom, M., Fatty acid, cholesterol, and proximate analyses of some ready-to-eat foods, *J. Am. Diet. Assoc.,* 50(5), 392—396, 1970.

251. Stansby, M. E. and Olcott, H. S., Composition of fish, in *Industrial Fishery Technology,* Reinhold, New York, 1963, 339—349.

252. Steffens, W., Chemische Zusammensetzung und Nahrwert des Karpfenfleisches, *Die Nahrung,* 18(8), 789—794, 1974.

253. Suarez, M. L., Massieu, G., Cravioto, R. O., and Garcis, J. G., Nuevos datos sobre contenido en aminoacidos indispensables en alimentos Mexicanos, *Ciencia,* 14, 19—30, 1954.

254. Sugimura, K., Taira, H., Hoshino, N., Ebisawa, H., and Hagahara, T., The amino acid content of fish muscle protein, *Bull. Jpn. Soc. Sci. Fish.,* 20(6), 520—524, 1954.

255. Sulit, J. I., Navarro, O. B., San Juan, R. C., and Caldito, E. B., Proximate chemical composition of various species of Philippine market fishes, *Philipp. J. Fish.,* 1—3, 109—122, 1951.

256. Sullivan, L. J. and Seagran, H. L., Technological investigations of pond-reared fish. I. Product development from buffalofish, *Fish. Ind. Res.,* 2(2), 29—42, 1963.

257. Suyama, M., Koike, J., and Suzuki, K., Studies on the buffering capacity of muscles of some marine animals, *Bull. Jpn. Soc. Sci. Fish.,* 24(4), 281—284, 1958.

258. Suyama, M. and Sedine, Y., Studies on the amino acid composition of shell-fish proteins, *Bull. Jpn. Soc. Sci. Fish.,* 31(8), 634—637, 1965.

259. Srasti, K., The mineral contents of bilis, a marine fish of Malaya, *Philipp. J. Sci.,* 83(4), 365—379, 1954.

260. Taarland, T. and Mathiesen, E., Nutritional values and vitamins of Norwegian fish and fish products, *Tidsskr. Hermetikind.,* 44(11), 405—411, 1958.

261. Takagi, I. and Simidu, W., Studies on muscle of aquatic animals. XXXV. Seasonal variation of chemical composition and extractive nitrogens in some species of shellfish, *Bull. Jpn. Soc. Sci. Fish.,* 29(1), 66—70, 1963.

262. Tamura, E., Nishihara, A., Isobe, S. and Matsuno, N., Amino acid contents in Japanese Foods, *Ann. Rep. Nat. Inst. Nutr. (Tokyo),* 32—34, 1957.

263. Tamura, E., Nishihara, A., Isobe, S., Matsuno, N., and Baba, H., Amino acid contents in protein and the extract of the edible portion of shellfish, *Ann. Rep. Nat. Inst. Nutr. (Tokyo),* 36—37, 1957.

264. Tamura, S., Kenmochi, K., Suzuki, T., and Asouda, H., Amino acid composition of Japanese foods, *J. Jpn. Soc. Food Nutr.,* 20, 14—20, 1967.

265. Tanikawa, E. and Suno, M., Studies on the complete utilization of squid. V. Nutritive and digestibility of squid meat, *Bull. Fac. Fish. Hokkaido Univ.,* 3—4, 75—80, 1952.

266. Tanikawa, E. and Yoshitani, S., Studies on the nutritive value of the meat of the sea cucumber. III. A comparison of the chemical components of the meat of the sea cucumber with the meat of other marine animals, *Bull. Fac. Fish. Hokkaido Univ.,* 5—6, 346—347, 1954.

267. Tanikawa, E., Wasaka, T., and Nagasawa, Y., Studies on the muscle meat of *Paralithodes camtschatica* (Til.), *Bull. Fac. Fish. Hokkaido Univ.,* 9, 227—257, 1959.

268. Tanikawa, E., Akiba, M., and Ishiko, H., Chemical studies on the meat of "Suketodara" ( *Theragra chalcogramma*), *Bull. Fac. Fish., Hokkaido Univ.,* 11, 162, 1960.

269. Teeri, A. E., Joughlin, M. E., and Jossely, D., Nutritive value of fish. 1. Nicotinic acid, riboflavin, vitamin $B_{12}$, and amino acids of various salt-water species, *Food Res.,* 22, 145—150, 1957.

270. Teixeria e Silva, H. M., Composicao quimica e valor nutritivao dos principias pescados maritimos encontrados no mercado de Sao Paulo, *Bol. Ind. Anim.,* 14, 141—152, 1954.

271. Templeman, W. and Andrews, G. L., Jellied condition in the America plaice, *J. Fish. Res. Board Can.,* 13(2), 147—182, 1956.

272. Teply, L. J., Derse, P. H., Krieger, C. H., and Elvehjem, C. A., Nutritive value of canned foods, *J. Agric. Food Chem.*, 1, 1204—1207, 1953.
273. Thomas, M. H. and Calloway, D. H., Nutritional value of dehydrated foods, *J. Am. Diet. Assoc.*, 39(2), 105—116, 1961.
274. Thompson, M. H., unpublished data, Pascagoua Laboratories, Pascagoua, Miss., 1960.
275. Thompson, M. H., Proximate composition of Gulf of Mexico industrial fish, *Fish. Ind. Res.*, 3(2), 29—67, 1966.
276. Thompson, M. H. and Farragut, R. N., unpublished data, Pascagoua Laboratories, Paçagoua, Miss., 1971.
277. Thompson, M. H. and Farragut, R. N., Amino acid composition of the Chesapeake Bay blue crab, *Callinectes sapidus, Comp. Biochem. Physiol.*, 17, 1065—1078, 1966.
278. Thompson, M. H. and Farragut, R. N., unpublished data on brown shrimp, Pasagoua Laboratories, Pascagoua, Miss., undated.
279. Thurston, C. E., Changes in composition of sole during refrigeration, *Commer. Fish. Rev.*, 20(8), 21—22, 1958.
280. Thurston, C. E., Variation in composition of southeastern Alaska pink salmon, *Food Res.*, 24, 619—625, 1959.
281. Thurston, C. E. and Groninger, H. S., Composition changes in Puget Sound pink salmon during storage in ice and refrigerated brine, *J. Agric. Food Chem.*, 7(4), 282—284, 1959.
282. Thurston, C. E., Stansby, M. E., Karrick, N. L., Miyauchi, D. T., and Clegg, N. C., Composition of certain species of fresh-water fish. II. Comparative data for 21 species of lake and river fish, *Food Res.*, 24, 493—502, 1959.
283. Thurston, C. E. and MacMaster, P. P., Variations in chemical composition of different parts of halibut flesh, *Food Res.*, 25, 229—236, 1960.
284. Thurston, C. E., Proximate composition and sodium and potassium contents of four species of commercial bottom fish, *J. Food Sci.*, 26, 495—596, 1961.
285. Thurston, C. E., Proximate composition of nine species of rockfish, *Food Res.*, 26, 38—42, 1961.
286. Thurston, C. E., Proximate composition of nine species of sole and flounder, *J. Agric. Food Chem.*, 9(4), 313—316, 1961.
287. Thurston, C. E. and Newman, H. W., Proximate composition changes in sockeye salmon (*Oncorhynchus nerka*) during spawning migration, *Fish. Ind. Res.*, 2(1), 15—22, 1962.
288. Tomala, A., Squid as a raw material for the fishing industry, *Biul. Zjed. Gosp. Ryb.*, 8(9), 47—52, 1971.
289. Tooley, P. J. and Lawrie, R. A., Effect of deep fat frying on the availability of lysine in fish fillets, *J. Food Techol.*, 9(2), 247—253, 1974.
290. Treichler, R., Lee, C. F., and Jarvis, N. D., Chemical Composition of Some Canned Fishery Products, U. S. Department of Interior Fishery Leaflet No. 295, U. S. Government Printing Office, Washington, D.C., 1948.
291. Tu, Y., *Nutritive value of Foods*, Won Yit, Hong Kong, 1969, 11—12.
292. Tully, J. P., British Columbia oysters are a valuable food, *Prog. Rep. Pac. Biol. Stn. Fish. Exp. Stn.*, 23, 18—21, 1946.
293. Tully, J. P., The nutritive value of marine products. XIV. Proximate analysis of fresh British Columbia oysters, *J. Biol. Board Can.*, 2(5), 447, 1936.
294. Valanju, N. N. and Sohonie, K., The studies in the nutritive value of Bombay fish. V. The digestibility and the biological value of fish proteins, *Indian J. Med. Res.*, 45, 125—132, 1957.
295. Valenzuela, A., Composition and nutritive value of Philippine food fishes, *Philipp. J. Sci.*, 36, 235—242, 1928.
296. Van Wyk, G. F., South African fish products. VIII. Composition of the flesh of cape fishes, *J. Soc. Chem. Ind.*, 12, 367—371, 1944.
297. Velarde, E., Determinación de valor nutritivo de la proteina de marina de pescado, *Bol. Soc. Quim Peru*, 37(1), 10—15, 1971.
298. Venkataraman, R. and Chari, S. T., Studies on oysters and clams: biochemical variations, *Indian J. Med. Res.*, 39, 533—541, 1951.
299. Venkataraman, R. and Chari, S. T., Amino acid composition of some marine fishes, *Indian J. Med. Res.*, 45(1), 77—80, 1957.
300. Villadelmar, M. L., Suarez Sata, M. L., Massieu, H., Guzman, G., and Cravioto, R. O., Determinación de aminoacidos indispensables en 24 alimentos Mexicanos, *Ciencia*, 16, 17—23, 1956—1957.
301. Walford, L. A., The sea as potential source of protein food, *Adv. Protein Chem.*, 10, 289—316, 1955.
302. Walker, M., Wenkman, N. S., and Miller, C. D., Composition of some Hawaii fish, *Hawaii Med. J.*, 18, 144—145, 1958.
303. Wangler, J. G., Seasonal variations of physical characteristics and chemical composition of fish from Middle Atlantic states, *Commer. Fish. Rev.*, 22(7), 17—20, 1960.

304. **Watson, V. K. and Fellers, C. R.**, Nutritive value of the blue crab *(Callinectes sapidus)* and sand crab *(Platyonichus ocellatus* Lateille), *Am. Fish. Soc. Trans.*, 65, 342—349, 1935.
305. **Webb, N. B., Thomas, F. B., Busta, F. F., and Monroe, R. J.**, Variations in proximate composition of North Carolina scallop meats, *J. Food Sci.*, 34, 471—474, 1969.
306. **Whipple, D. V.**, Vitamins A, D, and B in oysters — effect of cooking upon vitamins A and $B_1$, *J. Nutr.*, 9(2), 163—173, 1935.
307. **White, F. D.**, The nutritive value of marine products. IX. Proximate analysis of British Columbia canned pilchard, *J. Biol. Board Can.*, 2(5), 461—462, 1936.
308. **Willimott, S. G.**, Malayan food composition table, *Dep. Agric. Straights Settlements Fed. Malaya States Sci. Ser.*, 23, 1—34, 1949.
309. **Yarolavtseva, L. D.**, Technochemical properties of some Indian Ocean fishes, *Ryb. Khoz. (Moscow)*, 1, 60—64, 1966.
310. **Ziecik, M. and Nodzynski, J.**, Chemical and weight composition of the comestible parts, the waste and the gonads of the flounder (*Pleuronectes flesus*) caught in the zone of the Bay of Gdansk — in the annual cycle, *Zeszyty Nauk Wyzsz. Szk. Roln. Olsztynic*, 18, 263—295, 1964.
311. **National Marine Fisheries Service, National Oceanic and Atmospheric Administration, U.S. Department of Commerce**, *Fishery Statistics of the United States 1972*, Statistical Digest No. 66, U. S. Government Printing Office, Washington, D. C., 1975, 34.

# MILK AND MILK BY-PRODUCTS

John J. Jonas and Jerry F. Proctor

## INTRODUCTION

In foods, the purpose of supplementation is to bring about a meaningful interrelationship among constituents in such a fashion that obvious benefits are obtained in the resulting composite product. Benefits resulting from supplementation in the food systems could be related to the following criteria:

1. Nutritional
2. Organoleptic
3. Visual and tactile sensory
4. Food technological
5. Economical
6. Consumer acceptance

In foods supplemented with dairy products or dairy by-products, the supplementary relationship is justified, in most cases, by nutritional benefits. Foods, however, are more than a blend of nutritive components balanced optimally for meeting physiological energy and nutrient needs of humans; they are expected to fullfil expectations for pleasurable eating, sensory esthetics, appetizing appearance, and hygienic requirements. All these requirements have to be built into a dairy supplemented food system by food production methods of sound technology and economy at a price level commensurate to the food purchasing power of the consumer. Food supplementation with dairy products should also take into consideration the particular specific dictates of regional food habits, ethnic food preferences, age groups, and the physiological or reproductive state of the potential consumers to be served. Finally, in the area of dairy supplementation, there are highly specific nutritional limitations connected with genetic or environmental factors prevalent in certain population groups, i.e., phenylketonuria and lactose intolerance.

The concept of food supplementation leads us into an arena where numerous directional forces are operative. These could result occasionally in beneficial, sometimes self-defeating, and, under certain conditions, even undesirable finished-product characteristics. Food supplementation can only be considered successful if the resulting system satisfies at least the majority of the criteria discussed above without adding deleterious characteristics. A supplemented food should have viable, positive merits for the consumers. Failure to comply with a single criterion is usually enough to offset all the other potentially beneficial features of the supplemented system.

Two examples deserve some reflection in illustrating the role of counteracting forces when food supplementation is explored with dairy products. The first example refers to a bread supplementation development that stands as resolved at present, whereas the second example illustrates an unresolved situation.

Bread supplementation with dried milk powder is a nutritionally desirable goal because it improves the protein quality of this important and inexpensive staple. However, this goal was achieved only after the disadvantageous loaf deformation of milk powder-fortified bread dough could be avoided during the baking process. At first, researchers had to understand the cause and eliminate the unfavorable interaction between the bread dough and milk systems. Then commercially mature technology had to be devised and disseminated in the baking trade. After the acceptance of the new technology, the baking trade became ready to serve the public with a nutritionally improved bread that satisfied visual, organoleptic and sensory requirements as well as consumer interests at a reasonable cost.

The second example illustrates a condition that is not yet fully resolved. The beneficial, protein-supplementing effect of whey powder in cereal diets, due to whey protein's high lysine, methionine, and cysteine contribution, is easily affected by the significant lactose content of whey when the target consumer group is lactose intolerant. Although research has charted options to avoid this difficulty, product development technology is not yet supplying the desired products in quantity at reasonable cost.

Thus we see that dairy food supplementation requires a meaningful understanding and interplay among process-oriented technology, public acceptance-oriented marketing, and physiologically oriented nutrition/medical sciences. Satisfactory combinations with dairy foods should result in food systems of great significance to public health. It is the role of a responsible food industry to collaborate with nutritionists and health care professionals to develop technologically available and economically sound and locally adapted food supplementation systems.

## ROLE OF DAIRY INGREDIENTS IN FOOD SYSTEMS

Food supplementation with dairy products was originated at the household level where excess milk product and by-products were used for cooking and baking. These early historical aspects, discussed by Hulse,[110] are not considered in this review. The present discussion is focused rather on the milk ingredients in processed foods as they appear on the present-day markets.

Milk products and by-products in industrially prepared foods are intended to improve their nutritional values, to enhance consumer appeal, and to contribute technologically valuable functionality features. Most of present and future development is geared to increasing the performance value of the milk ingredients for manufactured foods. This may require some chemical or physical modification of the dairy ingredients. Care should also be exercised by food technologists to see that these modifications remain within the limits of food safety.

Modified dairy ingredients, when designed to meet specific functionality requirements of the food manufacturer, could supply not only the inherent benefits of the dairy raw materials, but also improve economy and convenience. Introduction of these new functionally designed, industrially oriented dairy ingredients into international trade would tend to reduce the economic pressures of overproduction in dairy areas and be of benefit to the food industries in the nondairying countries as well.

The industrially oriented products of dairy origin have been traditionally marketed to baby food manufacturers, bakeries, meat processors, confectioners, and other processed food industries. Manufacturers of prepackaged foods, frozen foods, and various convenience food items are also potential users of dairy ingredients. A close and technologically meaningful working relationship between the industrially oriented dairy producer and the food processor will be the source of new, functionally designed dairy ingredients. Because of these developmental processes, the dairy industry will present its industrial products in a diversified form that will be able to satisfy the numerous demands of food manufacturers. The nutrient composition of the various milk products and by-products is fundamental with respect to their use in food and food commodity manufacture.

### Nutrient Composition of Milk Products and Milk By-Products

The most commonly known and commercially available dairy products and dairy by-products are alphabetically listed in Table 1.* The nutrient content is expressed both on a g/100 g basis in terms of nutrients and in grams per common serving measure of the food item. The data were compiled by U.S. Department of Agriculture (USDA) under the leadership of Posati and Orr.[213] The original reference contains the full analysis of 122 dairy items. Table 1, in an abbreviated fashion, lists 38 products denoted as Table 1, Items 1 through 38. The following products are covered:

Item 1. Butter, regular
Item 2. Cheese, Blue
Item 3. Cheese, Camembert
Item 4. Cheese, Cheddar
Item 5. Cheese, cottage, creamed
Item 6. Cheese, cottage, dry curd
Item 7. Cheese, cream
Item 8. Cheese, Mozzarella
Item 9. Cheese, Parmesan, grated
Item 10. Cheese, Swiss
Item 11. Cheese, American, pasteurized process
Item 12. Cheese, spread, American, pasteurized process
Item 13. Cream, light, coffee or table, fluid
Item 14. Cream, medium, 25% fat, fluid
Item 15. Cream, sour, cultured
Item 16. Filled milk, with blend of hydrogenated vegetable oils, fluid
Item 17. Filled milk, with lauric acid oil, fluid
Item 18. Ice cream, vanilla, regular, (approximately 10% fat)
Item 19. Coffee whitener, (nondairy) powdered
Item 20. Dessert topping, (nondairy) powdered
Item 21. Milk, whole, 3.3% fat, fluid
Item 22. Milk, lowfat, 2% fat, fluid
Item 23. Milk, lowfat, 2% fat, protein fortified, fluid
Item 23. Milk, skim, fluid
Item 25. Milk, skim, protein fortified, fluid
Item 26. Milk, buttermilk, cultured, fluid
Item 27. Milk, dry, whole
Item 28. Milk, dry, nonfat, regular
Item 29. Milk, condensed, sweetened, canned
Item 30. Milk, evaporated, skim, canned
Item 31. Milk, chocolate, whole, fluid
Item 32. Milk, human, whole, mature, fluid
Item 33. Whey, acid, fluid
Item 34. Whey, acid, dry
Item 35. Whey, sweet, fluid
Item 36. Whey, sweet, dry
Item 37. Yogurt, plain
Item 38. Yogurt, plain, with skim milk solids added

## Organoleptic Role of Milk Products And Milk By-Products in Food Supplementation

Flavor and textural contributions of dairy supplements to food systems in general

---

* All tables will appear at the end of the text.

can be considered positive in value. The contributing features are mostly mild in flavor and smooth in body and feel.

The flavor of dairy-based supplements can be enhanced by microbiological fermentation as in cultured dairy products and cheeses; by enzymatic treatments, as in proteolytic hydrolysates of dairy proteins, in lipolytically processed dairy fats, or in lactase-treated milk sugar products. Controlled heat treatments of various dairy ingredients will produce Malliard (browning) reaction, resulting in a broad enhancement of flavors. Controlled caramelization of dairy proteins and carbohydrates is applied in dairy-based candy manufacture as the flavor-enhancing step. The controlled browning reaction in bread crust of bread that contains nonfat dried milk or whey also adds appealing color and flavor notes.

Cultured dairy products, when applied as supplements in food systems, contribute mild, acid flavors through their lactic acid content. A long list of volatile flavor bodies of extremely pleasing nature lend food products containing cottage cheese, buttermilk, yogurt, and sour cream excellent organoleptic properties. These flavors carry through during both the cooking and the baking processing of foods.

Flavor formation by proteolytic and lipolytic enzymic modifications of dairy supplements is based on the formation of amino acids, peptides and their degradation products from proteins, aldehydes, ketones, lactones, and free fatty acids from butterfat. The main dairy carbohydrate, lactose, is also a significant flavor modifier through its mild sweetness and its flavor accentuation. Thermally treated lactose is the source of various acids, aldehydes, furfural derivates and maltol — all significant flavor contributors.

Certain dairy by-products that represent fractions of milk or whey have great supplementing potential, but could be sources of negative flavor effects. The dairy protein concentrates and isolates are especially subject to this fault. The characteristic flavor of casein is often found "gluey".[214] This "off flavor" is very objectionable, and it is perceptible at significant dilution levels in supplemented systems that might require delicate or bland flavor. The origin of this flavor defect is technologically caused because native casein, as present in milk, is perfectly bland. It was found that small quantities of residual lactose and butter fat will cause flavor deterioration of casein during processing and storage. Careful manufacturing techniques and protective packaging are required to prevent the off-flavor formation.[215]

Textural contributions of dairy supplements to food systems originate very often from the viscous nature of the dairy proteins, the pH sensitivity of the proteins, and the subsequent curd formation. The "whipability" of many dairy systems is also a powerful tool in textural modifications when used in conjunction with other food systems. On whipping, air is imbibed in small bubbles and the dairy proteins, predominantly casein and certain whey proteins (lactalbumin and lactoglobulin) form a strong foam wall (lamella) structure around the air particles, resulting in light, foamed textures.

The proteins of dairy systems are instrumental in the fat emulsification process, thus modifying the organoleptic properties of fats. Classical examples are margarine, which contains nonfat dried milk, ice cream, the various whipped toppings, and creams, as well as the great success of homogenized milk.

The pronounced hydrophobic nature of casein, especially enhanced by rennin treatment, is the key to the textural property of cheeses. The heat-caused melting, flow, and resetting of cheese is of great significance in the formulated food industry. The enzymatically modified fat-protein combinations in cheeses could contribute distinctive flavor varieties to manufactured foods such as soups, frozen casserole dishes, soufflés, dips, and sauces.

### General Technological Role of Dairy Supplements in Foods

Technologically valuable contributions of dairy supplements in food can be many-fold, and the efficacy can be maximized by skillful modifications if so desired for specific uses. The food manufacturer prefers dairy supplement products that are adjusted to his particular functional requirements. The basic justification for the use of functionally designed dairy ingredients in food formulation is to provide the public with manufactured foods of the best overall food values.

The food ingredient demands of the food industry offer the dairy industry potential new markets. Since the 1950s there has been an upsurge in the prepared food industry. Prepackaged foods, either frozen or dried and ready for instant cooking, are becoming very popular. The preparation of these foodstuffs has brought about a close working relationship between the food and dairy industries. To cope with the demand of food manufacturers, the dairy industry is presenting its products in novel forms, for both retail and institutionally oriented food manufacturers.

Functionally designed dairy ingredients should be produced in such a fashion that the most desirable food value attributes are preserved. Furthermore, they should be developed to the maximum functional effectiveness and should be available for the food processor in the most economical and convenient form. There is little doubt that milk proteins are by far the most unique and also give the most opportunity for successful commercial application. The milk proteins also enjoy an unchallenged position in terms of intrinsic food values that are not equally shared by some of the other major dairy components such as milk fat or lactose.

In the protein field, for example, only casein was traditionally available for food use. Now buyers have a broad selection of acid-precipitated caseins, spray-dried caseins, soluble caseins, lactalbumins, and casein-lactalbumin coprecipitates. Each of these products has a particular use in food manufacture.

The food industry also requires cheeses for flavoring. The recent availability of spray-dried cheese powders offers a simpler and more versatile method of incorporating cheese flavor into its products.

Consumer trade acceptance of whey as a food supplement continues to grow worldwide. The supply of whey products is increasing because the dairy industry recognized the nutritional and economic values of whey ingredients when processed in a sanitary fashion to produce edible whey powder. Furthermore, the environmental pollution caused by the release of whey in the waterways is ecologically unsound and legally prohibited. Consequently, both arguments forced dairy plants to recover whey solids in a gainful manner. New processes and products will further widen the utility of whey. Rising prices of milk powder encourage the substitution of whey for higher priced ingredients. The major route of upgrading whey for human use is through the concentration of its protein contents. Whey can be demineralized, and, thus it gains more flexibility in food applications than the spray-dried whey itself.

Such whey protein concentrates powerfully improved protein quality when used to supplement vegetable protein-containing foods. The significance of this application is particularly valuable for developing countries where there is a serious animal protein shortage. A 35% protein product containing partially delactosed and demineralized whey product at 10% addition level is capable of significantly improving the amino acid composition of a wheat- rice-, or corn-based cereal food.

Lactose is recognized for making positive nutritional contributions in population groups that are not prone to lactose intolerance. Lactose is considered by many to be the preferred carbohydrate for modifying infant food formulations. It has also been found that lactose in a diet improves the utilization of calcium and other minerals, although the mechanism of action remains debatable.[6,27] Lactose, in an enzyme-hydrolyzed form, can be converted into food-grade syrups consisting of glucose and galactose. This sugar mixture would not be objectionable for the lactase deficient consumer.

Dairy supplementation with the intent of balancing the calcium-phosphorus intake is of great public health importance and is expected to gain in importance. Dairy products are the single high-calcium food sources of the American dietary. About 75% of the calcium intake in the U.S. is of dairy origin.

The food-supplementing value of milk was enhanced significantly by the practice of vitamin D fortification. In this way, most of the vitamin D in the American diet comes from milk, and in the case of some infants and small children, milk may be the only source of vitamin D.

Dairy supplements as sources of micronutrients (vitamins other than D, and trace minerals) enjoy a unique status. The acceptance of cultured dairy products as food supplements is expected to increase because of their unique, mildly acid flavor and, possibly, their reduced lactose contents. They may also have some unique nutritional benefits. The distinctive flavor of these products is an asset in low-fat dairy foods and is helpful when milk fats are being substituted with polyunsaturated oils.

In general, the response of the consumer toward dairy supplementation is positive. It supports the quality oriented consumer's choice, which is associated with traditional richness of dairy products. However, the changing dietary habits and consumer preoccupation with high cholesterol contents of dairy fats cast a shadow of high-fat cream- and butter-based supplementation. Protein-based supplementation is, beyond doubt, the strongest among the options of the dairy products.

## AN OVERVIEW OF THE LITERATURE OF DAIRY SUPPLEMENTS IN FOOD SYSTEMS

The most important supplementing effect of milk and milk by-products on the various food systems is reviewed in a tabular form. In Table 2, major recent literature surveys have been selected from the world literature. By means of this table, the reader can easily find key references concerning the nutritional, food technological, organoleptic, and economical contributions of dairy supplements in various food systems.

The structure of the table is simple. Only food applications that use dairy materials as supplements in practical food manufacturing are listed. These applications are

1.  Dairy supplementation in general
2.  Baby food and clinical nutrition products
3.  Beverages
4.  Cereals, baked, and pasta products
5.  Dessert and candy products
6.  Fatty products
7.  Food aid items and foods for developing countries
8.  Meat products
9.  Whipables and emulsion products

The basic parameters in terms of which the rationale of the supplementation is justified are

1.  Nutritional effects
2.  Food technological effects
3.  Organoleptic properties
4.  Economics and statistics

A complete, comprehensive coverage of the pertinent literature is not considered to be practical because the abundant data might obscure clarity and impede fast information recovery. The reader who requires for research, patent search, or for other purposes a complete coverage, is referred to the annotated bibliographies of *Dairy Science Abstracts,* issued by the Commonwealth Bureau of Dairy Science and Technology, Shinfield, Reading RG2, 9AT, U.K. The use of dairy products in foods is systematically reviewed in short, well-documented publications by Dairy Research, Inc., in the U.S.[54,109a,109b]

## DAIRY PRODUCTS USED IN FOOD SUPPLEMENTATION

Food supplements of dairy origin could be classified according to their chemical nature in five major groups: proteins, fats, carbohydrates, minerals, and vitamins. Another category that will be treated separately is cultured dairy products. These dairy products are available for food supplementation in numerous forms and concentrations; they can be in their native liquid condition or in partially dehydrated, jellied, semisolid, or fully dehydrated and powdered forms. In a minority of cases, the dairy supplements represent unfractionated milks or cultured milks, but more often these products are enriched fractions of original milk constituents. For instance, whole milk can be considered as a food supplement, as native whole milk, as concentrated milk, or as dried milk. By the physical removal of the emulsified milk fats in the form of cream, skim milk is obtained from the native milk. The skim milk is recovered for commercial use at various solids levels.

Further fractions of milk such as casein, lactalbumin, coprecipitated milk proteins, lipids, or lactose are commercially available at various enrichment levels as concentrates and isolates, mostly in dehydrated form for practical storage-life consideration.

In order to illustrate the generic correlations among the milk products used as food supplements, the major technological steps and the resulting products are shown in Figure 1. In the subsequent section, the basic rationale of the use of the individual dairy ingredients will be discussed.

In order to illustrate the generic correlations among the milk products used as food supplements, the major technological steps and the resulting products are shown in Figure 1. In the subsequent section, the basic rationale of the us of the individual dairy ingredients will be discussed.

### Milk Proteins in Foods

The various types of milk proteins designed for food supplementation are listed in Table 3.

*Status of Milk Protein Isolates as Food Supplements*

Consumption of casein and whey products, as well as the contribution of protein by these materials in the U.S., is shown in Table 4. Casein, caseinates, and whey solids consumed as components of human food contributed approximately 173,628,000 lb of high-quality protein to the American diet in 1974.

Borst[38] has reported that the main reason for the growth in use of casein in foods lies in its functionality. The fast growth of casein uses might become self limiting because of exhaustion of the supply and consequent price increases. There is a significant tendency in Scotland, Australia, and New Zealand to initiate increased production. It is advisable to tap the casein resources in Argentina by upgrading the quality of their production.

Casein and whey products have a wide range of functionality, which is extremely

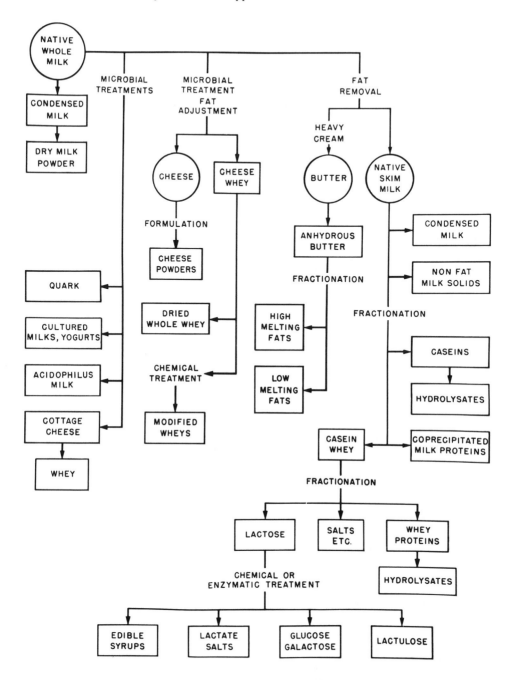

FIGURE 1.   Milk and major milk by-products.

useful in food technology.[156] The caseins and caseinates offer high concentrations of proteins with exceptional water-binding capacity, fat-emulsifying properties, whipping ability, ability to develop viscosity, and solubility in neutral or alkaline solutions. Perhaps most important, all this is provided by a product that is very bland. The milk protein coprecipitate products exhibit much the same properties as casein, but have somewhat limited solubility. Whey protein differs considerably in its functionality from casein and coprecipitated milk protein: whey protein concentrates offer a high-quality protein that absorbs little water and thus develops minimal viscosity in solution, is soluble in acid solutions, and has fat-emulsifying capacity, whipping ability, and bland flavor. The chemistry of milk proteins in food processing was reviewed by Morr[175,176] and that of the whey proteins and whey protein concentrates by Smith.[238]

The current importance of milk proteins to the food industry in the U.S. is illustrated by the change in the market for imported casein. In 1960, New Zealand and Australia constituted only a little over 29% of the total imports, which were nearly all consumed in industrial applications, whereas in 1969 these two countries accounted for 68.5% of the imports, most of which found their way into foods.

A recent marketing research report by Hammonds and Call[97] lists major uses of casein in various food products. Coprecipitates have found their greatest use and acceptance in the baking industry, where a high-quality, functional, carbohydrate-free milk protein is required.

The principal determinants of expanded utilization and production of milk protein concentrates, caseins, and whey proteins are economic and regulatory rather than technological. Milk marketing economics control the relative product flow. For example, it was not economically attractive in the early 1970s for manufacturers in the U.S. to produce casein or caseinate from the domestic milk supply. As a consequence, the U.S. is totally dependent on imported material to meet the U.S. food processors' demand for this functional protein. The relatively new, coprecipitated milk protein products likewise are not produced domestically but are available only as imported products, principally from Australia and New Zealand.

In projecting the future for dairy products, Neilsen[192] expressed his view that the expansion of the use of milk in foods might be accomplished through the use of milk components as ingredients in other products. Milk proteins have the highest food supplementing potential among the isolated milk components.

Milk proteins are of great importance for supplementing the diets of humans. In addition to supplying the essential amino acids, milk proteins have particular aspects that attract the interest of the nutritionist and food scientist. These specific features have been discussed by Alais and Blanc[4] and cover the following points:

1. The facility of enzymatic digestion of casein.
2. The existence of phospho-peptone residues.
3. The presence of immunoglobulins and an antitryptic factor.
4. The bonding of calcium and phosphorous to the micellar proteins that increase their availability.
5. The metabolism of iron via lactoferrin.

For practical food supplementation, the supply of essential amino acids and calcium are the most important merits of the milk proteins.

*Nutritional Supplementary Value of Milk Protein*
The support in nutritional values that different proteins may give to each other on the basis of their amino acid composition can be referred to as their supplementary value. Protein concentrates rich in certain amino acids will improve diets deficient in essential amino acids, provided they supply the missing ones. The biological value of such mixtures is greater than the average values of the separate protein components. In extremely favorable conditions, a protein source might meet the complete amino acid requirement and thus might represent an ideal protein with the highest biological value.

This ideal protein is not necessarily better than an adequately supplemented protein blend. In fact, under practical feeding conditions, based on a single protein-containing food ingredient, an ideal amino acid composition profile might be rarely obtained, whereas proteins with surplusses in various essential amino acids are abundantly available. Rationally designed blends of these proteins can be applied in food formulations, however. These blends will possess high biological values by supplying the proper amino acid requirements through mutual supplementary action.

One of the great nutritional advantages of including milk proteins in the diet is that it can have a most valuable supplementary effect in enhancing the value of the protein of the rest of the diet. Smith[239] gave a concise discussion of the experimental work leading to the assessment of the supplementary value of milk proteins. The supplementary relationships between, for instance, milk and cereals or potatoes, or between bread and cheese (where milk proteins contribute lysine, tryptophan, and other essential amino acids and raise the biological value of the mixed proteins) are well demonstrated. Kon and collaborators from the National Institute for Research in Dairying (Reading, England) conducted pioneering studies on this field in the late 1930 and 1940s.

The work of Henry and Kon[105] (Table 5) showed that the relatively low nutritive value of bread protein could be raised to the high value of cheese if half the bread protein were replaced by cheese protein. Similarly, the value of potato protein was very significantly increased when it was supplemented with the protein of dried milk.

Most of the work on the supplementary value of milk protein has been done with rats as the experimental animal, but there is every indication that the results should apply in principle to man. In fact, in experiments with young men as the subjects, it was found that when only one fifth of the protein of a purely vegetable diet was replaced by cheese, the biological value of the total protein of the diet was greatly increased.[239] Similarly, Mitra and Verman,[173] in nitrogen balance experiments with Indian subjects found higher biological values for the proteins of rice-milk diets than for the proteins of rice-pulse diets. When they studied the effect of varying the proportion of milk to rice, they obtained maximum values when milk supplied 25% of the protein of the mixture. Indeed, since rice contains about 7.5% protein with a lysine content of 4.4% and dried skimmed milk contains 36% protein with a lysine content of 8.0%, it can be calculated that supplementation of rice with 7% of its weight of dried skimmed milk will result in a quarter of the total protein in the mixture being milk protein and the lysine content of the total protein being about 5.3%.

It was also found in animal experiments that supplementary relationships are only manifested if the different proteins are given simultaneously or within a short-time interval, since the constituent amino acids must be available together to combine into body proteins. There are indications that this concept is valid in human nutrition, too.

The practical nutritional qualities of isolated milk proteins have been extensively studied.[53,77,78,105,189] One important consideration in expanded protein utilization is the ability of casein, milk protein coprecipitate and, more particularly, whey protein concentrates to complement and supplement vegetable proteins, which are the most important staple foods in developing countries. Figure 2 shows the increase in balanced protein [meets the Food and Agricultural Organization (FAO) profile] in cereal products when supplemented with 10% whey protein concentrate. Furthermore, Table 6 shows the effect on protein efficiency ratio (PER) when increasing amounts of whey protein are added to a commercial isolated soy protein. These data demonstrate that a relatively small quantity of whey protein is capable of improving the amino acid balance of the final protein mixture for human needs.

Economic and nutritional considerations require the quantification of the ratios of the proteins used in mutual supplementation. The determination of the ratios is accom-

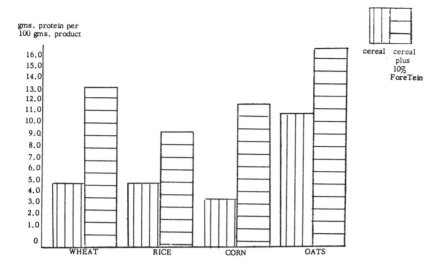

FIGURE 2.    Improvement in the amino acid balance of cereals by the addition of whey protein. The quantity of protein, which meets the FAO's recommended amino acid profile, is increased by the addition of 10% whey protein concentrate (ForeTein®) to wheat, rice, corn, and oats. These data demonstrate that a relatively small quantity of whey protein is capable of improving the amino acid composition of the respective protein balance mixture for human needs.

ForeTein® is a specially processed, edible whey product in which the protein has been concentrated through partial lactose removal and demineralization; ForeTein® contains 35% protein. (From **Foremost Foods Company**, ForeTein®, A High Protein Demineralization Whey Protein, 1970. Reprinted by the permission of the copyright owner — Foremost Foods, San Francisco.)

plished by calculations based on the respective amino acid compositions of the proteins selected and the amino acid compositions required in the particular food item.

*Calculating Optimum Supplementation Between Two Proteins Based on Their Amino Acid Content*

As an example, wheat flour supplementation by means of whey protein is being selected for macaroni production. The calculations and tabulations of the data for this example are illustrated by the recent paper of Schoppert et al.[228] The same authors also report on the experimental verification of the calculations in terms of biological testing.

Table 7 shows the amino acid analyses for the FAO protein and ordinary macaroni as reported in the literature and the data calculated from these values. The calculations are based on the assumption that the reference protein has the "ideal balance" of essential amino acids for nutritional quality — in other words, that particular proportion of essential amino acids that the body can use best for building proteins.

In calculating, the essential amino acid values of the reference protein (g/100 g as shown in the first column of Table 7) are converted to ratios of each acid compared to essential amino acid in the smallest amount (tryptophan). These ratios are given in the second column of Table 7. Common macaroni is handled in a similar way in the third and fourth columns. It will be noted that both protein sources are now on a common basis with respect to tryptophan (columns 2 and 4). Thus if it is assumed that the second column in Table 7 represents the best spectrum of essential amino acid ratios that the body can use to build proteins, the relative protein nutritional value for common macaroni can be calculated. This is done by first comparing each essential amino acid ratio of macaroni against the same acid ratio of the reference. That which is least compared to the corresponding ratio of the reference is the "limiting essential amino acid". Reference to the second and fourth columns of Table 7 reveals that lysine is the limiting essential amino acid of macaroni when the reference protein is that of the FAO. This means that the other essential amino acids of macaroni will be used "best" only insofar as their "ideal" ratio with respect to lysine will allow. Thus, to calculate how much of each essential amino acid will be best used, the content of the limiting amino acid (g/100 g) is multiplied in turn by the ideal ratio of each acid and divided by the ideal ratio of the limiting acid. The results of this calculation for each essential amino acid are given in the fifth column of Table 7. The sum of these results is 2.598 g. That means that 2.598 g of the 12.7 g of total protein in 100 g of macaroni are essential amino acids in "ideal balance". Thus 20.5% of the total protein of common macaroni can be "best" used by the body.

When the heat-coagulated whey protein fraction is added to the flour in the ratio of 1:5 (which results in a 20% protein macaroni), similar calculations (contained in Table 8) show that the limiting essential amino acid is shifted from lysine in the common macaroni to the sulfur groups in the enriched macaroni, and the percentage of the protein of macaroni that is in the recommended "ideal" essential amino acid balance is almost doubled due to enrichment. Thus the essential amino acid patterns of the durum wheat and whey proteins complement each other with a consequent increase in the quality of the combined proteins over the wheat alone.

The near doubling of the balanced essential amino acid content gives promise of a substantial increase in the biological value of the enriched macaroni. This expectation was borne out in subsequent biological testing, as shown in Table 9. PER data showed a highly significant improvement in the quality of the protein in pasta and indicated that the durum-whey protein blend is highly complementary, i.e., the PER of the blend is better than the sum of their individual contributions. The resultant 21.6% protein product has a twofold nutritional advantage in that the consumer will get a better protein than ordinarily found in pasta. Further, the data of Table 9 indicate that there is no significant difference in the PER assay of pasta enriched with insolubilized whey protein and casein when subjected to statistical analyses. Thus fortification with heat-coagulated acid whey proteins satisfies the criterion established by the research that the enriched product would have a PER that is equal to 95% of that of casein.

The most comprehensive discussion of the food supplementing value of whey proteins was written by Forsum.[78] The subsequent section is based on her work, demonstrating two examples.

Although the high nutritive value of whey proteins has been known since the early days of the scientific study of protein nutrition, new dimensions of uses are emerging for this whey protein through the advent of large-scale protein separation techniques. It is recognized that the iological function of whey proteins in milk is most likely nutritional and supplementary to that of casein. The casein is a unique phospho-protein designed to support the bone development of the offspring through its calcium and phosphorus contribution. Its amino acid profile is not optimal for the growth of muscle tissue. However, the amino acids supplied by whey proteins supplement the amino acid balance of casein for optimal growth and development of the young. Thus whey proteins are well utilizable in "humanized" infant foods. It is well known that human milk contains relatively little casein as compared with cow's milk. The ratio of casein to whey protein in human milk is 2:3, as compared with 4:1 in cow's milk. Tomarelli, et al.[251] reported high nutritive value of bovine casein and whey proteins mixed, simulating human milk composition. These findings found application in the formulation of bovine milk-based human infant feeding.

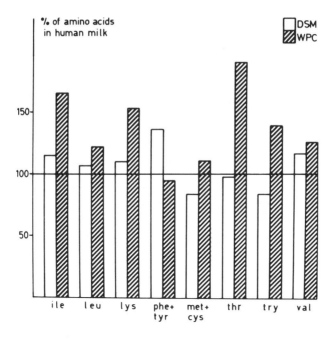

FIGURE 3. Essential amino acid content of dried skim milk (DSM) and whey protein concentrate (WPC) expressed in percent of the FAO human milk amino-acid reference pattern, 1973. (From Forsum, E., in *Protein Nutritional Quality of Foods and Feeds,* Vol. 1, Part 2, Friedman, M., Ed., Marcel Dekker, New York, 1975, 462. With permission.)

### Whey Proteins in Weaning Foods

The formulation of weaning foods depends on soluble animal protein resources and, more particularly, milk products. Traditionally, skim milk powder was used to balance the weaning formulations for best essential amino acid composition. As the price of skim milk powder limited its use, whey protein preparations gained increasing consideration.

When the essential amino acid compositions of whey protein concentrate (WPC) and dry milk solids (DSM) were compared with that of the essential amino acid contents of human milk (Figure 3), it was found that the surplus of several essential amino acids, especially lysine, threonine, and tryptophan, was greater in WPC than in DSM. Since vegetable proteins often are limited by these amino acids, this suggests that WPC would be more useful than DSM as an animal protein source in protein-rich weaning foods.

Forsum[78] studied the effect on the protein quality of three protein-rich weaning foods, CSM® (corn soy milk), Faffa®, and Superamine®, when protein from DSM was replaced by protein from WPC. CSM® is manufactured by the Lauhoff Grain Company (Danville, Ill.) and its composition in g/100 g is precooked corn flour, 64; defatted soyflour, 24; DSM, 5; soy oil, 5; and vitamins and minerals, 2. Faffa® is manufactured by the Ethiopian Nutrition Institute (Addis Ababa, Ethiopia) and its composition in g/100 g is wheat flour, 57; defatted soy flour, 18; chick pea flour, 10; DSM, 5; sugar, 8; and vitamins and minerals, 2. Superamine® is manufactured by S. N. Sempac (Alger, Algeria) and its composition in g/100 g is chick pea flour, 38; durum wheat flour, 28; lentil flour, 18; dried skim milk, 10; sugar, 5; and vitamins and minerals, 1. In these formulas protein from DSM constitutes 9 to 18% of the total protein. The protein quality was evaluated by chemical and biological methods. Theoretically, this change of animal protein source increased the chemical scores of CSM®, Faffa®, and Superamine® by 4 to 5 units.

As shown in Table 10, considerable improvements in PER and net protein utilization (NPU) were obtained when DSM was replaced by WPC in Superamine® and CSM®. In Superamine®, the PER value was increased by 43% and the NPU value by 14%, while the NPU of CSM® was increased by 17% as a result of this change in animal protein source. Only a slight improvement in the quality of Faffa protein was observed when DSM protein was replaced by WPC protein, the increase in PER as well as NPU being 7%. It should be noted that a dry 29% whey protein concentrate recently has been approved as an optional ingredient in CSM®.

Utilization of whey protein concentrate in emergency food mixtures based on Swedish ingredients has also been studied.[1] The mixtures contained mainly wheat supplemented by protein sources to satisfy the recommendations of the Protein Advisory Group (PAG) of the FAO/WHO for protein-rich weaning foods. Chemical and biological testing of mixtures containing 5 to 10% WPC showed the whey proteins to be of value for the protein quality of the mixture.[1] When these mixtures were used for preparation of bread or porridge, the presence of WPC was not found to impair the appearance or palatability of the product. Furthermore, field testing by Abrahamson et al.[2] of emergency foods containing WPC in Afghanistan and West Africa showed that the product was well accepted and tolerated.[220] Similar results were obtained by Rodier et al.[220] in the field testing of a soy-whey beverage, which showed that such a beverage will probably be acceptable in preschool feeding programs in most parts of the developing world.

Interesting aspects of the utilization of whey proteins in human nutrition have been published by Hutton.[113] This paper deals with technological, environmental, and nutritional, as well as agricultural and economic viewpoints of whey protein utilization. The outstanding ability of the whey proteins to boost food value of cereal proteins is stressed.

### Whey Proteins in Treatment of Phenylketonuria

Another special supplementing application of whey proteins is reported on by Forsum.[78] The amino acid compositions of two whey protein concentrates (WPC) produced by large-scale gel filtration and ultrafiltration are shown in Table 11.[80] It is seen that the contents of essential amino acids are high, and of special interest are the high contents of lysine, threonine, tryptophan, and cysteine. The contents of phenylalanine and tyrosine, however, are comparatively low. The low content of phenylalanine could be utilized in the dietary treatment of phenylketonuria (PKU). Most food proteins contain comparatively high amounts of phenylalanine and thus a child with PKU cannot tolerate a normal diet. This necessitates the use of special formulas based on synthetic amino acids without phenylalanine, or protein hydrolysates from which phenylalanine has been removed. Since these low-phenylalanine formulas are expensive and unpalatable, it is desirable that the natural protein source used should have a low-phenylalanine content but an otherwise well-balanced amino acid composition.

Hambraeus et al.[95] reported on the use of whey protein-containing formulas in the dietary treatment of PKU. In one test with a girl suffering from hyperphenylalaninemia, a formula based on a gel-filtered WPC was used as the sole source of nitrogen.[96] This resulted in a higher nitrogen retention but a lower level of phenylalanine in the blood than with the conventional treatment. These findings are not only of interest in connection with PKU, but also show that the whey proteins are of high-nutritive quality for humans.

Nutritional and biochemical studies of whey products was contained by Forsum and Hambraeus throughout the 1970s. During processing, whey often is subjected to heat treatments that might decrease the biological availability of lysine by the Maillard reaction. This reaction is likely to occur in whey products because of their high lactose content. Since an extensive Maillard reaction would impair the supplementary value of the whey protein, the availability of lysine is an important parameter when nutritional value of whey products is evaluated. Forsum and Hambraeus[79] found that, as a result of heat treatment, little impairment occurred to the biological value of whey products. In all whey products evaluated, the available lysine was considerably higher than 340 mg/g nitrogen, which is the content recommended by the FAO.[71]

### Whey Proteins in Cereals

The supplementary values of milk and whey products for creals, such as wheat flour and rice as well as gelatins, were compared with that of soy protein by Lohrey and Humphries.[149] All milk proteins, because of their relatively high lysine and tryptophan contents, may be expected to have excellent supplementary value for cereals, especially wheat products such as white flour, which contain a low percentage of lysine. With 4% casein in the mixture (equivalent to the 25% supplementary protein level), the PER was almost twice that of flour and the lysine content was increased by about 40%. This level of casein can readily and economically be incorporated into flour. Supplementing the flour with 10% casein (50% of the total protein) increased the PER and lysine content approximately two and one half times. On a protein basis, even better results were obtained with milk powders, coprecipitates, and especially whey proteins. Using such products at 25 and 50% supplementary protein levels, adjusted PERs of about 2.0 and 3.2, respectively, have been attained. Soy protein has proven inferior to milk proteins as a supplement to wheat flour.[149]

Trials with rice protein have indicated the superior quality of this protein relative to wheat protein. The PER values for ground rice and skim milk powder were significantly higher than those for wheat flour and skim milk powder at the 25% level of supplementation (approximately 7% skim milk powder in the mixture). With an adjusted PER of 2.57, the rice and skim milk powder mixture was of similar value to casein for growth and efficiency of protein utilization. At the 50% supplementation level, the ground rice and skim milk powder mixture had a PER only slightly higher than that of the comparable mixture of flour and skim milk powder. The differences between soy protein and skim milk powder as supplements to rice were not significant. In contrast to the results obtained with wheat flour, increasing the supplementary level of both skim milk powder and soy concentrate from 25 to 50% did not significantly increase the PERs in the case of rice, presumably because of the superior quality of rice protein.

Supplementing gelatin with whey protein at levels equivalent to 25 and 40% soluble whey powder in the mixture improved the PER from −1.0 to 1.3 and 2.2, respectively. The supplementation had an even more dramatic effect on the appearance of the rats, those on the diets containing gelatin as the sole protein were moribund after 28 days, while those on the soluble whey powder/gelatin mixtures were alert and normal in appearance although they grew only slowly by comparison. The chemical score of the gelatin was increased from 0 to 41 and 68, respectively, by supplementation with 25 and 40% soluble whey powder. Tryptophan was the limiting amino acid at the lower level and methionine and cystine at the higher level. Even at the higher level, the only amino acid that met the provisional amino acid requirements was lysine. It seems, therefore, that while supplementation of gelatin with soluble whey powder improves its nutritive value, the addition of whey proteins to gelatin products could not be justified on the basis of the subsequent nutritional value of the mixture.

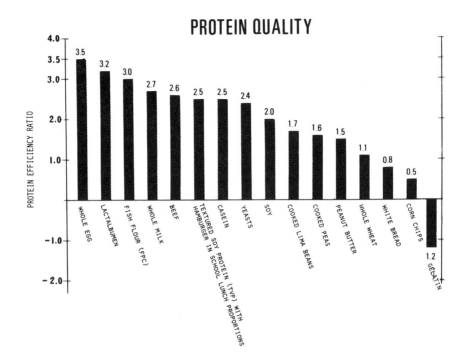

FIGURE 4.    Protein quality of various types of foods.

Although the supplementary value of whey proteins for products low in sulfur-containing amino acids has not been tested, their amino acid profile suggests that they would be valuable for this purpose. Because their total content of essential amino acids is high, whey proteins should prove valuable ingredients in baby foods formulated with vegetable and cereal products and in special diets such as those for renal dialysis patients, where a minimal amount of high-quality protein is desirable.

*Measures of the Nutritive Value of Proteins*

Whole milk protein has a slightly higher quality than meat due to the presence of more sulfur-containing amino acids in lactoglobulin and lactalbumin (about one fifth to one quarter of the total protein in milk). The most prevalent milk protein, casein, by itself is equivalent in protein quality to that of most other animal proteins and, along with lactalbumin, is generally considered as the standard reference protein for biological assay. The proteins of eggs are so well-proportioned in their amino acid composition that whole egg protein is sometimes also taken as a reference standard for comparing the quality of protein based upon amino acid composition.[34a]

Regardless of the species, the amino acid composition of the proteins in muscle tissue foods is relatively constant and of such balance and quality that red meats, fish, and poultry rank only slightly below eggs and milk protein in their ability to affect tissue synthesis. The proteins in legumes and nuts are of somewhat lesser quality than animal proteins because the amounts of methionine and lysine are below optimum levels. Cereal proteins rate generally lower, and certain proteins such as gelatin are significantly inferior (see Figure 4). The measurement of protein quality is generally accomplished by biological assay. The protein to be tested is fed to experimental animals, and its capacity to maintain the nitrogen balance or to promote growth is measured. The methods employed vary and are accordingly designated as biological value (BV), protein efficiency ratio (PER), net protein retention (NPR), and net protein utilization

(NPU). The combined measure of both quality and quantity of the protein in a diet is the net dietary protein value (NDPV) which is defined as intake of N × 6.25 × NPU. For a complete discussion of protein quality, the works of Munro and Allison,[180] Hegarty,[102] and Tomarelli[250] should be consulted.

A newer method being employed is the "slope-ratio" method, which employs a multidose protein assay. Three or four levels of the test and standard proteins are fed, but only doses falling on the curve-response linear portion are used to compute the assay value. The slope of the response curve for the test protein is expressed as a percentage of the standard protein (lactalbumin). For a discussion of the comparative values of these different techniques, the interested reader should consult Rosenfield[222] (see Table 12).

Utilizable protein is a concept that recognizes inherent interrelationships between the quality and quantity of protein in a given food. The value of utilizable protein is calculated by multiplying a food's crude protein content by the ratio of either NPR, NPU, or slope-ratio values of the particular protein in relation to either casein or lactalbumin. By utilizing amino acid patterns of a given food, it is also possible to make estimates of a protein's relative nutritive value. The most widely used of these calculations is the FAO amino acid pattern as contrasted in Table 12 with various other parameters. In addition, proteins may be rated in relation to milk or egg protein or lactalbumin, as also illustrated in Table 12.

Figure 4 illustrates the relative value of a food ingredient in an array of many food proteins when PER is used as the criterion for evaluation. For the PER assay a specific casein preparation, the Animal Nutrition Research Council (ANRC), casein has been used as the standard for approximately 20 years. This casein's PER is considered to be 2.5, and the test protein's PER, as determined by simultaneous assay, is adjusted accordingly. Most often, the results are reported as PER values although they may be stated as a relative percentage of the casein control.

New concepts for the rapid determination of protein quality have been the subject of the National Science Foundation's conference at the University of Nebraska in 1977.[186a] Conclusions of this conference stated (1) that the new, alternative, rapid, in vivo or in vitro protein quality test methods must be interrelated to the current PER bioassay and (2) that rapid methology for measuring protein quality is now needed by the food industry for quality assurance programs and as a tool to support product and process development work. This conference did not recommend a specific rapid test for the replacement of PER, but it urged continued research on this subject. The present status of the measurement of protein quality indicates that interest in rapid methods of protein quality assessment has become more prevalent in recent years, due to a great extent to some of the trends that are now occurring in food regulation.

Various methods of estimating the nutritive value of a protein ingredient or a food product have been developed and are used throughout various stages of product development. When it comes to determining the quality of the protein in a product to be used to legally document a protein quality claim, however, PER is the only officially recognized method.

In recent years, the U.S. Food and Drug Administration (FDA), either in regulations or proposed regulations dealing with food labeling, has included sections that affect the labeling of the protein contribution of a product, depending upon its quality as measured by PER. For example, in the FDA regulation dealing with the current nutrition labeling program, it is stated that:

"The U.S. Recommended Daily Allowance (RDA) of protein in a food product is 45 grams if the protein efficiency ratio (PER) of the total protein in the product is equal to or greater than that of casein, and 65 grams if the PER of the total protein in the product is less than that of casein. Total protein with a PER less than 20 percent of the PER of casein may not be stated on the label in terms of percentage U.S. RDA, and the statement of protein content in grams per serving (portion) shall be modified by the statement 'not significant source of protein' immediately adjacent to the protein content statement regardless of the actual amount of protein present.''[69b]

This regulation affects how protein may be declared as a percent of the U.S. RDA in a serving of food product depending upon its PER. For example, if a product supplies 4.5 g of protein in a serving and the PER of the protein is equal to or better than that of casein, it may be labeled as providing 10% of the RDA of protein in a serving. If, however, its PER is less than but at least 20% of that of casein, then it would be labeled as providing only 6% of the U.S. RDA of protein in a serving. If the PER were less than 20% of casein, it would have to be labeled as "not a significant source of protein", with this statement immediately adjacent to the protein content statement. Therefore, this regulation introduced protein quality as a factor in making protein claims very much a part of today's food labeling and relates it quantitatively to casein as a standard.

### Casein as a Nutritional Standard

The high digestibility and duplicatable biological value of casein lead to its selection as a standard in animal feeding experiments for the determination of protein efficiency ratio (PER). A specially blended casein composed of high-nitrogen edible casein in equal parts from winter, spring, and summer milk production, has been approved by the ANRC as a reference protein for use in biological assay for nutritive value of protein-containing material. The specifications of this product are described in Table 13.

Furthermore, this standardized protein derived from milk is free of nucleic acids and thus is not subject to the nutritional limitations of yeast and other microbial proteins. It is likewise free of antinutritional factors like those contained in certain vegetable proteins, e.g., the antitrypsin factor of soybean products.

### Factors Affecting Protein Nutritive Values

Lysine in milk proteins is vulnerable to heat processing in the presence of reducing carbohydrates. The ε-amino group on the lysine reacts easily with the carbonyls of the reducing sugars, resulting in a Schiff base that is not utilizable in the normal digestive process. Thus a portion of the valuable lysine is made unavailable for nutritional purposes. Heat-damaged dairy proteins usually have a reduced content of available lysine and are thus less useful for protein supplementation. Nutritional damage to dairy proteins is not significant when heat treatments are equivalent to those used in the pasteurization and ultrahigh-heat-short-time techniques. Sterilization of evaporated milks might lead to the loss of lysine and methionine availability. Heat-caused denaturation of the whey proteins in milk does not significantly affect their nutritional value for the laboratory rat or for the human infant, but it is substantially reduced for young calves.

The nutritive value of proteinaceous foods, even dry foods, changes progressively with time, depending on storage conditions. This depreciation of protein value does not level off. The rate of deterioration is accelerated by high humidity and high temperature. Generally, the protein value decreases less rapidly when the products are stored at 68°F and 40% RH than when stored at 86°F or 104°F and 50% RH. This impairment is reflected in a reduced growth as tested on experimental rats by the bioassay method.

Spray drying or roller drying can damage the nutritional value of dairy proteins or dairy powders. Spray-dried skim milk powder might lose 10% of its total lysine availability, and roller dried skim milk powder might lose up to 30%. Overheated roller drying conditions could lead to a 10% loss in methionine. Since the biological value of milk proteins is limited by their methionine and cysteine contents, any heat damage in these amino acids could be more destructive of nutritional value. Loss of lysine due to its relative overabundance in dairy proteins does not impair significantly the nutrition value of the dairy product per se; when the dairy product is used as a supplement in a mixed diet, however, any loss of lysine must be recognized in planning amino acid-balanced diets.

DeGroot and Slump[57] have investigated the effects of alkali treatment on food proteins under varying conditions of pH, temperature, and time. Their study showed that the exposure of several high-protein products to aqueous alkali resulted in the formation of the amino acid lysinoalanine. When the alkali treatment was made more severe, the protein's lysinoalanine content increased, and these were attended by decreased net protein utilization and protein digestibility.

The biological effects of this unnatural amino acid were investigated by Woodard et al.[282] These authors stated conclusively that lysinoalanine feeding in rats results in cytomegalic lesions. Ashquisth and co-workers reported on the chemistry of isopeptide crosslinks, their occurrence and importance in protein structure.[25] The heat-induced amino acid crosslinks formed in milk proteins were also studied by Klostermeyer and Reimerdes.[133] The amino acid crosslink formation very likely influences the nutritional properties of the proteins.

Besides the rat, other species have been found to resist the development of cytomegaly. Thus it is assumed that the rat's reaction is a species-specific laboratory curiosity. Generally, at present, the amino acid crosslink formation is not considered to be a threat to human health. Past experience in human pathology with cytomegaly is not described in the literature, even though alkali-treated corn protein has been a staple of the diet in many countries for centuries.

*Technology and Food Use of Milk Proteins*

Technological innovations in manufacturing isolated milk proteins have created new products with wide ranges of adaptability to food systems. This new orientation relegates to the past the traditional dairy industry approach that processed surplus skim milk to nonedible casein for the adhesives industry. The new trend calls for processing skim milk to yield a new line of edible, proteinaceous products with specific, technologically valuable functional properties. The present market demand clearly indicates a trend for using more dairy proteins in foods. This increased demand requires the production of edible caseins, lactalbumins, milk protein coprecipitates, microbiologically or chemically modified dairy proteins, and whey proteins through an efficient whey recovery system.

A short general survey of products based on milk proteins covering the present technology and certain future aspects was written by Buchanan.[39] It was concluded in that paper that an expanding range of milk protein products, because of their versatile functional properties and their contribution to nutrition, are sure to play a most useful role in food supplementation. The patent literature of milk-based protein food supplements was published by Noyes[194] covering the period of 1960 to 1969.

The current milk protein manufacturing processes are discussed by Richert.[218] In this paper, industrial production of acid caseins, coprecipitates, and whey proteins is described through flow diagrams and discussion of important operating variables. Variables in continuous casein manufacture include type of acid, pH, precipitation temperature, heating temperature and time, and washing techniques. Precipitation, ultrafiltration, gel filtration, and electrodialysis have been developed to commercial scale for whey fractionation. Ultrafiltration variables include membrane area and geometry, static pressure, flow rate, feed composition, temperature, pH, and membrane characteristics. Performance of gel filtration depends upon bed volume and geometry, feed composition, feed volume per cycle, wash volume per cycle, temperature, flow rates, pH, and gel properties. Electrodialysis is affected by membrane area and geometry, electrical potential, feed composition, flow rates, temperature, membrane characteristics, and brine stream.[218]

## Caseins

Most of the casein produced for edible purposes is acid-precipitated casein. The acid used can be sulfuric, or hydrochloric, or lactic acid produced by fermentation of lactose in the skim milk. The degree of purity desired is obtained by optimizing the level of acidity and the coagulating temperature, as well as the efficiency of washing the coagulum with water. Furthermore, the sanitation conditions of the processing and storage are of great significance for the commercial value of edible caseins.

The traditional edible casein, produced by acid precipitation, without proper purification, is easily manufactured. This product has a gluey flavor that imposes limitations on its use in some foods.[215,214] However, its use in less flavor-sensitive food applications, such as bread and cereal fortification, has been suggested by Clausi et al.[46]

Casein and soy flour combinations also can be converted to a fine fibrous form. The fibers, when bonded together, result in a texture resembling meat.[55,226,249] Industry also produces sodium caseinate by dissolving casein in the presence of sodium hydroxide and drying it by the spray process. Casein for food industrial application can also be obtained by rennet coagulation, but this product is somewhat different in its chemical composition from casein and could be referred to as calcium-phospho-paracaseinate.

## Whey Proteins

Traditionally produced lactalbumin is water insoluble but is of high nutritional value. Its established uses have been limited to nonfunctional applications, or nutritional protein supplementation, as in pasta products.[228] For example, addition of 4% lactalbumin to common cereals will double the protein efficiency ratio (PER) of the cereal protein. In spite of these nutritional benefits, its food applicability is limited because of its gritty texture. However, undenatured whey proteins, recovered under controlled heat treatment, are dispersible, have excellent whip-imparting properties, are efficient water binders, and are useful in many foods.[278]

Native lactalbumins can interact with other proteins when heated. Such interactions might result in a great increase in the water-binding capacity of the lactalbumin. The theoretical background and practical application of complexes formed between lactalbumin and other proteins is discussed by Wingerd.[279]

Lactalbumins and lactoglobulins in the future will be produced by the currently developing membrane technology. These products are very promising as to their colloid chemical functionalities.

By controlling the ash content of the whey proteins and using electrodialysis, demineralized and delactosed whey concentrates have been made available commercially for food use.[13] Further developments include using whey proteins as additives to sweet cream for improved whipping performance[181] and as functional additives in ice creams to achieve slow melting.[182] Reference is made to an excellent review on the use of whey proteins by Mann.[158]

## Dairy Protein Coprecipitates

The highest nutritional efficiency in the dairy protein field can be obtained by balanced blends of casein and the whey proteins. Such preparations possess an excellent amino acid profile and render highly nutritious protein supplements.

Depending on the method of preparation, the solubility, water-binding, and viscosity-building capability of the products can be regulated for the best food technological performance. The first attempts to produce coprecipitates for food use were made by D'yachenko et al. in the U.S.S.R.[62] This work considered coprecipitation of casein and serum proteins in the presence of calcium chloride and envisioned use of the recovered proteins in bread baking, macaroni products, soups, vegetable purees, and other locally important food items. In the U.S., Engel and Singleton[68] worked out a continuous process for producing a dairy protein coprecipitate.

In Australia, Muller and Hayes[179] systematically studied the effects of pH, and calcium and sodium tripolyphosphates on the coprecipitation process and reported recovery of products that are excellently suitable for production of a milk biscuit. This application uses spray-dried, coprecipitated milk proteins in a dry blend with flour and other additives to prepare a hot biscuit mix for home use.

New techniques are described for rehydrating or rendering soluble, high-calcium phosphate caseins to increase their application in food systems by Roeper of the New Zealand Dairy Research Institute.[221] One of the most valuable properties of high-calcium phosphate casein products is their excellent flavor stability. These products do not readily develop musty off-flavors like acid casein and retain their initial bland flavor for at least 1 to 2 years under normal storage conditions. Hydrated, curd-like forms of the high calcium phosphate caseins are suitable for cheese pastes and spreads. In this form, the protein is in an insoluble — but — fully hydrated in form and able to be blended with natural cheeses as part of the processed cheese manufacture. The PER of the high-calcium phosphate caseins is 2.4 to 2.5.

The activities of the Australian recombining plants in Southeast Asia are described by Strange and Singh.[247] The Japanese food industry is very active in introducing coprecipitates for the manufacture of recombined dairy prodcts.[263] Another Japanese work reports on a coprecipitate that is stable at low pH values, such as those occurring in natural fruit juices. This development opens up the possibility of developing protein-fortified fruit drinks.[39] Coprecipitates are important in preparation of lactose-free baby food formulations, useful in the diets of lactose intolerant infants. Recently Russian scientists combined dairy proteins with blood proteins and suggested a milk-blood coprecipitation process.[206] The resulting product is dark in color but, according to the reports, has a pleasant flavor and is useful in a variety of foods. The above data illustrate only a few highlights. Detailed review articles have been published in France by Genin,[84] in the U.S. by Fox,[81] and most recently by Muller in Australia.[177]

In the manufacture of marshmallows and nougats, milk proteins or coprecipitates are important because of their whip imparting properties. In caramels, fudges, and similar candies, milk proteins contribute to flavor, body, and color. To obtain a smooth textural quality, milk protein characteristics must be such that during cooking conditions of candy, when coagulation of the milk protein takes place, protein aggregates formed will be small.

Color formation is controlled by the simultaneous presence of reducing sugars and proteins. Similarly, the characteristic milk caramel flavor is developed as a result of chemical interactions between reducing sugars and proteins.

The significance of milk proteins in chocolate manufacturing is highly complex and processing details are kept confidential. Apparently, the most essential feature in this application is development of flavor-stabilizing compounds that might be powerful antioxidants.

In the meat industry dairy proteins can be used to increase the waterbinding capacity of chopped meats. In sausage processing, the finely dispersed milk protein curd also acts as a binding agent, yielding the desirable chewy texture. Additional attributes of dairy proteins in sausage formulations include the control of shrinkage during storage and formation under slicing.

### Modified Dairy Proteins

The modified dairy proteins have been listed in Table 3. Included are caseinate salts, lactalbumin phosphates, microbiologically and enzymatically modified proteins, membrane and gel filtration-processed milk protein concentrates and, finally, protein hydrolysates.

Caseinate salts — The method of manufacture and characterization of concentrates from all milk proteins, obtained in a form of sodium, calcium, ammonium and sodium-calcium salts, and milk protein concentrate are discussed by Chojnowski et al.[45] The chemical composition, biological protein value, solubility, water-binding capacity, water absorption, buffer capacity, critical coagulation point, thermal stability, relative viscosity and stabilizing capability of emulsions have been determined. The rationally designed powdered milk protein concentrates maximize their food-supplementing value, and thus they can increase the extent of milk protein utilization in food industry. The economical use might contribute to alleviation of the shortage of this highly valued and relatively inexpensive animal protein in many countries.

Among the caseinate salts, sodium caseinate is by far the most significant as a food supplement. The caseinate salt group also has a unique standing from the legal point of view. For instance, in the U.S. it is declared as a food chemical derived from milk rather than as a dairy product. The caseinate salts enjoy an exempt position with regard to the Filled Milk Act and, consequently, can be used in conjunction with vegetable fats without violating the above law. The best quality of sodium caseinate is made from freshly precipitated casein, followed by solubilization with sodium carbonate or sodium hydroxide. The resulting colloidal solution of sodium caseinate is then spray dried. In this form it has an acceptable flavor and possesses excellent water-binding, whip-imparting, and emulsion-stabilizing capabilities. Sodium caseinate disperses well in water or melted fats. Upon addition of warm water during processing, sodium caseinate dispersions hydrate, and the resulting colloidal solution forms a base for subsequent emulsions.

Caseinates in emulsion technology — The rationale of sodium caseinate application in emulsion technology is based on its manifold chemical reactivity. The reactivity of caseinates resides in the unique distribution of the electrical charges on the polymeric molecule, its hydrogen-bonding capability, and its richness of hydrophilic and lipophilic bonding sites. The complex colloid chemical performance of caseinate can be accentuated by its reactivity with lecithins and carrageenans. In homogenized emulsion systems the caseinate molecule is anchored to the surface of fat droplets and acts synergistically with synthetic emulsifiers contributing to formation of encapsulating layers.

The encapsulating layers on the outside surface of emulsified fat particles are instrumental in stabilizing emulsions toward heat effects or toward detrimental effects of freezing. In this way emulsions prepared with sodium caseinate are resistant against the heat shock of pasteurization and will show increased freeze-thaw tolerance during frozen storage. The structure of encapsulating layers remains unharmed by heat during the spray-drying process. This property of caseinates is essential to the preparation of dried emulsions.

Dried emulsions are rehydratable without the coalescence of fat particles. On the other hand, caseinate layers of dried emulsions in the rehydrated state are sensitive to the mechanical shearing action of whipping devices commonly used in food processing such as the kitchen whisks, the wire whips and rotors, and mixers, as well as the dashers of ice cream machines. This shearing action causes whipping in the presence of air. On whipping, the caseinate encapsulating layer rearranges to a foam lamella system that possesses high tolerance and stability under many conditions. In this highly complex mechanical and physicochemical process, very fine textured whips are formed. The whipped forms of fat or protein-rich food formulations are highly palatable and suitable for many commercial applications. This concept is widely used in the preparation of toppings, cream substitutes, and numerous desserts.[122]

**Caseinates in meat products** — Use of sodium caseinate in the meat industry is in the most advanced stage of development in Germany and in several other European countries. The rationale for use of caseinates is based on the water-binding and fat-emulsifying capability of the caseinate salts in sausage meat emulsions.[232] The effect of cations on the water binding of caseinates in meat emulsions is elucidated in the investigations of Brendl and Klein.[35] These authors found that Ca, Mg, and Zn ions reduce the useful water binding of caseinates.

The stabilizing and texture-building properties of caseinate salts are recognized as effective meat binders. The subject of meat binders was very thoroughly reviewed by Saffle in 1968.[225] He concluded that there are no guidelines to clearly indicate and predict the useful effects of the various nonmeat additives on formulation and stability of mean emulsions. In recent years, vegetable proteins have gained more emphasis as meat binders than the dairy proteins. It is very likely that the relative high price of dairy ingredients compared to functionally designed vegetable protein products has tipped the balance for the dairy industry.

Another problem connected with use of dairy proteins in meats has been a legal one. Most food control authorities require that the added dairy proteins be quantitatively detectable in the meat products. Active research work was instituted towards this goal in Europe. Successful development of practical analytical methods in West Germany lead to approval for use of sodium caseinates in sausage products. In 1970, Olsman[196] described an analytical method that differentiates between casein and meat proteins by means of a urea-starch gel electrophoresis technique. By this method, 0.25% casein can be readily determined in various heated, mixed, and processed meat products.

Recently in Norway, further new analytical developments have been published for the detection of sodium caseinate in raw and heated meat products. A method by Nordal and Rossebo[193] distinguishes sodium caseinate in meat products from additives such as dry milk powders. Caseinate addition levels in the range of 0.2 to 0.4% can be determined in processed meats.

Calcium caseinate for supplementation of cereal products was found by Humphries and Roeper[111] more satisfactory than sodium caseinate or nonfat milk solids in wheat, pasta, and bread products. Mixed calcium, potassium, and sodium caseinates were used as the protein source of space food formulations by Dymsza et al.[63]

### Lactalbumin Phosphates

The colloidal effectiveness of lactalbumin is greatly enhanced in lactalbumin phosphate products that have been developed mainly in the U.S. Between 1966 and 1971, several patents were issued to McKee and Tucker[170] and Ellinger and Schwartz[64,67] that describe the preparation and application of these chemically modified dairy proteins. The authors recommend broad usage of these products in cake mixes, meats, self-raising flour bread and pizza as a replacement for nonfat milk solids. Further application also suggested for replacement of sodium caseinates in coffee whiteners, mellorines, and whipped toppings.

Lactalbumin phosphates are precipitated from whey under acid conditions in the presence of certain condensed phosphates. Although there is some evidence that this precipitation involves chemical reactions, it is presently throught to be mainly one of cation-anion interaction. The lactalbumin phosphates contain both the lactalbumin and the beta lactoglobulin of the milk in undenatured form and thus is highly advantageous over the denatured, nonhydrating whey protein.

### Microbiologically and Enzymatically Modified Dairy Proteins

Cottage cheeses, cheeses and cheese powders, the highly popular quark of Germany and rennet-treated milks are the topics for discussion in this category. In recent years, demand for high-protein foods has gained wide publicity, mainly because of their alleged value in limited calorie foods. Medical and regulatory aspects of protein-fortified foods are in the process of development. Nutrition labeling required of fortified foods may focus even greater attention on protein.

**Cottage cheese as food ingredient** — The different cottage cheese types occupy a key position in food formulation. Dairy proteins recovered as cottage cheese can vary in a broad spectrum with respect to flavor and consistency, depending upon starting material and treatment used.

In Anglo-Saxon countries, creamed cottage cheese is the most popular item of this class; however, the European dairy industry has explored a wider range of products in this category. Quark and "Frisch Käse" are used in Germany, while "Fromage Frais" is used in France. Annual per capita consumption of these cheese varieties is 5.2 kg in Germany and 3.4 kg in France. The high-nutritional value and the extensive versatility of cottage cheeses await a more pronounced use of this product as an ingredient by the food industry.[165]

The basic idea for introducing microbiologically precipitated and modified dairy proteins hinges on the possibility of improving the rather pasty and occasionally bland-tasting characteristics of the quark and Fromage Frais dairy protein concentrates. By suitable modifications and processing, these raw materials become smooth, creamy, and light textured. Their blandness can be considered an advantage because the microbiologically precipitated dairy proteins are compatible with many sweeteners and fruit flavors. Furthermore, their mouthfeel and body can be readily modified by addition of homogenized fat emulsions. Light, textured qualities can also be introduced by whipping.

The perishable nature of cottage cheeses was considered as a major disadvantage in formulated food use; however, by suitable formulations, freeze/thaw-stable features can be created, thereby rendering these products as valuable ingredients in frozen food systems.

An entirely different approach to the texturized cottage cheeses has been suggested by the U.S. Department of Agriculture USDA.[14] This group developed a new milk food ingredient by frying milk curd. This high-protein modified milk ingredient is reported to have meat-like texture and can be flavored and sweetened to suit various tastes. The product can thus be used in a meat flavored gravy. Further application research was reported on use of this modified milk ingredient in snacks, hors d'oeuvres and confections.[15,281] Pinkston further elaborated on the concept[205] and proposed puffed snacks from milk curd using starch-containing formulations. Flavor of the oil-fried dough can be enhanced by dusting the bite size puffed material with cheese powders or barbecue flavor.

**The use of quark** — Quark, or quarg, is an old word with new meanings in the English language. Webster recognizes it as an archaic work meaning "to croak" and as a constituent of elementary particles in nuclear physics.[270a] In the dairy field it refers to an edible milk protein product, commonly used in Germany. In its original German meaning, quark is a fresh, uncured cheese in bulk form without the familiar form-elements of cottage cheese. Quark is widely used in Europe because of its versatility and ease of preparation.[147] To produce quark, milk is coagulated exactly the way cottage cheese is made, but instead of cutting, cooking, and washing the curd particles, the whole coagulum is passed through a specially designed centrifuge. In this step, whey is separated from the solidified protein curd. The curd is then cooled and packaged in bulk. When the operation is carried out under good sanitary practices, the product has good shelf life under refrigeration until further processing takes place by the food manufacturer.

Outside the European Economic Community (EEC), in Eastern European countries, the U.S.S.R. is the leader in quark production for the food industry. It is estimated that 30 to 40 different food items, based on quark are commercialized in significant quantities. The quark is blended in these items with dairy or vegetable fat emulsions, and it is salted and mixed with spices or herbs.[155] Preservation and formulation experiences with quark have been reviewed by Schulz.[229] The Australian dairy industry also recognized the utility of quark and extended its applications in conjunction with seafoods and tangy dips, beyond its sweetened versions.

According to a survey conducted by Claydon and associates[47] at Kansas State University, the American consumer is likely to accept this product. Based on a limited market study, it was concluded that quark has considerable potential. As with yogurt, the most newly accepted dairy food in the U.S., advertising and promotion would be necessary for its acceptance.

**Renneted milk proteins** — Solubilized renneted milk proteins are used in Germany to a limited extent in some meat products. The use of rennet casein in foods was surveyed recently by Southward.[211]

### Protein Concentrates Prepared by Membrane and Gel Filtration Processes

The newly developed technology of reverse osmosis and gel filtration when applied to milk or whey, results in recovery of entirely new dairy protein concentrates.[106,117] These concentrates are basically different from the heat- or microbiologically separated products.

It is expected that, when reverse osmosis and gel filtration techniques are brought to commercial use in the dairy industry, they will replace many of the existing processes now used to produce dairy protein concentrates and make available to food processors concentrates with improved functional properties. The utility of these products for the food industry is now actively pursued, but has not yet reached commercial maturity. However, there have been many speculative aspects discussed in the literature during the last several years concerning potential uses of products made by membrane processes. Because of the complexity of this subject, the reader is referred to the works of McDonough,[168] Porter and Michaels,[212] Fenton-May,[70] and Jensen.[119]

### Milk Protein Hydrolysates

Milk protein hydrolysates, produced by either mineral acids or enzymes, have been used in the food industry for 30 to 40 years. Chemically, these products represent amino acid mixtures and, depending on the extent of the hydrolysis, contain a great variety of peptides. After hydrolysis, the reaction mixture is neutralized and purified, and in many instances the inorganic salts are removed by filtration or ion exchange. Often carbon treatments or adsorptive column fractionation techniques are also employed to remove color or undesirable flavors or to cause flavor resolutions. The flavoring spectrum of the hydrolysates covers a very wide range. Use levels are generally low and highly specific.

Organoleptically, there is a highly desirable appetite-increasing flavor or odor associated with these products. Because of the complex processing and sophisticated purification methods employed, however, the cost of dairy protein hydrolysates might be high. Nevertheless, certain unique flavor qualities can be obtained with the specially treated hydrolysates and this, in certain uses, will justify the price.

The use of hydrolysates in the diets of patients sensitive to protein intake has clinical value. Casein hydrolysates have been used for intravenous feeding of humans and have been used more recently for enteric feeding. Fundamental studies concerning the flavors of amino acids and peptides has been reviewed by Eriksen and Fagerson.[69a]

With regard to meat flavorings, Germany has special regulations[201] for use of dairy protein hydrolysates. Oberg and co-workers[195] proposed hydrolysing casein by means of trypsin. A patent was developed for other enzymatic hydrolysates[188] of dairy proteins with proteolytic enzymes and phosphatases. The effects of enzymatic hydrolysis on whey proteins when used as whipping and emulsifier aids was also investigated by Kuehler and Stine.[146] Baker and Bertok[29] found that certain peptides of casein that form stable foams tend to be antigenic.

The physical characteristics of currently available hydrolysates leave something to be desired, and adjustments to commercial requirements will be beneficial for their more general acceptance by the food industry. Most of the hydrolysates are highly water soluble but are also extremely hygroscopic and, therefore, have somewhat limited storage stability features unless extreme packaging protection is achieved.

Preparations of foods for children with PKU make use of casein hydrolysates from which the phenylalanine is removed by adsorption on activated carbon. The phenylalanine-free product is then supplemented with methionine, tyrosine, and tryptophan to compensate for the losses of these amino acids in the adsorption process. Vujinovic describes uses of these preparations in formulating foods for clinical purposes.[261]

Technological advantages of using hydrolyzed milk proteins in comminuted meat products are discussed by Pfaff.[202] Improvements in emulsifying and water-binding capacity were found in such products when nonmilk protein-containing products were used for comparison.

### Dairy Powders in Foods
*Technology and Uses of Milk Protein Concentrates*

The dairy powders are spray or roller dried dairy by-products that contain milk-derived proteins in conjunction with substantial amounts of lactose, fat, and residual milk minerals. These dairy powders could be best considered milk protein concentrates in comparison with the caseins, whey proteins, and coprecipitated milk proteins, which are milk protein isolates. The dairy powders category involves the various milks in dried form (whole, skim, and buttermilk powders), dried whey powders and their admixtures, and the cheese powders. Since the food supplementary value of these products is determined by their protein content, their discussion is justified under the milk protein group. However, whey powder, which is predominantly composed of lactose, also will be mentioned under the carbohydrate section.

The basic processing technology leading to dairy powders is essentially the same for all the members of this product group. It encompasses condensing, various fractionation steps, heat treatments, drying, sieving, conditioning for reconstitutibility, and packaging. Very specific combinations of the physical treatments, however, such as homogenization, time-temperature aspects of the heat treatment, determine the functional properties in different food systems.[94] The great majority of these processing specificities control the molecular conformation of the proteins and thus their solubilities, hydrating, and emulsifying properties.

Storage of dairy powders is generally not conducive to loss of nutritional values, provided the goods are kept in moisture-proof containers or bags, at temperatures not exceeding 20 to 25°C. The major components of the dairy powders are shown in Table 14.

The major food outlets of the dairy powders are carefully monitored by the American Dry Milk Institute in its annual census publication.[9] The global skim milk powder economic situation and outlook is discussed in two recent FAO publications.[74,74a]

Skim milk powder (nonfat milk solids) is economically the most important member of the dairy powder group. Types and levels of this commodity used in food products are analyzed in detail by Miller.[172]

Low-heat powder is used exclusively by confectioners and by dairies for making cottage cheese and in fluid products such as skim milk, buttermilk, chocolate drink, and half-and-half. High-heat dry milk is used in the manufacture of all other products except some baked goods that require medium-heat dry milk. Table 15 also shows the variation in the percentage of nonfat dry milk used in four main product categories and in specific products within each category.

Whole milk and buttermilk powders are of lesser economical significance in comparison to skim milk powder. Statistical and use information on these products is available from the publication of American Dry Milk Institute.[9]

Whey products, presently are widely used in food products in the U.S. Increasing availability of whey, coupled with development of professional sales/marketing forces by U.S. companies, has been instrumental in gaining acceptance of whey by food processors. Several general references on whey utilization in food products are available.[17,152,161-163,270,279] Based on the publications of the Whey Products Institute and USDA data, Lough summarized the whey supply and utilization picture in the U.S.[149a] Recent literature has described supplementing use of whey in dairy products,[32,82,236] bakery products,[16,51,92,93] candy products,[216,268] snacks,[116] meat products,[187] and beverages.[108,109] In addition, whey serves as a major component of milk-replacing blends that are enjoying increasing popularity in the baking industry.[128] Use of whey solids in conjunction with edible sulfhydryl reducing substances for production of extruded pasta products is the subject of a U.S. patent by Craig et al.[52]

Market-determined prices backed by U.S. government-supported prices for manufactured dairy products (nonfat dry milk, butter, and cheese) are instrumental in determining production for domestic cheese and whey. Whey production is directly determined by interaction of the forces of supply and demand in the U.S. cheese market. Cheese consumption has been increasing on a per capita basis in the U.S.[171] Table 16 gives production figures for 1966 to 1976 for hard cheese, cottage cheese, and the accompanying whey production. The 28.738 million pounds of fluid whey produced in 1974 in the U.S. converts to 1.720 million pounds of dry whey equal to 207 million pounds of high-quality protein.

Comparing these values to the whey consumption figure of 568,611,000 lb, dry whey gives an overall food-oriented utilization of 33%. Adding whey consumed as animal feed (535,643,000 lb) gives an overall utilization figure of 64%. It is estimated that approximately 70 to 74% of the fluid sweet whey in the U.S. is presently recovered and utilized while only 20% of the fluid acid whey is recovered as usable product. Thus the presently unused whey production in the U.S. is approximately 623,160,000 lb dry whey solids, equivalent to 75 million pounds of protein annually.

Effective whey utilization is required wherever cheese is manufactured. The U.S. dairy industry has a head-start in this field because actual policy decisions on part of the government and industry were made as early as the 1950s. Whether the world market could accommodate increasing supplies of the traditional products of dried whey, lactose, and lactalbumin, in view of escalating manufacturing costs and limitations in end-use application, became vital questions for Australia recently. As a result, a concentrated effort was taken by the Australian casein and cheese industry to utilize whey for food uses. Muller[178] reported on the future of whey utilization in Australia recently. The process offering the best prospect for initial fractionation of whey in manufacturing specialized edible products is ultrafiltration. The development of uses and markets for whey protein concentrate (WPC) depends on understanding its properties.

The high-nutritional value and solubility of WPC can be the basis for a number of uses. The manufacture of infant foods comes into this category as, in endeavouring to obtain a composition similar to that of human milk, processors need to increase the ratio of whey proteins to casein.

Another area which nutritional value is a factor of interest is in bread and baked goods, however, other functional properties become important in this field. WPC will only be acceptable in bread if proven to be more reliable than high-heat skim milk powder in effect on loaf volume and texture. Collaborative studies in Australia[178] are providing interesting differences between various forms of WPC in this respect. Current experiments have indicated that WPC from cheddar cheese whey can perform better than those from hydrochloric acid-precipitated casein whey. The reasons for this are being explored to learn more about the ill-understood loaf volume-depressant factor in skim milk and whey.

The good solubility of WPC over a wide pH range is a useful property being studied in the U.S. and New Zealand, where beverages containing up to 3% protein have been prepared over the pH range 2.5 to 7.0. Other products in which WPC appear useful are marshmallow and similar confectionery items, desserts of the soufflé type, meringues, frozen desserts, sherbets, and ice cream.

The ability of the whey proteins to gel on heating has been shown in Australian work [178] to be a useful property if WPC are used as an ingredient in yogurt — a finding likely to be applicable in a number of foods.

*Constraints in Milk Protein Concentrates, Isolates, and in Whey Production and Utilization*

**Economics** — An excellent summary of the economic factors involved in whey utilization can be found in work reported by Groves.[88] The amount of casein, coprecipitate, cheese/whey and nonfat dry milk produced in the U.S. is determined principally by economics, in that manufacturing milk will flow to the outlet of highest return to the producer. Government support pricing policy can play a major role in shifting this flow as desired. In the absence of deliberate government manipulation in favor of one product over another, the market determines actual production figures. Utilization of these protein sources is determined by several economic factors including market price (a function of production/distribution costs) vs. competitive protein sources; and technological/functional/nutritional properties of value to U.S. food producers.

**Energy** — The increasing cost of energy will favor less energy-intensive processes.[42] For example, the costs involved in spray drying many encourage greater utilization of fluid whey concentrates. Less energy-intensive membrane techniques such as reverse osmosis already have begun to play a role in whey utilization.

**Environment** — The concern with environmental quality will be a factor working in favor of increased whey utilization and recovery. The organic nutrients of whey, if they go unused, create an enormous burden on sewage systems and waterways. The biological oxygen demand (BOD) of whey ranges from 32,000 to 60,000 ppm. Specific values for cottage cheese whey are between 30,000 and 45,000 ppm, depending primarily on the specific cheese-making process used. Every 1000 gal/day of raw whey discharged as waste can impose a sewage load equal to that from 1800 people. Every 1000 gal of raw whey discharged directly into a stream requires for its oxidation the dissolved oxygen in over 4.500 million gallons of unpolluted water.[183] The newer membrane processes now being applied to whey can result in BOD reduction of raw whey up to 97% from an initial value of about 35,000 mg/ℓ to less than 1000 mg/ℓ.[166]

The U.S. Environmental Protection Agency (EPA) guidelines for dairy processing plant effluent water quality will be a strong force for consolidation of cheese operations into larger plants better able to meatthose guidelines.[68a] This consolidation will, in turn, increase the attractiveness of whey recovery and utilization.

Regulatory — Whey utilization is restricted by certain government regulations. Whey and whey products are presently excluded from a variety of consumer food items. For example, USDA regulations presently prohibit whey from being used in all but a small portion of the comminuted meats being produced in the U.S. Likewise, FDA regulations currently limit whey utilization in frozen desserts to 25% replacement of the milk solids. Another example is the FDA prohibition of whey or modified whey in macaroni products. In view of the highly complementary nature of whey and wheat protein, this restriction makes little nutritional sense. While some progress has recently been made in terms of less restrictive standards, significant market outlets remain closed to whey, and present regulations serve as a disincentive toward further whey utilization in food. Proposed new standards that could widen whey usage in foods were the subject of Congressional hearings in 1977.[113a]

Acceptance — Consumer and trade aceptance of whey as a food ingredient continues to grow in the U.S. One factor limiting even greater trade acceptance, however, is the large amount of lactose usually found in whey compared to amounts found in nonfat dry milk (73 and 55%, respectively). Its presence in whey can contribute to both functional and digestive problems in certain consumer applications.[112] Membrane separation techniques have been used to produce lactose-reduced whey protein concentrates.

### Significance of Dairy Powders in Foods

The dairy industry has enjoyed for some time an already existing channel to the food processing industry by means of merchandising its dried skim milk, whey, buttermilk, and cheese powders. These by-products of excellent functional quality and nutritional value are facing increasing competition from the vegetable protein sources, especially from soy products. The dairy industry will be able to retain this business sector only when high-quality products are maintained and the best efforts are put into practice to tailor products for specific applications.

Illustrative examples indicate the appearance of patented, versatile whey products. Collins[48] developed whey powders with high-oil adsorbing capabilities. Drews and Collins[59] described the use of these whey products in novel food applications. According to these patents, whey processed in a flowable particulate form is suitable to hold liquid fats. Its adaptation results in dry salad dressing with whey powder as carrier. Factors affecting use of dairy ingredients in baking have been thoroughly studied by Singleton and Robertson.[237]

Kinsella has proposed widening the functional uses of dairy by-products with respect to baking performance and their fortification with industrially accepted surfactants.[129] The chemistry of dairy powders with reference to baking has also been discussed in depth by Kinsella.[128] This work elucidates the scientific background of numerous functional features of dried milk, buttermilk, or whey ingredients in baked-food systems.

To ensure the food industry's satisfaction with the dairy powders, Kinsella[129] proposes intensive research activities in specific areas.

*Cheese Powders and Cheese Flavored Dairy Powders*

The industrial use of cheeses in foods has been favorably advanced by the production of cheese powders. These ingredients make it convenient for food manufacturers to put cheese flavors into baked goods and convenience items, and their use is widening considerably. Cheese powders are produced by dispersing the selected cheese type in skim milk or, preferably, in whey as a 50% slurry.[114] This slurry is heat treated for emulsification, homogenized, and finally spray dried. The expected storage life is about 1 year under suitable conditions. Spray-dried cheese powders can be produced at various flavor levels and with salt addition to suit the food manufacturers. In addition, other compatible ingredients such as WPC, whey, or other dairy ingredients may be blended.

Starting in 1960, cheese-flavored powders were developed. These products have gained broad acceptance by the food manufacturers because of good flavoring strength and relatively low costs in comparison to cheese powders. Many foods such as salad dressings, soups, and various kinds of baked goods are flavored by cheese. Aged cheese usually is used for this purpose but this item is expensive because of long storage.

Disclosures of U.S. patents by Watts and Nelson[266] and Knight[134] demonstrate the possibility of creating a low-cost composition with high flavoring strength that can be produced without aging. The products are made by inoculating a fluid, aqueous culture medium based on homogenized milk, skim milk and whey, with spores of *Penicillium roqueforti*. The mix is fermented for a few days. The fermentation liquid is then heat treated, condensed or dried, and used in a liquid or solid form, respectively.

### Dairy Fats in Food

As regard to the utility of all dairy products in the food industry, butter occupies the least unique position as a food supplement. Apart from flavor and the prestige of butter flavor, milk fat has little rational advantage over the other edible fats. Consequently, in practical applications there is a distinct trend away from milk fat except for organoleptic preferences. The penetration of milk fat into other foods on the principles of supplementation are few and restricted by a number of constraining factors. These factors are cost, health considerations, and physical-chemical properties.

The combined momentum of the cost-health constraints has slowed down the incentive of technological research in favor of butterfat and has accelerated the butterfat replacement activities. Thus butter became replaced by margarine and the anhydrous milk fat by other edible vegetable fats such as cooking oils and shortening. The cream-based dairy products are being replaced by the "filled" milk products such as vegetable fat-based coffee creamers, various whipped toppings, and mellorine type, or "filled", ice creams. It is highly probable that the momentum of the cost factor will be prevailing in the future. Even under optimum climatic and agronomic conditions for dairying such as those prevailing in New Zealand, butterfat is more expensive than competing vegetable oils. In other parts of the world, the disparity is even more emphasized and is further burdened by man-made legislative and economic barriers.

Analyzing the health constraint, with respect to the present and future, brings to the surface the controversial, animal fat-caused coronary heart disease theory. This controversial health issue, disregarding its scientific merits, has influenced the dietary habits of certain sections of the consuming population.

Another closely related constraining factor was based on the hypothesis that xanthin oxidase in homogenized milk is a significant factor in the etiology of atherosclerosis. The concept holds that this enzyme is absorbed from the intestinal tract along with the small particles of homogenized milk fat, circulates, and is deposited in the arterial and myocardial cells, where it reacts with the plasmal moiety of cell membranes. The resulting lesions represent the first damage to the arterial cells; cholesterol and fibrin infiltration in the arterial wall and scarring of the myocardium are thought to occur subsequently.

This concept was investigated by Carr et al.[43] at the request of the Food and Drug Administration in 1975. The report concludes that the evidence supporting the hypothesis is inconclusive because the absorption of xanthine oxidase is negligible in the plasma, and none occurs in the lymphatic system. Later on, Clifford[21] did not find hardening of arteries in rabbits treated with massive doses of xanthin oxidase. The net result of the controversial issue was the increasing replacement of butter fat by polyunsaturated vegetable fats in the diets of consumers.

Recent developments in dairy science have brought a new dimension that focuses on the potential solution of the fat problems. New feed management methods resulting in a milk with a more highly polyunsaturated milk fat content are being developed. The origin of this new, imaginative approach will be discussed in depth at the end of this chapter. At present, conventional butter (standardized at an 80% fat minimum), butter oil, anhydrous milk fat, and ghee in India[137] are essentially the only commercialized forms of dairy fat. Thus this important food resource lacks the versatility of the chemically modified, competing vegetable oils. The technological options for the modification of butter fat are in the hands of dairy scientists. The latitude of their potential activities could be as broad as were the explorations of the lipid chemists' with respect to improvements of vegetable fat resources. Vegetable fat producers adjusted the properties of their products to the food processors' requirements and to the consumer's convenience by means of deodorization, fractionation, hydrogenation, interesterification, and purposeful blending. This technology is adaptable to dairy fats, and by its use increased versatility of butter-based fats can be demonstrated for the potential uses. Whether these approaches could turn the tide in favor of increased milk fat usage will depend on the relative future strength of the other two constraining factors, namely cost and health.

During the late 1960s, technological developments emerged that might propose new options for the use of dairy fats (Table 17). An attempt will be made to highlight some of these new concepts and to generate ideas toward new application opportunities.

*Butterfat Fractionation*

Butterfat can be separated into high-, medium-, and low-melting fractions. This is achieved by melting butter oil and letting crystallization take place first at a higher and then at a somewhat lower temperature. At the selected temperature, the solidified part of the fat can be easily separated from the liquid portion by pressing. The liquid portion, on further cooling, will again exhibit partial crystallization. Repeated separation of the solidified portion will result in a lower-melting solid fraction. Because these subsequent fractions have different compositions and functional properties, their applicability in food formulations will be wider than that of the unfractionated butter oil.

The high-melting butter components are superior for use in chocolate and ice cream manufacture and spray-dried butter emulsions, whereas, the lower-melting fractions blended with unfractionated butter will crease spreadability in table use. Swedish investigators[23] described the manufacturing operations of the fractionation process both for butter oil and for fresh cream processing.[24]

Anhydrous milk fat is suitable for bulk distribution and has favorable storage characteristics. It can be used for reconstituted liquid dairy products, and its reformulation for special-purpose butters or shortenings is envisioned.

The butter fractionation process might be the starting point of making milk fat just as versatile to the food industry as the vegetable fat producers made their various raw materials. A review on milk fat fractionation was recently issued in Germany.[260]

### Cultured Emulsified Vegetable and Dairy Fat Blends

The Swedish milk fat industry recently has taken the initiative on this controversial step. By the end of 1969, a new milk fat-vegetable fat blend called Bregott® was launched. This is a butter-like product with a ratio of 80% milk fat to 20% high-quality polyunsaturated vegetable oils. It is spreadable even at refrigerated temperatures, and is standardized to contain about 80% fat, 16% maximum water, and 1.4% salt. Bregott® is fortified with vitamins A and D, and its storage stability is satisfactory for retail distribution.[12]

### Spray-Dried Butter

Spray-dried butter brings convenience to the bakery since it is supplied in a storage-stable, free-flowing form. Furthermore, it gives the dry cake mix industry the opportunity to use butter fat.[11] Recent work on this product has been done at the University of Wisconsin. Spray-dried butter can be produced from heavy cream and butter oil in the presence of milk solids.[34]

The moisture content has to be reduced to 0.1% in spray-dried butter.[229,231] Spray-dried butter rehydrates readily to an emulsion that is organoleptially indistinguishable from cultured cream butter. The origin of spray-dried butter goes back to Hansen in Australia.[99] His product was made from butter oil by adding sodium caseinate, emulsifiers, and citrate salts. Subsequent German and U.S. developments avoided use of nondairy additives. Evaluation of these products in cake baking gave satisfactory results; however, addition of suitable emulsifiers might be useful for better baking performance.

### High Heat-Treated Butter

This approach was studied in Russia and in the U.S.; its final utility remains to be seen. Heat-treated butters have better keeping qualities than ordinary butter. In Eastern European countries, such products are used in conjunction with processed meat products.

### Polyunsaturated Fats via the Cow

McGillivray[169] gave an excellent summary and evaluation of this bioengineering approach. The modification of the composition of milkfat has been developed in Australia through feeding cows with suitably protected polyunsaturated fats. According to McGillivray:*

"It is well known that the diet of dairy cows frequently contains a high proportion of polyunsaturated vegetable fats, but that these are hydrogenated during the normal processes of rumen digestion. The Australian development involves encapsulating suitable polyunsaturated vegetable fats in a coating which protects them from bio-hydrogenation in the rumen, but which permits normal digestion in the abomasum and intestines. In a number of trials, these protected feeds were fed to cows at the rate of 1500 g per day, which appeared to be equivalent to half to two-thirds of the total fat in the diet. This resulted in a substantial increase in the degree of polyunsaturation of the milkfat. The increase in polyunsaturation in the milkfat is at the expense of the saturate fatty acid $C_{14}$, $C_{16}$, and $C_{18}$, all of which are reduced by about one-third.

---

\*   From McGillivray, W. A., in *Milk Products of the Future,* Rothwell, S., Ed., Society of Dairy Technology, Wembley, England, 1976, 37-41. With permission.

The milkfats produced are substantially softer than normal and, although this is advantageous for some purposes, it is likely to create problems in processing and packing. Because of the high degree of polyunsaturation and relatively low levels of natural antioxidants, the milkfat is also highly susceptible to oxidative rancidity, and special precautions must be taken in the handling and processing of milk from cows fed these protected fats. Suitable antioxidants must be added to these 'polyunsaturated' butters and related products. The feeding of protected fats must, of course, be continued throughout lactation, the fatty acid composition of the milkfat rapidly reverting to normal on cessation of feeding.

The original methods of preparing and encapsulating fat would probably be uneconomical commercially, but the process is being rapidly simplified and cheapened. Large quantities of protected lipids are now being produced both in Australia and New Zealand, with a view of carrying out semi-commercial trials in the near future.

This bio-engineering approach to changing the composition of ruminant milkfat was developed originally with a view to producing 'polyunsaturated' butters and other dairy products which would compete with 'polyunsaturated' margarines and other fats. Even on the most optimistic estimates, protected lipids will be relatively expensive to produce, and 'polyunsaturated' milkfats might be expected to cost up to U.S. $0.45 per kg more to produce than normal milkfat. However, the technique of feeding protected lipids to ruminants would appear to have much wider application than this, and the real interest in the process in the dairy industry is likely to be the production of a variety of speciality 'monounsaturated' and 'polyunsaturated' fats which could extend the end usage of milks and which could usefully, and possibly more economically, augment the fractionation process referred to earlier for producing the softer-type milkfats.''

### Nutritive and Supplementary Value of Dairy Fat

The nutritive value of milk fat rests entirely on its energy, vitamin A content, and content other fat-soluble vitamins. Milk fat is almost completely digestible, and its food technological features, texture, and palatability increase its food value. There are, however, neither unique nutritional nor food technological values in butter that would predicate its preferred use in food manufacture or cooking over other fats suitably prepared. In fact, over the years we have seen the opposite trend: butter has been replaced gradually by other edible fats in spreads, baked goods, whipables, and even in dairy cream-based products.

There are strong tendencies to associate the occurrence of coronary diseases in man with dietary intake of animal fats. These statements lead to deep-seated controversies, which stand unresolved a this time.

### Dairy Carbohydrates in Foods

The major dairy carbohydrate is lactose. Lactose can be modified chemically to result in closely related products with different physical or food technological properties (Table 18). Upon hydrolysis, lactose can be transformed to a glucose-galactose mixture, which is usually recovered as a syrup of somewhat sweeter taste and of higher solubility than lactose.[271] Lactose, on alkaline inversion, can be transformed into lactulose which is a 4-*O*-β-D-galactopyranosyl-D-fructose; this product has different nutritional properties than lactose and is considerably sweeter.

### Lactose

Lactose is presently the target of a considerable nutritional controversy, relating to its intolerance by certain individuals. Nevertheless, lactose deserves to be discussed from the food technological point of view because it has valuable properties when used with discretion by the food technologist.

Lactose as a food supplement is considered on the basis of some of its physical, chemical, and organoleptical properties. Nickerson,[190] in analyzing the food uses of lactose, arrives at the following motivational priority listing:

1.    Relative sweetness
2.    Browning capability in foods
3.    Alteration of crystallization patterns

4.    Flavor accentuation
5.    Fermentation and nutritive attributes

**Relative sweetness of lactose** — Sweetness perception studies on food carbohydrates conducted 50 years ago assigned a very low sweetness level to lactose in comparison to sucrose, glucose, fructose, etc. Recent studies conducted in a broader concentration range of customary sugar levels in various food systems, however, indicated that lactose is about one half to one quarter as sweet as sucrose in the respective concentration range of 0.5 to 20.0% solids (Table 19). The somewhat lower sweetness level of lactose can be advantageous in the preparation of desserts where a more balanced sweetness might increase the overall organoleptic appeal of the products.

**Controlled browning of lactose under heat treatment** — Lactose, a reducing sugar in contrast to sucrose, will undergo browning in the presence of amino acids or proteins. Guy[91] has shown that browning is improved if lactose alone is added to the formula of baked goods such as yellow cakes, but even greater color is produced if milk proteins from whey or nonfat milk solids are present to interact with lactose. Jelen and Jadlav[118] used lactose for controlled color development in french fried potatoes.

**Solubility and crystallization habit of lactose in food systems** — In food systems where concentrated sugar solutions are involved, textured properties are greatly influenced by the solubility and crystallization properties of the constituent carbohydrates. Lactose as a supplement in such foods results in useful effects that are exploited to great advantage. In blends of lactose and sucrose, the crystal habits of both sugars is changed, and softer, smoother crystals are produced. This approach appears appropriate for improving qualities of certain candy and confectionary products when lactose is used as a supplement.[191] In dry whipped toppings, lactose-containing formulations render a favorable encapsulating layer around the emulsified fat globules.[83b]

**Lactose as flavor enhancer** — In low-fat fluid milk products, extensive research was carried out during the 1950's to improve the flavor acceptability by the addition of nonfat milk solids. From the work of Pangborn and Dunkley, it became apparent that the actual flavor changes were caused by the added lactose.[198] The flavor-enhancing effects of lactose in cocoa-containing products was also extensively studied, both in liquid and solid food systems by Arnott and Bulloch[22] and Goller and Kube.[85] It seems that lactose can be used to supplement other foods to accentuate flavors and thus increase consumer acceptance. Full potential of this approach requires sharply targeted application work and, in many cases, changes in the legal definitions of certain standardized food items.

**Specific attributes of lactose in fermentation and nutrition** — Since lactose is not fermented by baker's or brewer's yeast, in contrast to glucose, added lactose in baked goods, beer, or wine could influence the properties of the finished goods. For instance, breads supplemented by small quantities of lactose have unique toasting properties because the lactose remains available for browning after the bread dough fermentation. Similarly, in beer, added lactose survives the yeast fermentation and, through its low sweetness level, balances the bitter flavor notes. Foods in which a substantial portion of the lactose is fermented to lactic acid will be discussed under the heading of "Cultured Dairy Products as Food Supplements."

*Enzymatically Hydrolyzed Lactose*

A new technology is in emergence which could be instrumental for a gainful utilization of large quantities of lactose in the food industry. It is projected that about 300 million pounds of lactose in the U.S. alone could be converted into food-grade syrups and sweeteners by the use of enzymatic treatments with $\beta$-galactosidase and glucoseiso-merase. The overall economy and large-scale industrial feasibility of this operation has yet to be determined. Vigorous research activity in the related industries promises larger-scale trials in the near future according to Shukla.[234]

Lactase ($\beta$-galactosidase) is the enzyme that hydrolyzes lactose into glucose and galactose.[277] This hydrolysate could be exposed to another enzyme (glucose isomerase), which transforms glucose to fructose, a ten times sweeter sugar than lactose. Such resulting syrups would be suitable for the replacement of the sucrose in large-scale food applications. This new technology is a good answer to the solution of the lactose intolerance and environmental pollution problems.

### Nutritional Aspects of Milk Carbohydrates
### Galactose and Galactosemia

Congenital galactosemia is a genetically transmitted disease characterized by inability to metabolize galactose or the galactose portion of lactose. This disease affects approximately one baby out of 40,000 due to the lack of the enzyme, which is responsible for the transformation of galactose to glucose in the genetically normal human infant. As a consequence of this in-born metabolic error in the enzyme machinery of the body, galactose builds up in the liver, and the babies become ill and frequently die. Almost all surviving galactosemics are mentally retarded, and the only way to treat the disease is to recognize it quickly and remove all galactose and lactose from the patients diet. Obviously, since babies drink only milk, we cannot do this without special dietary preparations. There are several products for the feeding of galactosemic infants available.[50] Guidelines for the nutritional regimens to be used in the treatment of galactosemia have been recommended by Koch and coworkers.[136]

The faulty metabolism is due to a defect in the enzyme galactose-1-phosphate-uridyl-transferase that is necessary to convert galactose-1-phosphate to utilizable glucose. Accumulation of galactose-1-phosphate in body tissue is thought to be responsible for damage to the developing brain, liver, lens of the eye, and other organs. The damage caused in the lens of the eye manifests itself as a "galactose-cataract". The weanling rat is extremely sensitive to this disease when maintained on a lactose-containing diet. This must result from the galactose part of the lactose, because if the rats are fed either galactose or human milk alone, they also develop cataracts, they do not if they are fed glucose alone.[33]

### Nutritional Aspects of Lactose

Reviews on the physiological nutritional effects of lactose appeared during the 1950s by Duncan[60] and Atkinson et al.[27] The essential findings at that time were that young mammals can tolerate large quantities of lactose, but the tolerance decreases with age. Observations as to the dietary origin of lactose or galactose cataracts were discussed, but the topic was left unresolved. Specific physiological effects of lactose and galactose had been found that have not been observed with other sugars. Lactose-containing dairy products were recommended as an effective supplement to the diet of babies and growing children.

Lactose, from a nutritional point of view, has been the target of a considerable controversy since 1969. This is based on the indigestibility of lactose by persons and population groups lacking the necessary enzymes. Where there is no deficiency in the digestive enzyme systems of the consuming individuals, however, lactose has unique nutritional contributions. For instance, the supplementation of cow's milk in infant formulations has proved to result in more desirable body composition for the growing human body than unsupplemented cow's milk diet. Lactose favorably influences the microflora of the human digestive system. It has also been observed by Ali and Evans[6] that the utilization of calcium is improved by lactose in the diet.

*Lactose Intolerance*

Human infants and adults of certain ethnic groups suffer from deficiency of β-galactosidase. The physiological implications are currently being examined by various agencies, such as the U.S. Office of Child Development and the Protein Advisory Group of the Food and Agricultural Organization (FAO) of the United Nations. The following excerpt from the Protein Advisory Group (PAG) of the FAO addresses this issue:

"During the last few years, reports have appeared in the world medical literature on the occurrence of low intestinal lactase (exact term: β-galactosidase) activity on large groups of apparently healthy, non-white populations in different parts of the world. Some of the reports and many articles in the lay press have concluded that milk consumption by these people may lead to untoward reactions in the form of gastrointestinal disturbances ('milk intolerance') and may interfere with proper utilization of milk nutrients.

It would be highly inappropriate, on the basis of present evidence, to discourage programmes to improve milk supplies and increase milk consumption among children because of the fear of milk intolerance."[213]

Both the Food and Nutrition Board of the National Academy of Sciences/National Research Council and the American Academy of Pediatrics have published statements indicating that milk should remain in the diet of children. Both groups agreed that the incidence of severe symptoms resulting from lactose intolerance is far too low to warrant any recommendation to reduce or eliminate milk from the diet. People who would experience severe enough symptoms to warrant elimination of milk from the diet should either eat low-lactose dairy foods such as cheese and cultured dairy foods or drink smaller quantities of milk more frequently and with other foods.[143a]

The background of the lactose intolerance problem is discussed by Shukla.[234] The enzyme lactase is a specific β-galactosidase and acts only upon the carbohydrate lactose by breaking the beta $1 \rightarrow 4$ glycosidic linkage, thus liberating the monomeric sugars glucose and galactose. This action takes place primarily in the small intestine. The monosaccharides then enter the bloodstream and finally reach the liver cells, where they are metabolized. The enzyme is not present in the intestine of the embryo or the fetus until the middle of the last stage of gestation; the activity attains a maximum immediately after birth (Figure 5). Within 1.5 to 3 years, the activity approaches a low level for human beings.

The symptoms of lactose intolerance are the same whether an individual lacks sufficient β-galactosidase activity or has ingested an amount of lactose that exceeds the hydrolytic capacity of the available β-galactosidase in the intestine. Data collected seem to indicate that many more groups all over the world are intolerant to lactose than are tolerant. The real lactose tolerance is actually confined to northern Europeans, approximatel 90% of whom tolerate lactose, and the members of two nomadic, pastoral tribes of Africa, of whom about 80% are tolerant. The tolerant group, therefore, represents a minority of the human species. Kretschmer[144] concludes that lactose tolerance is a genetically transmissible and dominant character. This would suggest that the offspring from tolerant-intolerant parents would be tolerant and that more tolerant populations should emerge in the future. The implications of lactose intolerance in a sound nutritional policy and milk-based food product development should be considered in the future. This is not to say that milk and milk products should be discarded from our diets. For most people, even after the age of four, drinking moderate amounts of milk has no adverse effects and is actually nutritionally beneficial. The attempts to reduce the lactose content of milk powders, concentrated cheese whey, and yogurt, however, are definitely in the interest of human nutrition in general. A review on the clinical aspects of lactose intolerance is available by Rosensweig.[223] Original clinical work is reported by a number of authors associated with Cornell,[244a] Johns Hopkins,[30a] Universities and the Massachusetts Institute of Technology.[83a]

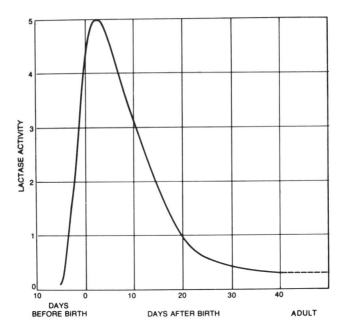

FIGURE 5. Lactase activity curve before and after birth in rats. The enzyme activity is expressed in relative units. The shape of the curve is found to be the same for all the species. (Reprinted with permission from Kretschmer, N., *Sci. Am.,* 227(10), 73, 1972. Copyright© 1972 by Scientific American, Inc. All rights reserved.)

## New Dairy Products with Lactase Treatments

The use of β-galactosidase[132] as a solution to the problems of lactose intolerance, whey utilization, and lactose crystallization, as well as a means for producing sweetener for the dairy and food industry, has been well recognized.[107,209] A great variety of product development work has been done by investigators all over the world attempting to alleviate the lactose intolerance problem in dairy products.[132,140-142,275]

The question of reducing the lactose content of market milk, sweet whey, and acid whey takes on a different dimension, including the issues of flavor, government regulation, and especially economics and industrial feasibility. It is reasoned that the application of immobilized β-galactosidase and the process technology of bioreactors should be an answer to such questions. A two-enzyme reactor, using β-galactosidase in one stage and the glucose isomerase in another, may be a good route to take for dairies large enough to install an ultrafiltration and reverse-osmosis system coupled to such a reactor. This system will be to produce whey protein concentrate, food syrups, and sweeteners while alleviating sewage disposal problems.

Frozen milk concentrates in which the lactose was enzymatically cleaved have been produced on a considerable scale for reconstitution as a fluid milk beverage, mostly for use on ships and by the services.[245,246] Crystallization of lactose in the frozen concentrate is a problem from the standpoint of difficulty in reconstitution, but more importantly because of its effect on the stability of proteins therein. Lactose hydrolysis prevents the formation of lactose crystals; hence, the protein stability is increased.[252]

Another use of β-galactosidase lies in new possibilities for breadmaking.[207,208] Skim milk solids are used in bread contributing about 1.5% lactose based on weight of flour used. The lactose so incorporated is not yeast fermentable and imparts no additional sweetness overall. Hydrolysis by β-galactosidase to glucose and galactose would make the former available for fermentation and the latter for the formation of crust color.

A sample of skim milk solids devoid of lactose would prove to be more suitable for protein efficiency ratio determinations, a necessity that may arise when whey proteins are formulated to supplement the quality of cereal proteins in simulated and specialty food products.

Lactose intolerance as a factor for nutritionally sound dairy product design and commercialization is discussed by Mauron.[167] It is the role of the responsible food industry to collaborate everywhere with the nutritionist and health services in order to develop technologically and economically sound as well as locally adapted solutions to problems like that of lactose intolerance.

### Lactulose and Other Oligosaccharides of Milk

The presence in milk of carbohydrates other than lactose has become evident through the advent of chromatographic analytical and preparative methods.[60] The most imporant finding on this field of dairy chemistry was the discovery of the "bifidus factor", its significance in infant nutrition and its relationship to lactulose and other oligosaccharides of milk. Milk preparations enriched with lactulose and other bifidus-active oligosaccharides have clinical value in supporting predominantly *Lactobacillus bifidus* intestinal flora in human infants. Thus this development contributed significantly to the supplementation of baby food preparation and achieving a nutritionally and physiologically more perfect simulation of the human milk.[3] Food supplementing applications of whey products mainly based on their lactose contents have been summarized by Webb at the 1970 Whey Utilization Conference* as follows:

"Whey can make valuable contributions in food processing. Lactose, the dominant component, is responsible for most of the flavor intensification observed when whey or lactose is added to many food formulas. The high lactose content seems to enhance flavor in somewhat the same manner that monosodium glutamate contributes to food flavor. There is also an improvemnt in the physical attriute of flavor in the creation of a pleasant 'mouth feel'.

Whey acts as a tenderizer in those foods where a soft or delicate structure is desired. This is in contrast to the firm adhesiveness of skim milk containing products which are lower in lactose and higher in protein. The tenderizing properties of whey are especially noticeable in the mild brittleness of cookies, the cake-like texture of baked goods, and the delicate gel structure which may be obtained in starch pudding mixes. As in cookies, whey produces a tender crispness in pie or pizza crust. In many products, whey helps retain moisture and freshness because of its high lactose content and because the lactose may often be present in the food in amorphous condition.

The color produced in foods containing whey is an attractive golden brown developed during heating in the presence of lactose and the nitrogenous components of whey. This color is especially sought after in the crust of bread, rolls, and cake, as well as on the surface of breaded meat, fish, and similar items that contain whey in the batter mix with which they may be covered."

Lactulose is not metabolized in the upper intestinal tract because the small intestine of man contains no enzymes capable of splitting it into its component monosaccharides. It therefore reaches the colon virtually unchanged. There it is degraded by intestinal bacteria into low-molecular weight organic acids, mainly lactic and acetic acids. The reduction of fecal pH might be regarded as the major mechanism whereby lactulose reduces blood ammonia levels and improves symptoms in patients with portosystematic encelopathy.[143] A commercially feasible process to produce lactulose was developed by Guth and Tumerman.[90]

### Lactobionic Acid, Lactic Acid and Salts

A number of derivatives of lactose with potential food technological or nutritional supplementing capabilities have been prepared and developed commercially to a lim-

---

* From Webb, B. H., Utilization of Whey in Foods and Feed, in Proc. Whey Utilization Conf., ARS-73-69, Agricultural Research Service, U.S. Department of Agriculture, Washington, D.C., 1970, 102—111.

ited extent. Mainly, the salts of lactobionic acid and lactic acid can be placed into this group. Lactobionic acid is made by the electrolytic or microbial oxidation of lactose. Its calcium salt is flavorless and highly soluble in water.

Lactic acid salts are made by fermentation of the lactose content of whey. The most commonly used is calcium lactate — a good nutritional source of calcium.

### Whey as a Source of Lactose and Its Use in Foods

The predominance of lactose in whey is the reason why this highly versatile industrial food ingredient of dairy origin is being discussed in the dairy carbohydrate section. Whey, as an industrial dairy ingredient, is much more than a source of lactose; it is even much more than a dairy waste product in the eyes of the food technologist. Dried whey is really a family of products with many food technological features, some of which are native, with others developed by the whey processor with food-industrial utility in mind.

It can be said that the diversification of whey powder for many food uses is one of the best examples of how a dairy ingredient with proper functionality can obtain an important supplementing position in manufactured foods. "The production and marketing of edible grade whey", writes Weisberg,[272] "has been one of the real successes in the past decade. This product has moved from a very small volume production on the order of a few million pounds, to a few hundred million pounds."[272] The successful graduation of dried whey from the status of an obscure dairy waste product to a profitable, functionally designed dairy ingredient targeted for food use was the result of many factors. A study of this development is enlightening for bringing other dairy ingredients along the same road to full acceptance. The elements of this development were:

1. Basic processing improvements to obtain a sanitary product.
2. Rigorous quality control for uniformity.
3. Establishment of a diversified line of products in response to realistic needs.
4. Imaginative application research conducted in cooperation with the various branches of the food industry.
5. Increasing the functionality features through additives.
6. Realistic pricing policy.

Descriptions of the many successful applications of the various whey products in the food industry are so numerous that, for reasons of practicality, reference is made to the most important recent major reviews of subject.[13,125,138,150,152,153,159,160,269,270,274]

The progress of whey utilization is well recorded in the series of Proceedings of the Whey Products Conferences (1970, 1972, and 1974) published by the Agricultural Research Service, U.S.D.A.[253-256,276] These publications review legal, technological, commercial, application, and, to a certain extent, basic scientific problems. The progress both on food and feed aspects of whey are also recorded.

Lactose, more often as a pure sugar rather than a component of dried whey, is used extensively as a carrier or extender in pharmaceuticals (e.g., in pills) or in flavor concentrates. For this purpose, lactose itself is practically tasteless, colorless, and stable. It absorbs pigment and supplements natural flavors. The properties of pharmaceutical-grade lactose are defined in the *Pharmacopeia of the United States of America*.[203]

Since the protein of whey is not coagulated at high acidity, whey may be used to make fruit-flavored dairy products. Whey will improve the body and flavor of sherbets, jams, fruit drinks, tomato beverages, or tomato soup. Whey can contribute whipping properties that will permit the incorporation of air upon whipping of food mixes, particularly for a whey-sugar mixture. Some examples of foods in which whey may be utilized are shown in Table 20.

It is sometimes pointed out that whey powders contain the main proportion of the skim milk nutrients, practically all the lactose and vitamins present in the milk, and a significant part of the minerals and proteins. However, it is the unbalanced relative proportion of these nutrients in the whey solids that complicates the use of dried whey products in human and animal nutrition from a nutritional point of view. The high mineral content is a problem when whey is utilized in baby foods, and the low protein content is a problem in the manufacture of whey protein products.

### Milk Minerals and Micronutrients as Food Supplements

The discussion of milk minerals and micronutrients will be restricted to those which, at the customary dietary intake or food technological application level, contribute significantly to the daily nutrient requirement of man. Data supplying information on milk salt constituents, certain trace elements, and vitamins in milk have been compiled by Johnson in 1974;[120] and in dairy products by Posati and Orr in 1976[213] (see Table 1).

The significance of milk as a supplier of minerals or vitamins for the diet of a large population group is best illustrated in terms of these critical nutrients and their percentage share in the American diet (Table 21). These data illustrate the singularity of milk as a supplementary source of key mineral and vitamin nutrients for the human diet. The public health aspect of the relative richness of most milk products in calcium and phosphorus is particularly important because there is no other comparable calcium food source available in the American diet. Thus the high calcium and phosphorus occurrences in milk underline the food supplementing power of dairy products.

The dietary iron contribution of milk products is low, which deserves corrective fortification. The precedent history of vitamin D fortification of milk should be considered as a model for the iron fortification. Native milk contains inadequate quantity of viamin D with respect to the requirements of the human body and growing child.

On the other hand, milk, fortified with synthetic vitamin D in the process of ordinary milk pasteurization-homogenization, became a standard source of this important vitamin. Most of the vitamin D in the American diet comes from milk even though the vitamin is added to this natural foodstuff.

Milk also provides other major or trace elements of nutritional significance. Among these, magnesium, copper, cobalt, and zinc deserve some consideration as potential supplementary sources.[34a]

### The Effect of Customary Technological Processing on the Vitamins of Dairy Products

Various time and temperature relations are used in dairy product heat processing to achieve sanitary standards and some preservation. The heat treatments may vary as to their basic technology, but all processes aim to preserve milk nutrients. Vitamins A, D, and riboflavin are usually not affected by heat processing. Thiamine and vitamin $B_{12}$ may suffer a 10 to 20% loss under the conditions of pasteurization or ultra-high-temperature short-time treatment. Vitmin $B_6$ is the most prone to heat-caused destruction leading to nutritional deficiency, especially during storage times beyond 180 days.[26,34a,137,210]

In the designing of food formulations when the supplementing capability of dairy products is considered, it should be remembered that fat-free products will not supply the fat-soluble vitamins, and fat-enriched protein poor fractions will be proportionately impoverished in the water-soluble vitamins. Similarly, calcium is present in the aqueous phase of milk products and not in the fat-enriched phase because calcium is supplied in the form of either colloidal calcium phosphate, calcium caseinate, or casein in which calcium is bound to the phosphorylated proteins.

*Dairy Products and Dietary Calcium Consumption*

The contribution of dairy products to the dietary calcium intake in the U.S. is especially significant in view of declining per capita dairy consumption. Calcium is one of the major mineral nutrients consumed in amounts less than those recommended. It has been determined that 30% of the American public consumes 20 to 40% less than the currently recommended 800 mg calcium per day. This may, in part, account for a trend toward decreased bone density with advanced age, which has been noted by researchers in recent years. A high phosphorus intake due to increased red meat and soft drink consumption may also be involved. A decrease in bone density may in turn be linked to higher incidences of osteoporosis and periodontal disease.

It has been estimated that about 6 milion spontaneous fractures due to osteoporosis occur anually in the U.S. among people 45 or more years old. Almost 5 million of these fractures occur in women. The unfortunate thing about bone disorders is that most of the calcium has been withdrawn from the skeleton before deficiency symptoms are detected, which means that it is too late for corrective measures to have any significant influence. An insufficient intake of calcium-containing food in the teenage years, especially among young women, sets the stage for greater bone problems with increasing age. Child bearing plus the stress of lactation coupled with poor dietary habits leads to poor skeletal health. A 10-year study on the clinical manifestation of inadequate bone health emphasizes the importance of maintaining proper calcium intake throughout life.[5]

Several factors have been suggested as affecting dietary calcium absorption and utilization. Among these are nutrients common to milk such as lactose, lysine, and phosphopeptides of casein. Hence, information now available points toward the efficacy of milk in the management and prevention of bone demineralization and certain nutritional disease states, as well as being a critical food for the general nutritional health of normal individuals.

*Calcium in Bone Health*[186]

Dietary regimens for the prevention or treatment of bone disease, particularly osteoporosis and periodontal disease, must be designed to result in a state of positive calcium balance. It must be remembered, however, that since osteoporosis involves the loss of bone matrix and minerals rather than minerals alone, nutrients other than calcium, (e.g., protein, vitamin C, and vitamin D) also must be provided in adequate amounts.

A suitable approach for achieving this must involve certain principles. First, there must be an adequate amount of calcium in the diet; amounts higher than the present recommended daily allowance (RDA) of 800 mg have been suggested as optimum intake for the prevention of bone disease in man. Second, there should be an adequate supply of substances that promote calcium absorption from the intestines, such as vitamin D and lactose. Third, substances inhibiting calcium absorption should be eliminated, e.g., oxalic and phytic acids. Last but not least, the total daily calcium allowance should be distributed in several smaller portions since it is well documented that the rate of calcium absorption increases inversely with the amount of calcium ingested at any one time.

The current RDA for calcium must be reevaluated for most adults and particularly for the elderly, not only in light of balance study data and absorption rates but also in terms of the bone density data now available. In addition, some of the dietary components recently suggested to affect calcium utilization (such as fiber) and the adverse effects of reduced physical activity associated with illness and/or aging must also be given consideration. It may be prudent to add another age-sex category to the present RDA for those over 60 years of age to reflect a higher calcium allowance.

The main dietary sources of calcium continue to be milk and milk products (excluding butter), which were estimated in 1976 to have contributed 75% of the total calcium available for civilian consumption. It is indeed a challenge to meet the calcium RDA with the exclusion of dairy foods from the diet.

Since the symptoms and clinical implications of advanced osteoporosis and periodontal disease may be severe and irreversible, emphasis should be placed not on treatment but on preventive measures initiated long before the disease becomes established. The dietary measures outlined above certainly constitute one course of action directed toward the prevention of the etiologically multifaceted osteoporosis as well as periodontal disease.

### Cultured Dairy Products as Food Supplements

The justification for using cultured dairy products as food supplements is twofold. Cultured dairy products might supply either (1) viable microorganisms to the diet of man which are supportive to the human physiology and are implantable into and symbiotic with human intestinal environment, or (2) nutrients, contained in dairy or cultured dairy products, that are instrumental for the maintenance of the microflora of the human digestive system. Not all cultured dairy products equally possess the qualities to satisfy one or the other of the above possibilities. Moreover, these goals, not excluding each other, can rarely be built into the same product. For instance, the kinds of bacteria commonly used in modern dairy practice for the production of buttermilk or yogurt are not implantable to the human gut. These bacteria do not survive in significant number in the respective products during commercial storage. On the other hand, cultured dairy products containing viable and implantable bacterial cultures such as *L. acidophilus* are not suitable for food product development because of limitations in taste appeal to certain population groups.

The search for palatable cultured dairy products with viable and implantable bacteria has accompanied humanity for millenia. The answer to this problem in the majority of cases was a local one based on specific, coincidental, environmental-microbiological interrelationships, food handling practices, and flavor preferences. Thus the review of the various cultured dairy foods seems like a study of regional food habits. Although microbiological classification of various cultured products would be the most accurate from scientific point of view, a regional survey seems sufficient for practical descriptive purposes. (Table 22).

Table 22 indicates that the use of cultured milks is widespread and extremely diversified. The unique health aspects, great food technological advantages, organoleptic variability, and good preservation capability are all inherent consequences of the bacterial acidulation.

The future of cultured milks might well become as diversified as their background history indicates, provided the dairy industry manages to preserve the original intrinsic values of the native products and couples these with necessary sanitation standards. Among the cultured dairy products, yogurt, because of popularity, and acidophilus milk, because of high nutritional-physiological effectiveness, deserve discussion as food supplements.

#### Yogurt as Food Supplement

Economic and consumption statistics on yogurt indicate an extremely fast growth since the end of 1950s in Europe and since end of 1960s in the U.S.[145] The monetary value of the yogurt market in America was $125 million in 1974, but the per capita consumption was still low at 0.68 kg/person/year. This is an insignificant fraction in comparison to 13.7 kg/person/year in the Netherlands, 7.5 kg/person/year in Switzerland, and 6.1 kg/person/year in France. By the end of 1986, however, the U.S. per capita consumption is expected to reach about the present level of France. These statistical figures suggest that consuption of yogurt is expected to grow rather explosively, and thus it will gain importance as a potential food-supplementing factor. The potential supplementing relationship of cultured dairy products and fruit juices and concentrates is covered by a patent review of the Noyes Data Corp.[199]

*Nutritive Value of Yogurt*

Essentially, yogurt shares with milk most of the basic nutritional values inherent in the caloric and protein quality features of unfermented dairy counterparts. However, fermentation by the various cultures introduces new, biochemically and nutritionally significant elements. The nutritional appraisal of these elements sometimes leads to controversial issues and certain unresolved scientific problems. Kon has summarized the nutritional aspects of the cultured milk products from a global perspective.[137] Writes Kon:*

"The ideas of Metchnikoff about the health-giving properties of soured and fermented milks still linger and it is not easy to separate cold facts from fancy. There is no doubt that souring and fermentation have played, and are still playing, a most important part in making milk safer and more wholesome in many parts of the world where these products are prepared traditionally. Souring inhibits and later destroys many pathogenic bacteria, particularly typhoid and paratyphoid organisms and noxious coliforms, so that outbreaks of intestinal disease, so common with untreated milk in hot countries, are much less likely with fermented products. Souring cannot be relied on to control all pathogenic organisms: for example, the tuberculosis and the brucellosis microorganisms survive for days if not weeks in fermented milks of quite high acidity.

The belief is still widespread that fermented milks owe their healthfulness not only to the depression of pathogens but also to the establishment of a specific lactic acid flora in the intestine. As yet, there is only very little evidence that particular organisms of various fermented milks, even those specially prepared for the purpose, can establish themselves and thrive in the gut. There is no doubt that, in the presence of the fermentable sugar, lactose, a special flora develops by selection from organisms normally present in the gut, in which lactic acid producers predominate, but it is so far not proved that these organisms develop better with cultured than with ordinary milk. However, claims of the positive healing effects of fermented milks cannot easily be swept aside, and it may be that they are specifically beneficial in certain conditions. The great and undisputed value of fermented milks is that for vast populations they are still the best practical means of milk preservation.

When it comes to the more strictly nutritive effects of fermentation, generalization is difficult because of the variety of treatments and conditions in which fermented milks are made. The change of lactose into lactic acid or alcohol, or both, decreases slightly the calorie content of the product, but not by more than 3 or 4 percent with most sour milks. Vitamins on the whole survive quite well and, with certain products, bacterial activity even leads to increases. In Leningrad, for example, the starters used increase appreciably the riboflavin and thiamine content of sour milk preparations. Proteolytic changes in some types of fermentation, for example, in kefir and kumiss are probably of little consequence since there is no evidence that the simpler protein fragments, together with the unchanged protein, do not have the same nutritive value as the original milk protein. It stands to reason that prolonged heating before fermentation, as in the traditional preparation of certain types of yogurt, must have an effect on heat-labile components.

Many traditional products could be improved hygienically and nutritionally by the use of more advanced techniques, but it is easier to plan such changes on paper than to carry them out in practice. Moreover, local methods with all their limitations have proved their worth through centuries of experience, and are successful where more ambitious schemes might fail. It is not the minutiae of shortcomings that count in these products, but their ability to supplement the remainder of the diet. In this connection, experiments on rats have shown, for what they are worth, that dahi, khoa, kheer, and channa were as satisfactory in supplementing a poor Indian rice diet as the milk from which they were made."

The health food aspects and the potential dietetic and therapeutic values of cultured

---

* From Kon, S. K., *Milk and Milk Products in Human Nutrition,* 2nd ed., Food and Agricultural Organization of the United Nations, Rome, 1972, 47. With permission.

dairy products are highly controversial issues. The view represented by Auclair and Mocquot from France is quoted below.*

"At the beginning of the century, Metchnikoff, in his famous study, 'The Prolongation of Life', put forth the idea that the consumption of fermented milks such as yogurt contributed to good health and long life. This idea once launched, in spite of the controversies which have been raised for the last 60 years because of the lack of a basis of irrefutable scientific argument, has survived, has been revived, and will certainly continue to hold ground for some long time.

The history of acidophilus milk in the United States shows what importance was attached to this idea in the past. It is the same for koumiss, a fermented milk officially recognized as an integral part of the treatment of tuberculosis and other diseases in sanatoria in Russia. It is generally admitted now that the bacteria of yogurt *Streptococcus thermophilus* and *Lactobacillus bulgaricus* are not only incapable of being implanted permanently in man's intestine, but also that they disappear almost completely during the intestinal transit. However the exploitation of the motivations of the consumers by arguments of health, and the search for expansion at any price explain why fermented milks with a dietetic application, have been the subject to much publicity.

A good example of this can be seen in Japan where, alongside with classical yogurts, numerous new products have been developed such as fermented milks with *Lactobacillus casei* and the acid milk drinks containing active lactic acid bacteria. In 1971, 17 million portions of these kinds of products were sold. In several European countries, there are at present fermented milks on the market which are said to contain *Lactobacillus acidophilus, Bifidobacterium bifidum* and *Streptococcus thermophilus,* and yogurts which contain *Lactobacillus acidophilus* or *Lactobacillus casei* var. *rhamnosus.* For example, this is the case in France where a firm prepares a fermented milk which contains the classical bacteria of yogurt, *Lactobacillus bulgaricus* and *Streptococcus thermophilus* (which, from a technological point of view, produce the desired acidification), and which is in addition inoculated with a frozen concentrated suspension of *Lactobacillus casei* var. *rhamnosus.*

The complexity of the normal intestinal flora of man, the virtual impossibility of carrying out experiments in this field, and the prudence that has to be observed when transposing to man the results obtained on animals, make it practically impossible at the present time for these commercial assertions to be based on sound scientific arguments. For instance, it should be pointed out that it has never been proven that there has ever been any lasting implantation of a given bacteria in an animal with a complex microbial flora. It is obviously insufficient to show that, after ingestion of certain lactobacilli, these are found in the feces and from that conclude that these germs have been implanted in the intestinal flora. Moreover, even if it could be permanently implanted, the role that is attributed to them as a microbiological barrier against undesirable microorganisms is still far from proven.

In other words, from the strictly scientific point of view, there is nothing at present which makes it possible to assert that fermented milks, containing certain bacteria, are any better for the health of the consumer than a classical yogurt. In fact, many of these products, particularly in France, are prepared and sold by the pharmaceutical industry' Even if recently the dairy industry has become interested in their preparation, it seems likey that their expansion depends on whether or not they are supported by the medical profession.

It is logical that this should be so, for it is very likely that their principal benefit for the consumer lies in their use in the treatment of certain pathological conditions, particularly in the case of intestinal infections."

*Acidophilus Milk and Lactobacillus Acidophilus Cultures as Nutritional Supplements*

The potential correlations between the nutritional effects of cultured products and the food supplementing capability of uniquely recognized dairy products with viable cultures gained a better understanding when the complete ecology of the lactic acid bacteria became apparent.[227]

Sandine and co-authors[227] illustrated the ecology of the lactic acid bacteria considering the interrelationships of plants, certain lactic bacteria, food or cultured dairy product, man, and soil. Green plants (Figure 6), in particular, serve as a natural reservoir for lactic acid bacteria; from then selected strains may be isolated and used to manufacture fermented foods. The organisms are recycled through man to the soil and back to the plants. Woman plays a special role as a source of lactobacilli, which colonize the intestinal tracts of the newborn, especially in the breast-fed infant.

---

*    From Auclair, J. and Mocquot, G., Cultured milk, in *Milk Products of the Future,* Rothwell, T., Ed.
     Society of Dairy Technology, Wembley, England, 1974, 33-36. With permission.

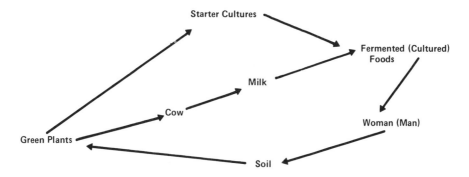

FIGURE 6. Ecology of the lactic acid bacteria. (From Sandune, W. E., Muralidhara, K. S., Elliker, P. R., and England, D. C., *J. Milk Food Technol.*, 35, 697, 1972. With permission.)

The lactic acid bacteria consist of rod- and spherical-shaped organisms *(Lactobacillus* and *Streptococcus* genera) in the family Lactobacteriaceae. They are widely distributed in nature and are easily isolated from mammals' mucous surfaces, green plants, milk, and fermenting foods. In man the lactobacilli are found in the mouth, lower intestine, and vagina. Because lactic acid is a principal end product of their carbohydrate (lactose, glucose, etc.) fermentation, they have been used by man for thousands of years in food preservation. This was at first done unknowingly as fermentations were allowed to proceed under the total influence of the natural food flora. More recently, man has learned to select certain species of these bacteria and use them under controlled conditions to produce the desired quality and stability in food products. Today, these bacteria are indispensable in the manufacture of many products such as silage, sausage, sauerkraut, sour-dough bread, yogurt, sour cream, rye bread, buttermilk, thousands of cheeses, and other fermented products peculiar to certain countries.[227]

For many years, studies on the implantation of lactobacilli in the intestinal tract have indicated preponderantly beneficial results when *L. acidophilus* was fed. This area of study has been the subject of many publications and the topic of numerous reviews.[217,227] It has been suggested that the most satisfactory result is obtained from the ingestion of $1 \times 10^8$ to $1 \times 10^9$ viable *L. acidophilus* organisms daily; ingestion of excessive numbers may induce mild diarrhea. Factors affecting the implantation of lactobacilli in the intestine have been reviewed.[101]

In spite of the beneficial roles ascribed to the ingestion of *L. acidophilus,* little has been done to include this bacterium as a dietary component, particularly in the U.S. The unappetizing flavor of regular acidophilus milk discourages its consumption for purposes other than an urgent need to correct an intestinal malady; consequently, it is essentially unavailable to the public. There are a number of products containing *L. acidophilus* that are dispensed as pharmaceuticals. These are often dried preparations. Also, there are a number of products available in health food stores, but viable lactobacilli in these products vary considerably, and the cost is relatively high. Efforts have been made to include *L. acidophilus* in the culture used to make yogurt; the merits of ingesting *L. acidophilus* by this means are not well documented. "Biogurt" has been used more in Europe than in the U.S. in an effort to promote the ingestion of *L. acidophilus* through yogurt.

A successful product has been marketed, in Japan by the Yakult Company that contains high numbers of lactobacilli including *L. acidophilus.* The product is acidic, with a pleasing background flavor that is appetizing. Research on this product at various Japanese medical schools attests to many beneficial effects in the intestinal tract from the ingestion of this product. Such studies have been directed toward alteration of intestinal flora by the Yakult strain of *L. acidophilus,* the strains' antagonism to intestinal pathogens, the reduction in intestinal gas production, and other subjects relating to beneficial results from the ingestion of *L. acidophilus.*[183]

The Japanese work was best summarized by Mitsuoka[174] and Mutai et al.[183] in 1971. Mitsuoka made studies on the significance the intestinal flora bears to the host. Particular emphasis was given to a taxonomic study dealing with the species and biotypes and the ecology in human and animal intestines. The results indicated that *L. acidophilus, L. salivarius,* and *L. fermenti* are indigenous in human and animal intestines. In general, the biotypes of the intestinal lactobacilli indicate animal species specificity. Furthermore, using germ-free chickens, it became apparent that whether an ingested lactobacillus will become established in the intestine or not depends greatly on the strain. Nonintestinal strains of lactobacilli could not become established in the intestine, and even with the intestinal strains, only the biotypes specific to the animal species could become established. These facts should also be considered when discussing the intestinal implantation of the lactobacilli employed in fermented milk. Mitsuoka concluded that the scientific merits of the apparent beneficial effects of intestinal bacteria have to be analyzed on the basis of the correct bacterial taxonomy.[174]

Mutai et al.[183] reported on the reasons of the wide commercial success of the live, lactobacilli-containing milks in Japan and discussed their potential physiological merits. For effectiveness, these beverages should contain enteric *lactobacillus* strains of human origin that must resist digestive fluids and reach the intestines in viable form and be able to multiply there to some extent. It must be harmless to humans, food for lactic acid production, and stable to its own metabolic products. Finally, it must have a good taste. The most suitable strains for the preparation of the beverage Yakult® are *L. jugurti* and *L. casei.* Guidelines for preparation and quality control criteria are thoroughly discussed by Mutai accompanied by shipping and storage conditions that maintain the viability of the bacteria.

Many of the sociological and nutritional impacts that affect today's diet suggest that replenishment of the intestinal lactobacilli could have beneficial effects for modern man, according to Speck.[242] There are, however, considerations that must be met. The first would be to have the microorganisms available in sufficient quantities but at a reasonable price. Further, additional information and consideration need to be directed toward the strain(s) of *L. acidophilus* that should be ingested. There is little that could be expected from ingesting a strain that would not survive passage to and residence in the intestinal tract. Also, there may be other species of lactobacilli that could be introduced beneficially. The study of the most advantageous carrier for the lactobacilli is also necessary to make available dietary adjuncts with costs comparable to those of other products used as normal dietary components. In spite of extensive studies that have been reported on various beneficial effects that can be derived from consuming *L. acidophilus,* additional work in collaboration with the medical profession is indicated. This seems desirable, not only to have the expertise of professional medical input, but to attain the necessary competent microbiological control of the cultures tested. Such a research effort is indicated for more objective clinical evaluation of feeding trials. In such trials it is necessary to use current knowledge of lactobacilli, factors that affect their viability and resistance, and qualities that would make them a valuable adjunct to the diet. Finally, the intimate association of lactobacilli with the intestine in the healthy individual would indicate that these microorganisms could be considered as appropriate to fill roles as important to human health as do many nutrients. As such, some of their specific microbial components may rightfully be classified as nutrients rather than medicants in the future.

Table 1
## NUTRIENT COMPOSITION OF MILK PRODUCTS AND BY-PRODUCTS

Item 1: Butter (Regular)[a]

| Nutrients | Units | Amount in 100 g (edible portion) | Amount in edible portion of common measures of food (approximate measure and weight) | | Amount in edible portion of 1 lb of food as purchased (refuse:0) |
|---|---|---|---|---|---|
| | | | 1 pat = 5 g[b] | 1 stick (net wt) 4 oz = 113.4 g[c] | |
| Proximate | | | | | |
| Water | g | 15.87 | 0.79 | 18.00 | 71.99 |
| Food energy | kcal | 717 | 36 | 813 | 3,251 |
| | kJ | 3,000 | 150 | 3,402 | 13,607 |
| Protein (N × 6.38) | g | 0.85 | 0.04 | 0.96 | 3.86 |
| Total lipid (fat) | g | 81.11 | 4.06 | 91.98 | 367.92 |
| Carbohydrate (total) | g | 0.06 | Trace | 0.07 | 0.27 |
| Fiber | g | 0 | 0 | 0 | 0 |
| Ash | g | 2.11 | 0.10 | 2.39 | 9.57 |
| Minerals | | | | | |
| Calcium | mg | 24 | 1 | 27 | 107 |
| Iron | mg | 0.16 | 0.01 | 0.18 | 0.73 |
| Magnesium | mg | 2 | Trace | 2 | 10 |
| Phosphorus | mg | 23 | 1 | 26 | 103 |
| Potassium | mg | 26 | 1 | 29 | 118 |
| Sodium | mg | 826 | 41 | 937 | 3,749 |
| Zinc | mg | 0.05 | Trace | 0.06 | 0.23 |
| Vitamins | | | | | |
| Ascorbic acid | mg | 0 | 0 | 0 | 0 |
| Thiamin | mg | 0.005 | Trace | 0.006 | 0.023 |
| Riboflavin | mg | 0.034 | 0.002 | 0.039 | 0.154 |
| Niacin | mg | 0.042 | 0.002 | 0.048 | 0.191 |
| Pantothenic acid | mg | —[d] | — | — | — |
| Vitamin B$_6$ | mg | 0.003 | Trace | 0.003 | 0.014 |
| Folacin | μg | 3 | Trace | 3 | 13 |
| Vitamin B$_{12}$ | μg | — | — | — | — |
| Vitamin A[e] | RE | 754 | 38 | 855 | 3,420 |
| | IU | 3,058 | 153 | 3,468 | 13,871 |
| Lipids | | | | | |
| Fatty acids[f] | | | | | |
| Saturated (total) | g | 50.49 | 2.52 | 57.25 | 229.02 |
| 4:0 | g | 2.63 | 0.13 | 2.98 | 11.93 |
| 6:0 | g | 1.56 | 0.08 | 1.77 | 7.06 |
| 8:0 | g | 0.91 | 0.04 | 1.03 | 4.11 |
| 10:0 | g | 2.03 | 0.10 | 2.31 | 9.23 |
| 12:0 | g | 2.28 | 0.11 | 2.58 | 10.33 |
| 14:0 | g | 8.16 | 0.41 | 9.25 | 37.00 |
| 16:0 | g | 21.33 | 1.07 | 24.19 | 96.77 |
| 18:0 | g | 9.83 | 0.49 | 11.15 | 44.59 |
| Monounsaturated (total) | g | 23.43 | 1.17 | 26.57 | 106.26 |
| 16:1 | g | 1.82 | 0.09 | 2.06 | 8.24 |
| 18:1 | g | 20.40 | 1.02 | 23.14 | 92.56 |
| 20:1 | g | | | | |
| 22:1 | g | | | | |
| Polyunsaturated (total) | g | 3.01 | 0.15 | 3.42 | 13.66 |
| 18:2 | g | 1.83 | 0.09 | 2.08 | 8.31 |
| 18:3 | g | 1.18 | 0.06 | 1.34 | 5.35 |
| 18:4 | g | | | | |
| 20:4 | g | | | | |
| 20:5 | g | | | | |
| 22:5 | g | | | | |
| 22:6 | g | | | | |
| Cholesterol | mg | 219 | 11 | 248 | 993 |
| Phytosterols | mg | | | | |
| Amino acids | | | | | |
| Tryptophan | g | 0.012 | 0.001 | 0.014 | 0.054 |
| Threonine | g | 0.038 | 0.002 | 0.044 | 0.174 |
| Isoleucine | g | 0.051 | 0.003 | 0.058 | 0.233 |
| Leucine | g | 0.083 | 0.004 | 0.094 | 0.378 |
| Lysine | g | 0.067 | 0.003 | 0.076 | 0.306 |
| Methionine | g | 0.021 | 0.001 | 0.024 | 0.097 |
| Cystine | g | 0.008 | Trace | 0.009 | 0.036 |

Table 1 (continued)
## NUTRIENT COMPOSITION OF MILK PRODUCTS AND BY-PRODUCTS

### Item 1: Butter (Regular)[a]

| Nutrients | Units | Amount in 100 g (edible portion) | 1 pat = 5 g[b] | 1 stick (net wt) 4 oz = 113.4 g[c] | Amount in edible portion of 1 lb of food as purchased (refuse: 0) |
|---|---|---|---|---|---|
| Phenylalanine | g | 0.041 | 0.002 | 0.047 | 0.186 |
| Tyrosine | g | 0.041 | 0.002 | 0.047 | 0.186 |
| Valine | g | 0.057 | 0.003 | 0.065 | 0.258 |
| Arginine | g | 0.031 | 0.002 | 0.035 | 0.140 |
| Histidine | g | 0.023 | 0.001 | 0.026 | 0.105 |
| Alanine | g | 0.029 | 0.001 | 0.033 | 0.133 |
| Aspartic acid | g | 0.064 | 0.003 | 0.073 | 0.292 |
| Glutamic acid | g | 0.178 | 0.009 | 0.202 | 0.807 |
| Glycine | g | 0.018 | 0.001 | 0.020 | 0.082 |
| Proline | g | 0.082 | 0.004 | 0.093 | 0.373 |
| Serine | g | 0.046 | 0.002 | 0.052 | 0.210 |

The "Amount in edible portion of common measures of food (approximate measure and weight)" heading spans the "1 pat = 5 g" and "1 stick (net wt) 4 oz = 113.4 g" columns.

### Item 2: Cheese (Blue)

| Nutrients | Units | Amount in 100 g (edible portion) | 1 oz = 28 g[e] | 1 cup (crumbled, not packed) = 135 g | Amount in edible portion o 1 lb of food as purchased (refuse: 0) |
|---|---|---|---|---|---|
| Proximate | | | | | |
| Water | g | 42.41 | 12.02 | 57.25 | 192.37 |
| Food energy | kcal | 353 | 100 | 477 | 1,601 |
| | kJ | 1,478 | 419 | 1,995 | 6,702 |
| Protein (N × 6.38) | g | 21.40 | 6.07 | 28.89 | 97.07 |
| Total lipid (fat) | g | 28.74 | 8.15 | 38.80 | 130.36 |
| Carbohydrate (total) | g | 2.34 | 0.66 | 3.16 | 10.61 |
| Fiber | g | 0 | 0 | 0 | 0 |
| Ash | g | 5.11 | 1.45 | 6.90 | 23.18 |
| Minerals | | | | | |
| Calcium | mg | 528 | 150 | 712 | 2,393 |
| Iron | mg | 0.31 | 0.09 | 0.42 | 1.41 |
| Magnesium | mg | 23 | 7 | 31 | 104 |
| Phosphorus | mg | 387 | 110 | 523 | 1,757 |
| Potassium | mg | 256 | 73 | 346 | 1,163 |
| Sodium | mg | 1,395 | 396 | 1,884 | 6,329 |
| Zinc | mg | 2.66 | 0.75 | 3.59 | 12.07 |
| Vitamins | | | | | |
| Ascorbic acid | mg | 0 | 0 | 0 | 0 |
| Thiamin | mg | 0.029 | 0.008 | 0.039 | 0.132 |
| Riboflavin | mg | 0.382 | 0.108 | 0.516 | 1.733 |
| Niacin | mg | 1.016 | 0.288 | 1.372 | 4.609 |
| Pantothenic acid | mg | 1.729 | 0.490 | 2.334 | 7.843 |
| Vitamin $B_6$ | mg | 0.166 | 0.047 | 0.224 | 0.753 |
| Folacin | μg | 36 | 10 | 49 | 165 |
| Vitamin $B_{12}$ | μg | 1.217 | 0.345 | 1.643 | 5.520 |
| Vitamin A | RE | 228 | 65 | 308 | 1,034 |
| | IU | 721 | 204 | 973 | 3,270 |
| Lipids | | | | | |
| Fatty acids | | | | | |
| Saturated (total) | g | 18.68 | 5.30 | 25.22 | 84.74 |
| 4:0 | g | 0.66 | 0.19 | 0.89 | 2.99 |
| 6:0 | g | 0.36 | 0.10 | 0.49 | 1.64 |
| 8:0 | g | 0.25 | 0.07 | 0.33 | 1.12 |
| 10:0 | g | 0.60 | 0.17 | 0.81 | 2.73 |
| 12:0 | g | 0.49 | 0.14 | 0.66 | 2.23 |
| 14:0 | g | 3.30 | 0.94 | 4.46 | 14.99 |
| 16:0 | g | 9.16 | 2.60 | 12.37 | 41.55 |

The "Amount in edible portion of common measures of food (approximate measures and weight)" heading spans the "1 oz = 28 g" and "1 cup (crumbled, not packed) = 135 g" columns.

Table 1 (continued)
NUTRIENT COMPOSITION OF MILK PRODUCTS AND BY-PRODUCTS
Item 2: Cheese (Blue)

| Nutrients | Units | Amount in 100 g (edible portion) | Amount in edible portion of common measures of food (approximate measures and weight) | | Amount in edible portion of 1 lb of food as purchased (refuse: 0) |
|---|---|---|---|---|---|
| | | | 1 oz = 28 g | 1 cup (crumbled, not packed) = 135 g | |
| 18:0 | g | 3.24 | 0.92 | 4.37 | 14.68 |
| Monounsaturated (total) | g | 7.78 | 2.21 | 10.51 | 35.31 |
| 16:1 | g | 0.82 | 0.23 | 1.10 | 3.70 |
| 18:1 | g | 6.63 | 1.88 | 8.94 | 30.06 |
| 20:1 | g | | | | |
| 22:1 | g | | | | |
| Polyunsaturated (total) | g | 0.80 | 0.23 | 1.08 | 3.63 |
| 18:2 | g | 0.54 | 0.15 | 0.72 | 2.43 |
| 18:3 | g | 0.26 | 0.08 | 0.36 | 1.20 |
| 18:4 | g | | | | |
| 20:4 | g | | | | |
| 20:5 | g | | | | |
| 22:5 | g | | | | |
| 22:6 | g | | | | |
| Cholesterol | mg | 75 | 21 | 102 | 341 |
| Phytosterols | mg | | | | |
| Amino acids | | | | | |
| Tryptophan | g | 0.313 | 0.089 | 0.422 | 1.418 |
| Threonine | g | 0.786 | 0.223 | 1.062 | 3.567 |
| Isoleucine | g | 1.126 | 0.319 | 1.520 | 5.106 |
| Leucine | g | 1.922 | 0.545 | 2.595 | 8.719 |
| Lysine | g | 1.855 | 0.526 | 2.504 | 8.414 |
| Methionine | g | 0.585 | 0.166 | 0.789 | 2.652 |
| Cystine | g | 0.108 | 0.030 | 0.145 | 0.488 |
| Phenylalanine | g | 1.089 | 0.309 | 1.470 | 4.939 |
| Tyrosine | g | 1.297 | 0.368 | 1.751 | 5.884 |
| Valine | g | 1.559 | 0.442 | 2.105 | 7.073 |
| Arginine | g | 0.712 | 0.202 | 0.962 | 3.232 |
| Histidine | g | 0.759 | 0.215 | 1.025 | 3.445 |
| Alanine | g | 0.645 | 0.183 | 0.871 | 2.927 |
| Aspartic acid | g | 1.438 | 0.408 | 1.942 | 6.524 |
| Glutamic acid | g | 5.189 | 1.471 | 7.005 | 23.536 |
| Glycine | g | 0.407 | 0.115 | 0.549 | 1.844 |
| Proline | g | 2.104 | 0.596 | 2.840 | 9.542 |
| Serine | g | 1.122 | 0.318 | 1.515 | 5.091 |

Item 3: Cheese (Camembert)

| Nutrients | Units | Amount in 100 g (edible portion) | Amount in edible portion of common measures of food (approximate measure and weight) | | Amount in edible portion of 1 lb of food as purchased (refuse:0) |
|---|---|---|---|---|---|
| | | | 1 oz = 28 g | 1 wedge (net wt) 1⅓ oz = 38 g | |
| Proximate | | | | | |
| Water | g | 51.80 | 14.68 | 19.68 | 234.96 |
| Food energy | kcal | 300 | 85 | 114 | 1,359 |
| | kJ | 1,254 | 355 | 476 | 5,687 |
| Protein (N × 6.38) | g | 19.80 | 5.61 | 7.52 | 89.81 |
| Total lipid (fat) | g | 24.26 | 6.88 | 9.22 | 110.04 |
| Carbohydrate (total) | g | 0.46 | 0.13 | 0.18 | 2.09 |
| Fiber | g | 0 | 0 | 0 | 0 |
| Ash | g | 3.68 | 1.04 | 1.40 | 16.69 |
| Minerals | | | | | |
| Calcium | mg | 388 | 110 | 147 | 1,758 |
| Iron | mg | 0.33 | 0.09 | 0.12 | 1.50 |
| Magnesium | mg | 20 | 6 | 8 | 91 |
| Phosphorus | mg | 347 | 98 | 132 | 1,572 |
| Potassium | mg | 187 | 53 | 71 | 846 |
| Sodium | mg | 842 | 239 | 320 | 3,818 |

Table 1 (continued)
## NUTRIENT COMPOSITION OF MILK PRODUCTS AND BY-PRODUCTS

### Item 3: Cheese (Camembert)

| Nutrients | Units | Amount in 100 g (edible portion) | Amount in edible portion of common measures of food (approximate measure and weight) | | Amount in edible portion of 1 lb of food as purchased (refuse:0) |
|---|---|---|---|---|---|
| | | | 1 oz = 28 g^ | 1 wedge (net wt) 1⅓ oz = 38 g | |
| Zinc | mg | 2.38 | 0.68 | 0.90 | 10.80 |
| Vitamins | | | | | |
| Ascorbic acid | mg | 0 | 0 | 0 | 0 |
| Thiamin | mg | 0.028 | 0.008 | 0.011 | 0.127 |
| Riboflavin | mg | 0.488 | 0.138 | 0.185 | 2.214 |
| Niacin | mg | 0.630 | 0.179 | 0.239 | 2.858 |
| Pantothenic acid | mg | 1.364 | 0.387 | 0.518 | 6.187 |
| Vitamin B$_6$ | mg | 0.227 | 0.064 | 0.086 | 1.030 |
| Folacin | μg | 62 | 18 | 24 | 282 |
| Vitamin B$_{12}$ | μg | 1.296 | 0.367 | 0.492 | 5.879 |
| Vitamin A | RE | 252 | 71 | 96 | 1,143 |
| | IU | 923 | 262 | 351 | 4,187 |
| Lipids | | | | | |
| Fatty acids | | | | | |
| Saturated, total | g | 15.26 | 4.33 | 5.80 | 69.22 |
| 4:0 | g | 0.49 | 0.14 | 0.19 | 2.24 |
| 6:0 | g | 0.28 | 0.08 | 0.11 | 1.28 |
| 8:0 | g | 0.26 | 0.07 | 0.10 | 1.18 |
| 10:0 | g | 0.59 | 0.17 | 0.22 | 2.68 |
| 12:0 | g | 0.44 | 0.12 | 0.17 | 2.00 |
| 14:0 | g | 2.69 | 0.76 | 1.02 | 12.18 |
| 16:0 | g | 7.23 | 2.05 | 2.75 | 32.78 |
| 18:0 | g | 2.52 | 0.72 | 0.96 | 11.45 |
| Monounsaturated, total | g | 7.02 | 1.99 | 2.67 | 31.86 |
| 16:1 | g | 0.88 | 0.25 | 0.34 | 4.01 |
| 18:1 | g | 5.75 | 1.63 | 2.19 | 26.09 |
| 20:1 | g | | | | |
| 22:1 | g | | | | |
| Polyunsaturated, total | g | 0.72 | 0.20 | 0.28 | 3.29 |
| 18:2 | g | 0.45 | 0.13 | 0.17 | 2.04 |
| 18:3 | g | 0.27 | 0.08 | 0.10 | 1.24 |
| 18:4 | g | | | | |
| 20:4 | g | | | | |
| 20:5 | g | | | | |
| 22:5 | g | | | | |
| 22.6 | g | | | | |
| Cholesterol | mg | 72 | 20 | 27 | 327 |
| Phytosterols | mg | | | | |
| Amino acids | | | | | |
| Tryptophan | g | 0.307 | 0.087 | 0.117 | 1.394 |
| Threonine | g | 0.717 | 0.203 | 0.272 | 3.252 |
| Isoleucine | g | 0.968 | 0.275 | 0.368 | 4.392 |
| Leucine | g | 1.840 | 0.522 | 0.699 | 8.348 |
| Lysine | g | 1.766 | 0.501 | 0.671 | 8.010 |
| Methionine | g | 0.565 | 0.160 | 0.215 | 2.562 |
| Cystine | g | 0.109 | 0.031 | 0.041 | 0.493 |
| Phenylalanine | g | 1.105 | 0.313 | 0.420 | 5.011 |
| Tyrosine | g | 1.145 | 0.325 | 0.435 | 5.195 |
| Valine | g | 1.279 | 0.362 | 0.486 | 5.800 |
| Arginine | g | 0.701 | 0.199 | 0.267 | 3.181 |
| Histidine | g | 0.683 | 0.194 | 0.259 | 3.097 |
| Alanine | g | 0.819 | 0.232 | 0.311 | 3.716 |
| Aspartic acid | g | 1.288 | 0.365 | 0.489 | 5.842 |
| Glutamic acid | g | 4.187 | 1.187 | 1.591 | 18.990 |
| Glycine | g | 0.379 | 0.107 | 0.144 | 1.717 |
| Proline | g | 2.346 | 0.665 | 0.892 | 10.642 |
| Serine | g | 1.114 | 0.316 | 0.423 | 5.054 |

Table 1 (continued)
## NUTRIENT COMPOSITION OF MILK PRODUCTS AND BY-PRODUCTS

Item 4: Cheese (Cheddar)

| Nutrients | Units | Amount in 100 g (edible portion) | Amount in edible portion of common measures of food (approximate measure and weight) | | Amount in edible portion of 1 lb of food as purchased (refuse:0) |
| | | | 1 oz = 28 g[i] | 1 cup (shredded, not packed) = 113 g | |
|---|---|---|---|---|---|
| **Proximate** | | | | | |
| Water | g | 36.75 | 10.42 | 41.53 | 166.70 |
| Food energy | kcal | 403 | 114 | 455 | 1,826 |
| | kJ | 1,685 | 478 | 1,904 | 7,642 |
| Protein (N × 6.38) | g | 24.90 | 7.06 | 28.14 | 112.95 |
| Total lipid (fat) | g | 33.14 | 9.40 | 37.45 | 150.32 |
| Carbohydrate (total) | g | 1.28 | .36 | 1.45 | 5.81 |
| Fiber | g | 0 | 0 | 0 | 0 |
| Ash | g | 3.93 | 1.11 | 4.44 | 17.83 |
| **Minerals** | | | | | |
| Calcium | mg | 721 | 204 | 815 | 3.272 |
| Iron | mg | 0.68 | 0.19 | 0.77 | 3.08 |
| Magnesium | mg | 28 | 8 | 31 | 126 |
| Phosphorus | mg | 512 | 145 | 579 | 2,323 |
| Potassium | mg | 98 | 28 | 111 | 446 |
| Sodium | mg | 620 | 176 | 701 | 2,815 |
| Zinc | mg | 3.11 | 0.88 | 3.51 | 14.11 |
| **Vitamins** | | | | | |
| Ascorbic acid | mg | 0 | 0 | 0 | 0 |
| Thiamin | mg | 0.027 | 0.008 | 0.031 | 0.122 |
| Riboflavin | mg | 0.375 | 0.106 | 0.424 | 1.701 |
| Niacin | mg | 0.080 | 0.023 | 0.090 | 0.363 |
| Pantothenic acid | mg | 0.413 | 0.117 | 0.467 | 1.873 |
| Vitamin $B_6$ | mg | 0.074 | 0.021 | 0.084 | 0.336 |
| Folacin | μg | 18 | 5 | 21 | 83 |
| Vitamin $B_{12}$ | μg | 0.827 | 0.234 | 0.935 | 3.751 |
| Vitamin A | RE | 303 | 86 | 342 | 1,374 |
| | IU | 1,059 | 300 | 1,197 | 4,804 |
| **Lipids** | | | | | |
| Fatty acids | | | | | |
| Saturated (total) | g | 21.09 | 5.98 | 23.83 | 95.67 |
| 4:0 | g | 1.05 | 0.30 | 1.18 | 4.74 |
| 6:0 | g | 0.53 | 0.15 | 0.60 | 2.40 |
| 8:0 | g | 0.28 | 0.08 | 0.32 | 1.27 |
| 10:0 | g | 0.60 | 0.17 | 0.68 | 2.72 |
| 12:0 | g | 0.54 | 0.15 | 0.61 | 2.46 |
| 14:0 | g | 3.33 | 0.94 | 3.76 | 15.10 |
| 16:0 | g | 9.80 | 2.78 | 11.08 | 44.47 |
| 18:0 | g | 4.01 | 1.14 | 4.53 | 18.17 |
| Monounsaturated (total) | g | 9.39 | 2.66 | 10.61 | 42.60 |
| 16:1 | g | 1.00 | 0.28 | 1.14 | 4.56 |
| 18:1 | g | 7.90 | 2.24 | 8.93 | 35.86 |
| 20:1 | g | | | | |
| 22:1 | g | | | | |
| Polyunsaturated (total) | g | 0.94 | 0.27 | 1.06 | 4.27 |
| 18:2 | g | 0.58 | 0.16 | 0.65 | 2.62 |
| 18:3 | g | 0.36 | 0.10 | 0.41 | 1.65 |
| 18:4 | g | | | | |
| 20:4 | g | | | | |
| 20:5 | g | | | | |
| 22:5 | g | | | | |
| 22:6 | g | | | | |
| Cholesterol | mg | 105 | 30 | 119 | 476 |
| Phytosterols | mg | | | | |
| **Amino acids** | | | | | |
| Tryptophan | g | 0.320 | 0.091 | 0.362 | 1.452 |
| Threonine | g | 0.886 | 0.251 | 1.001 | 4.019 |
| Isoleucine | g | 1.546 | 0.438 | 1.746 | 7.010 |
| Leucine | g | 2.385 | 0.676 | 2.695 | 10.817 |
| Lysine | g | 2.072 | 0.588 | 2.342 | 9.400 |
| Methionine | g | 0.652 | 0.185 | 0.737 | 2.956 |

Table 1 (continued)
NUTRIENT COMPOSITION OF MILK PRODUCTS AND BY-PRODUCTS

Item 4: Cheese (Cheddar)

| Nutrients | Units | Amount in 100 g (edible portion) | 1 oz = 28 g$^i$ | 1 cup (shredded, not packed) = 113 g | Amount in edible portion of 1 lb of food as purchased (refuse:0) |
|---|---|---|---|---|---|
| Cystine | g | 0.125 | 0.035 | 0.141 | 0.567 |
| Phenylalanine | g | 1.311 | 0.372 | 1.482 | 5.948 |
| Tyrosine | g | 1.202 | 0.341 | 1.358 | 5.453 |
| Valine | g | 1.663 | 0.471 | 1.879 | 7.542 |
| Arginine | g | 0.941 | 0.267 | 1.063 | 4.266 |
| Histidine | g | 0.874 | 0.248 | 0.988 | 3.966 |
| Alanine | g | 0.703 | 0.199 | 0.794 | 3.187 |
| Aspartic acid | g | 1.600 | 0.454 | 1.808 | 7.258 |
| Glutamic acid | g | 6.092 | 1.727 | 6.884 | 27.635 |
| Glycine | g | 0.429 | 0.122 | 0.485 | 1.947 |
| Proline | g | 2.806 | 0.796 | 3.171 | 12.729 |
| Serine | g | 1.456 | 0.413 | 1.645 | 6.603 |

Item 5: Cheese (Cottage, Creamed)

| Nutrients | Units | Amount in 100 g (edible portion) | 4 oz = 113 g | 1 cup (unpacked) = 210 g$^i$ | Amount in edible portion of 1 lb of food as purchased (refuse:0) |
|---|---|---|---|---|---|
| **Proximate** | | | | | |
| Water | g | 78.96 | 89.22 | 165.82 | 358.16 |
| Food energy | kcal | 103 | 117 | 217 | 469 |
| | kJ | 433 | 489 | 908 | 1,962 |
| Protein (N × 6.38) | g | 12.49 | 14.11 | 26.33 | 56.66 |
| Total lipid (fat) | g | 4.51 | 5.10 | 9.47 | 20.46 |
| Carbohydrate (total) | g | 2.68 | 3.03 | 5.63 | 12.16 |
| Fiber | g | 0 | 0 | 0 | 0 |
| Ash | g | 1.36 | 1.54 | 2.86 | 6.17 |
| **Minerals** | | | | | |
| Calcium | mg | 60 | 68 | 126 | 272 |
| Iron | mg | 0.14 | 0.16 | 0.29 | 0.64 |
| Magnesium | mg | 5 | 6 | 11 | 24 |
| Phosphorus | mg | 132 | 149 | 277 | 598 |
| Potassium | mg | 84 | 96 | 177 | 382 |
| Sodium | mg | 405 | 457 | 850 | 1,836 |
| Zinc | mg | 0.37 | 0.42 | 0.78 | 1.68 |
| **Vitamins** | | | | | |
| Ascorbic acid | mg | Trace | Trace | Trace | Trace |
| Thiamin | mg | 0.021 | 0.024 | 0.044 | 0.095 |
| Riboflavin | mg | 0.163 | 0.184 | 0.342 | 0.739 |
| Niacin | mg | 0.126 | 0.142 | 0.265 | 0.572 |
| Pantothenic acid | mg | 0.213 | 0.241 | 0.447 | 0.966 |
| Vitamin B$_6$ | mg | 0.067 | 0.076 | 0.141 | 0.304 |
| Folacin | µg | 12 | 14 | 26 | 55 |
| Vitamin B$_{12}$ | µg | 0.623 | 0.704 | 1.308 | 2.826 |
| Vitamin A | RE | 48 | 54 | 101 | 218 |
| | IU | 163 | 184 | 342 | 739 |
| **Lipids** | | | | | |
| **Fatty Acids** | | | | | |
| Saturated (total) | g | 2.85 | 3.22 | 5.99 | 12.94 |
| 4:0 | g | 0.14 | 0.16 | 0.30 | 0.66 |
| 6:0 | g | 0.03 | 0.04 | 0.07 | 0.15 |
| 8:0 | g | 0.04 | 0.04 | 0.08 | 0.16 |
| 10:0 | g | 0.08 | 0.09 | 0.17 | 0.37 |
| 12:0 | g | 0.07 | 0.08 | 0.15 | 0.33 |
| 14:0 | g | 0.47 | 0.53 | 0.99 | 2.14 |
| 16:0 | g | 1.36 | 1.54 | 2.86 | 6.18 |

Table 1 (continued)
NUTRIENT COMPOSITION OF MILK PRODUCTS AND BY-PRODUCTS

Item 5: Cheese (Cottage, Creamed)

| Nutrients | Units | Amount in 100 g (edible portion) | Amount in edible portion of common measures of food (approximate measure and weight) | | Amount in edible portion of 1 lb of food as purchased (refuse:0) |
|---|---|---|---|---|---|
| | | | 4 oz = 113 g | 1 cup (unpacked) = 210 g$^j$ | |
| 18:0 | g | 0.52 | 0.58 | 1.08 | 2.33 |
| Monounsaturated (total) | g | 1.28 | 0.45 | 2.70 | 5.83 |
| 16:1 | g | 0.16 | 0.18 | 0.34 | 0.73 |
| 18:1 | g | 1.06 | 1.19 | 2.22 | 4.79 |
| 20:1 | g | | | | |
| 22:1 | g | | | | |
| Polyunsaturated (total) | g | 0.14 | 0.16 | 0.29 | 0.63 |
| 18:2 | g | 0.10 | 0.11 | 0.21 | 0.45 |
| 18:3 | g | 0.04 | 0.04 | 0.08 | 0.18 |
| 18:4 | g | | | | |
| 20:4 | g | | | | |
| 20:5 | g | | | | |
| 22:5 | g | | | | |
| 22:6 | g | | | | |
| Cholesterol | mg | 15 | 17 | 31 | 68 |
| Phytosterols | mg | | | | |
| Amino acids | | | | | |
| Tryptophan | g | 0.139 | 0.157 | 0.292 | 0.630 |
| Threonine | g | 0.554 | 0.626 | 1.163 | 2.513 |
| Isoleucine | g | 0.734 | 0.830 | 1.542 | 3.330 |
| Leucine | g | 1.284 | 1.451 | 2.697 | 5.825 |
| Lysine | g | 1.010 | 1.141 | 2.121 | 4.582 |
| Methionine | g | 0.376 | 0.425 | 0.789 | 1.705 |
| Cystine | g | 0.116 | 0.131 | 0.243 | 0.524 |
| Phenylalanine | g | 0.673 | 0.761 | 1.414 | 3.055 |
| Tyrosine | g | 0.666 | 0.752 | 1.398 | 3.019 |
| Valine | g | 0.773 | 0.874 | 1.624 | 3.508 |
| Arginine | g | 0.570 | 0.644 | 1.196 | 2.584 |
| Histidine | g | 0.415 | 0.469 | 0.872 | 1.883 |
| Alanine | g | 0.648 | 0.732 | 1.361 | 2.939 |
| Aspartic acid | g | 0.846 | 0.956 | 1.776 | 3.836 |
| Glutamic acid | g | 2.706 | 3.057 | 5.682 | 12.272 |
| Glycine | g | 0.272 | 0.307 | 0.571 | 1.234 |
| Proline | g | 1.447 | 1.635 | 3.038 | 6.562 |
| Serine | g | 0.701 | 0.792 | 1.472 | 3.179 |

Item 6: Cheese (Cottage, Dry Curd)

| Nutrients | Units | Amount in 100 g (edible portion) | Amount in edible portion of common measures of food (approximate measure and weight) | | Amount in edible portion of 1 lb of food as purchased (refuse:0) |
|---|---|---|---|---|---|
| | | | 4 oz = 133 g | 1 cup (unpacked) = 145 g | |
| Proximate | | | | | |
| Water | g | 79.77 | 90.14 | 115.67 | 361.84 |
| Food energy | kcal | 85 | 96 | 123 | 384 |
| | kJ | 354 | 400 | 513 | 1,606 |
| Protein (N × 6.38) | g | 17.27 | 19.52 | 25.04 | 78.34 |
| Total lipid (fat) | g | 0.42 | 0.48 | 0.61 | 1.90 |
| Carbohydrate (total) | g | 1.85 | 2.09 | 2.68 | 8.39 |
| Fiber | g | 0 | 0 | 0 | 0 |
| Ash | g | 0.69 | 0.78 | 1.00 | 3.13 |
| Minerals | | | | | |
| Calcium | mg | 32 | 36 | 46 | 144 |
| Iron | mg | 0.23 | 0.26 | 0.33 | 1.04 |
| Magnesium | mg | 4 | 4 | 6 | 18 |
| Phosphorus | mg | 104 | 118 | 151 | 472 |
| Potassium | mg | 32 | 37 | 47 | 147 |

Table 1 (continued)
## NUTRIENT COMPOSITION OF MILK PRODUCTS AND BY-PRODUCTS

### Item 6: Cheese (Cottage, Dry Curd)

| Nutrients | Units | Amount in 100 g (edible portion) | Amount in edible portion of common measures of food (approximate measure and weight) | | Amount in edible portion of 1 lb of food as purchased (refuse:0) |
|---|---|---|---|---|---|
| | | | 4 oz = 133 g | 1 cup (unpacked) = 145 g | |
| Sodium* | mg | 13 | 14 | 19 | 58 |
| Zinc | mg | 0.47 | 0.55 | 0.68 | 2.13 |
| Vitamins | | | | | |
| Ascorbic acid | mg | 0 | 0 | 0 | 0 |
| Thiamin | mg | 0.025 | 0.028 | 0.036 | 0.113 |
| Riboflavin | mg | 0.142 | 0.160 | 0.206 | 0.644 |
| Niacin | mg | 0.155 | 0.175 | 0.225 | 0.703 |
| Pantothenic acid | mg | 0.163 | 0.184 | 0.236 | 0.739 |
| Vitamin B$_6$ | mg | 0.082 | 0.093 | 0.119 | 0.372 |
| Folacin | μg | 15 | 17 | 21 | 67 |
| Vitamin B$_{12}$ | μg | 0.825 | 0.932 | 1.196 | 3.742 |
| Vitamin A | RE | 8 | 9 | 12 | 36 |
| | IU | 30 | 34 | 44 | 136 |
| Lipids | | | | | |
| Fatty acids' | | | | | |
| Saturated (total) | g | 0.273 | 0.308 | 0.396 | 1.238 |
| 4:0 | g | 0.018 | 0.021 | 0.026 | 0.083 |
| 6:0 | g | 0.003 | 0.003 | 0.004 | 0.014 |
| 8:0 | g | 0.005 | 0.005 | 0.007 | 0.020 |
| 10:0 | g | 0.009 | 0.010 | 0.012 | 0.039 |
| 12:0 | g | 0.006 | 0.006 | 0.008 | 0.025 |
| 14:0 | g | 0.042 | 0.047 | 0.060 | 0.188 |
| 16:0 | g | 0.131 | 0.148 | 0.189 | 0.592 |
| 18:0 | g | 0.045 | 0.051 | 0.065 | 0.203 |
| Monounsaturated (total) | g | 0.110 | 0.124 | 0.160 | 0.499 |
| 16:1 | g | 0.012 | 0.014 | 0.018 | 0.055 |
| 18:1 | g | 0.093 | 0.105 | 0.135 | 0.423 |
| 20:1 | g | | | | |
| 22:1 | g | | | | |
| Polyunsaturated (total) | g | 0.015 | 0.017 | 0.022 | 0.069 |
| 18:2 | g | 0.011 | 0.012 | 0.016 | 0.050 |
| 18:3 | g | 0.004 | 0.005 | 0.006 | 0.019 |
| 18:4 | g | | | | |
| 20:4 | g | | | | |
| 20:5 | g | | | | |
| 22:5 | g | | | | |
| 22:6 | g | | | | |
| Cholesterol | mg | 7 | 8 | 10 | 30 |
| Phytosterols | mg | | | | |
| Amino acids | | | | | |
| Tryptophan | g | 0.192 | 0.217 | 0.279 | 0.872 |
| Threonine | g | 0.766 | 0.866 | 1.111 | 3.475 |
| Isoleucine | g | 1.015 | 1.147 | 1.472 | 4.604 |
| Leucine | g | 1.776 | 2.007 | 2.575 | 8.055 |
| Lycine | g | 1.397 | 1.578 | 2.025 | 6.336 |
| Methionine | g | 0.520 | 0.587 | 0.754 | 2.357 |
| Cystine | g | 0.160 | 0.180 | 0.232 | 0.724 |
| Phenylalanine | g | 0.931 | 1.052 | 1.350 | 4.224 |
| Tyrosine | g | 0.920 | 1.040 | 1.334 | 4.175 |
| Valine | g | 1.069 | 1.208 | 1.550 | 4.850 |
| Arginine | g | 0.788 | 0.890 | 1.142 | 3.573 |
| Histidine | g | 0.574 | 0.648 | 0.832 | 2.603 |
| Alanine | g | 0.896 | 1.012 | 1.299 | 4.064 |
| Apartic acid | g | 1.169 | 1.321 | 1.696 | 5.304 |
| Glutamic acid | g | 3.741 | 4.227 | 5.424 | 16.969 |
| Glycine | g | 0.376 | 0.425 | 0.546 | 1.707 |
| Proline | g | 2.000 | 2.260 | 2.901 | 9.074 |
| Serine | g | 0.969 | 1.095 | 1.405 | 4.396 |

Table 1 (continued)
## NUTRIENT COMPOSITION OF MILK PRODUCTS AND BY-PRODUCTS

Item 7: Cheese (Cream)

| Nutrients | Units | Amount in 100 g (edible portion) | Amount in edible portion of common measures of food (approximate measure and weight) | | Amount in edible portion of 1 lb of food as purchased (refuse: 0) |
|---|---|---|---|---|---|
| | | | 1 oz = 28 g" | 1 package (net wt) 3 oz = 85 g | |
| Proximate | | | | | |
| Water | g | 53.75 | 15.24 | 45.69 | 243.81 |
| Food energy | kcal | 349 | 99 | 297 | 1,583 |
| | kJ | 1,461 | 414 | 1,242 | 6,626 |
| Protein (N × 6.38) | g | 7.55 | 2.14 | 6.42 | 34.25 |
| Total lipid (fat) | g | 34.87 | 9.39 | 29.64 | 158.17 |
| Carbohydrate (total) | g | 2.66 | 0.75 | 2.26 | 12.07 |
| Fiber | g | 0 | 0 | 0 | 0 |
| Ash | g | 1.17 | 0.33 | 1.00 | 5.31 |
| Minerals | | | | | |
| Calcium | mg | 80 | 23 | 68 | 362 |
| Iron | mg | 1.20 | 0.34 | 1.02 | 5.44 |
| Magnesium | mg | 6 | 2 | 5 | 29 |
| Phosphorus | mg | 104 | 30 | 89 | 474 |
| Potassium | mg | 119 | 34 | 101 | 542 |
| Sodium | mg | 296 | 84 | 251 | 1,340 |
| Zinc | mg | 0.54 | 0.15 | 0.46 | 2.45 |
| Vitamins | | | | | |
| Ascorbic acid | mg | 0 | 0 | 0 | 0 |
| Thiamin | mg | 0.017 | 0.005 | 0.014 | 0.077 |
| Riboflavin | mg | 0.197 | 0.056 | 0.167 | 0.894 |
| Niacin | mg | 0.101 | 0.029 | 0.086 | 0.458 |
| Pantothenic acid | mg | 0.271 | 0.077 | 0.230 | 1.229 |
| Vitamin $B_6$ | mg | 0.047 | 0.013 | 0.040 | .213 |
| Folacin | µg | 13 | 4 | 11 | 60 |
| Vitamin $B_{12}$ | µg | 0.424 | 0.120 | 0.360 | 1.923 |
| Vitamin A | RE | 437 | 124 | 371 | 1,982 |
| | IU | 1,427 | 405 | 1,213 | 6,473 |
| Lipids | | | | | |
| Fatty acids | | | | | |
| Saturated (total) | g | 21.97 | 6.23 | 18.67 | 99.64 |
| 4:0 | g | 1.00 | 0.28 | 0.85 | 4.52 |
| 6:0 | g | 0.29 | 0.08 | 0.25 | 1.33 |
| 8:0 | g | 0.34 | 0.10 | 0.28 | 1.52 |
| 10:0 | g | 0.67 | 0.19 | 0.57 | 3.03 |
| 12:0 | g | 0.46 | 0.13 | 0.40 | 2.11 |
| 14:0 | g | 3.60 | 1.02 | 3.06 | 16.34 |
| 16:0 | g | 10.54 | 2.99 | 8.96 | 47.80 |
| 18:0 | g | 4.04 | 1.15 | 3.44 | 18.35 |
| Monounsaturated (total) | g | 9.84 | 2.79 | 8.36 | 44.62 |
| 16:1 | g | 0.98 | 0.28 | 0.84 | 4.46 |
| 18:1 | g | 8.38 | 2.38 | 7.12 | 38.02 |
| 20:1 | g | | | | |
| 22:1 | g | | | | |
| Polyunsaturated (total) | g | 1.26 | 0.36 | 1.08 | 5.74 |
| 18:2 | g | 0.77 | 0.22 | 0.66 | 3.51 |
| 18:3 | g | 0.49 | 0.14 | 0.42 | 2.22 |
| 18:4 | g | | | | |
| 20:4 | g | | | | |
| 20:5 | g | | | | |
| 22:5 | g | | | | |
| 22:6 | g | | | | |
| Cholesterol | mg | 110 | 31 | 93 | 498 |
| Phytosterols | mg | | | | |
| Amino acids | | | | | |
| Tryptophan | g | 0.067 | 0.019 | .057 | 0.306 |
| Threonine | g | 0.321 | 0.091 | .273 | 1.455 |
| Isoleucine | g | 0.399 | 0.113 | .339 | 1.809 |
| Leucine | g | 0.731 | 0.207 | .622 | 3.317 |
| Lysine | g | 0.676 | 0.192 | .574 | 3.065 |

Table 1 (continued)
NUTRIENT COMPOSITION OF MILK PRODUCTS AND BY-PRODUCTS

Item 7: Cheese (Cream)

| Nutrients | Units | Amount in 100 g (edible portion) | Amount in edible portion of common measures of food (approximate measure and weight) | | Amount in edible portion of 1 lb of food as purchased (refuse: 0) |
|---|---|---|---|---|---|
| | | | 1 oz = 28 g<sup>m</sup> | 1 package (net wt) 3 oz = 85 g | |
| Methionine | g | 0.181 | 0.051 | .154 | 0.821 |
| Cystine | g | 0.066 | 0.019 | .056 | 0.301 |
| Phenylalanine | g | 0.419 | 0.119 | .356 | 1.900 |
| Tyrosine | g | 0.360 | 0.102 | .306 | 1.632 |
| Valine | g | 0.443 | 0.125 | .376 | 2.008 |
| Arginine | g | 0.286 | 0.081 | .243 | 1.299 |
| Histidine | g | 0.271 | 0.077 | .230 | 1.229 |
| Alanine | g | 0.230 | 0.065 | .195 | 1.041 |
| Aspartic acid | g | 0.533 | 0.151 | .453 | 2.416 |
| Glutamic acid | g | 1.714 | 0.486 | 1.457 | 7.773 |
| Glycine | g | 0.149 | 0.042 | .127 | 0.676 |
| Proline | g | 0.689 | 0.195 | .585 | 3.124 |
| Serine | g | 0.398 | 0.113 | .338 | 1.804 |

Item 8: Cheese (Mozzarella)

| Nutrients | Units | Amount in 100 g (edible portion) | Amount in edible portion of common measures of food (approximate measure and weight) 1oz = 28 g | Amount in edible portion of 1 lb of food as purchased (refuse: 0) |
|---|---|---|---|---|
| Proximate | | | | |
| Water | g | 54.14 | 15.35 | 245.58 |
| Food energy | kcal | 281 | 80 | 1,276 |
| | kJ | 1,178 | 334 | 5,341 |
| Protein (N × 6.38) | g | 19.42 | 5.51 | 88.09 |
| Total lipid (fat) | g | 21.60 | 6.12 | 97.98 |
| Carbohydrate (total) | g | 2.22 | 0.63 | 10.07 |
| Fiber | g | 0 | 0 | 0 |
| Ash | g | 2.62 | 0.74 | 11.88 |
| Minerals | | | | |
| Calcium | mg | 517 | 147 | 2,345 |
| Iron | mg | 0.18 | 0.05 | 0.82 |
| Magnesium | mg | 19 | 5 | 84 |
| Phosphorus | mg | 371 | 105 | 1,681 |
| Potassium | mg | 67 | 19 | 304 |
| Sodium | mg | 373 | 106 | 1,692 |
| Zinc | mg | 2.21 | 0.63 | 10.02 |
| Vitamins | | | | |
| Ascorbic acid | mg | 0 | 0 | 0 |
| Thiamin | mg | 0.015 | 0.004 | 0.068 |
| Riboflavin | mg | 0.243 | 0.069 | 1.102 |
| Niacin | mg | 0.084 | 0.024 | 0.381 |
| Pantothenic acid | mg | 0.064 | 0.018 | 0.290 |
| Vitamin B<sub>6</sub> | mg | 0.056 | 0.016 | 0.254 |
| Folacin | µg | 7 | 2 | 32 |
| Vitamin B<sub>12</sub> | µg | 0.654 | 0.185 | 2.967 |
| Vitamin A | RE | 241 | 68 | 1,093 |
| | IU | 792 | 225 | 3,593 |
| Lipids | | | | |
| Fatty acids | | | | |
| Saturated (total) | g | 13.15 | 3.73 | 59.66 |
| 4:0 | g | 0.80 | 0.23 | 3.65 |
| 6:0 | g | 0.45 | 0.13 | 2.02 |
| 8:0 | g | 0.26 | 0.07 | 1.17 |
| 10:0 | g | 0.58 | 0.16 | 2.64 |
| 12:0 | g | 0.69 | 0.20 | 3.13 |
| 14:0 | g | 2.19 | 0.62 | 9.93 |
| 16:0 | g | 5.33 | 1.51 | 24.18 |
| 18:0 | g | 2.44 | 0.69 | 11.08 |
| Monounsaturated (total) | g | 6.57 | 1.86 | 29.82 |

Table 1 (continued)
NUTRIENT COMPOSITION OF MILK PRODUCTS AND BY-PRODUCTS

Item 8: Cheese (Mozzarella)

| Nutrients | Units | Amount in 100 g (edible portion) | Amount in edible portion of common measures of food (approximate measure and weight) 1oz = 28 g | Amount in edible portion of 1 lb of food as purchased (refuse: 0) |
|---|---|---|---|---|
| 16:1 | g | 0.60 | 0.17 | 2.71 |
| 18:1 | g | 5.65 | 1.60 | 25.62 |
| 20:1 | g | | | |
| 22:1 | g | | | |
| Polyunsaturated (total) | g | 0.76 | 0.22 | 3.47 |
| 18:2 | g | 0.39 | 0.11 | 1.78 |
| 18:3 | g | 0.37 | 0.10 | 1.69 |
| 18:4 | g | | | |
| 20:4 | g | | | |
| 20:5 | g | | | |
| 22:5 | g | | | |
| 22:6 | g | | | |
| Cholesterol | mg | 78 | 22 | 356 |
| Phytosterols | mg | | | |
| Amino acids | | | | |
| Tryptophan | g | —[d] | — | — |
| Threonine | g | 0.740 | 0.210 | 3.355 |
| Isoleucine | g | 0.931 | 0.264 | 4.225 |
| Leucine | g | 1.893 | 0.537 | 8.588 |
| Lysine | g | 1.972 | 0.559 | 8.947 |
| Methionine | g | 0.542 | 0.154 | 2.458 |
| Cystine | g | 0.116 | 0.033 | 0.525 |
| Phenylalanine | g | 1.014 | 0.287 | 4.598 |
| Tyrosine | g | 1.123 | 0.318 | 5.095 |
| Valine | g | 1.215 | 0.344 | 5.509 |
| Arginine | g | 0.834 | 0.236 | 3.783 |
| Histidine | g | 0.731 | 0.207 | 3.314 |
| Alanine | g | 0.594 | 0.168 | 2.692 |
| Aspartic acid | g | 1.406 | 0.399 | 6.379 |
| Glutamic acid | g | 4.545 | 1.288 | 20.614 |
| Glycine | g | 0.371 | 0.105 | 1.684 |
| Proline | g | 2.000 | 0.567 | 9.071 |
| Serine | g | 1.132 | 0.321 | 5.136 |

Item 9: Cheese (Parmesan, Grated)[n]

| Nutrients | Units | Amount in 100 g (edible portion) | Amount in edible portion of common measures of food (approximate measure and weight) 1 Tbsp = 5g | 1 oz = 28 g | Amount in edible portion of 1 lb of food as purchased (refuse: 0) |
|---|---|---|---|---|---|
| Proximate | | | | | |
| Water | g | 17.66 | 0.88 | 5.01 | 80.11 |
| Food energy | kcal | 456 | 23 | 129 | 2,068 |
| | kJ | 1,908 | 95 | 541 | 8,653 |
| Protein (N × 6.38) | g | 41.56 | 2.08 | 11.78 | 188.52 |
| Total lipid (fat) | g | 30.02 | 1.50 | 8.51 | 136.17 |
| Carbohydrate (total) | g | 3.74 | 0.19 | 1.06 | 16.96 |
| Fiber | g | 0 | 0 | 0 | 0 |
| Ash | g | 7.02 | 0.35 | 1.99 | 31.84 |
| Minerals | | | | | |
| Calcium | mg | 1,376 | 69 | 390 | 6,240 |
| Iron | mg | 0.95 | 0.05 | 0.27 | 4.31 |
| Magnesium | mg | 51 | 3 | 14 | 230 |
| Phosphorus | mg | 807 | 40 | 229 | 3,661 |
| Potassium | mg | 107 | 5 | 30 | 486 |
| Sodium | mg | 1,862 | 93 | 528 | 8,444 |
| Zinc | mg | 3.19 | 0.16 | 0.90 | 14.47 |
| Vitamins | | | | | |

Table 1 (continued)
NUTRIENT COMPOSITION OF MILK PRODUCTS AND BY-PRODUCTS

Item 9: Cheese (Parmesan, Grated)[n]

| Nutrients | Units | Amount in 100 g (edible portion) | Amount in edible portion of common measures of food (approximate measure and weight) | | Amount in edible portion of 1 lb of food as purchased (refuse: 0) |
|---|---|---|---|---|---|
| | | | 1 Tbsp = 5 g | 1 oz = 28 g | |
| Ascorbic acid | mg | 0 | 0 | 0 | 0 |
| Thiamin | mg | 0.045 | 0.002 | 0.013 | 0.204 |
| Riboflavin | mg | 0.386 | 0.019 | 0.109 | 1.751 |
| Niacin | mg | 0.315 | 0.016 | 0.089 | 1.429 |
| Pantothenic acid | mg | 0.527 | 0.026 | 0.149 | 2.390 |
| Vitamin B$_6$ | mg | 0.105 | 0.005 | 0.030 | 0.476 |
| Folacin | μg | 8 | Trace | 2 | 36 |
| Vitamin B$_{12}$ | μg | —[d] | — | — | — |
| Vitamin A | Re | — | — | — | — |
| | IU | 701 | 35 | 199 | 3,180 |
| Lipids | | | | | |
| Fatty acids | | | | | |
| Saturated (total) | g | 19.07 | 0.95 | 5.41 | 86.51 |
| 4:0 | g | 1.51 | 0.08 | 0.43 | 6.85 |
| 6:0 | g | 0.56 | 0.03 | 0.16 | 2.56 |
| 8:0 | g | 0.30 | 0.02 | 0.09 | 1.37 |
| 10:0 | g | 0.75 | 0.04 | 0.21 | 3.42 |
| 12:0 | g | 1.02 | 0.05 | 0.29 | 4.60 |
| 14:0 | g | 3.38 | 0.17 | 0.96 | 15.34 |
| 16:0 | g | 8.10 | 0.40 | 2.30 | 36.72 |
| 18:0 | g | 2.68 | 0.13 | 0.76 | 12.13 |
| Monounsaturated (total) | g | 8.73 | 0.44 | 2.48 | 39.62 |
| 16:1 | g | 0.46 | 0.02 | 0.13 | 2.08 |
| 18:1 | g | 7.74 | 0.39 | 2.19 | 35.09 |
| 20:1 | g | | | | |
| 22:1 | g | | | | |
| Polyunsaturated (total) | g | 0.66 | 0.03 | 0.19 | 3.00 |
| 18:2 | g | 0.32 | 0.02 | 0.09 | 1.43 |
| 18:3 | g | 0.34 | 0.02 | 0.10 | 1.56 |
| 18:4 | g | | | | |
| 20:4 | g | | | | |
| 20:5 | g | | | | |
| 22:5 | g | | | | |
| 22:6 | g | | | | |
| Cholesterol | mg | 79 | 4 | 22 | 357 |
| Phytosterols | mg | | | | |
| Amino acids | | | | | |
| Tryptophan | g | 0.560 | 0.028 | 0.159 | 2.541 |
| Threonine | g | 1.531 | 0.077 | 0.434 | 6.944 |
| Isoleucine | g | 2.202 | 0.110 | 0.624 | 9.987 |
| Leucine | g | 4.013 | 0.201 | 1.138 | 18.202 |
| Lysine | g | 3.843 | 0.192 | 1.090 | 17.433 |
| Methionine | g | 1.114 | 0.056 | 0.316 | 5.053 |
| Cystine | g | 0.274 | 0.014 | 0.078 | 1.241 |
| Phenylalanine | g | 2.234 | 0.112 | 0.633 | 10.135 |
| Tyrosine | g | 2.319 | 0.116 | 0.657 | 10.519 |
| Valine | g | 2.853 | 0.143 | 0.809 | 12.942 |
| Arginine | g | 1.531 | 0.077 | 0.434 | 6.944 |
| Histidine | g | 1.609 | 0.080 | 0.456 | 7.298 |
| Alanine | g | 1.218 | 0.061 | 0.345 | 5.525 |
| Aspartic acid | g | 2.599 | 0.130 | 0.737 | 11.790 |
| Glutamic acid | | 9.543 | 0.477 | 2.705 | 43.288 |
| Glycine | g | 0.723 | 0.036 | 0.205 | 3.280 |
| Proline | g | 4.860 | 0.243 | 1.378 | 22.043 |
| Serine | g | 2.404 | 0.120 | 0.681 | 10.903 |

Table 1 (continued)
## NUTRIENT COMPOSITION OF MILK PRODUCTS AND BY-PRODUCTS

Item 10: Cheese (Swiss)

| Nutrients | Units | Amount in 100 g (edible portion) | Amount in edible portion of common measures of food (approximate measure and weight) | | Amount in edible portion of 1 lb of food as purchased (refuse: 0) |
|---|---|---|---|---|---|
| | | | 1 in.³ = 15 g° | 1 oz = 28 g | |
| Proximate | | | | | |
| Water | g | 37.21 | 5.58 | 10.55 | 168.78 |
| Food energy | kcal | 376 | 56 | 107 | 1,704 |
| | kJ | 1,573 | 236 | 446 | 7,133 |
| Protein (N × 6.38) | g | 28.43 | 4.26 | 8.06 | 128.96 |
| Total lipid (fat) | g | 27.45 | 4.12 | 7.78 | 124.51 |
| Carbohydrate (total) | g | 3.38 | 0.51 | 0.96 | 15.33 |
| Fiber | g | 0 | 0 | 0 | 0 |
| Ash | g | 3.53 | 0.53 | 1.00 | 16.01 |
| Minerals | | | | | |
| Calcium | mg | 961 | 144 | 272 | 4,359 |
| Iron | mg | 0.17 | 0.02 | 0.05 | 0.77 |
| Magnesium | mg | 36 | 5 | 10 | 163 |
| Phosphorus | mg | 605 | 91 | 171 | 2,742 |
| Potassium | mg | 111 | 17 | 31 | 502 |
| Sodium | mg | 260 | 39 | 74 | 1,179 |
| Zinc | mg | 3.90 | 0.58 | 1.11 | 17.69 |
| Vitamins | | | | | |
| Ascorbic acid | mg | 0 | 0 | 0 | 0 |
| Thiamin | mg | 0.022 | 0.003 | 0.006 | 0.100 |
| Riboflavin | mg | 0.365 | 0.055 | 0.103 | 1.656 |
| Niacin | mg | 0.092 | 0.014 | 0.026 | 0.417 |
| Pantothenic acid | mg | 0.429 | 0.064 | 0.122 | 1.946 |
| Vitamin $B_6$ | mg | 0.083 | 0.012 | 0.024 | 0.376 |
| Folacin | µg | 6 | 1 | 2 | 29 |
| Vitamin $B_{12}$ | µg | 1.676 | 0.251 | 0.475 | 7.602 |
| Vitamin A | RE | 253 | 38 | 72 | 1,148 |
| | IU | 845 | 127 | 240 | 3,833 |
| Lipids | | | | | |
| Fatty acids | | | | | |
| Saturated (total) | g | 17.78 | 2.67 | 5.04 | 80.64 |
| 4:0 | g | 1.10 | 0.16 | 0.31 | 5.00 |
| 6:0 | g | 0.49 | 0.07 | 0.14 | 2.21 |
| 8:0 | g | 0.29 | 0.04 | 0.08 | 1.31 |
| 10:0 | g | 0.62 | 0.09 | 0.18 | 2.83 |
| 12:0 | g | 0.52 | 0.08 | 0.15 | 2.36 |
| 14:0 | g | 3.06 | 0.46 | 0.87 | 13.89 |
| 16:0 | g | 7.79 | 1.17 | 2.21 | 35.34 |
| 18:0 | g | 3.25 | 0.49 | 0.92 | 14.73 |
| Monounsaturated (total) | g | 7.27 | 1.09 | 2.06 | 33.00 |
| 16:1 | g | 0.88 | 0.13 | 0.25 | 3.99 |
| 18:1 | g | 6.02 | 0.90 | 1.71 | 27.29 |
| 20:1 | g | | | | |
| 22:1 | g | | | | |
| Polyunsaturated (total) | g | 0.97 | 0.15 | 0.28 | 4.41 |
| 18:2 | g | 0.62 | 0.09 | 0.18 | 2.81 |
| 18:3 | g | 0.35 | 0.05 | 0.10 | 1.60 |
| 18:4 | g | | | | |
| 20:4 | g | | | | |
| 20:5 | g | | | | |
| 22:5 | g | | | | |
| 22:6 | g | | | | |
| Cholesterol | mg | 92 | 14 | 26 | 416 |
| Phytosterols | mg | | | | |
| Amino acids | | | | | |
| Tryptophan | g | 0.401 | 0.060 | 0.114 | 1.819 |
| Threonine | g | 1.038 | 0.156 | 0.294 | 4.710 |
| Isoleucine | g | 1.537 | 0.231 | 0.436 | 6.973 |
| Leucine | g | 2.959 | 0.444 | 0.839 | 13.421 |
| Lysine | g | 2.585 | 0.388 | 0.733 | 11.723 |
| Methionine | g | 0.784 | 0.118 | 0.222 | 3.557 |
| Cystine | g | 0.290 | 0.043 | 0.082 | 1.314 |

Table 1 (continued)

NUTRIENT COMPOSITION OF MILK PRODUCTS AND BY-PRODUCTS

Item 10: Cheese (Swiss)

| Nutrients | Units | Amount in 100 g (edible portion) | Amount in edible portion of common measures of food (approximate measure and weight) | | Amount in edible portion of 1 lb of food as purchased (refuse: 0) |
|---|---|---|---|---|---|
| | | | 1 in.³ = 15 g° | 1 oz = 28 g | |
| Phenylalanine | g | 1.662 | 0.249 | 0.471 | 7.539 |
| Tyrosine | g | 1.693 | 0.254 | 0.480 | 7.681 |
| Valine | g | 2.139 | 0.321 | 0.606 | 9.702 |
| Arginine | g | 0.927 | 0.139 | 0.263 | 4.204 |
| Histidine | g | 1.065 | 0.160 | 0.302 | 4.831 |
| Alanine | g | 0.914 | 0.137 | 0.259 | 4.144 |
| Aspartic acid | g | 1.569 | 0.235 | 0.445 | 7.115 |
| Glutamic acid | g | 5.704 | 0.856 | 1.617 | 25.873 |
| Glycine | g | 0.508 | 0.076 | 0.144 | 2.304 |
| Proline | g | 3.690 | 0.553 | 1.046 | 16.736 |
| Serine | g | 1.640 | 0.246 | 0.465 | 7.438 |

Item 11: Cheese (American, Pasteurized Process)

| Nutrients | Units | Amount in 100 g (edible portion) | Amount in edible portion of common measures of food (approximate measure and weight) | | Amount in edible portion of 1 lb of food as purchased (refuse: 0) |
|---|---|---|---|---|---|
| | | | 1 in.³ = 17 5 gᵖ | 1 oz = 28 g | |
| Proximate | | | | | |
| Water | g | 39.16 | 6.85 | 11.10 | 177.63 |
| Food energy | kcal | 375 | 66 | 106 | 1,703 |
| | kJ | 1,571 | 275 | 445 | 7,127 |
| Protein (N × 6.38) | g | 22.15 | 3.88 | 6.28 | 100.47 |
| Total lipid (fat) | g | 31.25 | 5.47 | 8.86 | 141.75 |
| Carbohydrate (total) | g | 1.60 | 0.28 | 0.45 | 7.26 |
| Fiber | g | 0 | 0 | 0 | 0 |
| Ash | g | 5.84 | 1.02 | 1.66 | 26.49 |
| Minerals | | | | | |
| Calcium | mg | 616 | 108 | 174 | 2,792 |
| Iron | mg | 0.39 | 0.07 | .11 | 1.77 |
| Magnesium | mg | 22 | 4 | 6 | 101 |
| Phosphorus | mg | 745 | 130 | 211 | 3,379 |
| Potassium | mg | 162 | 28 | 46 | 735 |
| Sodium | mg | 1,430 | 250 | 406 | 6,488 |
| Zinc | mg | 2.99 | 0.52 | .85 | 13.56 |
| Vitamins | | | | | |
| Ascorbic acid | mg | 0 | 0 | 0 | 0 |
| Thiamin | mg | .027 | .005 | .008 | .122 |
| Riboflavin | mg | .353 | .062 | .100 | 1.601 |
| Niacin | mg | .069 | .012 | .020 | .313 |
| Pantothenic acid | mg | .482 | .084 | .137 | 2.186 |
| Vitamin $B_6$ | mg | .071 | .012 | .020 | .322 |
| Folacin | μg | 8 | 1 | 2 | 35 |
| Vitamin $B_{12}$ | μg | .696 | .122 | .197 | 3.157 |
| Vitamin A | RE | 290 | 51 | 82 | 1,315 |
| | IU | 1,210 | 212 | 343 | 5,487 |
| Lipids | | | | | |
| Fatty Acids | | | | | |
| Saturated (total) | g | 19.69 | 3.45 | 5.58 | 89.33 |
| 4:0 | g | 1.04 | .18 | .30 | 4.73 |
| 6:0 | g | .36 | .06 | .10 | 1.62 |
| 8:0 | g | .38 | .07 | .11 | 1.70 |
| 10:0 | g | .64 | .11 | .18 | 2.91 |
| 12:0 | g | .48 | .08 | .14 | 2.20 |
| 14:0 | g | 3.21 | .56 | .91 | 14.56 |
| 16:0 | g | 9.10 | 1.59 | 2.58 | 41.30 |
| 18:0 | g | 3.80 | .66 | 1.08 | 17.22 |
| Monounsaturated (total) | g | 8.95 | 1.57 | 2.54 | 40.60 |
| 16:1 | g | 1.03 | .18 | .29 | 4.66 |

Table 1 (continued)
## NUTRIENT COMPOSITION OF MILK PRODUCTS AND BY-PRODUCTS

### Item 11: Cheese (American, Pasteurized Process)

| Nutrients | Units | Amount in 100 g (edible portion) | Amount in edible portion of common measures of food (approximate measure and weight) | | Amount in edible portion of 1 lb of food as purchased (refuse: 0) |
|---|---|---|---|---|---|
| | | | 1 in.$^3$ = 17 5 g$^p$ | 1 oz = 28 g | |
| 18:1 | g | 7.51 | 1.31 | 2.13 | 34.07 |
| 20:1 | g | | | | |
| 22:1 | g | | | | |
| Polyunsaturated (total) | g | .99 | .17 | .28 | 4.49 |
| 18:2 | g | .61 | .11 | .17 | 2.75 |
| 18:3 | g | .38 | .07 | .11 | 1.74 |
| 18:4 | g | | | | |
| 20:4 | g | | | | |
| 20:5 | g | | | | |
| 22:5 | g | | | | |
| 22:6 | g | | | | |
| Cholesterol | mg | 94 | 17 | 27 | 428 |
| Phytosterols | mg | | | | |
| Amino Acids | | | | | |
| Tryptophan | g | .323 | .057 | .092 | 1.465 |
| Threonine | g | .719 | .126 | .204 | 3.260 |
| Isoleucine | g | 1.024 | .179 | .290 | 4.646 |
| Leucine | g | 1.958 | .343 | .555 | 8.882 |
| Lysine | g | 2.198 | .385 | .623 | 9.968 |
| Methionine | g | .573 | .100 | .162 | 2.598 |
| Cystine | g | .142 | .025 | .040 | .646 |
| Phenylalanine | g | 1.125 | .197 | .319 | 5.102 |
| Tyrosine | g | 1.212 | .212 | .344 | 5.496 |
| Valine | g | 1.326 | .232 | .376 | 6.016 |
| Arginine | g | .927 | .162 | .263 | 4.205 |
| Histidine | g | .903 | .158 | .256 | 4.094 |
| Alanine | g | .555 | 0.97 | .157 | 2.520 |
| Aspartic acid | g | 1.361 | .238 | .386 | 6.173 |
| Glutamic acid | g | 4.597 | .804 | 1.303 | 20.850 |
| Glycine | g | .365 | .064 | .103 | 1.654 |
| Proline | g | 2.253 | .394 | .639 | 10.220 |
| Serine | g | 1.069 | .187 | .303 | 4.850 |

### Item 12: Cheese Spread American, Pasteurized Process

| Nutrients | Units | Amount in 100 g (edible portion) | Amount in edible portion of common measures of food (approximate measure and weight) | | Amount in edible portion of 1 lb of food as purchased (refuse: 0) |
|---|---|---|---|---|---|
| | | | 1 oz = 28 g$^p$ | 1 jar (net wt) 5 oz = 142 g | |
| Proximate | | | | | |
| Water | g | 47.65 | 13.51 | 67.66 | 216.14 |
| Food energy | kcal | 290 | 82 | 412 | 1,318 |
| | kJ | 1,216 | 345 | 1,726 | 5,514 |
| Protein (N × 6.38) | g | 16.41 | 4.65 | 23.30 | 74.44 |
| Total lipid (fat) | g | 21.23 | 6.02 | 30.15 | 96.30 |
| Carbohydrate (total) | g | 8.73 | 2.48 | 12.40 | 39.60 |
| Fiber | g | 0 | 0 | 0 | 0 |
| Ash | g | 5.98 | 1.70 | 8.49 | 27.12 |
| Minerals | | | | | |
| Calcium | mg | 562 | 159 | 798 | 2,549 |
| Iron | mg | .33 | .09 | .47 | 1.50 |
| Magnesium | mg | 29 | 8 | 40 | 129 |
| Phosphorus | mg | 712 | 202 | 1,011 | 3,229 |
| Potassium | mg | 242 | 69 | 343 | 1,097 |
| Sodium | mg | 1,345 | 381 | 1,910 | 6,102 |
| Zinc | mg | 2.59 | 0.73 | 3.68 | 11.75 |
| Vitamins | | | | | |
| Ascorbic acid | mg | 0 | 0 | 0 | 0 |
| Thiamin | mg | 0.048 | .014 | 0.068 | .218 |

Table 1 (continued)
## NUTRIENT COMPOSITION OF MILK PRODUCTS AND BY-PRODUCTS

Item 12: Cheese Spread American, Pasteurized Process

| Nutrients | Units | Amount in 100 g (edible portion) | Amount in edible portion of common measures of food (approximate measure and weight) | | Amount in edible portion of 1 lb of food as purchased (refuse: 0) |
|---|---|---|---|---|---|
| | | | 1 oz = 28 g[r] | 1 jar (net wt) 5 oz = 142 g | |
| Riboflavin | mg | 0.431 | .122 | .612 | 1.955 |
| Niacin | mg | 0.131 | .037 | .186 | .594 |
| Pantothenic acid | mg | 0.686 | .194 | .974 | 3.112 |
| Vitamin $B_6$ | mg | 0.117 | .033 | .166 | .531 |
| Folacin | μg | 7 | 2 | 10 | 32 |
| Vitamin $B_{12}$ | μg | .400 | .113 | .568 | 1.814 |
| Vitamin A | RE | —[d] | — | — | — |
| | IU | 788 | 223 | 1,119 | 3,574 |
| Lipids | | | | | |
| Fatty acids | | | | | |
| Saturated (total) | g | 13.33 | 3.78 | 18.92 | 60.45 |
| 4:0 | g | .69 | .20 | .98 | 3.12 |
| 6:0 | g | .41 | .12 | .58 | 1.85 |
| 8:0 | g | .31 | .09 | .44 | 1.41 |
| 10:0 | g | .51 | .14 | .73 | 2.33 |
| 12:0 | g | .63 | .18 | .90 | 2.87 |
| 14:0 | g | 2.18 | .62 | 3.10 | 9.90 |
| 16:0 | g | 5.91 | 1.68 | 8.39 | 26.80 |
| 18:0 | g | 2.43 | .69 | 3.46 | 11.04 |
| Monounsaturated (total) | g | 6.22 | 1.76 | 8.83 | 28.21 |
| 16:1 | g | .56 | .16 | .80 | 2.54 |
| 18:1 | g | 5.22 | 1.48 | 7.41 | 23.68 |
| 20:1 | g | | | | |
| 22:1 | g | | | | |
| Polyunsaturated (total) | g | .62 | .18 | .89 | 2.83 |
| 18:2 | g | .40 | .11 | .57 | 1.82 |
| 18:3 | g | .22 | .06 | .32 | 1.01 |
| 18:4 | g | | | | |
| 20:4 | g | | | | |
| 20:5 | g | | | | |
| 22:5 | g | | | | |
| 22:6 | g | | | | |
| Cholesterol | mg | 55 | 6 | 78 | 250 |
| Phytosterols | mg | | | | |
| Amino acids | | | | | |
| Tryptophan | g | — | — | — | — |
| Threonine | g | .628 | .178 | .891 | 2.847 |
| Isoleucine | g | .833 | .236 | 1.183 | 3.780 |
| Leucine | g | 1.780 | .505 | 2.527 | 8.074 |
| Lysine | g | 1.507 | .427 | 2.140 | 6.837 |
| Methionine | g | .538 | .152 | .763 | 2.438 |
| Cystine | g | — | — | — | — |
| Phenylalanine | g | .931 | .264 | 1.322 | 4.223 |
| Tyrosine | g | .890 | .252 | 1.264 | 4.037 |
| Valine | g | 1.366 | .387 | 1.939 | 6.195 |
| Arginine | g | .545 | .155 | .774 | 2.473 |
| Histidine | g | .509 | .144 | .723 | 2.310 |
| Alanine | g | .602 | .171 | .855 | 2.730 |
| Aspartc acid | g | 1.103 | .313 | 1.567 | 5.005 |
| Glutamic acid | g | 3.475 | .985 | 4.934 | 15.762 |
| Glycine | g | .311 | .088 | .442 | 1.412 |
| Proline | g | 2.320 | .658 | 3.294 | 10.524 |
| Serine | g | 1.037 | .294 | 1.472 | 4.702 |

Table 1 (continued)
NUTRIENT COMPOSITION OF MILK PRODUCTS AND BY-PRODUCTS

Item 13: Cream (Light, Coffee or Table, Fluid)

| Nutrients | Units | Amount in 100 g (edible portion) | Amount in edible portion of common measures of food (approximate measure and weight) | | Amount in edible portion of 1 lb of food as purchased (refuse: 0) |
|---|---|---|---|---|---|
| | | | 1 Tbsp = 15 g | 1 cup = 240 g | |
| Proximate | | | | | |
| Water | g | 73.75 | 11.06 | 177.00 | 334.53 |
| Food energy | kcal | 195 | 29 | 469 | 886 |
| | kJ | 818 | 123 | 1,963 | 3,710 |
| Protein (N × 6.38) | g | 2.70 | 0.40 | 6.48 | 12.25 |
| Total lipid (fat) | g | 19.31 | 2.90 | 46.34 | 87.59 |
| Carbohydrate (total) | g | 3.66 | .55 | 8.78 | 16.60 |
| Fiber | g | 0 | 0 | 0 | 0 |
| Ash | g | 0.58 | .09 | 1.39 | 2.63 |
| Minerals | | | | | |
| Calcium | mg | 96 | 14 | 231 | 436 |
| Iron | mg | .04 | .01 | .10 | .18 |
| Magnesium | mg | 9 | 1 | 21 | 39 |
| Phosphorus | mg | 80 | 12 | 192 | 362 |
| Potassium | mg | 122 | 18 | 292 | 552 |
| Sodium | mg | 40 | 6 | 95 | 180 |
| Zinc | mg | .27 | .04 | .65 | 1.22 |
| Vitamins | | | | | |
| Ascorbic acid | mg | .76 | .11 | 1.82 | 3.45 |
| Thiamin | mg | .032 | .005 | .077 | .145 |
| Riboflavin | mg | .148 | .022 | .355 | .671 |
| Niacin | mg | .057 | .009 | .137 | .259 |
| Pantothenic acid | mg | .276 | .041 | .662 | 1.252 |
| Vitamin $B_6$ | mg | .032 | .005 | .077 | .145 |
| Folacin | μg | 2 | Trace | 6 | 10 |
| Vitamin $B_{12}$ | μg | .220 | .033 | .528 | .998 |
| Vitamin A | RE | 182 | 27 | 437 | 826 |
| | IU | 720 | 108 | 1,728 | 3,266 |
| Lipids | | | | | |
| Fatty acid | | | | | |
| Saturated (total) | g | 12.02 | 1.80 | 28.85 | 54.52 |
| 4:0 | g | .63 | .09 | 1.50 | 2.84 |
| 6:0 | g | .37 | .06 | .89 | 1.68 |
| 8:0 | g | .22 | .03 | .52 | .98 |
| 10:0 | g | .48 | .07 | 1.16 | 2.20 |
| 12:0 | g | .54 | .08 | 1.30 | 2.46 |
| 14:0 | g | 1.94 | .29 | 4.66 | 8.81 |
| 16:0 | g | 5.08 | .76 | 12.19 | 23.04 |
| 18:0 | g | 2.34 | .35 | 5.62 | 10.62 |
| Monounsaturated (total) | g | 5.58 | .84 | 13.38 | 25.30 |
| 16:1 | g | .43 | .06 | 1.04 | 1.96 |
| 18:1 | g | 4.86 | .73 | 11.66 | 22.04 |
| 20:1 | g | | | | |
| 22:1 | g | | | | |
| Polyunsaturated (total) | g | .72 | .11 | 1.72 | 3.25 |
| 18:2 | g | .44 | .06 | 1.05 | 1.98 |
| 18:3 | g | .28 | .04 | .67 | 1.27 |
| 18:4 | g | | | | |
| 20:4 | g | | | | |
| 20:5 | g | | | | |
| 22:5 | g | | | | |
| 22:6 | g | | | | |
| Cholesterol | mg | 66 | 10 | 159 | 300 |
| Phytosterols | mg | | | | |
| Amino acids | | | | | |
| Tryptophan | g | .038 | .006 | .091 | .173 |
| Threonine | g | .122 | .018 | .293 | .553 |
| Isoleucine | g | .163 | .025 | .392 | .741 |
| Leucine | g | .264 | .040 | .635 | 1.200 |
| Lysine | g | .214 | .032 | .514 | .971 |
| Methionine | g | .068 | .010 | .163 | .307 |
| Cystine | g | .025 | .004 | .060 | .113 |

Table 1 (continued)
NUTRIENT COMPOSITION OF MILK PRODUCTS AND BY-PRODUCTS

Item 13: Cream (Light, Coffee or Table, Fluid)

| Nutrients | Units | Amount in 100 g (edible portion) | Amount in edible portion of common measures of food (approximate measure and weight) 1 Tbsp = 15 g | 1 cup = 240 g | Amount in edible portion of 1 lb of food as purchased (refuse: 0) |
|---|---|---|---|---|---|
| Phenylalanine | g | .130 | .020 | .313 | .591 |
| Tyrosine | g | .130 | .020 | .313 | .591 |
| Valine | g | .181 | .027 | .434 | .820 |
| Arginine | g | .098 | .015 | .235 | .443 |
| Histidine | g | .073 | .011 | .176 | .332 |
| Alanine | g | .093 | .014 | .223 | .422 |
| Aspartic acid | g | .205 | .031 | .492 | .929 |
| Glutamic acid | g | .565 | .085 | 1.357 | 2.565 |
| Glycine | g | .057 | .009 | .137 | .259 |
| Proline | g | .262 | .039 | .628 | 1.186 |
| Serine | g | .147 | .022 | .352 | .666 |

Item 14: Cream (Medium, 25% Fat, Fluid)

| Nutrients | Units | Amount in 100 g (edible portion) | Amount in edile portion of common measures of food (approximate measure and weight) 1 Tbsp = 15 g | 1 cup = 239 g | Amount in edible portion of 1 lb of food as purchased (refuse: 0) |
|---|---|---|---|---|---|
| Proximate | | | | | |
| Water | g | 68.50 | 10.28 | 163.72 | 310.72 |
| Food energy | kcal | 244 | 37 | 583 | 1,106 |
| | kJ | 1,020 | 153 | 2,438 | 4,627 |
| Protein (N × 6.38) | g | 2.47 | 0.37 | 5.90 | 11.20 |
| Total lipid (fat) | g | 25.00 | 3.75 | 59.75 | 113.40 |
| Carbohydrate (total) | g | 3.48 | 0.52 | 8.32 | 15.78 |
| Fiber | g | 0 | 0 | 0 | 0 |
| Ash | g | 0.55 | .08 | 1.31 | 2.50 |
| Minerals | | | | | |
| Calcium | mg | 90 | 14 | 216 | 409 |
| Iron | mg | 0.04 | .01 | .10 | .18 |
| Magnesium | mg | 8 | | 20 | 38 |
| Phosphorus | mg | 71 | 11 | 169 | 320 |
| Potassium | mg | 114 | 7 | 274 | 519 |
| Sodium | mg | 37 | 6 | 88 | 168 |
| Zinc | mg | 0.26 | .04 | .62 | 1.18 |
| Vitamins | | | | | |
| Ascorbic acid | mg | .71 | .11 | 1.70 | 3.22 |
| Thiamin | mg | .029 | .004 | .069 | .132 |
| Riboflavin | mg | .136 | .020 | .325 | .617 |
| Niacin | mg | .052 | .008 | .124 | .236 |
| Pantothenic acid | mg | .270 | .040 | .645 | 1.225 |
| Vitamin B$_6$ | mg | .031 | .005 | .074 | .141 |
| Folacin | μg | 2 | Trace | 6 | 10 |
| Vitamin B$_{12}$ | μg | .218 | .033 | .521 | .989 |
| Vitamin A | RE | 232 | 35 | 554 | 1,052 |
| | IU | 942 | 141 | 2,251 | 4,273 |
| Lipids | | | | | |
| Fatty acids | | | | | |
| Saturated (total) | g | 15.56 | 2.33 | 37.19 | 70.59 |
| 4:0 | g | .81 | .12 | 1.94 | 3.68 |
| 6:0 | g | .48 | .07 | 1.15 | 2.18 |
| 8:0 | g | .28 | .04 | .67 | 1.27 |
| 10:0 | g | .63 | .09 | 1.50 | 2.84 |
| 12:0 | g | .70 | .10 | 1.68 | 3.18 |
| 14:0 | g | 2.51 | .38 | 6.01 | 11.40 |
| 16:0 | g | 6.58 | .99 | 15.72 | 29.83 |
| 18:0 | g | 3.03 | .45 | 7.24 | 13.74 |
| Monounsaturated (total) | g | 7.22 | 1.08 | 17.26 | 32.75 |
| 16:1 | g | .56 | .08 | 1.34 | 2.54 |

Table 1 (continued)
NUTRIENT COMPOSITION OF MILK PRODUCTS AND BY-PRODUCTS

Item 14: Cream (Medium, 25% Fat, Fluid)

| Nutrients | Units | Amount in 100 g (edible portion) | Amount in edile portion of common measures of food (approximate measure and weight) | | Amount in edible portion of 1 lb of food as purchased (refuse: 0) |
|---|---|---|---|---|---|
| | | | 1 Tbsp = 15 g | 1 cup = 239 g | |
| 18:1 | g | 6.29 | .94 | 15.03 | 28.53 |
| 20:1 | g | | | | |
| 22:1 | g | | | | |
| Polyunsaturated (total) | g | .93 | .14 | 2.22 | 4.21 |
| 18:2 | g | .56 | .08 | 1.35 | 2.56 |
| 18:3 | g | .36 | .06 | .87 | 1.65 |
| 18:4 | g | | | | |
| 20:4 | g | | | | |
| 20:5 | g | | | | |
| 22:5 | g | | | | |
| 22:6 | g | | | | |
| Cholesterol | mg | 88 | 13 | 209 | 397 |
| Phytosterols | mg | | | | |
| Amino acids | | | | | |
| Tryptophan | g | 0.035 | .005 | .083 | .158 |
| Threonine | g | .111 | .017 | .266 | .506 |
| Isoleucine | g | .149 | .022 | .357 | .678 |
| Leucine | g | .242 | .036 | .578 | 1.098 |
| Lysine | g | .196 | .029 | .468 | .889 |
| Methionine | g | .062 | .009 | .148 | .281 |
| Cystine | g | .023 | .003 | .055 | .104 |
| Phenylalanine | g | .119 | .018 | .285 | .541 |
| Tyrosine | g | .119 | .018 | .285 | .541 |
| Valine | g | .165 | .025 | .395 | .750 |
| Arginine | g | .089 | .013 | .214 | .406 |
| Histidine | g | .067 | .010 | .160 | .304 |
| Alanine | g | .085 | .013 | .204 | .386 |
| Aspartic acid | g | .187 | .028 | .448 | .850 |
| Glutamic acid | g | .517 | .078 | 1.236 | 2.346 |
| Glycine | g | .052 | .008 | .125 | .237 |
| Proline | g | .239 | .036 | .572 | 1.085 |
| Serine | g | .134 | .020 | .321 | .609 |

Item 15: Cream (Sour, Cultured)

| Nutrients | Units | Amount in 100 g (edible portion) (Mean ± SE) | Amount in edible portion of common measures of food (approximate measure and weight) | | Amount in edible portion of 1 lb of food as purchased (refuse: 0) |
|---|---|---|---|---|---|
| | | | 1 Tbsp = 12 g | 1 cup = 230 g | |
| Proximate | | | | | |
| Water | g | 70.95 | 8.51 | 163.18 | 321.83 |
| Food energy | kcal | 214 | 26 | 493 | 972 |
| | kJ | 897 | 108 | 2,062 | 4,067 |
| Protein (N × 6.38) | g | 3.16 | .38 | 7.27 | 14.33 |
| Total lipid (fat) | g | 20.96 | 2.52 | 48.21 | 95.08 |
| Carbohydrate (total) | g | 4.27 | .51 | 9.82 | 19.37 |
| Fiber | g | 0 | 0 | 0 | 0 |
| Ash | g | .66 | .08 | 1.52 | 2.99 |
| Minerals | | | | | |
| Calcium | mg | 116 | 14 | 268 | 528 |
| Iron | mg | .06 | .01 | .14 | .27 |
| Magnesium | mg | 11 | 1 | 26 | 51 |
| Phosphorus | mg | 85 | 10 | 195 | 385 |
| Potassium | mg | 144 | 17 | 331 | 653 |
| Sodium | mg | 53 | 6 | 123 | 242 |
| Zinc | mg | .27 | .03 | .62 | 1.22 |

Table 1 (continued)
## NUTRIENT COMPOSITION OF MILK PRODUCTS AND BY-PRODUCTS

### Item 15: Cream (Sour, Cultured)

| Nutrients | Units | Amount in 100 g (edible portion) (Mean ± SE) | Amount in edible portion of common measures of food (approximate measure and weight) | | Amount in edible portion of 1 lb of food as purchased (refuse: 0) |
|---|---|---|---|---|---|
| | | | 1 Tbsp = 12 g | 1 cup = 230 g | |
| Vitamins | | | | | |
| Ascorbic acid | mg | .86 | .10 | 1.98 | 3.90 |
| Thiamin | mg | .035 | .004 | .081 | .159 |
| Riboflavin | mg | .149 | .018 | .343 | .676 |
| Niacin | mg | .067 | .008 | .154 | .304 |
| Pantothenic acid | mg | .360 | .043 | .828 | 1.633 |
| Vitamin B$_6$ | mg | .016 | .002 | .037 | .073 |
| Folacin | μg | 11 | 1 | 25 | 49 |
| Vitamin B$_{12}$ | μg | .300 | .036 | .690 | 1.361 |
| Vitamin A | RE | 195 | 23 | 448 | 885 |
| | IU | 790 | 95 | 1,817 | 3,583 |
| Lipids | | | | | |
| Fatty acids | | | | | |
| Saturated (total) | g | 13.05 | 1.57 | 30.01 | 59.18 |
| 4:0 | g | .68 | .08 | 1.56 | 3.08 |
| 6:0 | g | .40 | .05 | .92 | 1.82 |
| 8:0 | g | .23 | .03 | .54 | 1.06 |
| 10:0 | g | .53 | .06 | 1.21 | 2.38 |
| 12:0 | g | .59 | .07 | 1.35 | 2.67 |
| 14:0 | g | 2.11 | .25 | 4.85 | 9.56 |
| 16:0 | g | 5.51 | .66 | 12.68 | 25.01 |
| 18:0 | g | 2.54 | .30 | 5.84 | 11.52 |
| Monounsaturated (total) | g | 6.05 | .73 | 13.92 | 27.46 |
| 16:1 | g | .47 | .06 | 1.08 | 2.13 |
| 18:1 | g | 5.27 | .63 | 12.13 | 23.92 |
| 20:1 | g | | | | |
| 22:1 | g | | | | |
| Polyunsaturated (total) | g | .78 | .09 | 1.79 | 3.53 |
| 18:2 | g | .47 | .06 | 1.09 | 2.15 |
| 18:3 | g | .30 | .04 | .70 | 1.38 |
| 18:4 | g | | | | |
| 20:4 | g | | | | |
| 20:5 | g | | | | |
| 22:5 | g | | | | |
| 22:6 | g | | | | |
| Cholesterol | mg | 44 | 5 | 102 | 201 |
| Phytosterols | mg | | | | |
| Amino Acids | | | | | |
| Tryptophan | g | —$^d$ | — | — | — |
| Threonine | g | — | — | — | — |
| Isoleucine | g | — | — | — | — |
| Leucine | g | — | — | — | — |
| Lysine | g | — | — | — | — |
| Methionine | g | — | — | — | — |
| Cystine | g | — | — | — | — |
| Phenylalanine | g | — | — | — | — |
| Tyrosine | g | — | — | — | — |
| Valine | g | — | — | — | — |
| Arginine | g | — | — | — | — |
| Histidine | g | — | — | — | — |
| Alanine | g | — | — | — | — |
| Aspartic acid | g | — | — | — | — |
| Glutamic acid | g | — | — | — | — |
| Glycine | g | — | — | — | — |
| Proline | g | — | — | — | — |
| Serine | g | — | — | — | — |

Table 1 (continued)
## NUTRIENT COMPOSITION OF MILK PRODUCTS AND BY-PRODUCTS

Item 16: Filled Milk (Containing Blend of Hydrogenated Vegetable Oils, Fluid)[q]

| Nutrients | Units | Amount in 100 g (edible portion) | Amount in edible portion of common measures of food (approximate measure and weight) | | Amount in edible portion of 1 lb of food as purchased (refuse:0) |
|---|---|---|---|---|---|
| | | | 1 cup = 244 g | 1 qt = 976 g | |
| Proximate | | | | | |
| Water | g | 87.67 | 213.92 | 855.66 | 397.67 |
| Food energy | kcal | 63 | 154 | 616 | 286 |
| | kJ | 264 | 645 | 2,579 | 1,199 |
| Protein (N × 6.38) | g | 3.33 | 8.12 | 32.50 | 15.10 |
| Total lipid (fat) | g | 3.46 | 8.44 | 33.77 | 15.70 |
| Carbohydrate (total) | g | 4.74 | 11.57 | 46.26 | 21.50 |
| Fiber | g | 0 | 0 | 0 | 0 |
| Ash | g | 0.80 | 1.95 | 7.81 | 3.63 |
| Minerals | | | | | |
| Calcium | mg | 128 | 312 | 1,247 | 580 |
| Iron | mg | .05 | 0.12 | .49 | .23 |
| Magnesium | mg | 13 | 32 | 130 | 60 |
| Phosphorus | mg | 97 | 236 | 946 | 440 |
| Potassium | mg | 139 | 339 | 1,357 | 631 |
| Sodium | mg | 57 | 138 | 553 | 257 |
| Zinc | mg | .36 | .088 | 3.51 | 1.63 |
| Vitamins | | | | | |
| Ascorbic acid | mg | .90 | 2.20 | 8.78 | 4.08 |
| Thiamin | mg | .030 | .073 | .293 | .136 |
| Riboflavin | mg | .123 | .300 | 1.200 | .558 |
| Niacin | mg | .087 | .212 | .849 | .395 |
| Pantothenic acid | mg | .301 | .734 | 2.938 | 1.365 |
| Vitamin B$_6$ | mg | .040 | .098 | .390 | .181 |
| Folacin | μg | 5 | 12 | 47 | 22 |
| Vitamin B$_{12}$ | μg | .342 | .834 | 3.338 | 1.551 |
| Vitamin A[r] | RE | 2 | 5 | 20 | 9 |
| | IU | 7 | 17 | 68 | 32 |
| Lipids | | | | | |
| Fatty acids | | | | | |
| Saturated (total) | g | .77 | 1.87 | 7.49 | 3.48 |
| 4:0 | g | | | | |
| 6:0 | g | | | | |
| 8:0 | g | Trace | .01 | .02 | .01 |
| 10:0 | g | Trace | .01 | .04 | .02 |
| 12:0 | g | .02 | .04 | .16 | .08 |
| 14:0 | g | .03 | .07 | .29 | .14 |
| 16:0 | g | .49 | 1.20 | 4.78 | 2.22 |
| 18:0 | g | .23 | .57 | 2.26 | 1.05 |
| Monounsaturated (total) | g | 1.78 | 4.35 | 17.41 | 8.09 |
| 16:1 | g | Trace | Trace | .01 | Trace |
| 18:1 | g | 1.78 | 4.35 | 17.42 | 8.10 |
| 20:1 | g | | | | |
| 22:1 | g | | | | |
| Polyunsaturated (total) | g | .75 | 1.83 | 7.32 | 3.40 |
| 18:2 | g | .72 | 1.75 | 6.99 | 3.25 |
| 18:3 | g | .03 | .07 | .26 | .12 |
| 18:4 | g | | | | |
| 20:4 | g | | | | |
| 20:5 | g | | | | |
| 22:5 | g | | | | |
| 22:6 | g | | | | |
| Cholesterol | mg | 2 | 4 | 18 | 8 |
| Phytosterols | mg | —[d] | — | — | — |
| Amino Acids | | | | | |
| Tryptophan | mg | .047 | .115 | .458 | .213 |
| Threonine | g | .150 | .367 | 1.467 | .682 |
| Isoleucine | g | .201 | .492 | 1.966 | .914 |
| Leucine | g | .326 | .796 | 3.184 | 1.480 |
| Lysine | g | .264 | .644 | 2.578 | 1.198 |
| Methionine | g | .084 | .204 | .815 | .379 |
| Cystine | g | .031 | .075 | .301 | .140 |

Table 1 (continued)
## NUTRIENT COMPOSITION OF MILK PRODUCTS AND BY-PRODUCTS

### Item 16: Filled Milk (Containing Blend of Hydrogenated Vegetable Oils, Fluid)[q]

| Nutrients | Units | Amount in 100 g (edible portion) | Amount in edible portion of common measures of food (approximate measure and weight) | | Amount in edible portion of 1 lb of food as purchased (refuse:0) |
|---|---|---|---|---|---|
| | | | 1 cup = 244 g | 1 qt = 976 g | |
| Phenylanine | g | .161 | .392 | 1.569 | .729 |
| Tyrosine | g | .161 | .392 | 1569 | .729 |
| Valine | g | .223 | .544 | 2.175 | 1.011 |
| Arginine | g | .121 | .294 | 1.177 | .547 |
| Histidine | g | .090 | .220 | .881 | .410 |
| Alanine | g | .115 | .280 | 1.121 | .521 |
| Aspartic acid | g | .253 | .616 | 2.466 | 1.146 |
| Glutamic acid | g | .697 | 1.701 | 6.806 | 3.163 |
| Glycine | g | .070 | 172 | .688 | .320 |
| Proline | g | .323 | .787 | 3.148 | 1.463 |
| Serine | g | .181 | .442 | 1.768 | .822 |

### Item 17: Filled Milk (Containing Lauric Acid Oil, Fluid)[s]

| Nutrients | Units | Amount in 100 g (edible portion) | Amount in edible portion of common measures of food (approximate measure and weight) | | Amount in edible portion of 1 lb of food as purchased (refuse:0) |
|---|---|---|---|---|---|
| | | | 1 cup = 244 g | 1 qt = 976 g | |
| Proximate | | | | | |
| Water | g | 87.73 | 214.06 | 856.24 | 397.94 |
| Food energy | kcal | 63 | 153 | 611 | 284 |
| | kJ | 262 | 639 | 2,558 | 1,189 |
| Protein (N × 6.38) | g | 3.33 | 8.12 | 32.50 | 15.10 |
| Total lipid (fat) | g | 3.40 | 8.30 | 33.18 | 15.42 |
| Carbohydrate (total) | g | 4.74 | 11.57 | 46.26 | 21.50 |
| Fiber | g | 0 | 0 | 0 | 0 |
| Ash | g | .80 | 1.95 | 7.81 | 3.63 |
| Minerals | | | | | |
| Calcium | mg | 128 | 312 | 1,247 | 580 |
| Iron | mg | .05 | .12 | .49 | .23 |
| Magnesium | mg | 13 | 32 | 130 | 60 |
| Phosphorus | mg | 97 | 236 | 946 | 440 |
| Potassium | mg | 139 | 339 | 1,357 | 631 |
| Sodium | mg | 57 | 138 | 553 | 257 |
| Zinc | mg | .36 | .83 | 3.51 | 1.63 |
| Vitamins | | | | | |
| Ascorbic acid | mg | .90 | 2.20 | 8.78 | 4.08 |
| Thiamin | mg | .030 | .073 | .293 | .136 |
| Riboflavin | mg | .123 | .300 | 1.200 | .558 |
| Niacin | mg | .087 | .212 | .849 | .395 |
| Pantothenic acid | mg | .301 | .734 | 2.938 | 1.365 |
| Vitamin B$_6$ | mg | .040 | .098 | .390 | .181 |
| Folacin | μg | 5 | 12 | 47 | 22 |
| Vitamin B$_{12}$ | μg | .342 | .834 | 3.338 | 1.551 |
| Vitamin A[r] | RE | 2 | 5 | 20 | 9 |
| | IU | 7 | 17 | 68 | 32 |
| Lipids | | | | | |
| Fatty acids | | | | | |
| Saturated (total) | g | 3.10 | 7.67 | 30.27 | 14.07 |
| 4:0 | g | | | | |
| 6:0 | g | | | | |
| 8:0 | g | .17 | .42 | 1.69 | .78 |
| 10:0 | g | .13 | .32 | 1.27 | .59 |
| 12:0 | g | 2.05 | 5.00 | 19.98 | 9.29 |
| 14:0 | g | .40 | .97 | 3.89 | 1.81 |
| 16:0 | g | .19 | .47 | 1.87 | .87 |
| 18:0 | g | .15 | .36 | 1.44 | .67 |
| Monounsaturated (total) | g | .10 | .24 | .97 | .45 |
| 16:1 | g | | | | |
| 18:1 | g | .10 | .24 | .97 | .45 |

Table 1 (continued)
## NUTRIENT COMPOSITION OF MILK PRODUCTS AND BY-PRODUCTS

### Item 17: Filled Milk (Containing Lauric Acid Oil, Fluid)[s]

| Nutrients | Units | Amount in 100 g (edible portion) | Amount in edible portion of common measures of food (approximate measure and weight) | | Amount in edible portion of 1 lb of food as purchased (refuse:0) |
|---|---|---|---|---|---|
| | | | 1 cup = 244 g | 1 qt = 976 g | |
| 20:1 | g | | | | |
| 22:1 | g | | | | |
| Polyunsaturated (total) | g | .01 | .02 | .10 | .05 |
| 18:2 | g | .01 | .02 | .08 | .04 |
| 18:3 | g | 0 | 0 | 0 | 0 |
| 18:4 | g | | | | |
| 20:4 | g | | | | |
| 20:5 | g | | | | |
| 22:5 | g | | | | |
| 22:6 | g | | | | |
| Cholesterol | mg | 2 | 4 | 18 | 8 |
| Phytosterols | mg | —[d] | — | — | — |
| Amino acids | | | | | |
| Tryptophan | g | .047 | .115 | .458 | .213 |
| Threonine | g | .150 | .367 | 1.467 | .682 |
| Isoleucine | g | .201 | .492 | 1.966 | .914 |
| Leucine | g | .326 | .796 | 3.184 | 1.480 |
| Lysine | g | .264 | .644 | 2.578 | 1.198 |
| Methionine | g | .084 | .204 | .815 | .379 |
| Cystine | g | .031 | .075 | .301 | .140 |
| Phenylalanine | g | .161 | .392 | 1.569 | .729 |
| Tyrosine | g | .161 | .392 | 1.569 | .729 |
| Valine | g | .223 | .544 | 2.175 | 1.011 |
| Arginine | g | .121 | .294 | 1.177 | .547 |
| Histidine | g | .090 | .220 | .881 | .410 |
| Alanine | g | .115 | .280 | 1.121 | .521 |
| Aspartic acid | g | .253 | .616 | 2.466 | 1.146 |
| Glutamic acid | g | .697 | 1.701 | 6.806 | 3.163 |
| Glycine | g | .070 | .172 | .688 | .320 |
| Proline | g | .323 | .787 | 3.148 | 1.463 |
| Serine | g | .181 | .442 | 1.768 | .822 |

### Item 18: Ice Cream [Vanilla, Regular (Ca. 10% Fat) Hardened]

| Nutrients | Units | Amount in 100 g (edible portion) | Amount in edible portion of common measures of food (approximate measure and weight) | | Amount in edible portion of 1 lb of food as purchased (refuse: 0) |
|---|---|---|---|---|---|
| | | | 1 cup (8 fl oz) = 133 g | ½ gal = 1,064 g | |
| Proximate | | | | | |
| Water | g | 60.80 | 80.86 | 646.91 | 275.79 |
| Food energy | kcal | 202 | 269 | 2,153 | 918 |
| | kJ | 847 | 1,126 | 9,012 | 3,842 |
| Protein (N × 6.38) | g | 3.61 | 4.80 | 38.41 | 16.38 |
| Total lipid (fat) | g | 10.77 | 14.32 | 114.59 | 48.85 |
| Carbohydrate (total) | g | 23.85 | 31.72 | 253.76 | 108.18 |
| Fiber | g | 0 | 0 | 0 | 0 |
| Ash | g | .97 | 1.29 | 10.32 | 4.40 |
| Minerals | | | | | |
| Calcium | mg | 132 | 176 | 1,406 | 599 |
| Iron | mg | .09 | .12 | .96 | .41 |
| Magnesium | mg | 14 | 18 | 148 | 63 |
| Phosphorus | mg | 101 | 134 | 1,075 | 458 |
| Potassium | mg | 193 | 257 | 2,052 | 875 |
| Sodium | mg | 87 | 116 | 929 | 396 |
| Zinc | mg | 1.06 | 1.41 | 11.28 | 4.81 |
| Vitamins | | | | | |
| Ascorbic acid | mg | .53 | .70 | 5.64 | 2.40 |
| Thiamin | mg | .039 | .052 | .415 | .177 |

Table 1 (continued)
## NUTRIENT COMPOSITION OF MILK PRODUCTS AND BY-PRODUCTS

### Item 18: Ice Cream [Vanilla, Regular (Ca. 10% Fat) Hardened]

| Nutrients | Units | Amount in 100 g (edible portion) | Amount in edible portion of common measures of food (approximate measure and weight) | | Amount in edible portion of 1 lb of food as purchased (refuse: 0) |
|---|---|---|---|---|---|
| | | | 1 cup (8 fl oz) = 133 g | ½ gal = 1,064 g | |
| Riboflavin | mg | .247 | .329 | 2.628 | 1.120 |
| Niacin | mg | .101 | .134 | 1.075 | .458 |
| Pantothenic acid | mg | .492 | .654 | 5.235 | 2.232 |
| Vitamin $B_6$ | mg | .046 | .061 | .489 | .209 |
| Folacin | μg | 2 | 3 | 22 | 10 |
| Tyrosine | g | .174 | .232 | 1.854 | .791 |
| Valine | g | .242 | .321 | 2.571 | 1.096 |
| Arginine | g | .131 | .174 | 1.391 | .593 |
| Histidine | g | .098 | .130 | 1.042 | .444 |
| Alanine | g | .124 | .166 | 1.324 | .565 |
| Aspartic acid | g | .274 | .364 | 2.914 | 1.242 |
| Glutamic acid | g | .756 | 1.005 | 8.043 | 3.429 |
| Glycine | g | .076 | .102 | .813 | .346 |
| Proline | g | .350 | .465 | 3.721 | 1.586 |
| Serine | g | .196 | .261 | 2.089 | .891 |

### Item 19: Coffee Whitener (Nondairy, Powdered)[r]

| Nutrients | Units | Amount in 100 g (edible portion) | Amount in edible portion of common measures of food (approximate measure and weight) | | Amount in edible portion of 1 lb of food as purchased (refuse:0) |
|---|---|---|---|---|---|
| | | | 1 tsp = 2 g | 1 cup = 94 g | |
| **Proximate** | | | | | |
| Water | g | 2.21 | 0.04 | 2.08 | 10.02 |
| Food energy | kcal | 546 | 11 | 514 | 2,479 |
| | kJ | 2,287 | 46 | 2.150 | 10,374 |
| Protein (N × 6.29) | g | 4.79 | .10 | 4.50 | 21.73 |
| Vitamin $B_{12}$ | μg | .470 | .625 | 5.001 | 2.132 |
| Vitamin A | RE | 100 | 133 | 1,064 | 454 |
| | IU | 408 | 543 | 4,341 | 1,851 |
| **Lipids** | | | | | |
| Fatty acids | | | | | |
| Saturated (total) | g | 6.70 | 8.92 | 71.33 | 30.41 |
| 4:0 | g | .35 | .46 | 3.72 | 1.58 |
| 6:0 | g | .21 | .28 | 2.20 | .94 |
| 8:0 | g | .12 | .16 | 1.28 | .55 |
| 10:0 | g | .27 | .36 | 2.87 | 1.22 |
| 12:0 | g | .30 | .40 | 3.22 | 1.37 |
| 14:0 | g | 1.08 | 1.44 | 11.52 | 4.91 |
| 16:0 | g | 2.83 | 3.77 | 30.14 | 12.85 |
| 18:0 | g | 1.30 | 1.74 | 13.89 | 5.92 |
| Monounsaturated (total) | g | 3.11 | 4.14 | 33.10 | 14.11 |
| 16:1 | g | .24 | .32 | 2.57 | 1.09 |
| 18:1 | g | 2.71 | 3.60 | 28.83 | 12.29 |
| 20:1 | g | | | | |
| 22:1 | g | | | | |
| Polyunsaturated (total) | g | .40 | .53 | 4.26 | 1.81 |
| 18:2 | g | .24 | .32 | 2.59 | 1.10 |
| 18:3 | g | .16 | .21 | 1.67 | 0.71 |
| 18:4 | g | | | | |
| 20:4 | g | | | | |
| 20:5 | g | | | | |
| 22:5 | g | | | | |
| 22:6 | g | | | | |
| Cholesterol | mg | 45 | 59 | 476 | 203 |
| Phytosterols | mg | | | | |
| Amino acids | | | | | |
| Tryptophan | g | .051 | .068 | .542 | .231 |

Table 1 (continued)
## NUTRIENT COMPOSITION OF MILK PRODUCTS AND BY-PRODUCTS

Item 19: Coffee Whitener (Nondairy, Powdered)[r]

| Nutrients | Units | Amount in 100 g (edible portion) | Amount in edible portion of common measures of food (approximate measure and weight) | | Amount in edible portion of 1 lb of food as purchased (refuse:0) |
|---|---|---|---|---|---|
| | | | 1 tsp = 2 g | 1 cup = 94 g | |
| Threonine | g | .103 | .217 | 1.734 | .739 |
| Isoleucine | g | .218 | .290 | 2.324 | .991 |
| Lucine | g | .354 | .470 | 3.763 | 1.604 |
| Lysine | g | .286 | .381 | 3.046 | 1.299 |
| Methionine | g | .091 | .120 | .963 | .411 |
| Cystine | g | .033 | .044 | .355 | .151 |
| Phenylalanine | g | .174 | .232 | 1.854 | .791 |
| Total lipid (fat) | g | 35.48 | .71 | 33.35 | 160.94 |
| Carbohydrate (total) | g | 54.88 | 1.10 | 51.59 | 248.94 |
| Fiber | g | 0 | 0 | 0 | 0 |
| Ash | g | 2.64 | .05 | 2.48 | 11.98 |
| Minerals | | | | | |
| Calcium | mg | 22 | Trace | 21 | 101 |
| Iron | mg | 1.15 | .02 | 1.08 | 5.22 |
| Magnesium | mg | 4 | Trace | 4 | 18 |
| Phosphorus | mg | 422 | 8 | 397 | 1,914 |
| Potassium | mg | 812 | 16 | 763 | 3,682 |
| Sodium | mg | 181 | 4 | 170 | 821 |
| Zinc | mg | .51 | .01 | .48 | 2.31 |
| Vitamins | | | | | |
| Ascorbic acid | mg | 0 | 0 | 0 | 0 |
| Thiamin | mg | 0 | 0 | 0 | 0 |
| Riboflavin[u] | mg | .165 | .003 | .155 | .748 |
| Niacin | mg | 0 | 0 | 0 | 0 |
| Pantothenic acid | mg | 0 | 0 | 0 | 0 |
| Vitamin B₆ | mg | 0 | 0 | 0 | 0 |
| Folacin | μg | 0 | 0 | 0 | 0 |
| Vitamin B₁₂ | μg | 0 | 0 | 0 | 0 |
| Vitamin A[v] | RE | 20 | Trace | 19 | 92 |
| | IU | 203 | 4 | 191 | 921 |
| Lipids | | | | | |
| Fatty acids | | | | | |
| Saturated (total) | g | 32.52 | .65 | 30.57 | 147.53 |
| 4:0 | g | | | | |
| 6:0 | g | | | | |
| 8:0 | g | 1.33 | .03 | 1.25 | 6.04 |
| 10:0 | g | 1.46 | .03 | 1.37 | 6.61 |
| 12:0 | g | 13.58 | .27 | 12.76 | 61.60 |
| 14:0 | g | 5.99 | .12 | 5.63 | 27.16 |
| 16:0 | g | 3.75 | .08 | 3.53 | 17.02 |
| 18:0 | g | 6.34 | .13 | 5.96 | 28.75 |
| Monounsaturated (total) | g | .97 | .02 | .91 | 4.39 |
| 16:1 | g | | | | |
| 18:1 | g | .97 | .02 | .91 | 4.39 |
| 20:1 | g | | | | |
| 22:1 | g | | | | |
| Polyunsaturated (total) | g | .01 | Trace | .01 | .06 |
| 18:2 | g | Trace | Trace | Trace | .02 |
| 18:3 | g | .01 | Trace | .01 | .05 |
| 18:4 | g | | | | |
| 20:4 | g | | | | |
| 20:5 | g | | | | |
| 22:5 | g | | | | |
| 22:6 | g | | | | |
| Cholesterol | mg | 0 | 0 | 0 | 0 |
| Phytosterols | mg | — | [d] — | — | — |
| Amino acids | | | | | |
| Tryptophan | g | .066 | .001 | .062 | .301 |
| Threonine | g | .203 | .004 | .190 | .919 |
| Isoleucine | g | .294 | .006 | .276 | 1.333 |
| Leucine | g | .473 | .009 | .445 | 2.145 |
| Lysine | g | .385 | .008 | .362 | 1.748 |

Table 1 (continued)
## NUTRIENT COMPOSITION OF MILK PRODUCTS AND BY-PRODUCTS

### Item 19: Coffee Whitener (Nondairy, Powdered)[c]

| Nutrients | Units | Amount in 100 g (edible portion) | Amount in edible portion of common measures of food (approximate measure and weight) | | Amount in edible portion of 1 lb of food as purchased (refuse:0) |
|---|---|---|---|---|---|
| | | | 1 tsp = 2 g | 1 cup = 94 g | |
| Methionine | g | .145 | .003 | .137 | .660 |
| Cystine | g | .021 | Trace | .019 | .093 |
| Phenylalanine | g | .257 | .005 | .241 | 1.164 |
| Tyrosine | g | .274 | .005 | .258 | 1.244 |
| Valine | g | .343 | .007 | .322 | 1.554 |
| Arginine | g | .190 | .004 | .178 | .860 |
| Histidine | g | .142 | .003 | .133 | .642 |
| Alanine | g | .150 | .003 | .141 | .680 |
| Aspartic acid | g | .339 | .007 | .319 | 1.537 |
| Glutamic acid | g | 1.088 | .022 | 1.023 | 4.936 |
| Glycine | g | .096 | .002 | .090 | .435 |
| Proline | g | .540 | .011 | .508 | 2.449 |
| Serine | g | .295 | .006 | .277 | 1.337 |

### Item 20: Dessert Topping (Nondairy, Powdered)[c]

| Nutrients | Units | Amount in 100 g (edible portion) | Amount in edible portion of common measures of food (approximate measure and weight) | | Amount in edible portion of 1 lb of food as purchased (refuse:0) |
|---|---|---|---|---|---|
| | | | Mount to prepare 1 Tbsp = 1.3 g | 1½ oz = 42.5 g | |
| **Proximate** | | | | | |
| Water | g | 1.47 | 0.02 | 0.62 | 6.67 |
| Food energy | kcal | 577 | 8 | 245 | 2,618 |
| | kJ | 2,415 | 31 | 1,027 | 10,956 |
| Protein (N × 6.29) | g | 4.90 | .06 | 2.08 | 22.23 |
| Total lipid (fat) | g | 39.92 | .52 | 16.97 | 181.08 |
| Carbohydrate (total) | g | 52.54 | .68 | 22.33 | 238.32 |
| Fiber | g | 0 | 0 | 0 | 0 |
| Ash | g | 1.17 | .02 | .50 | 5.31 |
| **Minerals** | | | | | |
| Calcium | mg | 17 | Trace | 7 | 75 |
| Iron | mg | — | — | — | — |
| Magnesium | mg | — | — | — | — |
| Phosphorus | mg | 74 | 1 | 31 | 333 |
| Potassium | mg | 166 | 2 | 71 | 753 |
| Sodium | mg | 122 | 2 | 52 | 551 |
| Zinc | mg | — | — | — | — |
| **Vitamins** | | | | | |
| Ascorbic acid | mg | 0 | 0 | 0 | 0 |
| Thiamin | mg | 0 | 0 | 0 | 0 |
| Riboflavin | mg | 0 | 0 | 0 | 0 |
| Niacin | mg | 0 | 0 | 0 | 0 |
| Pantothenic acid | mg | 0 | 0 | 0 | 0 |
| Vitamin B$_6$ | mg | 0 | 0 | 0 | 0 |
| Folacin | μg | 0 | 0 | 0 | 0 |
| Vitamin B$_{12}$ | μg | 0 | 0 | 0 | 0 |
| Vitamin A[v] | RE | 108 | 1 | 46 | 489 |
| | IU | 1,077 | 14 | 458 | 4,885 |
| **Lipids** | | | | | |
| Fatty acids | | | | | |
| Saturated (total) | g | 36.65 | .48 | 15.58 | 166.25 |
| 4:0 | g | | | | |
| 6:0 | g | | | | |
| 8:0 | g | .67 | .01 | .28 | 3.04 |
| 10:0 | g | .96 | .01 | .41 | 4.37 |
| 12:0 | g | 14.51 | .19 | 6.16 | 65.80 |
| 14:0 | g | 5.75 | .08 | 2.44 | 26.06 |

Table 1 (continued)
## NUTRIENT COMPOSITION OF MILK PRODUCTS AND BY-PRODUCTS

### Item 20: Dessert Topping (Nondairy, Powdered)[r]

| Nutrients | Units | Amount in 100 g (edible portion) | Amount in edible portion of common measures of food (approximate measure and weight) | | Amount in edible portion of 1 lb of food as purchased (refuse:0) |
|---|---|---|---|---|---|
| | | | Mount to prepare 1 Tbsp = 1.3 g | 1½ oz = 42.5 g | |
| 16:0 | g | 5.43 | .07 | 2.31 | 24.62 |
| 18:0 | g | 9.41 | .12 | 4.00 | 42.67 |
| Monounsaturated (total) | g | .60 | .01 | .26 | 2.72 |
| 16:1 | g | | | | |
| 18:1 | g | .60 | .01 | .26 | 2.72 |
| 20:1 | g | | | | |
| 22:1 | g | | | | |
| Polyunsaturated (total) | g | .45 | .01 | .19 | 2.03 |
| 18:2 | g | .45 | .01 | .19 | 2.03 |
| 18:3 | g | | | | |
| 18:4 | g | | | | |
| 20:4 | g | | | | |
| 20:5 | g | | | | |
| 22:5 | g | | | | |
| 22:6 | g | | | | |
| Cholesterol | mg | 0 | 0 | 0 | 0 |
| Phytosterols | mg | — | — | — | — |
| Amino acids | | | | | |
| Tryptophan | g | .068 | .001 | .029 | .307 |
| Threonine | g | .207 | .003 | .088 | .940 |
| Isoleucine | g | .301 | .004 | .128 | 1.364 |
| Leucine | g | .484 | .006 | .206 | 2.194 |
| Lysine | g | .394 | .005 | .168 | 1.788 |
| Methionine | g | .149 | .002 | .063 | .675 |
| Cystine | g | .021 | Trace | .009 | .095 |
| Phenylalanine | g | .263 | .003 | .112 | 1.191 |
| Tyrosine | g | .280 | .004 | .119 | 1.272 |
| Valine | g | .351 | .005 | .149 | 1.590 |
| Arginine | g | .194 | .003 | .082 | .880 |
| Histidine | g | .145 | .002 | .062 | .657 |
| Alanine | g | .153 | .002 | .065 | .696 |
| Aspartic acid | g | .347 | .005 | .147 | 1.572 |
| Glutamic acid | g | 1.113 | .014 | .473 | 5.050 |
| Glycine | g | .098 | .001 | .042 | .445 |
| Proline | g | .552 | .007 | .235 | 2.505 |
| Serine | g | .301 | .004 | .128 | 1.368 |

### Item 21: Milk (Whole, 3.3% Fat, Fluid)[w,x]

| Nutrients | Units | Amount in 100 g (edible portion) | Amount in edible portion of common measures of food (approximate measure and weight) | | Amount in edible portion of 1 lb of food as purchased (refuse:0) |
|---|---|---|---|---|---|
| | | | 1 cup = 244 g | 1 qt = 976 g | |
| Proximate | | | | | |
| Water | g | 87.99 | 214.70 | 858.78 | 399.12 |
| Food energy | kcal | 61 | 150 | 600 | 279 |
| | kJ | 257 | 627 | 2,510 | 1,166 |
| Protein (N × 6.38) | g | 3.29 | 8.03 | 32.11 | 14.92 |
| Total lipid (fat)[y] | g | 3.34 | 8.15 | 32.60 | 15.15 |
| Carbohydrate (total) | g | 4.66 | 11.37 | 45.48 | 21.14 |
| Fiber | g | 0 | 0 | 0 | 0 |
| Ash | g | .72 | 1.76 | 7.03 | 3.27 |
| Minerals | | | | | |
| Calcium | mg | 119 | 291 | 1.165 | 542 |
| Iron | mg | .05 | .12 | .49 | .23 |
| Magnesium | mg | 13 | 33 | 131 | 61 |
| Phosphorus | mg | 93 | 228 | 912 | 424 |
| Potassium | mg | 152 | 370 | 1,479 | 687 |
| Sodium | mg | 49 | 120 | 478 | 222 |

Table 1 (continued)
NUTRIENT COMPOSITION OF MILK PRODUCTS AND BY-PRODUCTS

Item 21: Milk (Whole, 3.3% Fat, Fluid)[w,x]

| Nutrients | Units | Amount in 100 g (edible portion) | Amount in edible portion of common measures of food (approximate measure and weight) | | Amount in edible portion of 1 lb of food as purchased (refuse:0) |
|---|---|---|---|---|---|
| | | | 1 cup = 244 g | 1 qt = 976 g | |
| Zinc | mg | .38 | .93 | 3.71 | 1.72 |
| Vitamins | | | | | |
| Ascorbic acid | mg | .94 | 2.29 | 9.17 | 4.26 |
| Thiamin | mg | .038 | .093 | .371 | .172 |
| Riboflavin | mg | .162 | .395 | 1.581 | .735 |
| Niacin | mg | .084 | .205 | .820 | .381 |
| Pantothenic acid | mg | .314 | .766 | 3.065 | 1.424 |
| Vitamin B$_6$ | mg | .042 | .102 | .410 | .191 |
| Folacin | μg | 5 | 12 | 49 | 23 |
| Vitamin B$_{12}$ | μg | .357 | .871 | 3.484 | 1.619 |
| Vitamin A[z] | RE | 31 | 76 | 303 | 141 |
| | IU | 126 | 307 | 1,230 | 572 |
| Lipids | | | | | |
| Fatty acids | | | | | |
| Saturated (total) | g | 2.08 | 5.07 | 20.29 | 9.43 |
| 4:0 | g | .11 | .26 | 1.06 | .49 |
| 6:0 | g | .06 | .16 | .63 | .29 |
| 8:0 | g | .04 | .09 | .36 | .17 |
| 10:0 | g | .08 | .20 | .82 | .38 |
| 12:0 | g | .09 | .23 | .92 | .42 |
| 14:0 | g | .34 | .82 | 3.28 | 1.52 |
| 16:0 | g | .88 | 2.14 | 8.57 | 3.98 |
| 18:0 | g | .40 | .99 | 3.95 | 1.84 |
| Monounsaturated (total) | g | .96 | 2.35 | 9.42 | 4.38 |
| 16:1 | g | .08 | .18 | .73 | .34 |
| 18:1 | g | .84 | 2.05 | 8.20 | 3.81 |
| 20:1 | g | Trace | | | |
| 22:1 | g | Trace | | | |
| Polyunsaturated (total) | g | .12 | .30 | 1.21 | .56 |
| 18:2 | g | .08 | .18 | .74 | .34 |
| 18:3 | g | .05 | .12 | .47 | .22 |
| 18:4 | g | Trace | | | |
| 22:4 | g | Trace | | | |
| 20:5 | g | Trace | | | |
| 22:5 | g | Trace | | | |
| 22:6 | g | Trace | | | |
| Cholesterol | mg | 14 | 33 | 133 | 62 |
| Phytosterols | mg | Trace | | | |
| Amino acids | | | | | |
| Tryptophan | g | .046 | .113 | .453 | .211 |
| Threonine | g | .149 | .362 | 1.449 | .674 |
| Isoleucine | g | .199 | .486 | 1.943 | .903 |
| Leucine | g | .322 | .786 | 3.146 | 1.462 |
| Lysine | g | .261 | .637 | 2.547 | 1.184 |
| Methionine | g | .083 | .201 | .805 | .374 |
| Cystine | g | .030 | .074 | .297 | .138 |
| Phenylalanine | g | .159 | .388 | 1.550 | .720 |
| Tyrosine | g | .159 | .388 | 1.550 | .720 |
| Valine | g | .220 | .537 | 2.149 | .999 |
| Arginine | g | .119 | .291 | 1.163 | .540 |
| Histidine | g | .089 | .218 | .871 | .405 |
| Alanine | g | .113 | .277 | 1.107 | .515 |
| Aspartic acid | g | .250 | .609 | 2.436 | 1.132 |
| Glutamic acid | g | .689 | 1.681 | 6.724 | 3.125 |
| Glycine | g | .070 | .170 | .679 | .316 |
| Proline | g | .319 | .778 | 3.110 | 1.446 |
| Serine | g | .179 | .437 | 1.746 | .812 |

Table 1 (continued)
## NUTRIENT COMPOSITION OF MILK PRODUCTS AND BY-PRODUCTS

Item 22: Milk (Lowfat, 2% Fat, Fluid)[x]

| Nutrients | Units | Amount in 100 g (edible portion) | Amount in edible portion of common measures of food (approximate measure and weight) | | Amount in edible portion of 1 lb food as purchased (refuse:0) |
|---|---|---|---|---|---|
| | | | 1 cup = 244 g | 1 qt = 976 g | |
| Proximate | | | | | |
| Water | g | 89.21 | 217.67 | 870.69 | 404.66 |
| Food energy | kcal | 50 | 121 | 485 | 225 |
| | kJ | 208 | 507 | 2,029 | 943 |
| Protein (N × 6.38) | g | 3.33 | 8.12 | 32.50 | 15.10 |
| Total lipid (fat) | g | 1.92 | 4.68 | 18.74 | 8.71 |
| Carbohydrate (total) | g | 4.80 | 11.71 | 46.85 | 21.77 |
| Fiber | g | 0 | 0 | 0 | 0 |
| Ash | g | .74 | 1.81 | 7.22 | 3.36 |
| Minerals | | | | | |
| Calcium | mg | 122 | 297 | 1,187 | 552 |
| Iron | mg | .05 | .12 | .49 | .23 |
| Magnesium | mg | 14 | 33 | 133 | 62 |
| Phosphorus | mg | 95 | 232 | 928 | 431 |
| Potassium | mg | 154 | 377 | 1,507 | 700 |
| Sodium | mg | 50 | 122 | 487 | 226 |
| Zinc | mg | .39 | .95 | 3.81 | 1.77 |
| Vitamins | | | | | |
| Ascorbic acid | mg | .95 | 2.32 | 9.27 | 4.31 |
| Thiamin | mg | .039 | .095 | .381 | .177 |
| Riboflavin | mg | .165 | .403 | 1.610 | .748 |
| Niacin | mg | .086 | .210 | .839 | .390 |
| Pantothenic acid | mg | .320 | .781 | 3.123 | 1.452 |
| Vitamin $B_6$ | mg | .043 | .105 | .420 | .195 |
| Folacin | μg | 5 | 12 | 50 | 23 |
| Vitamin $B_{12}$ | μg | .364 | .888 | 3.553 | 1.651 |
| Vitamin A[**] | RE | 57 | 140 | 561 | 259 |
| | IU | 205 | 500 | 2,000 | 930 |
| Lipids | | | | | |
| Fatty acids[f] | | | | | |
| Saturated (total) | g | 1.20 | 2.92 | 11.66 | 5.42 |
| 4:0 | g | .06 | .15 | .61 | .28 |
| 6:0 | g | .04 | .09 | .36 | .17 |
| 8:0 | g | .02 | .05 | .21 | .10 |
| 10:0 | g | .05 | .12 | 47 | .22 |
| 12:0 | g | .05 | .13 | .53 | .24 |
| 14:0 | g | .19 | .47 | 1.88 | .88 |
| 16:0 | g | .50 | 1.23 | 4.93 | 2.29 |
| 18:0 | g | .23 | .57 | 2.27 | 1.06 |
| Monounsaturated (total) | g | .56 | 1.35 | 5.41 | 2.52 |
| 16:1 | g | .04 | .10 | .42 | .20 |
| 18:1 | g | .48 | 1.18 | 4.71 | 2.19 |
| 20:1 | g | | | | |
| 22:1 | g | | | | |
| Polyunsaturated (total) | g | .07 | .17 | .70 | .32 |
| 18:2 | g | .04 | .11 | .42 | .20 |
| 18:3 | g | .03 | .07 | .27 | .13 |
| 18:4 | g | | | | |
| 20:4 | g | | | | |
| 20:5 | g | | | | |
| 22:5 | g | | | | |
| 22:6 | g | | | | |
| Cholesterol | mg | 8 | 18 | 73 | 34 |
| Phytosterols | mg | | | | |
| Amino Acids | | | | | |
| Tryptophan | g | .047 | .115 | .458 | .213 |
| Threonine | g | .150 | .367 | 1.467 | .682 |
| Isoleucine | g | .201 | .492 | 1.966 | .914 |
| Leucine | g | .326 | .796 | 3.184 | 1.480 |
| Lysine | g | .264 | .644 | 2.578 | 1.198 |
| Methionine | g | .084 | .204 | .815 | .379 |

Table 1 (continued)
## NUTRIENT COMPOSITION OF MILK PRODUCTS AND BY-PRODUCTS

### Item 22: Milk (Lowfat, 2% Fat, Fluid)[x]

| Nutrients | Units | Amount in 100 g (edible portion) | Amount in edible portion of common measures of food (approximate measure and weight) | | Amount in edible portion of 1 lb food as purchased (refuse:0) |
|---|---|---|---|---|---|
| | | | 1 cup = 244 g | 1 qt = 976 g | |
| Cystine | g | .031 | .075 | .301 | .140 |
| Phenylalanine | g | .161 | .392 | 1.569 | .729 |
| Tyrosine | g | .161 | .392 | 1.569 | .729 |
| Valine | g | .223 | .544 | 2.175 | 1.011 |
| Arginine | g | .121 | .294 | 1.177 | .547 |
| Histidine | g | .090 | .220 | .881 | .410 |
| Alanine | g | .115 | .280 | 1.121 | .521 |
| Aspartic acid | g | .253 | .616 | 2.466 | 1.146 |
| Glutamic acid | g | .697 | 1.701 | 6.806 | 3.163 |
| Glycine | g | .070 | .172 | .688 | .320 |
| Proline | g | .323 | .787 | 3.148 | 1.463 |
| Serine | g | .181 | .442 | 1.768 | .822 |

### Item 23: Milk (Lowfat 2% Fat, Protein Fortified, Fluid)[x,bb]

| Nutrients | Units | Amount in 100 g (edible portion) | Amount in edible portion of common measures of food (approximate measure and weight) | | Amount in edible portion of 1 lb of food as purchased (refuse: 0) |
|---|---|---|---|---|---|
| | | | 1 cup = 246 g | 1 qt = 984 g | |
| Proximate | | | | | |
| Water | g | 87.71 | 215.77 | 863.07 | 397.85 |
| Food energy | kcal | 56 | 137 | 546 | 252 |
| | kJ | 232 | 572 | 2,286 | 1,054 |
| Protein (N × 6.38) | g | 3.95 | 9.72 | 38.87 | 17.92 |
| Total lipid (fat) | g | 1.98 | 4.87 | 19.48 | 8.98 |
| Carbohydrate (total) | g | 5.49 | 13.80 | 54.02 | 24.90 |
| Fiber | g | 0 | 0 | 0 | 0 |
| Ash | g | .87 | 2.14 | 8.56 | 3.95 |
| Minerals | | | | | |
| Calcium | mg | 143 | 352 | 1,408 | 649 |
| Iron | mg | .06 | .15 | .59 | .27 |
| Magnesium | mg | 16 | 40 | 158 | 73 |
| Phosphorus | mg | 112 | 276 | 1,102 | 508 |
| Potassium | mg | 182 | 447 | 1,788 | 824 |
| Sodium | mg | 59 | 145 | 579 | 267 |
| Zinc | mg | .45 | 1.11 | 4.43 | 2.04 |
| Vitamins | | | | | |
| Ascorbic acid | mg | 1.12 | 2.76 | 11.02 | 5.08 |
| Thiamin | mg | .045 | .111 | .443 | .204 |
| Riboflavin | mg | .194 | .477 | 1.909 | .880 |
| Niacin | mg | .101 | .248 | .994 | .458 |
| Pantothenic acid | mg | .376 | .925 | 3.700 | 1.706 |
| Vitamin $B_6$ | mg | .051 | .125 | .502 | .231 |
| Folacin | μg | 6 | 15 | 59 | 27 |
| Vitamin $B_{12}$ | μg | .428 | 1.053 | 4.212 | 1.941 |
| Vitamin A[aa] | RE | 57 | 140 | 561 | 259 |
| | IU | 203 | 500 | 2,000 | 922 |
| Lipids | | | | | |
| Fatty acids | | | | | |
| Saturated (total) | g | 1.23 | 3.03 | 12.13 | 5.59 |
| 4:0 | g | .06 | .16 | .63 | .29 |
| 6:0 | g | .04 | .09 | .37 | .17 |
| 8:0 | g | .02 | .05 | .22 | .10 |
| 10:0 | g | .05 | .12 | .49 | .22 |
| 12:0 | g | .06 | .14 | .55 | .25 |
| 14:0 | g | .20 | .49 | 1.96 | .90 |
| 16:0 | g | .52 | 1.28 | 5.12 | 2.36 |
| 18:0 | g | .24 | .59 | 2.36 | 1.09 |
| Monounsaturated (total) | g | .57 | 1.41 | 5.63 | 2.59 |

Table 1 (continued)
NUTRIENT COMPOSITION OF MILK PRODUCTS AND BY-PRODUCTS

Item 23: Milk (Lowfat 2% Fat, Protein Fortified, Fluid)[x,bb]

| Nutrients | Units | Amount in 100 g (edible portion) | Amount in edible portion of common measures of food (approximate measure and weight) | | Amount in edible portion of 1 lb of food as purchased (refuse: 0) |
|---|---|---|---|---|---|
| | | | 1 cup = 246 g | 1 qt = 984 g | |
| 16:1 | g | .04 | .11 | .44 | .20 |
| 18:1 | g | .50 | 1.22 | 4.90 | 2.26 |
| 20:1 | g | | | | |
| 22:1 | g | | | | |
| Polyunsaturated (total) | g | .07 | .18 | .72 | .33 |
| 18:2 | g | .04 | .11 | .44 | .20 |
| 18:3 | g | .03 | .07 | .28 | .13 |
| 18:4 | g | | | | |
| 20:4 | g | | | | |
| 20:5 | g | | | | |
| 22:5 | g | | | | |
| 22:6 | g | | | | |
| Cholesterol | mg | 8 | 19 | 76 | 35 |
| Phytosterols | mg | | | | |
| Amino acids | | | | | |
| Tryptophan | g | .056 | .137 | .548 | .253 |
| Threonine | g | .178 | .439 | 1.755 | .809 |
| Isoleucine | g | .239 | .588 | 2.352 | 1.084 |
| Leucine | g | .387 | .952 | 3.808 | 1.755 |
| Lysine | g | .313 | .771 | 3.083 | 1.421 |
| Methionine | g | .099 | .244 | .975 | .449 |
| Cystine | g | .037 | .090 | .359 | .166 |
| Phenylalanine | g | .191 | .469 | 1.876 | .865 |
| Tyrosine | g | .191 | .469 | 1.876 | .865 |
| Valine | g | .264 | .650 | 2.601 | 1.199 |
| Arginine | g | .143 | .352 | 1.407 | .649 |
| Histidine | g | .107 | .263 | 1.054 | .486 |
| Alanine | g | .136 | .335 | 1.340 | .618 |
| Aspartic acid | g | .300 | .737 | 2.949 | 1.359 |
| Glutamic acid | g | .827 | 2.035 | 8.139 | 3.752 |
| Glycine | g | .084 | .206 | .822 | .379 |
| Proline | g | .383 | .941 | 3.765 | 1.736 |
| Serine | g | .215 | .528 | 2.114 | .974 |

Item 24: Milk (Skim, Fluid)[x]

| Nutrients | Units | Amount in 100 g (edible portion) | Amount in edible portion of common measures of food (approximate measure and weight) | | Amount in edible portion of 1 lb of food as purchased (refuse:0) |
|---|---|---|---|---|---|
| | | | 1 cup = 245 g | 1 qt = 980 g | |
| Proximate | | | | | |
| Water | g | 90.80 | 222.46 | 889.84 | 411.87 |
| Food energy | kcal | 35 | 86 | 342 | 158 |
| | kJ | 146 | 358 | 1,432 | 663 |
| Protein (N × 6.38) | g | 3.41 | 8.35 | 33.42 | 15.47 |
| Total lipid (fat) | g | .18 | .44 | 1.76 | .82 |
| Carbohydrate (total) | g | 4.85 | 11.88 | 47.53 | 22.00 |
| Fiber | g | 0 | 0 | 0 | 0 |
| Ash | g | .76 | 1.86 | 7.45 | 3.45 |
| Minerals | | | | | |
| Calcium | mg | 123 | 302 | 1,209 | 560 |
| Iron | mg | .04 | .10 | .39 | .18 |
| Magnesium | mg | 11 | 28 | 111 | 52 |
| Phosphorus | mg | 101 | 247 | 989 | 458 |
| Potassium | mg | 166 | 406 | 1,623 | 751 |
| Sodium | mg | 52 | 126 | 505 | 234 |
| Zinc | mg | .40 | .98 | 3.92 | 1.81 |

Table 1 (continued)
## NUTRIENT COMPOSITION OF MILK PRODUCTS AND BY-PRODUCTS

### Item 24: Milk (Skim, Fluid)[z]

| Nutrients | Units | Amount in 100 g (edible portion) | Amount in edible portion of common measures of food (approximate measure and weight) | | Amount in edible portion of 1 lb of food as purchased (refuse:0) |
|---|---|---|---|---|---|
| | | | 1 cup = 245 g | 1 qt = 980 g | |
| Vitamins | | | | | |
| Ascorbic acid | mg | .98 | 2.40 | 9.60 | 4.44 |
| Thiamin | mg | .036 | .088 | .353 | .163 |
| Riboflavin | mg | .140 | .343 | 1.372 | .635 |
| Niacin | mg | .088 | .216 | .862 | .399 |
| Pantothenic acid | mg | .329 | .806 | 3.224 | 1.492 |
| Vitamin B$_6$ | mg | .040 | .098 | .392 | .181 |
| Folacin | μg | 5 | 13 | 51 | 24 |
| Vitamin B$_{12}$ | μg | .378 | .926 | 3.704 | 1.715 |
| Vitamin A$^{aa}$ | RE | 61 | 149 | 598 | 277 |
| | IU | 204 | 500 | 2,000 | 926 |
| Lipids | | | | | |
| Fatty acids | | | | | |
| Saturated (total) | g | 117 | .287 | 1.146 | .531 |
| 4:0 | g | .009 | .023 | .901 | .042 |
| 6:0 | g | .001 | .003 | .013 | .006 |
| 8:0 | g | .002 | .005 | .019 | .009 |
| 10:0 | g | .004 | .009 | .036 | .017 |
| 12:0 | g | .003 | .006 | .025 | .011 |
| 14:0 | g | .017 | .042 | .168 | .078 |
| 16:0 | g | .053 | .129 | .517 | .239 |
| 18:0 | g | .019 | .046 | .185 | .086 |
| Monounsaturated (total) | g | .047 | .116 | .462 | .214 |
| 16:1 | g | .007 | .016 | .065 | .030 |
| 18:1 | g | .038 | .093 | .374 | .173 |
| 20:1 | g | | | | |
| 22:1 | g | | | | |
| Polyunsaturated (total) | g | .007 | .016 | .064 | .030 |
| 18:2 | g | .005 | .011 | .046 | .021 |
| 18:3 | g | .002 | .005 | .018 | .009 |
| 18:4 | g | | | | |
| 20:4 | g | | | | |
| 20:5 | g | | | | |
| 22:5 | g | | | | |
| 22:6 | g | | | | |
| Cholesterol | mg | 2 | 4 | 18 | 8 |
| Phytosterols | mg | | | | |
| Amino acids | | | | | |
| Tryptophan | g | .048 | .118 | .471 | .218 |
| Threonine | g | .154 | .377 | 1.509 | .698 |
| Isoteucine | g | .206 | .505 | 2.022 | .936 |
| Leucine | g | .334 | .818 | 3.274 | 1.515 |
| Lysine | g | .270 | .663 | 2.650 | 1.227 |
| Methionine | g | .086 | .210 | .838 | .388 |
| Cystine | g | .032 | .077 | .309 | .143 |
| Phenylalanine | g | .165 | .403 | 1.613 | .747 |
| Tyrosine | g | .165 | .403 | 1.613 | .747 |
| Valine | g | .228 | .559 | 2.237 | 1.035 |
| Arginine | g | .123 | .302 | 1.210 | .560 |
| Histidine | g | .092 | .227 | .906 | .419 |
| Alanine | g | .118 | .288 | 1.152 | .533 |
| Aspartic acid | g | .259 | .634 | 2.535 | 1.173 |
| Glutamic acid | g | .714 | 1.749 | 6.998 | 3.239 |
| Glycine | g | .072 | .177 | .707 | .327 |
| Proline | g | .330 | .809 | 3.237 | 1.498 |
| Serine | g | .185 | .454 | 1.818 | .841 |

Table 1 (continued)
## NUTRIENT COMPOSITION OF MILK PRODUCTS AND BY-PRODUCTS

Item 25: Milk (Skim, Protein Fortified, Fluid)[x,bb]

| Nutrients | Units | Amount in 100 g (edible portion) | Amount in edible portion of common measures of food (approximate measure and weight) | | Amount in edible portion of 1 lb of food as purchased (refuse:0) |
|---|---|---|---|---|---|
| | | | 1 cup = 246 g | 1 qt = 984 g | |
| Proximate | | | | | |
| Water | g | 89.36 | 219.83 | 879.30 | 405.34 |
| Food energy | kcal | 41 | 100 | 400 | 184 |
| | kJ | 170 | 418 | 1,673 | 771 |
| Protein (N × 6.38) | g | 3.96 | 9.74 | 38.97 | 17.96 |
| Total lipid (fat)[cc] | g | .25 | .62 | 2.46 | 1.13 |
| Carbohydrate (total) | g | 5.56 | 13.68 | 54.71 | 25.22 |
| Fiber | g | 0 | 0 | 0 | 0 |
| Ash | g | .87 | 2.14 | 8.56 | 3.95 |
| Minerals | | | | | |
| Calcium | mg | 143 | 352 | 1,407 | 649 |
| Iron | mg | .06 | .15 | .59 | .27 |
| Magnesium | mg | 16 | 40 | 158 | 73 |
| Phosphorus | mg | 112 | 275 | 1,101 | 508 |
| Potassium | mg | 182 | 446 | 1,786 | 823 |
| Sodium | mg | 59 | 144 | 578 | 266 |
| Zinc | mg | .45 | 1.11 | 4.43 | 2.04 |
| Vitamins | | | | | |
| Ascorbic acid | mg | 1.12 | 2.76 | 11.02 | 5.08 |
| Thiamin | mg | .045 | .111 | .443 | .204 |
| Riboflavin | mg | .194 | .477 | 1.909 | .880 |
| Niacin | mg | .101 | .248 | .994 | .458 |
| Pantothenic acid | mg | .376 | .925 | 3.700 | 1.706 |
| Vitamin B_6 | mg | .050 | .123 | .492 | .227 |
| Folacin | μg | 6 | 15 | 59 | 27 |
| Vitamin B_{12} | μg | .427 | 1.050 | 4.202 | 1.937 |
| Vitamin A[aa] | RE | 61 | 149 | 598 | 277 |
| | IU | 203 | 500 | 2,000 | 922 |
| Lipids | | | | | |
| Fatty acids [dd] | | | | | |
| Saturated (total) | g | .162 | .400 | 1.598 | .737 |
| 4:0 | g | .013 | .032 | .126 | .058 |
| 6:0 | g | .002 | .004 | .017 | .008 |
| 8:0 | g | .003 | .007 | .026 | .012 |
| 10:0 | g | .005 | .013 | .051 | .023 |
| 12:0 | g | .003 | .009 | .034 | .016 |
| 14:0 | g | .024 | .059 | .235 | .108 |
| 16:0 | g | .073 | .180 | .721 | .332 |
| 18:0 | g | .026 | .065 | .259 | .119 |
| Monounsaturated (total) | g | .065 | .161 | .644 | .297 |
| 16:1 | g | .009 | .023 | .090 | .042 |
| 18:1 | g | .053 | .130 | .521 | .240 |
| 20:1 | g | | | | |
| 22:1 | g | | | | |
| Polyunsaturated (total) | g | .009 | .022 | .089 | .041 |
| 18:2 | g | .006 | .016 | .064 | .029 |
| 18:3 | g | .003 | .006 | .026 | 012 |
| 18:4 | g | | | | |
| 20:4 | g | | | | |
| 20:5 | g | | | | |
| 22:5 | g | | | | |
| 22:6 | g | | | | |
| Cholesterol | mg | 2 | 5 | 20 | 9 |
| Phytosterols | mg | | | | |
| Amino acids | | | | | |
| Tryptophan | g | .056 | .137 | .550 | .253 |
| Threonine | g | .179 | .440 | 1.759 | .811 |
| Isoleucine | g | .240 | .589 | 2.358 | 1.087 |
| Leucine | g | .388 | .954 | 3.817 | 1.760 |
| Lysine | g | .314 | .773 | 3.090 | 1.425 |
| Methionine | g | .099 | .244 | .977 | .450 |
| Cystine | g | .037 | .090 | .360 | .166 |
| Phenylalanine | g | .191 | .470 | 1.881 | .867 |

Table 1 (continued)
## NUTRIENT COMPOSITION OF MILK PRODUCTS AND BY-PRODUCTS

### Item 25: Milk (Skim, Protein Fortified, Fluid)[x,bb]

| Nutrients | Units | Amount in 100 g (edible portion) | Amount in edible portion of common measures of food (approximate measure and weight) | | Amount in edible portion of 1 lb of food as purchased (refuse:0) |
|---|---|---|---|---|---|
| | | | 1 cup = 246 g | 1 qt = 984 g | |
| Tyrosine | g | .191 | .470 | 1.881 | .867 |
| Valine | g | .265 | .652 | 2.608 | 1.202 |
| Arginine | g | .143 | .353 | 1.411 | .650 |
| Histidine | g | .107 | .264 | 1.057 | .487 |
| Alanine | g | .137 | .336 | 1.344 | .619 |
| Aspartic acid | g | .300 | .739 | 2.956 | 1.363 |
| Glutamic acid | g | .829 | 2.040 | 8.160 | 3.761 |
| Glycine | g | .084 | .206 | .825 | .380 |
| Proline | g | .384 | .944 | 3.774 | 1.740 |
| Serine | g | .215 | .530 | 2.119 | .977 |

### Item 26: Milk (Buttermilk, Cultured, Fluid)

| Nutrients | Units | Amount in 100 g (edible portion) | Amount in edible portion of common measures of food (approximate measures and weight) | | Amount in edible portion of 1 lb of food as purchased (refuse:0) |
|---|---|---|---|---|---|
| | | | 1 cup = 245 g | 1 qt = 980 g | |
| Proximate | | | | | |
| Water | g | 90.13 | 220.82 | 883.27 | 408.83 |
| Food energy | kcal | 40 | 99 | 396 | 183 |
| | kJ | 169 | 414 | 1,657 | 767 |
| Protein (N × 6.38) | g | 3.31 | 8.11 | 32.44 | 15.01 |
| Total lipid (fat) | g | .88 | 2.16 | 8.62 | 3.99 |
| Carbohydrate (total) | g | 4.79 | 11.74 | 46.94 | 21.73 |
| Fiber | g | 0 | 0 | 0 | 0 |
| Ash | g | .89 | 2.18 | 8.72 | 4.04 |
| Minerals | | | | | |
| Calcium | mg | 116 | 285 | 1,141 | 528 |
| Iron | mg | .05 | .12 | .49 | .23 |
| Magnesium | mg | 11 | 27 | 107 | 50 |
| Phosphorus | mg | 89 | 219 | 874 | 405 |
| Potassium | mg | 151 | 371 | 1,483 | 686 |
| Sodium[cc] | mg | 105 | 257 | 1,028 | 476 |
| Zinc | mg | .42 | 1.03 | 4.12 | 1.90 |
| Vitamins | | | | | |
| Ascorbic acid | mg | .98 | 2.40 | 9.60 | 4.44 |
| Thiamin | mg | .034 | .083 | .333 | .154 |
| Riboflavin | mg | .154 | .377 | 1.509 | .699 |
| Niacin | mg | .058 | .142 | .568 | .263 |
| Pantothenic acid | mg | .275 | .674 | 2.695 | 1.247 |
| Vitamin $B_6$ | mg | .034 | .083 | .333 | .154 |
| Folacin | µg | —[d] | — | — | — |
| Vitamin $B_{12}$ | µg | .219 | .537 | 2.146 | .993 |
| Vitamin A | RE | 8 | 20 | 78 | 36 |
| | IU | 33 | 81 | 323 | 150 |
| Lipids | | | | | |
| Fatty acids | | | | | |
| Saturated (total) | g | .55 | 1.34 | 5.37 | 2.48 |
| 4:0 | g | .03 | .07 | .28 | .13 |
| 6:0 | g | .02 | .04 | .17 | .08 |
| 8:0 | g | .01 | .02 | .10 | .04 |
| 10:0 | g | .02 | .05 | .22 | .10 |
| 12:0 | g | .02 | .06 | .24 | .11 |
| 14:0 | g | .09 | .22 | .87 | .40 |
| 16:0 | g | .23 | .57 | 2.27 | 1.05 |
| 18:0 | g | .11 | .26 | 1.04 | .48 |
| Monounsaturated (total) | g | .25 | .62 | 2.49 | 1.15 |
| 16:1 | g | .02 | .05 | .19 | .09 |

Table 1 (continued)
NUTRIENT COMPOSITION OF MILK PRODUCTS AND BY-PRODUCTS

Item 26: Milk (Buttermilk, Cultured, Fluid)

| Nutrients | Units | Amount in 100 g (edible portion) | Amount in edible portion of common measures of food (approximate measures and weight) | | Amount in edible portion of 1 lb of food as purchased (refuse:0) |
|---|---|---|---|---|---|
| | | | 1 cup = 245 g | 1 qt = 980 g | |
| 18:1 | g | .22 | .54 | 2.17 | 1.00 |
| 20:1 | g | | | | |
| 22:1 | g | | | | |
| Polyunsaturated (total) | g | .03 | .08 | .32 | .15 |
| 18:2 | g | .02 | .05 | .20 | .09 |
| 18:3 | g | .01 | .03 | .12 | .06 |
| 18:4 | g | | | | |
| 20.4 | g | | | | |
| 20:5 | g | | | | |
| 22:5 | g | | | | |
| 22:6 | g | | | | |
| Cholesterol | mg | 4 | 9 | 34 | 16 |
| Phytosterols | mg | | | | |
| Amino acids | | | | | |
| Tryptophan | g | .036 | 0.88 | .351 | .162 |
| Threonine | g | .158 | .386 | 1.546 | .715 |
| Isoleucine | g | .204 | .500 | 1.998 | .925 |
| Leucine | g | .329 | .807 | 3.229 | 1.494 |
| Lysine | g | .277 | .679 | 2.715 | 1.257 |
| Methionine | g | .081 | .198 | .793 | .367 |
| Cystine | g | .031 | .076 | .305 | .141 |
| Phenylalanine | g | .174 | .427 | 1.708 | .791 |
| Tyrosine | g | .139 | .339 | 1.358 | .628 |
| Valine | g | .243 | .596 | 2.385 | 1.104 |
| Arginine | g | .126 | .309 | 1.235 | .572 |
| Histidine | g | .095 | .233 | .930 | .431 |
| Alanine | g | .119 | .292 | 1.169 | .541 |
| Aspartic acid | g | .264 | .647 | 2.588 | 1.198 |
| Glutamic acid | g | .643 | 1.576 | 6.305 | 2.918 |
| Glycine | g | .073 | .178 | .712 | .329 |
| Proline | g | .334 | .819 | 3.274 | 1.516 |
| Serine | g | .172 | .422 | 1.688 | .781 |

Item 27: Milk (Dry, Whole)[″]

| Nutrients | Units | Amount in 100 g (edible portion) | Amount in edible portion of common measures of food (approximate measure and weight) | | Amount in edible portion of 1 lb of food as purchased (refuse:0) |
|---|---|---|---|---|---|
| | | | ¼ cup = 32 g | 1 cup = 128 g | |
| Proximate | | | | | |
| Water | g | 2.47 | 0.75 | 3.16 | 11.20 |
| Food energy | kcal | 496 | 159 | 635 | 2,249 |
| | kJ | 2,075 | 664 | 2,656 | 9,413 |
| Protein (N × 6.38) | g | 26.32 | 8.42 | 33.69 | 119.39 |
| Total lipid (fat) | g | 26.71 | 8.55 | 34.19 | 121.16 |
| Carbohydrate (total) | g | 38.42 | 12.29 | 49.18 | 174.27 |
| Fiber | g | 0 | 0 | 0 | 0 |
| Ash | g | 6.08 | 1.95 | 7.78 | 27.58 |
| Minerals | | | | | |
| Calcium | mg | 912 | 292 | 1,168 | 4,139 |
| Iron | mg | .47 | .15 | .60 | 2.13 |
| Magnesium | mg | 85 | 27 | 108 | 383 |
| Phosphorus | mg | 776 | 248 | 993 | 3,518 |
| Potassium | mg | 1,330 | 426 | 1,702 | 6,032 |
| Sodium | mg | 371 | 119 | 475 | 1,684 |
| Zinc | mg | 3.34 | 1.07 | 4.28 | 15.15 |
| Vitamins | | | | | |
| Ascorbic acid | mg | 8.64 | 2.76 | 11.06 | 39.19 |

Table 1 (continued)
## NUTRIENT COMPOSITION OF MILK PRODUCTS AND BY-PRODUCTS

Item 27: Milk (Dry, Whole)[ʰ]

| Nutrients | Units | Amount in 100 g (edible portion) | Amount in edible portion of common measures of food (approximate measure and weight) | | Amount in edible portion of 1 lb of food as purchased (refuse:0) |
|---|---|---|---|---|---|
| | | | ¼ cup = 32 g | 1 cup = 128 g | |
| Thiamin | mg | .283 | .091 | .362 | 1.284 |
| Riboflavin | mg | 1.205 | .386 | 1.542 | 5.466 |
| Niacin | mg | .646 | .207 | .827 | 2.930 |
| Pantothenic acid | mg | 2.271 | .727 | 2.907 | 10.301 |
| Vitamin B₆ | mg | .302 | .097 | .387 | 1.370 |
| Folacin | μg | 37 | 12 | 47 | 168 |
| Vitamin B₁₂ | μg | 3.253 | 1.041 | 4.164 | 14.756 |
| Vitamin A | RE | 280 | 90 | 358 | 1,270 |
| | IU | 922 | 295 | 1,180 | 4,182 |
| Lipids | | | | | |
| Fatty acids | | | | | |
| Saturated (total) | g | 16.74 | 5.36 | 21.43 | 75.94 |
| 4:0 | g | .87 | .28 | 1.11 | 3.93 |
| 6:0 | g | .24 | .08 | .31 | 1.09 |
| 8:0 | g | .27 | .09 | .34 | 1.22 |
| 10:0 | g | .60 | .19 | .76 | 2.70 |
| 12:0 | g | .61 | .20 | .79 | 2.79 |
| 14:0 | g | 2.82 | .90 | 3.61 | 12.79 |
| 16:0 | g | 7.52 | 2.41 | 9.63 | 34.12 |
| 18:0 | g | 2.85 | .91 | 3.65 | 12.94 |
| Monounsaturated (total) | g | 7.92 | 2.54 | 10.14 | 35.94 |
| 16:1 | g | 1.20 | .38 | 1.53 | 5.43 |
| 18:1 | g | 6.19 | 1.98 | 7.93 | 28.09 |
| 20:1 | g | | | | |
| 22:1 | g | | | | |
| Polyunsaturated(total) | g | 1.66 | .21 | .85 | 3.02 |
| 18:2 | g | .46 | .15 | .59 | 2.09 |
| 18:3 | g | .20 | .06 | .26 | .93 |
| 18:4 | g | | | | |
| 20:4 | g | | | | |
| 20:5 | g | | | | |
| 22:5 | g | | | | |
| 22:6 | g | | | | |
| Cholesterol | mg | 97 | 31 | 124 | 440 |
| Phytosterols | mg | | | | |
| Amino acids | | | | | |
| Tryptophan | g | .371 | .119 | .475 | 1.684 |
| Threoine | g | 1.188 | .380 | 1.521 | 5.389 |
| Isoleucine | g | 1.592 | .510 | 2.038 | 7.223 |
| Leucine | g | 2.578 | .825 | 3.300 | 11.695 |
| Lysine | g | 2.087 | .668 | 2.672 | 9.469 |
| Methionine | g | .660 | .211 | .845 | 2.994 |
| Cystine | g | .243 | .078 | .312 | 1.104 |
| Phenylalanine | g | 1.271 | .407 | 1.626 | 5.764 |
| Tyrosine | g | 1.271 | .407 | 1.626 | 5.764 |
| Valine | g | 1.762 | .564 | 2.255 | 7.990 |
| Arginine | g | .953 | .305 | 1.220 | 4.323 |
| Histidine | g | .714 | .228 | .914 | 3.237 |
| Alanine | g | .908 | .290 | 1.162 | 4.117 |
| Aspartic acid | g | 1.997 | .639 | 2.556 | 9.057 |
| Glutamic acid | g | 5.512 | 1.764 | 7.055 | 25.000 |
| Glycine | g | .557 | .178 | .713 | 2.526 |
| Proline | g | 2.549 | .816 | 3.263 | 11.564 |
| Serine | g | 1.432 | .458 | 1.832 | 6.493 |

Table 1 (continued)
NUTRIENT COMPOSITION OF MILK PRODUCTS AND BY-PRODUCTS

Item 28: Milk (Dry, Nonfat, Regular)[ff]

| Nutrients | Units | Amount in 100 g (edible portion) | Amount in edible portion of common measures of food (approximate measure and weight) | | Amount in edible portion of 1 lb of food as purchased (refuse:0) |
|---|---|---|---|---|---|
| | | | ¼ cup = 30 g | 1 cup = 120 g | |
| Proximate | | | | | |
| Water | g | 3.16 | 0.95 | 3.79 | 14.33 |
| Food energy | kcal | 362 | 109 | 435 | 1,644 |
| | kJ | 1,516 | 455 | 1,820 | 6,878 |
| Protein (N × 6.38) | g | 36.16 | 10.85 | 43.39 | 164.02 |
| Total lipid (fat) | g | .77 | .23 | .92 | 3.49 |
| Carbohydrate (total) | g | 51.98 | 15.59 | 62.38 | 235.78 |
| Fiber | g | 0 | 0 | 0 | 0 |
| Ash | g | 7.93 | 2.38 | 9.52 | 35.97 |
| Minerals | | | | | |
| Calcium | mg | 1,257 | 377 | 1,508 | 5,701 |
| Iron | mg | .32 | .10 | .38 | 1.45 |
| Magnesium | mg | 110 | 33 | 132 | 499 |
| Phosphorus | mg | 968 | 290 | 1,162 | 4,392 |
| Potassium | mg | 1,794 | 538 | 2,153 | 8,138 |
| Sodium | mg | 535 | 161 | 642 | 2,428 |
| Zinc | mg | 4.08 | 1.22 | 4.90 | 18.51 |
| Vitamins | | | | | |
| Ascorbic acid | mg | 6.76 | 2.03 | 8.11 | 30.66 |
| Thiamin | mg | .415 | .124 | .498 | 1.882 |
| Riboflavin | mg | 1.550 | .465 | 1.860 | 7.031 |
| Niacin | mg | .951 | .285 | 1.141 | 4.314 |
| Pantothenic acid | mg | 3.568 | 1.070 | 4.282 | 16.184 |
| Vitamin $B_6$ | mg | .361 | .108 | .433 | 1.637 |
| Folacin | μg | 50 | 5 | 60 | 227 |
| Vitamin $B_{12}$ | μg | 4.033 | 1.210 | 4.840 | 18.294 |
| Vitamin A[gg] | RE | 8 | 2 | 10 | 36 |
| | IU | 36 | 1 | 43 | 163 |
| Lipids | | | | | |
| Fatty acids[hh] | | | | | |
| Saturated (total) | g | .50 | .15 | .60 | 2.26 |
| 4:0 | g | .03 | .01 | .03 | .12 |
| 6:0 | g | .01 | Trace | .01 | .03 |
| 8:0 | g | .01 | Trace | .01 | .03 |
| 10:0 | g | .02 | Trace | .02 | .08 |
| 12:0 | g | .01 | Trace | .02 | .06 |
| 14:0 | g | .08 | .02 | .10 | .38 |
| 16:0 | g | .24 | .07 | .28 | 1.06 |
| 18:0 | g | .08 | .03 | .10 | .39 |
| Monounsaturated (total) | g | .20 | .06 | .24 | .91 |
| 16:1 | g | .02 | .01 | .03 | .10 |
| 18:1 | g | .17 | .05 | .20 | .76 |
| 20:1 | g | | | | |
| 22:1 | g | | | | |
| Polyunsaturated (total) | g | .03 | .01 | .04 | .14 |
| 18:2 | g | .02 | .01 | .02 | .09 |
| 18:3 | g | .01 | Trace | .01 | .05 |
| 18:4 | g | | | | |
| 20:4 | g | | | | |
| 20:5 | g | | | | |
| 22:5 | g | | | | |
| 22:6 | g | | | | |
| Cholesterol | mg | 20 | 6 | 24 | 89 |

Table 1 (continued)
## NUTRIENT COMPOSITION OF MILK PRODUCTS AND BY-PRODUCTS

### Item 28: Milk (Dry, Nonfat, Regular)[ff]

| Nutrients | Units | Amount in 100 g (edible portion) | Amount in edible portion of common measures of food (approximate measure and weight) | | Amount in edible portion of 1 lb of food as purchased (refuse:0) |
|---|---|---|---|---|---|
| | | | ¼ cup = 30 g | 1 cup = 120 g | |
| Phytosterols | mg | | | | |
| Amino acids | | | | | |
| Tryptophan | g | .510 | .153 | .612 | 2.314 |
| Threonine | g | 1.632 | .490 | 1.959 | 7.404 |
| Isoleucine | g | 2.188 | .656 | 2.625 | 9.924 |
| Leucine | g | 3.542 | 1.063 | 4.251 | 16.068 |
| Lysine | g | 2.868 | .860 | 3.441 | 13.009 |
| Methionine | g | .907 | .272 | 1.088 | 4.113 |
| Cystine | g | .334 | .100 | .401 | 1.517 |
| Phenylalanine | g | 1.746 | .524 | 2.095 | 7.918 |
| Tyrosine | g | 1.746 | .524 | 2.095 | 7.918 |
| Valine | g | 2.420 | .726 | 2.904 | 10.978 |
| Arginine | g | 1.309 | .393 | 1.571 | 5.939 |
| Histidine | g | .981 | .294 | 1.177 | 4.448 |
| Alanine | g | 1.247 | .374 | 1.496 | 5.656 |
| Aspartic acid | g | 2.743 | .823 | 3.292 | 12.443 |
| Glutamic acid | g | 7.572 | 2.272 | 9.086 | 34.347 |
| Glycine | g | .765 | .230 | .918 | 3.471 |
| Proline | g | 3.503 | 1.051 | 4.203 | 15.888 |
| Serine | g | 1.957 | .590 | 2.360 | 8.21 |

### Item 29: Milk (Condensed, Sweetened, Canned)

| Nutrients | Units | Amount in 100 g (edible portion) | Amount in edible portion of common measures of food (approximate measure and weight) | | Amount in edible portion of 1 lb of food as purchased (refuse:0) |
|---|---|---|---|---|---|
| | | | 1 fl oz = 38.2 g | 1 cup = 306 g | |
| Proximate | | | | | |
| Water | g | 27.16 | 10.88 | 83.11 | 123.20 |
| Food energy | kcal | 321 | 123 | 982 | 1,455 |
| | kJ | 1,342 | 513 | 4,108 | 6,089 |
| Protein (N × 6.38) | g | 7.91 | 3.02 | 24.20 | 35.88 |
| Total lipid (fat) | g | 8.70 | 3.32 | 26.62 | 39.46 |
| Carbohydrate (total) | g | 54.40 | 20.78 | 166.46 | 246.76 |
| Fiber | g | 0 | 0 | 0 | 0 |
| Ash | g | 1.83 | .70 | 5.60 | 8.30 |
| Minerals | | | | | |
| Calcium | mg | 284 | 108 | 868 | 1,286 |
| Iron | mg | .19 | .07 | .58 | .86 |
| Magnesium | mg | 26 | 10 | 78 | 116 |
| Phosphorus | mg | 253 | 97 | 775 | 1,149 |
| Potassium | mg | 371 | 142 | 1,136 | 1,685 |
| Sodium | mg | 127 | 49 | 389 | 576 |
| Zinc | mg | .94 | .36 | 2.88 | 4.26 |
| Vitamins | | | | | |
| Ascorbic acid | mg | 2.60 | .99 | 7.96 | 11.79 |
| Thiamin | mg | .090 | .034 | .275 | .408 |
| Riboflavin | mg | .416 | .159 | 1.273 | 1.887 |
| Niacin | mg | .210 | .080 | .643 | .953 |
| Pantothenic acid | mg | .750 | .286 | 2.295 | 3.402 |
| Vitamin B$_6$ | mg | .051 | .019 | .156 | .231 |
| Folacin | μg | 11 | 4 | 34 | 51 |
| Vitamin B$_{12}$ | μg | .444 | .170 | 1.359 | 2.014 |
| Vitamin A | RE | 81 | 31 | 248 | 367 |
| | IU | 328 | 125 | 1,004 | 1,488 |
| Lipids | | | | | |
| Fatty acids | | | | | |

Table 1 (continued)
## NUTRIENT COMPOSITION OF MILK PRODUCTS AND BY-PRODUCTS

### Item 29: Milk (Condensed, Sweetened, Canned)

| Nutrients | Units | Amount in 100 g (edible portion) | Amount in edible portion of common measures of food (approximate measure and weight) | | Amount in edible portion of 1 lb of food as purchased (refuse:0) |
| --- | --- | --- | --- | --- | --- |
| | | | 1 fl oz = 38.2 g | 1 cup = 306 g | |
| Saturated (total) | g | 5.49 | 2.10 | 16.79 | 24.88 |
| 4:0 | g | .28 | .11 | .86 | 1.28 |
| 6:0 | g | .17 | .06 | .51 | .76 |
| 8:0 | g | .10 | .04 | .30 | .44 |
| 10:0 | g | .07 | .03 | .22 | .33 |
| 12:0 | g | .18 | .07 | .55 | .82 |
| 14:0 | g | .78 | .30 | 2.40 | 3.55 |
| 16:0 | g | 2.40 | .92 | 7.33 | 10.87 |
| 18:0 | g | 1.21 | .46 | 3.70 | 5.48 |
| Monounsaturated (total) | g | 2.43 | .93 | 7.43 | 11.01 |
| 16:1 | g | .14 | .05 | .42 | .62 |
| 18:1 | g | 2.19 | .84 | 6.70 | 9.92 |
| 20:1 | g | | | | |
| 22:1 | g | | | | |
| Polyunsaturated (total) | g | .34 | .13 | 1.03 | 1.53 |
| 18:2 | g | .22 | .08 | .66 | .98 |
| 18:3 | g | .12 | .05 | .37 | .55 |
| 18:4 | g | | | | |
| 20:4 | g | | | | |
| 20:5 | g | | | | |
| 22:5 | g | | | | |
| 22:6 | g | | | | |
| Cholesterol | mg | 34 | 3 | 104 | 154 |
| Phytosterols | mg | | | | |
| Amino acids | | | | | |
| Tryptophan | g | .112 | .043 | .341 | .506 |
| Threonine | g | .357 | .136 | 1.093 | 1.620 |
| Isoleucine | g | .479 | .183 | 1.464 | 2.171 |
| Leucine | g | .775 | .296 | 2.371 | 3.515 |
| Lysine | g | .627 | .240 | 1.920 | 2.846 |
| Methionine | g | .198 | .076 | .607 | .900 |
| Cystine | g | .073 | .028 | .224 | .332 |
| Phenylalanine | g | .382 | .146 | 1.168 | 1.732 |
| Tyrosine | g | .382 | .146 | 1.168 | 1.732 |
| Valine | g | .529 | .202 | 1.620 | 2.401 |
| Arginine | g | .286 | .109 | .876 | 1.299 |
| Histidine | g | .214 | .082 | .656 | .973 |
| Alanine | g | .273 | .104 | .835 | 1.237 |
| Aspartic acid | g | .600 | .229 | 1.836 | 2.722 |
| Glutamic acid | g | 1.656 | .633 | 5.069 | 7.513 |
| Glycine | g | .167 | .064 | .512 | .759 |
| Proline | g | .766 | .293 | 2.345 | 3.475 |
| Serine | g | .430 | .164 | 1.316 | 1.951 |

### Item 30: Milk (Evaporated, Skim, Canned)[a]

| Nutrients | Units | Amount in 100 g (edible portion) | Amount in edible portion of common measures of food (approximate measure and weight) | | Amount in edible portion of 1 lb of food as purchased (refuse: 0) |
| --- | --- | --- | --- | --- | --- |
| | | | 1 fl oz = 3.9 g | ½ cup = 128 g | |
| Proximate | | | | | |
| Water | g | 79.40 | 25.33 | 101.24 | 360.16 |
| Food energy | kcal | 78 | 25 | 99 | 353 |
| | kJ | 326 | 104 | 416 | 1,479 |
| Protein (N × 6.38) | g | 7.55 | 2.41 | 9.63 | 34.25 |
| Total lipid (fat) | g | .20 | .06 | .26 | .91 |
| Carbohydrate (total) | g | 11.35 | 3.62 | 14.47 | 51.48 |
| Fiber | g | 0 | 0 | 0 | 0 |

Table 1 (continued)
## NUTRIENT COMPOSITION OF MILK PRODUCTS AND BY-PRODUCTS

Item 30: Milk (Evaporated, Skim, Canned)[a]

| Nutrients | Units | Amount in 100 g (edible portion) | Amount in edible portion of common measures of food (approximate measure and weight) | | Amount in edible portion of 1 lb of food as purchased (refuse: 0) |
|---|---|---|---|---|---|
| | | | 1 fl oz = 3.9 g | ½ cup = 128 g | |
| Ash | g | 1.50 | .48 | 1.91 | 6.80 |
| Minerals | | | | | |
| Calcium | mg | 290 | 92 | 369 | 1,313 |
| Iron | mg | .29 | .09 | .37 | 1.32 |
| Magnesium | mg | 27 | 9 | 34 | 122 |
| Phosphorus | mg | 195 | 62 | 248 | 884 |
| Potassium | mg | 332 | 106 | 423 | 1,504 |
| Sodium | mg | 115 | 37 | 147 | 522 |
| Zinc | mg | .90 | .29 | 1.15 | 4.08 |
| Vitamins | | | | | |
| Ascorbic acid | mg | 1.24 | .40 | 1.58 | 5.62 |
| Thiamin | mg | .045 | .014 | .057 | .204 |
| Riboflavin | mg | .309 | .099 | .394 | 1.402 |
| Niacin | mg | .174 | .056 | .222 | .789 |
| Pantothenic acid | mg | .738 | .235 | .941 | 3.348 |
| Vitamin $B_6$ | mg | .055 | .018 | .070 | .249 |
| Folacin | μg | 9 | 3 | 11 | 39 |
| Vitamin $B_{12}$ | μg | .239 | .076 | .305 | 1.084 |
| Vitamin A[b] | RE | 117 | 37 | 150 | 531 |
| | IU | 392 | 125 | 500 | 1,778 |
| Lipids | | | | | |
| Fatty acids[aa] | | | | | |
| Saturated (total) | g | .121 | .039 | .155 | .551 |
| 4:0 | g | .005 | .002 | .007 | .023 |
| 6:0 | g | .004 | .001 | .005 | .016 |
| 8:0 | g | .001 | Trace | .002 | .006 |
| 10:0 | g | .003 | .001 | .004 | .013 |
| 12:0 | g | .004 | .001 | .005 | .019 |
| 14:0 | g | .019 | .006 | .025 | .088 |
| 16:0 | g | .054 | .017 | .068 | .243 |
| 18:0 | g | .024 | .008 | .031 | .111 |
| Monounsaturated (total) | g | .062 | .020 | .079 | .280 |
| 16:1 | g | .004 | .001 | .005 | .019 |
| 18:1 | g | .056 | .018 | .071 | .252 |
| 20:1 | g | | | | |
| 22:1 | g | | | | |
| Polyunsaturated (total) | g | .006 | .002 | .008 | .029 |
| 18:2 | g | .004 | .001 | .006 | .020 |
| 18:3 | g | .002 | .001 | .003 | .009 |
| 18:4 | g | | | | |
| 20:4 | g | | | | |
| 20:5 | g | | | | |
| 22:5 | g | | | | |
| 22:6 | g | | | | |
| Cholesterol | mg | 4 | 1 | 5 | 16 |
| Phytosterols | mg | | | | |
| Amino acids | | | | | |
| Tryptophan | g | .107 | .034 | .136 | .483 |
| Threonine | g | .341 | .109 | .435 | 1.546 |
| Isoleucine | g | .457 | .146 | .582 | 2.072 |
| Leucine | g | .740 | .236 | .943 | 3.355 |
| Lysine | g | .599 | .191 | .763 | 2.716 |
| Methionine | g | .189 | .060 | .241 | .859 |
| Cystine | g | .070 | .022 | .089 | .317 |
| Phenylalanine | g | .364 | .116 | .465 | 1.653 |
| Tyrosine | g | .364 | .116 | .465 | 1.653 |
| Valine | g | .505 | .161 | .644 | 2.292 |
| Arginine | g | .273 | .087 | .349 | 1.240 |
| Histidine | g | .205 | .065 | .261 | .929 |
| Alanine | g | .260 | .083 | .332 | 1.181 |
| Aspartic acid | g | .573 | .183 | .730 | 2.598 |

Table 1 (continued)
## NUTRIENT COMPOSITION OF MILK PRODUCTS AND BY-PRODUCTS

### Item 30: Milk (Evaporated, Skim, Canned)[a]

| Nutrients | Units | Amount in 100 g (edible portion) | Amount in edible portion of common measures of food (approximate measure and weight) | | Amount in edible portion of 1 lb of food as purchased (refuse: 0) |
|---|---|---|---|---|---|
| | | | 1 fl oz = 3.9 g | ½ cup = 128 g | |
| Glutamic acid | g | 1.581 | .504 | 2.016 | 7.171 |
| Glycine | g | .160 | .051 | .204 | .725 |
| Proline | g | .731 | .233 | .932 | 3.317 |
| Serine | g | .411 | .131 | .524 | 1.863 |

### Item 31: Milk (Chocolate, Whole, Fluid)[x]

| Nutrients | Units | Amount in 100 g (edible portion) | Amount in edible portion of common measures of food (approximate measure and weight) | | Amount in edible portion of 1 lb of food as purchased (refuse:0) |
|---|---|---|---|---|---|
| | | | 1 cup = 250 g | 1 qt = 1,000 g | |
| Proximate | | | | | |
| Water | g | 82.30 | 205.75 | 823.00 | 373.31 |
| Food energy | kcal | 83 | 208 | 833 | 378 |
| | kJ | 349 | 872 | 3,488 | 1,582 |
| Protein (N × 6.38) | g | 3.17 | 7.92 | 31.70 | 14.38 |
| Total lipid (fat) | g | 3.39 | 8.48 | 33.90 | 15.38 |
| Carbohydrate (total) | g | 10.34 | 25.85 | 103.40 | 46.90 |
| Fiber | g | .06 | .15 | .60 | .27 |
| Ash | g | .80 | 2.00 | 8.00 | 3.63 |
| Minerals | | | | | |
| Calcim | mg | 112 | 280 | 1,121 | 508 |
| Iron | mg | .24 | .60 | 2.40 | 1.09 |
| Magnesium | mg | 13 | 33 | 130 | 59 |
| Phosphorus | mg | 100 | 251 | 1,005 | 456 |
| Potassium | mg | 167 | 417 | 1,669 | 757 |
| Sodium | mg | 60 | 149 | 596 | 270 |
| Zinc | mg | .41 | 1.02 | 4.10 | 1.86 |
| Vitamins | | | | | |
| Ascorbic acid | mg | .91 | 2.28 | 9.10 | 4.13 |
| Thiamin | mg | .037 | .092 | .370 | .168 |
| Riboflavin | mg | .162 | .405 | 1.620 | .735 |
| Niacin | mg | .125 | .313 | 1.250 | .567 |
| Pantothenic acid | mg | .295 | .738 | 2.950 | 1.338 |
| Vitamin B₆ | mg | .040 | .100 | .400 | .181 |
| Folacin | µg | 5 | 12 | 47 | 21 |
| Vitamin B₁₂ | µg | .334 | .835 | 3.340 | 1.515 |
| Vitamin A | RE | 29 | 72 | 290 | 132 |
| | IU | 121 | 302 | 1,210 | 549 |
| Lipids | | | | | |
| Fatty acids | | | | | |
| Saturated (total) | g | 2.10 | 5.26 | 21.04 | 9.54 |
| 4:0 | g | .10 | .25 | 1.01 | .46 |
| 6:0 | g | .06 | .15 | .60 | .27 |
| 8:0 | g | .04 | .09 | .35 | .16 |
| 10:0 | g | .08 | .20 | .78 | .36 |
| 12:0 | g | .09 | .22 | .88 | .40 |
| 14:0 | g | .32 | .79 | 3.15 | 1.43 |
| 16:0 | g | .89 | 2.22 | 8.89 | 4.03 |
| 18:0 | g | .47 | 1.16 | 4.66 | 2.11 |
| Monounsaturated (total) | g | .99 | 2.48 | 9.90 | 4.49 |
| 16:1 | g | .07 | .18 | .71 | .32 |
| 18:1 | g | .87 | 2.18 | 8.72 | 3.96 |
| 20:1 | g | | | | |
| 22:1 | g | | | | |
| Polyunsaturated (total) | g | .12 | .31 | 1.24 | .56 |
| 18:2 | g | .08 | .20 | .78 | .36 |
| 18:3 | g | .05 | .12 | .46 | .21 |
| 18:4 | g | | | | |

Table 1 (continued)
## NUTRIENT COMPOSITION OF MILK PRODUCTS AND BY-PRODUCTS

### Item 31: Milk (Chocolate, Whole, Fluid)[x]

| Nutrients | Units | Amount in 100 g (edible portion) | Amount in edible portion of common measures of food (approximate measure and weight) 1 cup = 250 g | 1 qt = 1,000 g | Amount in edible portion of 1 lb of food as purchased (refuse:0) |
|---|---|---|---|---|---|
| 20:4 | g | | | | |
| 20:5 | g | | | | |
| 22:5 | g | | | | |
| 22:6 | g | | | | |
| Cholesterol | mg | 12 | 30 | 122 | 55 |
| Phytosterols | mg | | | | |
| Amino acids | | | | | |
| Tryptophan | g | .045 | .112 | .447 | .203 |
| Threonine | g | .143 | .358 | 1.431 | .649 |
| Isoleucine | g | .192 | .479 | 1.918 | .870 |
| Leucine | g | .311 | .776 | 3.105 | 1.409 |
| Lysine | g | .251 | .629 | 2.514 | 1.140 |
| Methionine | g | .079 | .199 | .795 | .361 |
| Cystine | g | .029 | .073 | .293 | .133 |
| Phenylalanine | g | .153 | .383 | 1.530 | .694 |
| Tyrosine | g | .153 | .383 | 1.530 | .694 |
| Valine | g | .212 | .530 | 2.122 | .962 |
| Arginine | g | .115 | .287 | 1.148 | .521 |
| Histidine | g | .086 | .215 | .860 | .390 |
| Alanine | g | .109 | .273 | 1.093 | .496 |
| Aspartic acid | g | .240 | .601 | 2.405 | 1.091 |
| Glutamic acid | g | .664 | 1.660 | 6.638 | 3.011 |
| Glycine | g | .067 | .168 | .671 | .304 |
| Proline | g | .307 | .768 | 3.071 | 1.393 |
| Serine | g | .172 | .431 | 1.724 | .782 |

### Item 32: Milk (Human, Whole, Mature, Fluid)

| Nutrients | Units | Amount in 100 g (edible portion) | Amount in edible portion of common measures of food (approximate measure and weight) 1 fl oz = 30.8 g | 1 cup = 246 g | Amount in edible portion of 1 lb of food (refuse:0) |
|---|---|---|---|---|---|
| Proximate | | | | | |
| Water | g | 87.50 | 26.95 | 215.25 | 396.90 |
| Food energy | kcal | 70 | 21 | 171 | 316 |
| | kJ | 291 | 90 | 716 | 1,321 |
| Protein (N × 6.38) | g | 1.03 | .32 | 2.53 | 4.67 |
| Total lipid (fat) | g | 4.38 | 1.35 | 10.78 | 19.87 |
| Carbohydrate (total) | g | 6.89 | 2.12 | 16.95 | 31.25 |
| Fiber | g | 0 | 0 | 0 | 0 |
| Ash | g | .20 | .06 | .49 | .91 |
| Minerals | | | | | |
| Calcium | mg | 32 | 10 | 79 | 146 |
| Iron | mg | .03 | .01 | .07 | .14 |
| Magnesium | mg | 3 | 1 | 8 | 15 |
| Phosphorus | mg | 14 | 4 | 34 | 62 |
| Potassium | mg | 51 | 16 | 126 | 232 |
| Sodium | mg | 17 | 5 | 42 | 77 |
| Zinc | mg | .17 | .05 | .42 | .77 |
| Vitamins | | | | | |
| Ascorbic acid | mg | 5.00 | 1.54 | 12.30 | 22.68 |
| Thiamin | mg | .014 | .004 | .034 | .064 |
| Riboflvain | mg | .036 | .011 | .089 | .163 |
| Niacin | mg | .177 | .055 | .435 | .803 |
| Pantothenic acid | mg | .223 | .069 | .549 | 1.012 |
| Vitamin B$_6$ | mg | .011 | .003 | .027 | .050 |
| Folacin | μg | 5 | 2 | 13 | 24 |

Table 1 (continued)
## NUTRIENT COMPOSITION OF MILK PRODUCTS AND BY-PRODUCTS
### Item 32: Milk (Human, Whole, Mature, Fluid)

| Nutrients | Units | Amount in 100 g (edible portion) | Amount in edible portion of common measures of food (approximate measure and weight) 1 fl oz = 30.8 g | 1 cup = 246 g | Amount in edible portion of 1 lb of food (refuse:0) |
|---|---|---|---|---|---|
| Vitamin B$_{12}$ | μg | .045 | .014 | .111 | .204 |
| Vitamin A | RE | 64 | 20 | 157 | 290 |
|  | IU | 241 | 74 | 593 | 1,093 |
| Lipids |  |  |  |  |  |
| Fatty acids |  |  |  |  |  |
| Saturated (total) | g | 2.01 | .62 | 4.94 | 9.12 |
| 4:0 | g |  |  |  |  |
| 6:0 | g |  |  |  |  |
| 8:0 | g |  |  |  |  |
| 10:0 | g | .06 | .02 | .16 | .29 |
| 12:0 | g | .26 | .08 | 63 | 1.16 |
| 14:0 | g | .32 | .10 | .79 | 1.46 |
| 16:0 | g | .92 | .28 | 2.26 | 4.17 |
| 18:0 | g | .29 | .09 | .72 | 1.33 |
| Monounsaturated (total) | g | 1.66 | .51 | 4.08 | 7.52 |
| 16:1 | g | .13 | .04 | .32 | .59 |
| 18:1 | g | 1.48 | .46 | 3.63 | 6.69 |
| 20:1 | g | .04 | .01 | .09 | .18 |
| 22:1 | g | Trace |  |  |  |
| Polyunsaturated (total) | g | .50 | .15 | 1.22 | 2.26 |
| 18:2 | g | .37 | .12 | .92 | 1.70 |
| 18:3 | g | .05 | .02 | .13 | .24 |
| 18:4 | g |  |  |  |  |
| 20:4 | g | .03 | .01 | .06 | .12 |
| 20:5 | g | Trace |  |  |  |
| 22:5 | g | Trace |  |  |  |
| 22:6 | g | Trace |  |  |  |
| Cholesterol | mg | 14 | 4 | 34 | 63 |
| Phytosterols | mg |  |  |  |  |
| Amino acids |  |  |  |  |  |
| Tryptophan | g | .017 | .005 | .041 | .076 |
| Threonine | g | .046 | .014 | .112 | .207 |
| Isoleucine | g | .056 | .017 | .137 | .253 |
| Leucine | g | .095 | .029 | .233 | .429 |
| Lysine | g | .068 | .021 | .168 | .309 |
| Methionine | g | .021 | .006 | .052 | .095 |
| Cystine | g | .019 | .006 | .047 | .086 |
| Phenylalanine | g | .046 | .014 | .113 | .209 |
| Tyrosine | g | .053 | .016 | .129 | .239 |
| Valine | g | .063 | .019 | .156 | .287 |
| Arginine | g | .043 | .013 | .105 | .194 |
| Histidine | g | .023 | .007 | .057 | .105 |
| Alanine | g | .036 | .011 | .089 | .165 |
| Aspartic acid | g | .082 | .025 | .201 | .371 |
| Glutamic acid | g | .168 | .052 | .414 | .764 |
| Glycine | g | .026 | .008 | .064 | .119 |
| Proline | g | .082 | .025 | .203 | .374 |
| Serine | g | .043 | .013 | .107 | .197 |

### Item 33: Whey (Acid, Fluid)

| Nutrients | Units | Amount in 100 g (edible portion) | Amount in edible portion of common measures of food (approximate measure and weight) 1 cup = 246 g | 1 qt = 984 g | Amount in edible portion of 1 lb of food as purchased (refuse: 0) |
|---|---|---|---|---|---|
| Proximate |  |  |  |  |  |
| Water | g | 93.42 | 229.81 | 919.25 | 423.75 |
| Food energy | kcal | 24 | 59 | 235 | 108 |
|  | kJ | 100 | 246 | 982 | 453 |
| Protein (N × 6.38) | g | .76 | 1.87 | 7.48 | 3.45 |

Table 1 (continued)
## NUTRIENT COMPOSITION OF MILK PRODUCTS AND BY-PRODUCTS

### Item 33: Whey (Acid, Fluid)

| Nutrients | Units | Amount in 100 g (edible portion) | Amount in edible portion of common measures of food (approximate measure and weight) | | Amount in edible portion of 1 lb of food as purchased (refuse: 0) |
|---|---|---|---|---|---|
| | | | 1 cup = 246 g | 1 qt = 984 g | |
| Total lipid (fat) | g | .09 | .22 | .89 | .41 |
| Carbohydrate (total) | g | 5.12 | 12.60 | 50.38 | 23.22 |
| Fiber | g | 0 | 0 | 0 | 0 |
| Ash | g | .61 | 1.50 | 6.00 | 2.77 |
| Minerals | | | | | |
| Calcium | mg | 103 | 253 | 1,011 | 466 |
| Iron | mg | .08 | .20 | .79 | .36 |
| Magnesium | mg | 10 | 24 | 96 | 44 |
| Phosphorus | mg | 78 | 191 | 764 | 352 |
| Potassium | mg | 143 | 352 | 1,408 | 649 |
| Sodium | mg | 48 | 118 | 473 | 218 |
| Zinc | mg | .43 | 1.06 | 4.23 | 1.95 |
| Vitamins | | | | | |
| Ascorbic acid | mg | .06 | .15 | .59 | .27 |
| Thiamin | mg | .042 | .103 | .413 | .191 |
| Riboflavin | mg | .140 | .344 | 1.378 | .635 |
| Niacin | mg | .079 | .194 | .777 | .358 |
| Pantothenic acid | mg | .381 | .937 | 3.749 | 1.728 |
| Vitamin $B_6$ | mg | .042 | .103 | .413 | .191 |
| Folacin | μg | 2 | 5 | 22 | 10 |
| Vitamin $B_{12}$ | μg | .179 | .440 | 1.761 | .812 |
| Vitamin A | RE | 1 | 2 | 10 | 5 |
| | IU | 7 | 17 | 69 | 32 |
| Lipids | | | | | |
| Fatty acids | | | | | |
| Saturated (total) | g | .057 | .140 | .561 | .258 |
| 4:0 | g | .004 | .010 | .038 | .018 |
| 6:0 | g | .001 | .003 | .013 | .006 |
| 8:0 | g | .001 | .002 | .009 | .004 |
| 10:0 | g | .002 | .004 | .016 | .008 |
| 12:0 | g | .001 | .003 | .011 | .005 |
| 14:0 | g | .008 | .019 | .075 | .034 |
| 16:0 | g | .025 | .062 | .247 | .114 |
| 18:0 | g | .010 | .025 | .098 | .045 |
| Monounsaturated (total) | g | .025 | .061 | .244 | .113 |
| 16:1 | g | .004 | .011 | .043 | .020 |
| 18:0 | g | .019 | .047 | .187 | .086 |
| 20:1 | g | | | | |
| 22:1 | g | | | | |
| Polyunsaturated (total) | g | .004 | .009 | .035 | .016 |
| 18:2 | g | .003 | .008 | .030 | .014 |
| 18:3 | g | Trace | .001 | .005 | .002 |
| 18:4 | g | | | | |
| 20:4 | g | | | | |
| 20:5 | g | | | | |
| 22:5 | g | | | | |
| 22:6 | g | | | | |
| Cholesterol | mg | — | — | — | — |
| Phytosterols | mg | | | | |
| Amino acids | | | | | |
| Tryptophan | g | .016 | .038 | .154 | .071 |
| Threonine | g | .038 | .094 | .376 | .173 |
| Isoleucine | g | .038 | .093 | .370 | .171 |
| Leucine | g | .072 | .178 | .712 | .328 |
| Lysine | g | .065 | .161 | .642 | .296 |
| Methionine | g | .014 | .035 | .141 | .065 |
| Cystine | g | .014 | .034 | .135 | .062 |
| Phenylalanine | g | .025 | .062 | .246 | .113 |
| Tyrosine | g | .019 | .048 | .191 | .088 |
| Valine | g | .038 | .092 | .369 | .170 |
| Arginine | g | .021 | .052 | .209 | .096 |
| Histidine | g | .015 | .037 | .147 | .068 |

## Table 1 (continued)
## NUTRIENT COMPOSITION OF MILK PRODUCTS AND BY-PRODUCTS

### Item 33: Whey (Acid, Fluid)

| Nutrients | Units | Amount in 100 g (edible portion) | Amount in edible portion of common measures of food (approximate measure and weight) | | Amount in edible portion of 1 lb of food as purchased (refuse: 0) |
|---|---|---|---|---|---|
| | | | 1 cup = 246 g | 1 qt = 984 g | |
| Alanine | g | .033 | .081 | .322 | .149 |
| Aspartic acid | g | .074 | .183 | .733 | .338 |
| Glutamic acid | g | .136 | .334 | 1.336 | .616 |
| Glycine | g | .014 | .034 | .135 | .062 |
| Proline | g | .045 | .111 | .445 | .205 |
| Serine | g | .035 | .086 | .345 | .159 |

### Item 34: Whey (Acid, Dry)

| Nutrients | Units | Amount in 100 g (edible portion) | Amount in edible portion of common measures of food (approximate measure and weight) | | Amount in edible portion of 1 lb of food as purchased (refuse: 0) |
|---|---|---|---|---|---|
| | | | 1 Tbsp = 2.9 g | 1 cup = 57 g | |
| **Proximate** | | | | | |
| Water | g | 3.51 | 0.10 | 2.00 | 15.92 |
| Food energy | kcal | 339 | 10 | 193 | 1,538 |
| | kJ | 1,419 | 41 | 809 | 6,437 |
| Protein (N × 6.38) | g | 11.73 | .34 | 6.69 | 53.21 |
| Total lipid (fat) | g | .54 | .02 | .31 | 2.45 |
| Carbohydrate (total) | g | 73.45 | 2.11 | 41.87 | 333.17 |
| Fiber | g | 0 | 0 | 0 | 0 |
| Ash | g | 10.77 | .31 | 6.14 | 48.85 |
| **Minerals** | | | | | |
| Calcium | mg | 2,054 | 59 | 1,171 | 9,319 |
| Iron | mg | 1.24 | .04 | .71 | 5.62 |
| Magnesium | mg | 199 | 6 | 113 | 902 |
| Phosphorus | mg | 1,348 | 39 | 769 | 6,117 |
| Potassium | mg | 2,288 | 66 | 1,304 | 10,381 |
| Sodium | mg | 968 | 28 | 552 | 4,390 |
| Zinc | mg | 6.31 | .18 | 3.60 | 28.62 |
| **Vitamins** | | | | | |
| Ascorbic acid | mg | .90 | .03 | .51 | 4.08 |
| Thiamin | mg | .622 | .018 | .355 | 2.821 |
| Riboflavin | mg | 2.060 | .059 | 1.174 | 9.344 |
| Niacin | mg | 1.160 | .033 | .661 | 5.262 |
| Pantothenic acid | mg | 5.632 | .162 | 3.210 | 25.547 |
| Vitamin B$_6$ | mg | .620 | .018 | .353 | 2.812 |
| Folacin | μg | 33 | 1 | 19 | 151 |
| Vitamin B$_{12}$ | μg | 2.500 | .072 | 1.425 | 11.340 |
| Vitamin A | RE | 9 | Trace | 5 | 41 |
| | IU | 58 | 2 | 33 | 263 |
| **Lipids** | | | | | |
| Fatty acids[a] | | | | | |
| Saturated (total) | g | .34 | .01 | .20 | 1.55 |
| 4:0 | g | .02 | Trace | .01 | .11 |
| 6:0 | g | .01 | Trace | Trace | .04 |
| 8:0 | g | Trace | Trace | Trace | .02 |
| 10:0 | g | .01 | Trace | .01 | .04 |
| 12:0 | g | .01 | Trace | Trace | .03 |
| 14:0 | g | .05 | Trace | .03 | .21 |
| 16:0 | g | .15 | Trace | .09 | .68 |
| 18:0 | g | .06 | Trace | .03 | .27 |
| Monounsaturated (total) | g | .15 | Trace | .08 | .68 |
| 16:1 | g | .03 | Trace | .02 | .12 |
| 18:1 | g | .11 | Trace | .06 | .52 |
| 20:1 | g | | | | |
| 22:1 | g | | | | |
| Polyunsaturated (total) | g | .02 | Trace | .01 | .10 |
| 18:2 | g | .02 | Trace | .01 | .08 |
| 18:3 | g | Trace | Trace | Trace | .01 |

Table 1 (continued)
NUTRIENT COMPOSITION OF MILK PRODUCTS AND BY-PRODUCTS

Item 34: Whey (Acid, Dry)

| Nutrients | Units | Amount in 100 g (edible portion) | Amount in edible portion of common measures of food (approximate measure and weight) | | Amount in edible portion of 1 lb of food as purchased (refuse: 0) |
|---|---|---|---|---|---|
| | | | 1 Tbsp = 2.9 g | 1 cup = 57 g | |
| 18:4 | g | | | | |
| 20:4 | g | | | | |
| 20:5 | g | | | | |
| 22:5 | g | | | | |
| 22:6 | g | | | | |
| Cholesterol | mg | —[a] | — | — | — |
| Phytosterols | mg | | | | |
| Amino Acids | | | | | |
| Tryptophan | g | .241 | .007 | .137 | 1.092 |
| Threonine | g | .590 | .017 | .336 | 2.677 |
| Isoleucine | g | .581 | .017 | .331 | 2.635 |
| Leucine | g | 1.116 | .032 | .636 | 5.062 |
| Lysine | g | 1.008 | .029 | .574 | 4.570 |
| Methionine | g | .221 | .006 | .126 | 1.001 |
| Cystine | g | .211 | .006 | .121 | .959 |
| Phenylalanine | g | .386 | .011 | .220 | 1.751 |
| Tyrosine | g | .300 | .009 | .171 | 1.359 |
| Valine | g | .579 | .017 | .330 | 2.627 |
| Arginine | g | .327 | .009 | .187 | 1.484 |
| Histidine | g | .230 | .007 | .131 | 1.042 |
| Alanine | g | .506 | .015 | .288 | 2.293 |
| Aspartic acid | g | 1.149 | .033 | .655 | 5.212 |
| Glutamic acid | g | 2.096 | .060 | 1.195 | 9.507 |
| Glycine | g | .211 | .006 | .121 | .959 |
| Proline | g | .699 | .020 | .398 | 3.169 |
| Serine | g | .541 | .016 | .308 | 2.452 |

Item 35: Whey (Sweet, Fluid)

| Nutrients | Units | Amount in 100 g (edible portion) | Amount in edible portion of common measures of food (approximate measure and weight) | | Amount in edible portion of 1 lb of food as purchased (refuse: 0) |
|---|---|---|---|---|---|
| | | | 1 cup = 246 g | 1 qt = 984 g | |
| Proximate | | | | | |
| Water | g | 93.12 | 229.08 | 916.30 | 422.39 |
| Food energy | kcal | 27 | 66 | 263 | 121 |
| | kJ | 112 | 275 | 1,099 | 507 |
| Protein (N × 6.38) | g | .85 | 2.09 | 8.36 | 3.86 |
| Total lipid (fat) | g | .36 | .89 | 3.54 | 1.63 |
| Carbohydrate (total) | g | 5.14 | 12.64 | 50.58 | 23.32 |
| Fiber | g | 0 | 0 | 0 | 0 |
| Ash | g | .53 | 1.30 | 5.22 | 2.40 |
| Minerals | | | | | |
| Calcium | mg | 47 | 115 | 461 | 212 |
| Iron | mg | .06 | .15 | .59 | .27 |
| Magnesium | mg | 8 | 20 | 81 | 37 |
| Phosphorus | mg | 46 | 112 | 449 | 207 |
| Potassium | mg | 161 | 396 | 1,584 | 730 |
| Sodium | mg | 54 | 132 | 526 | 243 |
| Zinc | mg | .13 | .32 | 1.28 | .59 |
| Vitamins | | | | | |
| Ascorbic acid | mg | .10 | .25 | .98 | .45 |
| Thiamin | mg | .036 | .089 | .354 | .163 |
| Riboflavin | mg | .158 | .389 | 1.555 | .717 |
| Niacin | mg | .074 | .182 | .728 | .336 |
| Pantothenic acid | mg | .383 | .942 | 3.769 | 1.737 |
| Vitamin B$_6$ | mg | .031 | .076 | .305 | .141 |
| Folacin | μg | 1 | 2 | 8 | 4 |

Table 1 (continued)
## NUTRIENT COMPOSITION OF MILK PRODUCTS AND BY-PRODUCTS

### Item 35: Whey (Sweet, Fluid)

| Nutrients | Units | Amount in 100 g (edible portion) | Amount in edible portion of common measures of food (approximate measure and weight) | | Amount in edible portion of 1 lb of food as purchased (refuse: 0) |
|---|---|---|---|---|---|
| | | | 1 cup = 246 g | 1 qt = 984 g | |
| Vitamin B$_{12}$ | μg | .277 | .681 | 2.726 | 1.256 |
| Vitamin A | RE | 4 | 10 | 39 | 18 |
| | IU | 16 | 39 | 157 | 73 |
| Lipids | | | | | |
| Fatty acids | | | | | |
| Saturated (total) | g | .230 | .566 | 2.263 | 1.043 |
| 4:0 | g | .020 | .049 | .195 | .090 |
| 6:0 | g | .003 | .007 | .029 | .013 |
| 8:0 | g | .003 | .008 | .033 | .015 |
| 10:0 | g | .006 | .015 | .060 | .028 |
| 12:0 | g | .004 | .010 | .039 | .018 |
| 14:0 | g | .035 | .087 | .347 | .160 |
| 16:0 | g | .110 | .270 | 1.079 | .497 |
| 18:0 | g | .033 | .081 | .322 | .148 |
| Monounsaturated (total) | g | .100 | .246 | .984 | .454 |
| 16:1 | g | .011 | .027 | .109 | .050 |
| 18:1 | g | .084 | .208 | .831 | .383 |
| 20:1 | g | | | | |
| 22:1 | g | | | | |
| Polyunsaturated (total) | g | .011 | .028 | .112 | .051 |
| 18:2 | g | .008 | .021 | .083 | .038 |
| 18:3 | g | .003 | .007 | .028 | .013 |
| 18:4 | g | | | | |
| 20:4 | g | | | | |
| 20:5 | g | | | | |
| 22:5 | g | | | | |
| 22:6 | g | | | | |
| Cholesterol | mg | 2 | 5 | 20 | 9 |
| Phytosterols | mg | | | | |
| Amino acids | | | | | |
| Tryptophan | g | .013 | .033 | .132 | .061 |
| Threonine | g | .054 | .132 | .528 | .244 |
| Isoleucine | g | .047 | .116 | .465 | .215 |
| Leucine | g | .078 | .192 | .767 | .354 |
| Lysine | g | .068 | .166 | .666 | .307 |
| Methionine | g | .016 | .039 | .156 | .072 |
| Cystine | g | .017 | .041 | .164 | .076 |
| Phenylalanine | g | .027 | .066 | .264 | .121 |
| Tyrosine | g | .024 | .059 | .235 | .108 |
| Valine | g | .046 | .113 | .451 | .208 |
| Arginine | g | .025 | .061 | .243 | .112 |
| Histidine | g | .016 | .038 | .153 | .071 |
| Alanine | g | .039 | .097 | .387 | .178 |
| Aspartic acid | g | .083 | .205 | .821 | .378 |
| Glutamic acid | g | .148 | .363 | 1.454 | .670 |
| Glycine | g | .018 | .045 | .181 | .083 |
| Proline | g | .052 | .127 | .509 | .234 |
| Serine | g | .041 | .101 | .402 | .186 |

### Item 36: Whey (Sweet, Dry)

| Nutrients | Units | Amount in 100 g (edible portion) | Amount in edible portion of common measures of food | | Amount in edible portion of 1 lb of food as purchased (refuse:0) |
|---|---|---|---|---|---|
| | | | 1 Tbsp = 7.5 g | 1 cup = 145 g | |
| Proximate | | | | | |
| Water | g | 3.19 | 0.24 | 4.62 | 14.47 |
| Food energy | kcal | 353 | 26 | 512 | 1,600 |
| | kJ | 1,476 | 110 | 2,141 | 6,697 |

Table 1 (continued)
NUTRIENT COMPOSITION OF MILK PRODUCTS AND BY-PRODUCTS

Item 36: Whey (Sweet, Dry)

| Nutrients | Units | Amount in 100 g (edible portion) | Amount in edible portion of common measures of food | | Amount in edible portion of 1 lb of food as purchased (refuse: 0) |
| | | | 1 Tbsp = 7.5 g | 1 cup = 145 g | |
|---|---|---|---|---|---|
| Protein (N × 6.38) | g | 12.93 | .96 | 18.75 | 58.65 |
| Total lipid (fat) | g | 1.07 | .08 | 1.55 | 4.85 |
| Carbohydrate (total) | g | 74.46 | 5.56 | 107.97 | 337.75 |
| Fiber | g | 0 | 0 | 0 | 0 |
| Ash | g | 8.35 | .62 | 12.11 | 37.88 |
| Minerals | | | | | |
| Calcium | mg | 796 | 59 | 1,154 | 3,611 |
| Iron | mg | .88 | .07 | 1.28 | 3.99 |
| Magnesium | mg | 176 | 13 | 255 | 799 |
| Phosphorus | mg | 932 | 70 | 1,351 | 4,226 |
| Potassium | mg | 2,080 | 155 | 3,016 | 9,434 |
| Sodium | mg | 1,079 | 80 | 1,565 | 4,894 |
| Zinc | mg | 1.97 | .15 | 2.86 | 8.94 |
| Vitamins | | | | | |
| Ascorbic acid | mg | 1.49 | .11 | 2.16 | 6.76 |
| Thiamin | mg | .519 | .039 | .753 | 2.354 |
| Riboflavin | mg | 2.208 | .165 | 3.202 | 10.015 |
| Niacin | mg | 1.258 | .094 | 1.824 | 5.706 |
| Pantothenic acid | mg | 5.620 | .419 | 8.149 | 25.492 |
| Vitamin $B_6$ | mg | .584 | .044 | .847 | 2.649 |
| Folacin | μg | 12 | 1 | 17 | 53 |
| Vitamin $B_{12}$ | μg | 2.371 | .177 | 3.438 | 10.755 |
| Vitamin A | RE | 10 | 1 | 14 | 45 |
| | IU | 44 | 3 | 64 | 200 |
| Lipids | | | | | |
| Fatty acids""" | | | | | |
| Saturated (total) | g | .68 | .05 | .99 | 3.10 |
| 4:0 | g | .06 | Trace | .09 | .27 |
| 6:0 | g | .01 | Trace | .01 | .04 |
| 8:0 | g | .01 | Trace | .01 | .04 |
| 10:0 | g | .02 | Trace | .03 | .08 |
| 12:0 | g | .01 | Trace | .02 | .05 |
| 14:0 | g | .10 | .01 | .15 | .47 |
| 16:0 | g | .33 | .02 | .47 | 1.48 |
| 18:0 | g | .10 | .01 | .14 | .44 |
| Monounsaturated (total) | g | .30 | .02 | .43 | 1.35 |
| 16:1 | g | .03 | Trace | .05 | .15 |
| 18:1 | g | .25 | .02 | .36 | 1.14 |
| 20:1 | g | | | | |
| 22:1 | g | | | | |
| Polyunsaturated (total) | g | .03 | Trace | .05 | .15 |
| 18:2 | g | .02 | Trace | .04 | .11 |
| 18:3 | g | .01 | Trace | .01 | .04 |
| 18:4 | g | | | | |
| 20:4 | g | | | | |
| 20:5 | g | | | | |
| 22:5 | g | | | | |
| 22:6 | g | | | | |
| Cholesterol | mg | 6 | Trace | 9 | 27 |
| Phytosterols | mg | | | | |
| Amino Acids | | | | | |
| Tryptophan | g | .205 | .015 | .297 | .928 |
| Threonine | g | .817 | .061 | 1.184 | 3.705 |
| Isoleucine | g | .719 | .054 | 1.043 | 3.263 |
| Leucine | g | 1.186 | .088 | 1.719 | 5.378 |
| Lysine | g | 1.030 | .077 | 1.493 | 4.670 |
| Methionine | g | .241 | .018 | .350 | 1.094 |
| Cystine | g | .253 | .019 | .367 | 1.149 |
| Phenylalanine | g | .407 | .030 | .591 | 1.848 |
| Tyrosine | g | .363 | .027 | .526 | 1.646 |
| Valine | g | .697 | .052 | 1.011 | 3.162 |
| Arginine | g | .375 | .028 | .544 | 1.701 |

Table 1 (continued)
## NUTRIENT COMPOSITION OF MILK PRODUCTS AND BY-PRODUCTS

### Item 36: Whey (Sweet, Dry)

| Nutrients | Units | Amount in 100 g (edible portion) | Amount in edible portion of common measures of food | | Amount in edible portion of 1 lb of food as purchased (refuse: 0) |
|---|---|---|---|---|---|
| | | | 1 Tbsp = 7.5 g | 1 cup = 145 g | |
| Histidine | g | .237 | .018 | .344 | 1.076 |
| Alanine | g | .598 | .045 | .867 | 2.712 |
| Aspartic acid | g | 1.269 | .095 | 1.840 | 5.755 |
| Glutamic acid | g | 2.248 | .168 | 3.259 | 10.195 |
| Glycine | g | .280 | .021 | .406 | 1.269 |
| Proline | g | .786 | .059 | 1.140 | 3.567 |
| Serine | g | .622 | .046 | .902 | 2.822 |

### Item 37: Yogurt (Plain, Containing 8 g of Protein/8-oz Serving)[nn]

| Nutrients | Units | Amount in 100 g (edible portion) | Amount in edible portion of common measures of food (approximate measure and weight) | | Amount in edible portion of 1 lb of food as purchased (refuse:0) |
|---|---|---|---|---|---|
| | | | ½ container (net wt) 4 oz = 113 g | 1 container (net wt) 8 oz = 227 g | |
| **Proximate** | | | | | |
| Water | g | 87.90 | 99.68 | 199.53 | 398.71 |
| Food energy | kcal | 61 | 70 | 139 | 279 |
| | kJ | 257 | 291 | 583 | 1,166 |
| Protein (N × 6.38) | g | 3.47 | 3.94 | 7.88 | 15.74 |
| Total lipid (fat) | g | 3.25 | 3.68 | 7.38 | 14.75 |
| Carbohydrate (total) | g | 4.66 | 5.28 | 10.58 | 21.14 |
| Fiber | g | 0 | 0 | 0 | 0 |
| Ash | g | .72 | .82 | 1.63 | 3.27 |
| **Minerals** | | | | | |
| Calcium | mg | 121 | 137 | 274 | 547 |
| Iron | mg | .05 | .06 | .11 | .23 |
| Magnesium | mg | 12 | 13 | 26 | 53 |
| Phosphorus | mg | 95 | 108 | 215 | 430 |
| Potassium | mg | 155 | 175 | 351 | 701 |
| Sodium | mg | 46 | 53 | 105 | 210 |
| Zinc | mg | .59 | .67 | 1.34 | 2.68 |
| **Vitamins** | | | | | |
| Ascorbic acid | mg | .53 | .60 | 1.20 | 2.40 |
| Thiamin | mg | .029 | .033 | .066 | .132 |
| Riboflavin | mg | .142 | .161 | .322 | .644 |
| Niacin | mg | .075 | .085 | .170 | .340 |
| Pantothenic acid | mg | .389 | .441 | .883 | 1.765 |
| Vitamin $B_6$ | mg | .032 | .036 | .073 | .145 |
| Folacin | µg | 7 | 8 | 17 | 34 |
| Vitamin $B_{12}$ | µg | .372 | .422 | .844 | 1.687 |
| Vitamin A | RE | 30 | 34 | 68 | 136 |
| | IU | 123 | 139 | 279 | 558 |
| **Lipids** | | | | | |
| Fatty acids | | | | | |
| Saturated (total) | g | 2.10 | 2.38 | 4.76 | 9.51 |
| 4:0 | g | .10 | .11 | .22 | .44 |
| 6:0 | g | .07 | .08 | .15 | .30 |
| 8:0 | g | .04 | .05 | .10 | .19 |
| 10:0 | g | .09 | .10 | .21 | .42 |
| 12:0 | g | .11 | .13 | .25 | .50 |
| 14:0 | g | .34 | .39 | .78 | 1.55 |
| 16:0 | g | .89 | 1.00 | 2.01 | 4.02 |
| 18:0 | g | .32 | .36 | .72 | 1.44 |
| Monounsaturated (total) | g | .89 | 1.01 | 2.03 | 4.05 |
| 16:1 | g | .07 | .08 | .16 | .32 |
| 18:1 | g | .74 | .84 | 1.69 | 3.37 |
| 20:1 | g | | | | |
| 22:1 | g | | | | |

Table 1 (continued)
NUTRIENT COMPOSITION OF MILK PRODUCTS AND BY-PRODUCTS

Item 37: Yogurt (Plain, Containing 8 g of Protein/8-oz Serving)[nn]

| Nutrients | Units | Amount in 100 g (edible portion) | Amount in edible portion of common measures of food (approximate measure and weight) | | Amount in edible portion of 1 lb of food as purchased (refuse:0) |
|---|---|---|---|---|---|
| | | | ½ container (net wt) 4 oz = 113 g | 1 container (net wt) 8 oz = 227 g | |
| Polyunsaturated (total) | g | .09 | .10 | .21 | .42 |
| 18:2 | g | .06 | .07 | .15 | .30 |
| 18:3 | g | .03 | .03 | .06 | .12 |
| 18:4 | g | | | | |
| 20:4 | g | | | | |
| 20:5 | g | | | | |
| 22:5 | g | | | | |
| 22:6 | g | | | | |
| Cholesterol | mg | 13 | 14 | 29 | 58 |
| Phytosterols | mg | | | | |
| Amino acids | | | | | |
| Tryptophan | g | .020 | .022 | .044 | .089 |
| Threonine | g | .142 | .162 | .323 | .646 |
| Isoleucine | g | .189 | .215 | .430 | .859 |
| Leucine | g | .350 | .397 | .794 | 1.586 |
| Lysine | g | .311 | .353 | .706 | 1.411 |
| Methionine | g | .102 | .116 | .232 | .464 |
| Cystine | g | —[d] | — | — | — |
| Phenylaline | g | .189 | .215 | .430 | .859 |
| Tyrosine | g | .175 | .199 | .398 | .794 |
| Valine | g | .287 | .326 | .652 | 1.303 |
| Arginine | g | .104 | .118 | .237 | .474 |
| Histidine | g | .086 | .097 | .195 | .390 |
| Alanine | g | .148 | .168 | .337 | .674 |
| Aspartic acid | g | .275 | .312 | .625 | 1.248 |
| Glutamic acid | g | .679 | .770 | 1.542 | 3.081 |
| Glycine | g | .084 | .095 | .190 | .380 |
| Prline | g | .411 | .466 | .933 | 1.865 |
| Serine | g | .215 | .244 | .488 | .974 |

Item 38: Yogurt (Plain, Skim Milk, Containing 13g of Protein/8-oz Serving)[oo]

| Nutrients | Units | Amount in 100 g (edible portion) (Mean ± SE) | Amount in edible portion of common measures of food (approximate measure and weight) | | Amount in edible portion of 1 lb of food as purchased (refuse:0) |
|---|---|---|---|---|---|
| | | | ½ container (net wt) 4 oz = 113 g | 1 container (net wt) 8 oz = 227 g | |
| Proximate | | | | | |
| Water | g | 85.23 | 96.65 | 193.47 | 386.60 |
| Food energy | kcal | 56 | 63 | 127 | 253 |
| | kJ | 233 | 265 | 530 | 1,059 |
| Protein (N × 6.38) | g | 5.73 | 6.50 | 13.01 | 25.99 |
| Total lipid (fat) | g | 0.18 | .20 | .41 | .82 |
| Carbohydrate (total) | g | 7.68 | 8.71 | 17.43 | 34.84 |
| Fiber | g | 0 | 0 | 0 | 0 |
| Ash | g | 1.18 | 1.34 | 2.68 | 5.35 |
| Minerals | | | | | |
| Calcium | mg | 199 | 226 | 452 | 903 |
| Iron | mg | .09 | .10 | .20 | .41 |
| Magnesium | mg | 19 | 22 | 43 | 87 |
| Phosphorus | mg | 156 | 177 | 355 | 710 |
| Potassium | mg | 255 | 289 | 579 | 1,156 |
| Sodium | mg | 76 | 87 | 174 | 347 |
| Zinc | mg | .97 | 1.10 | 2.20 | 4.40 |
| Vitamins | | | | | |
| Ascorbic acid | mg | .87 | .99 | 1.98 | 3.95 |
| Thiamin | mg | .048 | .054 | .109 | .218 |
| Ribovlavin | mg | .234 | .265 | .531 | 1.061 |

Table 1 (continued)
## NUTRIENT COMPOSITION OF MILK PRODUCTS AND BY-PRODUCTS

Item 38: Yogurt (Plain, Skim Milk, Containing 13g of Protein/8-oz Serving)[oo]

| Nutrients | Units | Amount in 100 g (edible portion) (Mean ± SE) | ½ container (net wt) 4 oz = 113 g | 1 container (net wt) 8 oz = 227 g | Amount in edible portion of 1 lb of food as purchased (refuse:0) |
|---|---|---|---|---|---|
| Niacin | mg | .124 | .141 | .281 | .562 |
| Pantothenic acid | mg | .641 | .727 | 1.455 | 2.908 |
| Vitamin B$_6$ | mg | .053 | .060 | .120 | .240 |
| Folacin | μg | 12 | 14 | 28 | 55 |
| Vitamin B$_{12}$ | μg | .613 | .695 | 1.392 | 2.781 |
| Vitamin A | RE | 2 | 2 | 5 | 9 |
| | IU | 7 | 8 | 16 | 32 |
| Lipids | | | | | |
| Fatty acids[pp] | | | | | |
| Saturated (total) | g | .116 | .132 | .264 | .527 |
| 4:0 | g | .005 | .006 | .012 | .024 |
| 6:0 | g | .005 | .004 | .008 | .017 |
| 8:0 | g | .002 | .003 | .005 | .010 |
| 10:0 | g | .005 | .006 | .012 | .023 |
| 12:0 | g | .006 | .007 | .014 | .028 |
| 14:0 | g | .019 | .022 | .043 | .086 |
| 16:0 | g | .049 | .056 | .111 | .223 |
| 18:0 | g | .018 | .020 | .040 | .080 |
| Monounsaturated (total) | g | .049 | .056 | .012 | .0224 |
| 16:1 | g | .004 | .004 | .009 | .018 |
| 18:1 | g | .041 | .047 | .093 | .187 |
| 20:1 | g | | | | |
| 22:1 | g | | | | |
| Polyunsaturated (total) | g | .005 | .006 | .012 | .023 |
| 18:2 | g | .004 | .004 | .008 | .016 |
| 18:3 | g | .001 | .002 | .003 | .007 |
| 18:4 | g | | | | |
| 20:4 | g | | | | |
| 20:5 | g | | | | |
| 22:5 | g | | | | |
| 22:6 | g | | | | |
| Cholesterol | mg | 2 | 2 | 4 | 8 |
| Phytosterols | mg | | | | |
| Amino Acids | | | | | |
| Tryptophan | g | .032 | .037 | .073 | .147 |
| Threonine | g | .235 | .267 | .534 | 1.067 |
| Isoleucine | g | .313 | .354 | .709 | 1.418 |
| Leucine | g | .577 | .655 | 1.311 | 2.619 |
| Lysine | g | .514 | .583 | 1.166 | 2.330 |
| Methionine | g | .169 | .191 | .383 | .766 |
| Cystine | g | —[d] | — | — | — |
| Phenylalanine | g | .313 | .354 | .709 | 1.418 |
| Tyrosine | g | .289 | .328 | .656 | 1.312 |
| Valine | g | .474 | .538 | 1.076 | 2.151 |
| Arginine | g | .172 | .196 | .391 | .782 |
| Histidine | g | .142 | .161 | .322 | .644 |
| Alanine | g | .245 | .278 | .557 | 1.112 |
| Aspartic acid | g | .454 | .515 | 1.032 | 2.061 |
| Glutamic acid | g | 1.122 | 1.272 | 2.546 | 5.088 |
| Glycine | g | .138 | .157 | .314 | .627 |
| Proline | g | .679 | .770 | 1.541 | 3.080 |
| Serine | g | .355 | .402 | .805 | 1.609 |

[a]  Nutritive values apply to salted butter. Unsalted butter contains 11 mg of sodium per 100 g.
[b]  Weight applies to pat, which is 1 in.² and 1/3 in. high (90 pats = 1 lb).
[c]  One stick is approximately ½ cup.
[d]  Dashes denote lack of reliable data for a constituent believed to be present in measurable amount.
[e]  Values for vitamin A represent year-round average.
[f]  Values based on data for fat extracted from whole milk.
[g]  Based on specific gravity, 1 in.³ of cheese weighs 17.3 g.

Table 1 (continued)

**NUTRIENT COMPOSITION OF MILK PRODUCTS AND BY-PRODUCTS**

ʰ   Based on specific gravity, 1 in.³ of cheese weighs 17.1 g.

ⁱ   Based on specific gravity, 1 in.³ of cheese weighs 17.2 g.

ʲ   Weight applies to small curd. An unpacked cup of large-curd cottage cheese weighs 225 g.

ᵏ   Values are for unsalted product.

ˡ   Values based on data for fat extracted from cottage cheese containing 4.5% fat.

ᵐ   Based on specific gravity, 1 in.³ of cheese weighs 16.1 g.

ⁿ   Values were obtained by combining data for hard and grated samples on a moisture-free basis and recalculating results to a moisture content of 17.66%. Nutritive values shown do not apply to hard and shredded forms. Hard product contains approximately 29% water, and shredded product contains approximately 25% water.

ᵒ   Based on specific gravity.

ᵖ   Based on specific gravity, 1 in.³ of cheese weighs 17.5 g.

q   Product is made by combining fats or oils other than milk fat with milk solids, which may be milk, cream, or skim milk. The resulting product resembles milk. Vegetable oils include soybean, cottonseed, and/or safflower. Product may contain added vitamin D; refer to label for content.

ʳ   Values based on data for products without added vitamin A. Product may contain added vitamin A; refer to label for content.

ˢ   Product is made by combining fats or oils other than milk fat with milk solids, which may be milk, cream, or skim milk. The resulting product resembles milk. Lauric oils include modified coconut oil, hydrogenated coconut oil, and/or palm kernel oil. Products may contain added vitamin D; refer to label for content.

ᵗ   Values based on data for products containing lauric acid oil and sodium caseinate as ingredients. Lauric oils include modified coconut oil, hydrogenated coconut oil, and/or palm kernel oil.

ᵘ   Values based on data for products containing added riboflavin used for coloring. Product may not contain added riboflavin.

ᵛ   Contributed largely from β-carotene used for coloring.

ʷ   Values apply to pasteurized and raw products.

ˣ   If vitamin D is added, each quart contains 400 IU.

ʸ   Values based on all-market average. Minimum standards for fat vary in different states. Selection of values to be used in dietary calculations may need to be based on information at local level.

ᶻ   Values based on data for butter.

ᵃᵃ   Values based on addition of vitamin A to level of 2000 IU/qt.

ᵇᵇ   Product contains not less than 10% milk-derived nonfat solids. Values apply to products containing concentrated skim milk or nonfat dry milk as the added milk-derived ingredient(s).

ᶜᶜ   Includes data for samples to which solids were added but which were not protein fortified.

ᵈᵈ   Values based on data for fat extracted from skim milk.

ᵉᵉ   Values are for salted product. Unsalted product contains approximately 50 mg of sodium per 100 g.

ᶠᶠ   If vitamin D is added, each quart of milk, reconstituted according to label directions, contains 400 IU.

ᵍᵍ   Values based on data for products without added vitamin A. If vitamin A is added, each quart of milk, reconstituted according to label directions, contains 2000 IU.

ʰʰ   Values based on data for fat extracted from instantized product.

ⁱⁱ   If vitamin D is added, product contains 25 IU/fl oz.

ʲʲ   Values based on addition of vitamin A to level of 125 IU/fl oz. Product without added vitamin A contains 8 IU/100 g.

ᵏᵏ   Values based on data for fat extracted from evaporated whole milk.

ˡˡ   Values based on data for fat extracted from fluid acid whey.

ᵐᵐ   Values based on data for fat extracted from fluid sweet whey.

ⁿⁿ   Product is made with whole milk.

ᵒᵒ   Product is made with skim milk and contains added nonfat milk solids.

ᵖᵖ   Values based on data for fat extracted from plain yogurt made with whole milk.

From Posati, P. L. and Orr, M. L., Composition of Foods, Dairy and Egg Products, Agric. Handb. No. 8-1, Agricultural Research Service, U.S. Department of Agriculture, U.S. Government Printing Office, Washington, D.C., 1976.

Table 2

MAJOR REVIEW ARTICLES DEALING WITH THE RATIONALE OF DAIRY PRODUCT SUPPLEMENTATION IN GENERAL AND IN VARIOUS FOOD SYSTEMS

| Dairy supplementation directed to | Authors discussing rationale of supplementation in terms of | | | |
| --- | --- | --- | --- | --- |
| | Nutrition | Food technology | Organoleptic properties | Economics and statistics |
| General applications | Alyward, 1970[7] <br> Barnes, 1971[30] <br> Forsum, 1975[78] <br> Graham, 1974[87] <br> Guérin, 1974[89] <br> National Dairy Council 1965[184,185] <br> Phillips nd Briggs, 1975[204] <br> Porter, 1975[211] <br> Shukla, 1975[234] | Buchanan, 1970[39] <br> Buchanan, 1971[40] <br> Dairy Research Inc., 1972[54] <br> Davies, 1976[56] <br> Dennis, 1971[58] <br> Jonas, 1973[121] <br> Rocamora Ruiz, 1974[219] <br> Rothwell, 1974[224] <br> Schulz, 1969[230] <br> Shukla, 1975[234] | Eriksen and Fagerson, 1976[69a] <br> Nickerson, 1976[190] <br> Strokel et al., 1953[248] | Anonymous, 1974[18] <br> FAO, 1974[72] <br> FAO, 1975[73] <br> Hammonds and Call, 1970 and 1972[97,98] <br> Kinsella, 1972[129] <br> Singh, 1971[235] <br> Winkelmann, 1974[280] |
| Baby foods and clinical nutrition | Atkinson et al., 1957[27] <br> Corden, 1974[49] <br> Cuthberson, 1974[53] <br> Duncan, 1955[60] <br> Forsum, 1974[77] <br> Neumann and Jelliffe, 1977[189] | Cuthberson, 1974[53] <br> Forsum, 1974[77] <br> Henderson and Buchanan, 1973[104] <br> Wadsworth, 1974[262] | Corden, 1974[49] | Anonymous, 1976[20] <br> Neuman and Jelliffe, 1977[189] |
| Beverages | — | Holsinger et al., 1974[109] <br> Kosikowsky, 1968[139] <br> Pallansch, 1974[197] <br> Paul, 1975[199] | Mason and Katz, 1976[164] <br> Rodier et al., 1974[220] | — |
| Cereals, Baked and pasta products | Henry and Kon, 1946[105] <br> Hulse, 1974[110] <br> Webb, 1963[267] | Craig and Colmey, 1971[51] <br> Dürr and Neukom, 1972[61] | Jack and Haynes, 1951[115] | Hammonds and Call, 1972[98] |

Table 2 (continued)
## MAJOR REVIEW ARTICLES DEALING WITH THE RATIONALE OF DAIRY PRODUCT SUPPLEMENTATION IN GENERAL AND IN VARIOUS FOOD SYSTEMS

| Dairy supplementation directed to | Authors discussing rationale of supplementation in terms of | | | |
|---|---|---|---|---|
| | Nutrition | Food technology | Organoleptic properties | Economics and statistics |
| | | Hulse, 1974[110]; Kinsella, 1971[128]; Singleton and Robertson, 1966[237] | | |
| Dessert and candy products | Campbell, 1976[41] | Anonymous, 1967[10]; Frazeur, 1967[82]; Kinsella, 1970[127]; Mann, 1970[154]; Mann, 1971[157]; Steinitz, 1970[244] | Nickerson, 1976[190] | Anonymous, 1976[19]; Hammonds and Call, 1972[98] |
| Fatty products | Brink and Kritchevsky, 1968[36]; Harrap, 1973[100]; Kaunitz, 1975[124]; Kieseker, 1975[126] | Asbjörn, 1970[23,24]; Graeve, 1974[86]; Mann, 1968[151]; Smith, 1973[240]; Spurgeon, 1973[243] | Ericksen, 1976[69]; Forss, 1971[76]; Kinsella, 1975[130]; Mason and Katz, 1976[164]; Walker, 1973[265] | Asbjörn, 1970[23,24]; Smith, 1973[240] |
| Food aid items and foods for developing countries | Bender, 1971[31]; Mauron, 1972[167]; Weisberg, 1976[273] | Bookwalter et al., 1971[37]; Chapmann, 1968[44]; Weisberg, 1976[273,274] | Alyward, 1974[8]; Rodier et al., 1974[220] | Barnes, 1971[30]; Strange and Singh, 1971[247]; Weisberg, 1976[274] |
| Meat products | — | Brendl and Klein, 1972[35]; Saffle, 1968[225]; Schut, 1970[232] | — | Saffle, 1968[225]; Hammonds and Call, 1972[98] |
| Whipables and emulsion products | — | Kinsella, 1976[131]; Knightly, 1968[135]; Petrowski, 1976[200] | Walker, 1972[264] | Kinsella, 1976[131] |

*Note:* The author's names and dates listed refer to literature references in this chapter.

Table 3
MILK PROTEINS FOR FOOD SUPPLEMENTS

Milk protein isolates
  Isoelectric caseins
  Whey proteins (lactalbumin and lactoglobulins)
  Coprecipitated milk proteins
  Modified milk proteins
    Caseinate salts
    Lactalbumin phosphates
    Microbiologically or enzymatically modified proteins:
      Cottage cheese, cheese powders
      Quark
      Rennet-treated milks or proteins
    Proteins from membrane gel filtration processes
    Milk protein hydrolysates
Milk protein concentrates (dairy powders)
  Skim milk powder
  Whole milk powder
  Buttermilk powder
  Whey powder
  Cheese powder

Table 4
U.S. CONSUMPTION OF FOOD GRADE CASEIN AND WHEY
PRODUCTS (1,000 LB)[123,257,258]

|  | Casein | | Whey | |
| --- | --- | --- | --- | --- |
| Year | Total | Protein contribution | Total | Protein contribution |
| 1969 | 116,107 | 107,980 | — | — |
| 1970 | 135,288 | 126,423 | 292,952 | 35,154 |
| 1971 | 105,939 | 98,523 | 319,383 | 38,326 |
| 1972 | 105,401 | 98,023 | 376,652 | 45,198 |
| 1973 | 112,828 | 104,930 | 501,231 | 60,148 |
| 1974 | 113,328 | 105,395 | 568,611 | 68,233 |

Table 5
THE SUPPLEMENTARY VALUE OF MILK PROTEIN IN EXPERIMENTS
WITH RATS

|  | Biological value[a] |
| --- | --- |
| White bread alone | 52 |
| Cheese alone | 76 |
| Mixture — 50% of the protein from bread, 50% cheese | 75 |
| When the two sources of protein were given on alternate days | 67 |
| Potato | 71 |
| Dried skim milk | 89 |
| Mixture — 50% of the protein from potato, 50% from dried milk | 86 |
| When the two sources were given on different days | 81 |

[a]   Biological value is computed as the percentage of protein actually utilized in the body from that contained in the foodstuff.

From Henry, M. and Kon, S. K., *J. Dairy Res.*, 14, 330, 1946. With permission.

Table 6
EFFECT OF WHEY
PROTEIN
SUPPLEMENTATION ON
SOY PROTEIN VALUE[148]

| Source of protein | PER[a] |
|---|---|
| Whey protein | 3.4 |
| Isolated soy protein | 1.4 |
| Whey Protein | |
| Soy isolate (1:9) | 2.0 |
| Soy isolate (1:3) | 2.7 |
| Soy isolate (1:1) | 2.9 |
| Casein | 2.5 |

[a]  PER: protein efficiency ratio; grams gain per gram protein consumed.

Table 7
ESSENTIAL AMINO ACID CONTENT OF MACARONI
(12.7% PROTEIN) VS. FAO REFERENCE PROTEIN

| Essential amino acid | FAO reference protein (g/100 g) | FAO ideal essential amino acid ratios | Amino acid content of macaroni (g/100 g) | Macaroni essential amino acid ratios | FAO ideal essential amino acids in macaroni (g/100 g) |
|---|---|---|---|---|---|
| Isoleucine | 4.2 | 3.0 | 0.551 | 3.5 | 0.348 |
| Leucine | 4.8 | 3.4 | 0.852 | 5.4 | 0.394 |
| Lysine | 4.2 | 3.0 | 0.348 | 2.2 | 0.348 |
| Methionine + cystine | 4.2 | 3.0 | 0.473 | 3.0 | 0.348 |
| Phenylalanine + tyrosine | 5.6 | 4.0 | 0.936 | 6.0 | 0.464 |
| Threonine | 2.8 | 2.0 | 0.366 | 2.3 | 0.232 |
| Tryptophan | 1.4 | 1.0 | 0.157 | 1.0 | 0.116 |
| Valine | 4.2 | 3.0 | 0.588 | 3.7 | 0.348 |
| Total | | | | | 2.598 g |

Reprinted with permission from *J. Food Sci.,* 41, 1297-1300, 1976. Copyright© by Institute of Food Technologists, Chicago, Ill.

Table 8

INCREASE IN ESSENTIAL AMINO ACID CONTENT OF MACARONI AFTER
ENRICHMENT TO 21.6% PROTEIN

| Essential amino acid | Amino acid content of 100 g heat co-agulated whey protein | Amino acid content of 500 g durum | Content of 600 g amino acid en-riched pasta | Enriched macaroni essential amino acid ratios | FAO ideal es-sential amino acids in en-riched pasta (g/100 g) |
|---|---|---|---|---|---|
| Isoleucine | 5.92 | 1.740 | 7.66 | 3.0 | 1.062 |
| Leucine | 12.90 | 2.030 | 14.93 | 5.8 | 1.203 |
| Lysine | 9.71 | 1.740 | 11.45 | 4.4 | 1.062 |
| Methionine + cystine | 4.63 | 1.740 | 6.37 | 2.5 | 1.062 |
| Phenylalaine + tyrosine | 8.21 | 1.160 | 9.37 | 3.6 | 1.415 |
| Threonine | 4.75 | 1.160 | 5.91 | 2.3 | 0.708 |
| Tryptophan | 2.01 | 0.580 | 2.59 | 1.0 | 0.353 |
| Valine | 5.70 | 1.740 | 7.44 | 2.9 | 1.062 |
| Total | | | | | 7.927 g |

Reprinted with permission from *J. Food Sci.,* 41, 1297-1300, 1976. Copyright© by Institute of Food Technologists, Chicago, Ill.

Table 9

PER OF WHEY PROTEIN FRACTIONS AND MACARONI
PRODUCTS

| Dietary source of protein | Approx. protein content (%) | PER corrected test |
|---|---|---|
| ANRC casein | — | 2.50 |
| Common macaroni | 13 | 0.70 |
| Whey protein | 66 | 3.05 |
| Macaroni enriched with whey protein | 20 | 2.41 |

Reprinted with permission from *J. Food Sci.,* 41, 1297-1300, 1976. Copyright© by Institute of Food Technologists, Chicago, Ill.

## Table 11
## AMINO ACID COMPOSITION OF GEL-FILTERED AND ULTRAFILTERED WHEY PROTEIN CONCENTRATE (MG AMINO ACID/G TOTAL NITROGEN)

| Amino acid | Whey protein concentrate | |
| --- | --- | --- |
| | Ultrafiltered | Gel-filtered |
| Isoleucine | 461 | 474 |
| Leucine | 708 | 709 |
| Lysine | 617 | 630 |
| Methionine | 147 | 124 |
| Cysteine | 166 | 169 |
| Phenylalanine | 213 | 218 |
| Tyrosine | 201 | 210 |
| Threonine | 516 | 512 |
| Tryptophan | 160 | 147 |
| Valine | 423 | 435 |
| Arginine | 171 | 172 |
| Histidine | 122 | 131 |
| Alanine | 336 | 335 |
| Aspartic acid | 741 | 743 |
| Glutamic acid | 1217 | 1206 |
| Glycine | 124 | 126 |
| Proline | 441 | 451 |
| Serine | 391 | 381 |

From Forsum, E., Hambraevs, L., and Siddiqi, I. H., *J. Dairy Sci.*, 57(6), 659, 1974. With permission.

## Table 10
## NUTRITIVE VALUE OF SOME PROTEIN-RICH WEANING FOODS, WHEN ANIMAL PROTEIN IS SUPPLIED BY DRIED SKIM MILK (DSM) OR WHEY PROTEIN CONCENTRATE (WPC)

| Diet | PER | NPU |
| --- | --- | --- |
| Corn soy milk with | | |
| DSM | — | 71 |
| WPC | — | 83 |
| Faffa® with | 2.8 | 59 |
| DSM | | |
| WPC | 3.0 | 63 |
| Superamine® with | 2.3 | 59 |
| DSM | | |
| WPC | 3.3 | 67 |
| Reference casein | 3.2 | 61 |

From Forsum, E., in *Protein Nutritional Quality of Foods and Feeds*, Vol. 1, Part 2, Friedman, M., Ed., Marcel Dekker, New York, 1975, 463. With permission.

**Table 12**
## RELATIVE NUTRITIVE VALUE AND UTILIZABLE PROTEIN IN PROTEIN SOURCES

| | Protein content (%) | Relative nutritive value (%) | Utilizable[a] protein (%) | FAO amino acid pattern (%) | Milk protein (%) | Egg protein (%) | NPU (%) |
|---|---|---|---|---|---|---|---|
| Lactalbumin | 77.60 | 100 | 77.6 | — | — | — | — |
| Casein | 86.30 | 75 | 64.6 | 80 | 75 | 60 | 72 |
| Fish protein concentrate | 81.10 | 77 | 62.5 | 70 | 70 | 75 | 83 |
| Soya flour (heated) | 51.90 | 60 | 31.1 | 70 | 85 | 70 | 56 |
| Full-fat soya | 39.40 | 58 | 22.9 | | | | |
| Wheat gluten | 71.00 | 24 | 17.0 | 40 | 40 | 40 | 37 |
| Peanut flour | 48.40 | 54 | 26.1 | 60 | 80 | 70 | 48 |
| Rice flour (high protein) | 19.10 | 44 | 8.4 | 70 | 75 | 75 | 57 |
| White flour | 13.75 | 28 | 3.8 | 50 | 50 | 50 | 52 |
| Rice | 8.30 | 50 | 4.2 | 70 | 75 | 75 | 57 |
| Corn meal | 7.95 | 37 | 3.0 | 40 | 40 | 45 | 55 |

[a]    RNV × % protein.

From Hegsted, D. M., in *Protein Enriched Cereal Foods for World Needs,* Millner, M., Ed., American Association of Cereal Chemists, St. Paul, Minn., 1969, 41. With permission.

Table 13
ANRC[a] CASEIN

Typical Analysis (As Is)

| | |
|---|---|
| Moisture (%) | 6.8 |
| Ash (phosphorus-fixed) (%) | 2.07 |
| Acidity (as lactic) (%) | 0.16 |
| Protein (N × 6.38) (%) | 89.8 |
| pH (10% suspension) | 4.85 |
| Color, odor, appearance | Normal |
| Heavy metals (as Pb) | <20 ppm |

Approximate Vitamin Content($\mu$g/g)

| | |
|---|---|
| Biotin | 0.02 |
| Folic acid | 0.15 |
| Niacin | 0.05 |
| Pantothenic acid | 0.42 |
| Pyridoxine | 0.76 |
| Riboflavin | 7.53 |
| Thiamine | 0.25 |

Amino Acid Content (As Is) (%)

| | | | |
|---|---|---|---|
| Alanine | 2.6 | Lysine | 7.3 |
| Arginine | 3.6 | Methionine | 2.5 |
| Aspartic acid | 6.3 | Phenylalanine | 4.4 |
| Cystine | 0.3 | Proline | 10.1 |
| Glycine | 2.4 | Serine | 5.6 |
| Glutamic acid | 20.0 | Threonine | 4.3 |
| Histidine | 2.7 | Tryptophan | 1.1 |
| Isoleucine | 5.4 | Tyrosine | 5.6 |
| Leucine | 8.2 | Valine | 6.4 |

Mineral Content

| | | | |
|---|---|---|---|
| Manganese | 0.05% | Sodium | 35 ppm |
| Magnesium | <0.1 ppm | Potassium | 99 ppm |
| Iron | 17 ppm | Cobalt | <0.1 ppm |
| Copper | 19.2 ppm | Total phosphorous | 0.81% |
| Zinc | 12.1 ppm | Calcium | 0.06% |
| Mercury | <0.1 ppm | Chloride | 0.57% |

[a]    ANRC; Animal Nutrition Research Council.

From Sheffield-Humko Division, Kraft Inc., A.N.R.C. Reference Protein (brochure), Norwich, N.Y., 1960. With permission.

## Table 14
## MAJOR COMPONENTS IN VARIOUS DRIED DAIRY POWDERS

|  | Whole milk powder | Skim milk powder | Buttermilk powder | Whey powder |
|---|---|---|---|---|
| Carbohydrates (lactose) (%) | 38 | 52 | 50 | 72 |
| Proteins (%) | 26 | 36 | 34 | 13 |
| Lipids (%) | 27 | 1 | 5 | 2 |
| Ash Constituents (%) | 6 | 8 | 7 | 8 |
| Energy (cal) | 500 | 360 | 390 | 350 |

## Table 15
## PERCENTAGE OF NONFAT DRY MILK USED IN FOODS

| Food category and product | Range of amount of nonfat dry milk used |
|---|---|
| Confections | |
| Caramels | 5—9 |
| Fudge | 3—5.5 |
| Chocolate | 5—18 |
| Nougats | 3—5 |
| Meat products | |
| Frankfurts | 1—3.9 |
| Loaves | 1—3.9 |
| Bologna | 1—3.9 |
| Salami | 1—3 |
| Liver sausage | 1—3 |
| Minced ham | 1—3 |
| Bakery products and mixes | |
| Bread | 2—8 |
| Cake | 1—20 |
| Yeast doughnuts | 1—5 |
| Cake doughnuts | 1—5 |
| Refrigerator doughnuts | 1.5—3 |
| Rolls | 1—6 |
| Muffins | 1—5 |
| Cracker mix | 0.9 |
| Frozen baked goods | 5—7 |
| Dairy products | |
| Ice cream | 8—11 |
| Ice milk | 11—14 |
| Sherbet | 2.5 |
| Skim milk | 1—2 |
| Cottage cheese | 3—16 |
| Buttermilk | 1—8.5 |
| Chocolate drink | 6 |
| Half-and-half cream | 2 |

From Miller, E. B., Cooperative Marketing of Nonfat Dry Milk to Commercial Outlets, USDA Rep. 129, U.S. Department of Agriculture, Washington, D.C., 1965.

Table 16
## U.S. CHEESE AND WHEY PRODUCTION IN MILLIONS OF POUNDS[171,259]

| Years | Cheese | Sweet whey[a] | Cottage cheese | Acid whey[b] |
|-------|--------|---------------|----------------|--------------|
| 1966 | 1,918 | 15,344 | 861 | 4,305 |
| 1967 | 1,973 | 15,784 | 868 | 4,340 |
| 1968 | 2,002 | 16,016 | 901 | 4,505 |
| 1969 | 2,134 | 17,072 | 955 | 4,775 |
| 1970 | 2,281 | 18,248 | 1,039 | 5,195 |
| 1971 | 2,404 | 19,232 | 1,089 | 5,445 |
| 1972 | 2,664 | 21,312 | 1,115 | 5,575 |
| 1973 | 2,853 | 22,824 | 1,099 | 5,495 |
| 1974 | 2,981 | 23,848 | 978 | 4,890 |
| 1975 | 2,811 | 22,488 | 991 | 4,955 |
| 1976 | 3,326 | 26,408 | 1,020 | 5,100 |

[a]  Based on 8 lb of whey produced per pound of cheese.
[b]  Based on 5 lb of whey produced per pound of cottage cheese.

Table 17.
## DAIRY FATS FOR FOODS

| | |
|---|---|
| Commercial forms | Butter |
| | Butter oil |
| | Anhydrous milk fat and ghee |
| Potential new dairy fat varieties | Fractionated butter fat |
| | Cultured emulsified dairy and vegetable fat blends |
| | Spray-dried butter |
| | High heat-treated butter |
| | Polyunsaturated fat containing milk produced by the cow |

Table 18
## DAIRY CARBOHYDRATES AND DERIVATIVES FOR FOODS

Lactose
Hydrolyzed lactose
Lactulose and naturally occurring oligosaccharides of milk[a]
Lactobionic acid, lactic acid, and salts[b]
Whey as source of lactose

[a]  Among the minor carbohydrates of milk, several oligosaccharides of physiological importance have been found. These have not yet been explored as to their commercial utility, however. The subject of the various oligosaccharides and lactulose in milk products has been reviewed by Adachi and Patton (Reference 3).
[b]  Lactobionic acid is obtained from lactose by chemical or biological oxidation. Lactic acid and salts are produced from lactose or whey by fermentation. These products find limited use in the food and pharmaceutical industries.

## Table 19
### EFFECT OF CONCENTRATION ON RELATIVE SWEETNESS OF SUGARS (PERCENT CONCENTRATION TO GIVE EQUIVALENT SWEETNESS)

| Sucrose | Glucose | Fructose | Lactose | Lactose: sucrose |
|---------|---------|----------|---------|------------------|
| 0.5 | 0.9 | 0.4 | 1.9 | 4 |
| 1.0 | 1.8 | 0.8 | 3.5 | 3.5 |
| 2.0 | 3.6 | 1.7 | 6.5 | <3.5 |
| 2.0 | 3.8 | — | 6.5 | — |
| 2.0 | 3.2 | — | 6.0 | 3 |
| 5.0 | 8.3 | 4.2 | 15.7 | — |
| 5.0 | 8.3 | 4.6 | 14.9 | <3 |
| 5.0 | 7.2 | 4.5 | 13.1 | — |
| 10.0 | 13.9 | 8.6 | 25.9 | 2.5 |
| 10.0 | 14.6 | — | — | — |
| 10.0 | 12.7 | 8.7 | 20.7 | — |
| 15.0 | 17.2 | 12.8 | 27.8 | — |
| 15.0 | 20.0 | 13.0 | 34.6 | 2 |
| 20.0 | 21.8 | 16.7 | 33.3 | <2 |

From Nickerson, T. A., *J. Dairy Sci.,* 59, 582, 1976. With permission.

## Table 20
### EXAMPLES OF THE UTILIZATION OF WHEY IN FOODS

| Food | Quantity of whey solids (%) | Outstanding contributions of whey components besides low cost and good nutrition |
|------|------------------------------|----------------------------------------------------------------------------------|
| Baked goods/sweet goods, bread, crackers (percent of flour weight) | 3.0 | Flavor, texture, shorter dough time, improved keeping quality |
| Dry mixes | 10.0 | Tenderizing, color, flavor |
| Dry whey flow agent to absorb oils | 93.0 | Carrier for fats, oils |
| Ice cream | 2.7 | Flavor, acid and fruit stability |
| Sherbet | 4.0 | |
| Confections | 10.0 ⎫ | Flavor, body, moisture retention, whipping properties |
| Icings, frostings | 6.0 ⎬ | |
| Jams, apple butter | 4.0 ⎭ | |
| Water ice on a stick | 2.6 | Furnish Ca, P, lactic acid, retard tooth erosion |
| Batter mix (for frying) | 5.0 | Color, flavor |
| Whey-soy beverage, citrus flavor | 6.0 | Lactose acid (from cottage cheese whey), flavor |
| Whey-soy beverage, sterilized (35% total solids) | 16.5 | Flavor, body |
| Whey 2/3, soy 1/3, dried | 66.0 | Masks soy flavor |
| Whey-soy blends for food manufacture (use fat-free soy flour) | 40.0 | Masks soy flavor, high protein |

From Webb, B. H., in Proc. Whey Utilization Conf., ARS-73-69, Agricultural Research Service, U.S. Department of Agriculture, Washington, D.C., 1970, 102.

Table 21
SHARE OF SIGNIFICANT
MILK MINERALS AND
VITAMINS SUPPLIED TO
THE U.S. DIET BY DAIRY
PRODUCTS (EXCLUDING
BUTTER), 1975

| | |
|---|---|
| Calcium | 75.5% |
| Phosphorus | 34.7% |
| Magnesium | 21.1% |
| Riboflavin | 39.8% |
| Vitamin $B_{12}$ | 19.8% |
| Vitamin A value | 12.7% |
| Vitamin $B_6$ | 10.2% |
| Thiamine | 9.0% |

From Friend, B. and Marston, R., Nutrition Review, National Food Situation NFS-154, Economics Research Service, U.S. Department of Agriculture, Washington, D.C., 1975, 28.

Table 22
SOME CULTURED DAIRY FOODS

| Name of cultured product | Origin and use area | How consumed | Developmental stage |
|---|---|---|---|
| Sour milk curd | Eastern Europe, U.S.S.R. | As curd with potatoes and black bread | Homemade from unboiled milk; recently industrially made |
| Long milk (langmjölk, etc.) | Scandinavian countries | A beverage with bread | Home industry; at 10°C, storage life up to 10 months |
| Yogurt, (tarho, laban, dahi, etc.) | Southeast Europe, Middle East, Caucasus, Iran; origin: Bulgaria | In cooking with wheat flour and vegetables | About 30—40 varieties made in home industry; long-storage life in curd form or sun dried |
| Cultured yogurt (industrially made) | Industrial variety of *Lactobacillus bulgarious* and *Streptococcus thermophilus* fermentation | As spoonable curd with fruits | Modern mass production |
| Kefir | France, Caucasus | Beverage with alcohol content | Home industry based on lactic and yeast fermentation |
| Kumiss | U.S.S.R. (Western Siberia), Mare's milk | Beverage with 3% alcohol | Industrially developed and adjusted to bovine milk with sugar addition |
| Buttermilk (Europe) | Benelux, Denmark, France | Beverage, by-product from butter churning; consumed with bread and used in cooking vegetables | Industrially developed product |
| Cultured buttermilk (U.S.) | Industrial variety of *St. lactis* fermentation | Beverage of refreshing quality based on skim milk; losing popularity | Industrially produced from skim milk |

## Table 22 (continued)
## SOME CULTURED DAIRY FOODS

| Name of cultured product | Origin and use area | How consumed | Developmental stage |
|---|---|---|---|
| Acidophilus milk in U.S., yakult in Japan | *L. acidophilus* cultured milk, of sweet milk stored cold with viable *L. acidophilus* culture in U.S , Japan uses *L. casei* | Beverage used as milk; clinical value to reestablish gut microflora | Industrially produced; contains antibiotics acidophilin, lactolidin, lactolin, acidolin |

## REFERENCES

1. **Abrahamsson, L., Forsum, E., and Hambraeus, L.,** Nutritional evaluation of emergency food mixtures based on wheat supplemented by different protein concentrates, *Nutr. Rep. Int.,* 9, 169, 1974.
2. **Abrahamsson, L., Hambraeus, L., and Vahlquist, B.,** Swedish emergency food (SEF): an ongoing applied nutrition research program, *PAG Bull.,* 4(4), 26—30, 1974.
3. **Adachi, S. and Patton, S.,** Presence and significance of lactulose in milk products: review, *J. Dairy Sci.,* 44, 1375—1393, 1961.
4. **Alais, C. and Blanc, B.,** Milk protein: biochemical and biological aspects, *World Rev. Nutr. Diet.,* 20, 66—167, 1975.
5. **Albanese, A. A., Edelson, A. H., and Lorenza, E. J., Jr.,** Problems of bone health in the elderly, *N.Y. State J. Med.,* 75, 326—336, 1975.
6. **Ali, R., and Evans, J. L.,** Lactose and calcium metabolism: a review, *J. Agric. Univ. P.R.,* 57, 149, 1973.
7. **Alyward, F.,** The contribution of dairy science to the food industries, *J. Soc. Dairy Technol.,* 23, 122—129, 1970.
8. **Alyward, F.,** Milk and milk products in the less developed countries, in *Milk Products of the Future,* Rothwell, J., Ed., Society of Dairy Technology, Wembley, England, 1974, 66—69.
9. **Anon.,** *Census of Dry Milk Distribution and Production Trends,* American Dry Milk Institute, Chicago, Ill., 1975.
10. **Anon.,** Milk as component in chocolate, *Zucker Susswaren Wirtsch.,* 20(2), 69—73, 1967.
11. **Anon.,** Spray-dried butter: now it's available in new forms, *Dairy Ice Cream Field,* 151(6), 82—83, 1969.
12. **Anon.,** Sweden launches Bregott, *Dairy Ind.,* 35, 490, 1970.
13. **Anon.,** 35% Protein whey, *Food Process., (Chicago),* 31(10), F-19, 1970.
14. **Anon.,** Fried milk curd is new development by gov't. research service, *Cheese Rep.,* 94(23), 10, 1971.
15. **Anon.,** New high-protein food, *Dairy Ind. Newsl.,* 251(4), 2, 1971.
16. **Anon.,** Whey in the bakery world, *Baking Ind.,* 138(1707), 30—32, 1972a.
17. **Anon.,** Emphasis on whey utilization is growing as more profitable outlets are being sought, *Dairy Rec.,* 73(2), 28—30, 1972.
18. **Anon.,** Whey — an important potential protein source, *Mon., Bull. Agric. Econ. Stat.,* 23(4), 12—19, 1974.
19. **Anon.,** Candy sales rebound as high sugar prices ease, *Supermarketing,* 98, 100, and 101, September 1976.
20. **Anon.,** Baby needs see 65.2% milk modifier sales hikes in groceries, *Supermarketing,* 96, September 1976.
21. **Anon.,** No evidence of xanthin oxidase involvement in heart disease found, *Food Chem. News,* 17, April 11, 1977.
22. **Arnott, D. R. and Bulloch, D. H.,** Can lactose increase for your chocolate drink?, *Can. Dairy Ice Cream J.,* 42(1), 21, 1963.

23. Asbjörn, F., Anhydrous milk fat manufacturing technique and future applications, *Dairy Ind.*, 35(7), 424—428, 1970.

24. Asbjörn, F., Anhydrous milk fat fractionation offers new applications for milk fat, *Dairy Ind.*, 35(8), 502—505, 1970.

25. Ashquisth, R. S., Otterburn, M. S., and Sinclair, W. J., Isopeptide crosslinks — their occurrence and importance in protein structure, *Angew. Chem. Int. Ed. Engl.*, 514—520, July 1974.

26. Ashton, W. M., The components of milk, their nutritive value, and the effects of processing. I and II, *Dairy Ind.*, 37, 535—538; 606—602, and 611, 1972.

27. Atkinson, R. L., Kratzer, R. H., and Stewart, G. F., Lactose in animal and human feeding: a review, *J. Dairy Sci.*, 4, 1114—1132, 1957.

28. Auclair, J. and Mocquot, G., Cultured milks, in *Milk Products of the Future*, Rothwell, T., Ed., Society of Dairy Technology, Wembley, England, 1974, 33—36.

29. Baker, B. E. and Bertok, E. I., Studies on protein hydrolysis. VII. Anaphylaxis in guinea pigs produced by some fractions of antigenic casein hydrolysates, *J. Sci. Food Agric.*, 14, 498—501, 1963.

30. Barnes, S. F., The dairy industry and malnutrition, *Aust. J. Dairy Technol.*, 92—96, September 1971.

30a. Bayless, T. M., Rothfeld, B., Massa, C., Wise, L., Paige, D., and Bedine, M. S., Lactose and milk intolerance: clinical implications, *N. Engl. J. Med.*, 292, 1156—1159, 1975.

31. Bender, A. E., Proteins: their properties, characteristics and nutritional value, *J. Soc. Dairy Technol.*, 24(4), 131—134, 1971.

32. Bills, D. D., The right of whey, *Dairy Ice Cream Field*, 157(10), 148—151, 1974.

33. Birch, G. G., Lactose: one of nature's paradoxes, *J. Milk Food Technol.*, 35, 32—34, 1972.

34. Bondreau, A., Richardson, T., and Amundson, C. H., Spray-dried butter and loss of volatile fatty acids during spray drying, *Food Technol. (Chicago)*, 20, 668—671, 1966.

34a. Borgstrom, A. G. and Proctor, J. F., Nutrition: food composition and nutrient aspects of food processing, in *Encyclopedia of Food Technology*, Johnson, A. H. and Peterson, M. S., Eds., AVI Publishing, Westport, Conn., 1974, 623—653.

35. Brendl, J. and Klein, S., The effect of added milk protein on water binding capacity of meat, *Fleischwirtschaft*, 52(3), 339—340 and 343—344, 1972.

36. Brink, M. F. and Kritchevsky, D., *Symposium: Dairy Lipids and Lipid Metabolism*, AVI Publishing, Westport, Conn., 1968.

37. Bookwalter, G. N., Moser, H. A., Kwolek, W. F., Pfeifer, V. F., and Griffin, E. L., Jr., Storage stability of CSM: alternate formulations for corn-soy-milk, *J. Food Sci.*, 36, 731—736, 1971.

38. Borst, J. R., Milk proteins for use in the food industry, *Food Technol. Aust.*, 23(11), 544—551, 1971.

39. Buchanan, R. A., Dairy products in other food industries, *Milk Ind.*, 67(6), 38—41, 1970.

40. Buchanan, R. A., Scope for increasing the usage of dairy products in other foods, *Aust. J. Dairy Technol.*, 6—12, September, 1971.

41. Campbell, L. B., Dairy products and their alternates in chocolate and confections, *Candy Snack Ind.*, 39—44, January 1976.

42. Food Research Institute, Proceeding of the Whey Utilization Symposium, June 1974, Canada Department of Agriculture, Ottawa, 1974.

43. Carr, C. J., Talbot, J. M., and Fisher, K. D., A Review of the Significance of Bovine Milk Xanthine Oxidase in the Etiology of Atherosclerosis, Life Sciences Research Office, Federation of the American Societies for Experimental Biology, Bethesda, Md., 1975.

44. Chapman, L. P. J., The story of the New Zealand milk biscuit, *Dairy Ind.*, 33(6), 379—383 and 33(7), 468—472, 1968.

45. Chojnowski, W., Poznanski, S., Jakubowski, J., Bednarski, W., Smietana, Z., Jedrychowski, J., and Leman, J., Characterization of concentrates of all milk proteins, *Milchwissenschaft*, 30, 407—413, 1975.

46. Clausi, A. S., Wollink, W. L., and Michael E. W., Breakfast Cereal Process, U.S. Patent 3,318,705, May 9, 1967.

47. Claydon, T. J., Pinkston, P. J., and Roberts, H. A., Experiences with quarg on a pilot scale, *Am. Dairy Rev.*, 34(Suppl. 2), 32B—32C, 1972.

48. Collins, T. W., Preparation of a Flowable Particulate Composition, U.S. Patent 3,617,302, November 2, 1971.

49. Corden, W. M., The nutritional value of dairy products in present day health concepts, *Aust. J. Dairy Technol. Suppl.*, 9—13, June 1974.

50. Cow and Gate, Eds., *Handbook for the use of the Medical Profession*, Cow and Gate, Guildford, Surrey, England, 1970, 24.

51. Craig, T. W. and Colmey, J. C., Milk and milk byproducts for use in bakery products, *Baker's Dig.*, 45(1), 36—39, 1971.

52. **Craig, T. W., Henika, R. G., and Hoyer, W. H.**, Alimentary Paste Products, U.S. Patent 3,762,931, 1973.

53. **Cuthberson, W. F. J.**, Infant food formulations in *Milk Products of the Future*, Rothwell, J., Ed., Society of Dairy Technology, Wembley, England, 1974, 51—57.

54. **Dairy Research Inc.**, Use of Milk Proteins in Milk Products and Other Foods, Bibliography, November 1972, Dairy Research Inc., Rosemont, Ill., 1972.

55. **Dannert, R. D. and Manwaring, M. E.**, Protein Fiber Fabrication Process, U.S. Patent 3,794,731, 1974.

56. **Davies, J. G.**, The utilization of dairy products in the food industry, *Process Biochem.*, 11(8), 13—19, 24, October 1976.

57. **DeGroot, A P. and Slump, P.**, Effects of severe alkali treatment of proteins on amino acids composition and nutritive value, *J. Nutr.*, 98, 45—56, 1969.

58. **Dennis, R. A.**, The dairy complement in food processes, *Food Technol. N.Z.*, 6, 27—29, February 1971.

59. **Drews, H. J. and Collins, T. W.**, Dry Dressing Mix and Method for Manufacture, U.S. Patent 3,585,362, June 1, 1971.

60. **Duncan, D. L.**, The physiological effects of lactose, *Nutr. Abstr. Rev.*, 25, 309—320, 1955.

61. **Dürr, P. and Neukom, H.**, Enrichment of pasta products with milk proteins, *Lebensm. Wiss. Technol.*, 5(4), 132—136, 1972.

62. **D'yachenko, P. F., Vlodavets, I. N., and Bogomolova, E.**, Method for production of edible casein, *Molochn. Prom.*, 14(6), 33—36, 1953.

63. **Dymsza, H. A., Stoewsand, G. S., Donovan, P., Barrett, F. F., and Lachance, P. A.**, Development of nutrient — defined formula diets for space feeding, *Food Technol. (Chicago)*, 20, 1349—1952, 1966.

64. **Ellinger, R. H.**, Lactalbumin Phosphate as Protein Ingredient in Non-Butterfat Dairy Products, U.S. Patent 3,563,761, February 16, 1971.

65. **Ellinger, R. H. and Schwartz, M. G.**, Replacement of Sodium Caseinate, U.S. Patent 3,615,661, October 26, 1971.

66. **Ellinger, R. H. and Schwartz, M. G.**, Replacement of Sodium Caseinate, U.S. Patent 3,615,662, October, 26, 1971.

67. **Ellinger, R. H. and Schwartz, M. G.**, Replacement of Sodium Caseinate, U.S. Patent 3,620,757, November 16, 1971.

68. **Engel, M. E. and Singleton, A. D.**, Process for the Manufacture of Casein, U.S. Patent 3,361,567, January, 2, 1968.

68a. **EPA**, Dairy Product Processing Point Source Category, EPA-440/1-74-021-a, U.S. Environmental Protection Agency, Washington, D.C., May 1974.

69. **Eriksen, S.**, Flavors of milk and milk products. I. The role of lactones, *Milchwissenschaft*, 31, 549—550, 1976.

69a. **Eriksen, S. and Fagerson, I. S.**, Flavors of amino acids and peptides, *Flavours*, 13—16, January/February 1976.

69b. **Fed. Regist.**, Food label information panel, 38(49), 6960, March 14, 1973.

70. **Fenton-May, R. I.**, The Use of Reverse Osmosis and Ultrafiltration in the Food Industry, Ph.D. thesis, University of Wisconsin, Madison, 1971.

71. **FAO**, *Energy and Protein Requirements*, Nutr. Meet. Rep. Ser. No. 52, WHO Tech. Rep. Ser. No. 522, Food and Agricultural Organization of the United Nations, Rome, 1973.

72. **FAO**, Whey — an important protein source, *Mon. Bull. Agric. Econ. Stat.*, 23(4), 12—19, 1974.

73. **FAO**, The milk and milk product situation — mid-1975, *Mon. Bull. Agric. Econ. Stat.*, 24(9), 1—4, 1975.

74. **FAO**, Skim milk powder situation and outlook, *Mon. Bull. Agric. Econ. Stat.*, 25(7/8), 29—34, 1976.

74a. **FAO**, Review of national dairy policies in 1975-76, *Mon. Bull. Agric. Econ. Stat.*, 26(1), 13—18, 1977.

75. **Foremost Foods Company**, ForeTein®, A High Protein Demineralized Whey Protein, Foremost Foods Company, San Francisco, 1970.

76. **Forss, D. A.**, The flavor of dairy fats: a review, *J. Am. Oil Chem. Soc.*, 48, 702—710, 1971.

77. **Forsum, E.**, Nutritional evaluation of whey protein concentrates and their fractions, *J. Dairy Sci.*, 57(6), 665—670, 1974.

78. **Forsum, E.**, Whey proteins for food and feed supplement, in *Protein Nutritional Quality of Foods and Feeds*, Vol. 1, Part 2, Priedman, M., Ed., Marcel Dekker, New York, 1975, 433—470.

79. **Forsum, E. and Hambraeus, L.**, Nutritional and biochemical studies of whey products, *J. Dairy Sci.*, 60(3), 370—377, 1977.

80. Forsum, E., Hambraeus, L., and Siddiqi, I. H., Large scale fractionation of whey, *J. Dairy Sci.,* 57(6), 659—664, 1974.
81. Fox, K. K., Casein and whey products, in *By-Products from Milk,* 2nd ed., Webb, B. H. and Whittier, E. O., Eds., AVI Publishing, Westport, Conn., 1970, 338—340.
82. Frazeur, D. R., The use of wheys in frozen desserts, *Ice Cream Field Trade J.,* 149, 22, 23, 26, and 32, 1967.
83. Friend, B. and Marston, R., Nutrition Review, National Food Situation NFS-154, Economics Research Service, U.S. Department of Agriculture, Washington, D.C., 1975, 28—32.
83a. Garza, C. and Scrimshaw, N. S., Relationship of lactose intolerance to milk intolerance in young children, *Am. J. Clin. Nutr.,* 29, 192—196, 1976.
83b. General Foods Corporation, Whipable Compositions and Manufacture Thereof, British Patent 1,140,937, January 22, 1969.
84. Genin, G., Australian research on production of a new by-product of the dairy industry: coprecipitated casein and whey proteins, *Lait,* 46(458), 522—527, 1966.
85. Goller, H. J. and Kube, J., Lactose in chocolate manufacture, *Int. Rev. Sugar Confectionary,* 27(9), 391, 1974.
86. Graeve, K., Consideration of 'half-butter', *Molk. Ztg. Welt Milch,* 28(37), 1028—1030, 1974.
87. Graham, D. M., Alteration of nutritional value by processing and fortification of milk and milk products, *Cultured Dairy Prod. J.,* 18—22, November 1974.
88. Groves, F., An Economic Analysis of Whey Utilization, Staff Paper Series #48, University of Wisconsin, Madison, 1972.
89. Guérin, J. and Alais, C. H., Les caséinates dans les industries alimentaires utilization et analyse, *Ind. Aliment. Agric.,* 91, 343—348, April 1974.
90. Guth, J. H. and Tumerman, L., Method of Making Lactulose, U.S. Patent 3,546,206, December 8, 1970.
91. Guy, E. J., Lactose: review of its properties and uses in bakery products, *Bakers Dig.,* 45(2), 34—38 and 74, 1971.
92. Guy, E. J., Vettel, H. E., and Pallansch, M. J., Effect of cheese whey protein concentrates on the baking quality and rheological characteristics of sponge doughs made from hard red spring wheat flour, *Cereal Sci. Today,* 19, 551—556, 1974.
93. Habighurst, A. B., Replaces nonfat dry milk in wide range of foods, *Food Process (Chicago),* 33(7), 34, 1972.
94. Hall, C. W. and Hedrick, T. I., *Drying of Milk and Milk Products,* AVI Publishing, Westport, Conn., 1965.
95. Hambraeus, L., Wranne, L., and Loretsson, R., Whey protein formulas in the treatment of phenylketonuria in infants, *Nutr. Metab.,* 12, 151, 1970.
96. Hambraeus, L., Hardell, L. I., Forsum, E., and Loretsson, R., Use of a formula based on a whey protein concentrate in the feeding of an infant with hyperphenylalaninemia, *Nutr. Metab.,* 17, 84, 1974.
97. Hammonds, T. M. and Call, D. L., Utilization of protein ingredients in the U.S. food industry. A. E. Res. 320 and A. E. Res. 321, Cornell University, Ithaca, N.Y., 1970.
98. Hammonds, T. M. and Call, D. L., Protein use patterns, current and future, *Chemtech,* 156—162, March 1972.
99. Hansen, P. M. T., Manufacture of butter powder, *Aust. J. Dairy Technol.,* 18(2), 79—86, 1963.
100. Harrap, B. S., Recent developments in the production of dairy products with increased levels of polyunsaturation, *Aust. J. of Dairy Technol.,* 101—104, September 1973.
101. Hawley, H. B., Shepherd, P. A., and Wheater, D. M., Factors affecting the implantation and lactobacilli in the intestine, *J. Appl. Bacteriol.,* 22, 360, 1959.
102. Hegarty, P. V. J., Some biological considerations in the nutritional evaluation of foods, *Food Technol. (Chicago),* 29(4), 52, 54, 56, 58, 60, 62, and 64, 1975.
103. Hegsted, D. M., Nutritional value of cereal protein in relation to human needs, in *Protein Enriched Cereal Foods for World Needs,* Millner, M., Ed., American Association of Ceral Chemists, St. Paul, Minn., 1969, 38—48.
104. Henderson, J. O. and Buchanan, R. A., Manufacture of CFI: a sterilized dairy-based carbohydrate-free infant food, *Aust. J. Dairy Technol.,* 28, 7—11, 1973.
105. Henry, M. Kathleen and Kon, S. K., The supplementary relationship between the proteins of dairy products and those of bread and potato as affected by the method of feeding, *J. Dairy Res.,* 14, 330--339, 1946.
106. Holton, B. S., Ultrafiltration of whey and milk for protein recovery, in *Proc. 4th Int. Congr. Food Sci. Technol.,* Vol. 4, Marco, E. P., Instituto Nacional de Ciencia y Technologia de Alimentos, Valencia, Spain, 1974, 322—331.
107. Hood, L. F., Enzyme hydrolysis of lactose in dairy foods, *J. Dairy Sci.,* 54, 761, 1971.

108. Holsinger, V. H., Posati, L. P., DeVilbiss, E. D., and Pallansch, M. J., Fortifying soft drinks with cheese whey protein, *Food Technol. (Chicago)*, 27(2), 59—50 and 64—65, 1973.

109. Holsinger, V. H., Posati, L. P., and DeVilbiss, E. D., Whey beverages: a review, *J. Dairy Sci.*, 57, 849—859, 1974.

109a. Hugunin, A. G. and Ewing, N. L., Dairy-based ingredients for food products, Dairy Research, Inc., Rosemont, Ill., 1977, 1—24.

109b. Hugunin, A. G. and Lee, S. M., A Fresh Look at Dairy-Based Ingredients for Processed Foods, Dairy Research, Inc., Rosemont, Ill., 1977, 1—13.

110. Hulse, J. H., Protein enrichment in bread and baked products, in *New Protein Foods Volume 1A Technology*, Altschul, A. M., Ed., Academic Press, New York, 1974, 167—176.

111. Humphries, M. A. and Roeper, J., Calcium caseinate for fortification of cereal products, in *Proc. 19th Int. Dairy Congr. IE*, 778—779, 1974.

112. Hurt, H. D., Lactose intolerance, *Cultured Dairy Prod. J.*, 7(4), 7—10, 1972.

113. Hutton, J. T., Whey protein, *Act. Rep. Res. Dev. Assoc. Mil. Food Packag. Syst.*, 26(2), 102, 1974.

113a. Hutton, J. T., Casein and whey: let's set the record straight, *Food Eng.*, 49(11), 80—82, 1977.

114. Hynd, J., Utilization of milk proteins (a review), *J. Soc. Dairy Technol.*, 23(2), 95—99, 1970.

115. Jack, E. L. and Haynes, V. M., Consumer preference for bread containing different levels of non-fat dry milk solids, *Food Res.*, 16, 57—61, 1951.

116. Jaynes, H. D. and Chiang, C. T., High protein snack utilizes whey protein concentrate, *Food Prod. Dev.*, 8(9), 32—34, 1974.

117. Jelen, P., Utilization of cheese whey components in human foods, in *Proc. 4th Int. Congr. Food Sci. Technol.*, Vol. 4, Marco, E. P., Ed., Instituto Nacional de Ciencia y Technologia de Alimentos, Valencia, Spain, 1974, 281—288.

118. Jelen, P. and Jadlav, S. J., Color improvement of french-fried potatoes using lactose or cheese whey, *J. Food Sci.*, 39, 1269—1270, 1974.

119. Jensen, G. K., Sale of membrane filtration products from dairying to the food industry, *Maelkeritideude*, 88, 255—263, 1975.

120. Johnson, A. H., The composition of milk, in *Fundamentals of Dairy Chemistry*, Webb, B. H., Johnson, A. H., and Alford, J. A., Eds., AVI Publishing, Westport, Conn., 1974, 22—44.

121. Jonas, J. J., Utilization of dairy ingredients in other foods, *J. Milk Food Technol.*, 36, 323—332, 1973.

122. Jonas, J. J., Multi-Purpose Whipped Dessert and Method of Manufacture, U.S. Patent 4,012,533, March 15, 1977.

123. Jonas, J. J., Craig, T. W., Huston, R. L., Marth, E. H., Speckmann, E. W., Steiner, T. F., and Weisberg, S. M., Dairy products as food protein resources, *J. Milk Food Technol.*, 39, 778—795, 1976.

124. Kaunitz, H., Dietary lipids and arteriosclerosis, *J. Am. Oil Chem. Soc.*, 52, 293—297, 1975.

125. Keay, J., Experts point to expand role for whey as a valuable ingredient in many foods, *Mod. Dairy*, 50(3), 24—26, 1971.

126. Kieseker, F. G., Polyunsaturated milk fat products, *Aust. J. Dairy Technol.*, 7—10, March 1975.

127. Kinsella, J. E., Functional chemistry of milk products in candy and chocolate manufacture, *Manuf. Confect.*, 50(10), 45—48, 52 and 54, 1970.

128. Kinsella, J. E., The chemistry of dairy powders with reference to baking, in *Advances in Food Research*, Vol. 19, Chichester, C. O., Mrak, E. M., and Stewart, G. F., Eds., Academic Press, New York, 1971, 147—213.

129. Kinsella, J. E., Dairy foods: trends, research, and development, *J. Milk Food Technol.*, 35, 142—147, 1972.

130. Kinsella, J. E., Butter flavor, *Food Technol. (Chicago)*, 29(5), 82—98, 1975.

131. Kinsella, J. E., Functional properties of proteins in foods: a survey, *Crit. Rev. Food Sci. Nutr.*, 7(3), 219—280, 1976.

132. Kisza, J., Switka, J., Kruk, A., and Surazymski, A., Essai d'utilisation de la bêta-D-galactosidase pour la fabrication du lait condensé sucré, *Lait*, 53, 430—439, 1973.

133. Klostermeyer, H. and Reimerdes, E. H., Heat Induced Crosslinks in Milk Proteins and Consequences for the Milk System, Paper 56, 172nd Am. Chem. Soc. Meeting, Division of Agricultural and Food Chemistry, San Francisco, August 30 — September 3, 1976.

134. Knight, S. G., Process for Preparing Flavoring Compositions, U.S. Patent 3,100,153, August 6, 1963.

135. Knightly, W. H., The role of ingredients in the formulation of whipped toppings, *Food Technol. (Chicago)*, 22, 721—744, 1968.

136. Koch, R., Acosta, P., Ragsdale, N., and Donnell, G. N., Nutrition in the treatment of galactosemia, *J. Am. Diet. Assoc.*, 43, 216—222, 1963.

137. Kon, S. K., *Milk and Milk Products in Human Nutrition,* 2nd ed., Food and Agricultural Organization of United Nations, Rome, 1972, 47.

138. Kosikowski, F. V., Greater utilization of whey powder for human consumption and nutrition, *J. Dairy Sci.,* 50, 1343—1345, 1967.

139. Kosikowski, F. V., Nutritional beverages from acid whey powder, *J. Dairy Sci.,* 51, 1299—1301, 1968.

140. Kosikowski, F. V. and Wierzbicki, L. E., Low lactose yogurt from microbiological lactose (betagalactosidase) applications, *J. Dairy Sci.,* 54, 764, 1971.

141. Kosikowski, F. V., Wierzbicki, L. E., and Iwasaki, T., Low lactose milk from *Lactobacillus helveticus* derived from lactose, *J. Dairy Sci.,* 55, 670—671, 1972.

142. Kosikowski, F. V. and Wierzbicki, L. E., Lactose hydrolysis of raw and pasteurized milk by *Saccharomyces lactis* lactase, *J. Dairy Sci.,* 56, 146—148, 1973.

143. Kosman, M. E., Lactulose in portosystemic encephalopathy, *J. Am. Med. Assoc.,* 236, 2444—2445, 1976.

143a. Kowalski, R., Lactose intolerance, how wide spread?, *Nursing Care,* 30 and 34, May 1977.

144. Kretschmer, N., Lactose and lactase, *Sci. Am.,* 227(10), 71—78, 1972.

145. Kroger, M., Quality of yogurt, *J. Dairy Sci.,* 59, 344—350, 1976.

146. Kuehler, C. A. and Stine, C. M., Effect of enzymatic hydrolysis of some functional properties of whey protein, *J. Food Sci.,* 39, 379—382, 1974.

147. Lang, F. and Lang, A., Some major new European developments, *Milk Ind.,* 76, 28—30, 1975.

148. Lefaivre, J., Tremblay, L., and Julien, J. P., Rôle de complémanterité des protéines solubles du lait pour le protéines de la fève soya, *Can. Inst. Food Sci. Technol. J.,* 5(2), 87—92 and 5(4), 221, 1972.

149. Lohrey, E. E. and Humphries, M. D., The protein quality of some New Zealand milk products, *N.Z. J. Dairy Sci. Technol.,* 11, 147—154, 1976.

149a. Lough, H. W., Whey supply and utilization, *Am. Dairy Rev.,* 39(4), 34B, 34D, 34E, and 34F, 1977.

150. Mann, E. J., Whey processing and utilization, *Dairy Ind.,* 30, 966—967, 1965.

151. Mann, E. J., New forms of butterfat, *Dairy Ind.,* 33(12), 848—849, 1968.

152. Mann, E. J., Whey processing and utilization. I, *Dairy Ind.,* 34, 507—508, 1969.

153. Mann, E. J., Whey processing and utilization. II, *Dairy Ind.,* 34, 571—573, 1969.

154. Mann, E. J., Custards and related products, *Dairy Ind.,* 35(3), 156—157, 1970.

155. Mann, E. J., The quiet revolution in new uses for liquid milk, *Milk Ind.,* 67(6), 42—45, 1970.

156. Mann, E. J., Utilization of milk proteins, *J. Soc. Dairy Technol.,* 24(4), 145—150, 1971.

157. Mann, E. J., Jellied milks, milk desserts, and custards, *Dairy Ind.,* 36(7), 414—415, 1971.

158. Mann, E. J., Lactalbumin and its uses, *Dairy Ind.,* 36, 528—529, 1971.

159. Mann, E. J., Whey processing and utilization. I, *Dairy Ind.,* 36, 44—45, 1971.

160. Mann, E. J., Whey processing and utilization. II, *Dairy Ind.,* 36, 96—97, 1971.

161. Mann, E. J., Some aspects of whey utilization, *Dairy Ind.,* 38, 77—78, 1973.

162. Mann, E. J., Whey utilization. I, *Dairy Ind.,* 39, 303—304, 1974.

163. Mann, E. J., Whey utilization. II, *Dairy Ind.,* 39, 343—344, 1974.

164. Mason, M. E. and Katz, I., Flavor in new protein technologies, in *New Protein Foods,* Vol. 2, Part B, Altschul, A. M., Ed., Academic Press, New York, 1976, 142—158.

165. Mansvelt, J. W., Variations on the theme of cottage cheese, *Naarden News,* 22(231), 3, 1971.

166. Marshall, P. G., Dunkley, W. L., and Love, E., Fractionation and concentration of whey by reverse osmosis, *Food Technol. (Chicago),* 22(8), 37—44, 1968.

167. Mauron, J., Malabsorption due to lactose intolerance: reflections on the problem in the food industry, in *Proc. 9th Int. Congr. Nutrition, Mexico, 1972,* Vol. 1, S. Karger, Basel 1975, 187—197.

168. McDonough, F. E., Concentration and fractionation of whey by reverse osmosis, in Proc. Whey Utilization Conf., USDA-ARS-73-69, Agricultural Research Service, U.S. Department of Agriculture, Washington, D.C., 1970, 36—47.

169. McGillivray, W. A., Milkfat and its derivates, in *Milk Products of the Future,* Rothwell, J., Ed., Society of Dairy Technology, Wembley, England, 1976, 37—41.

170. McKee, J. E. and Tucker, J. W., Food Compositions Containing Undenatured Water-Soluble Lactalbumin Phosphates, U.S. Patent 3,299,843, August 30, 1966.

171. Milk Industry Foundation, Milk Facts, Washington, D.C., 1974.

172. Miller, E. B., Cooperative Marketing of Nonfat Dry Milk to Commercial Outlets, USDA. Rep. 129, U.S. Department of Agriculture, Washington, D.C., September 1965.

173. Mitra, K. and Verma, S. K., The biological value of the proteins of rice, pulse, and milk fed in different porportions to human subjects, *Indian J. Med. Res.,* 35, 23—28, 1947.

174. Mitsuoka, T., Bacteriology of fermented milk with special reference to the implantation of lactobacti in the intestine, in *Proc. 6th Int. Symp. Conversion and Manufacture of Foodstuffs by Microorganism,* Saikon Publishing, Tokyo, Japan, 1971, 169—180.

175. **Morr, C. V.**, Chemistry of milk proteins in food processing, *J. Dairy Sci.,* 58, 977—984, 1975.
176. **Morr, C. V.**, Whey protein concentrates: an update, *Food Technol. (Chicago),* 30(3), 18—22 and 42, 1976.
177. **Muller, L. L.**, Manufacture and uses of casein and coprecipitate (a review), *Dairy Sci. Abstr.,* 33, 659—674, 1971.
178. **Muller, L. L.**, Whey utilization in Australia, *Aust. J. Dairy Technol.,* 31, 92—97, 1976.
179. **Muller, L. L. and Hayes, J. F.**, The manufacture of a coprecipitate for baked goods, in *Proc. 18th Int. Dairy Congr. 1E,* Ramsay Wate Publishing, Melbourne, Australia, 1970, 429.
180. **Munro, H. N. and Allison, J. B.**, *Mammalian Protein Metabolism,* Vol. 2, Academic Press, New York, 1964.
181. **Mussellwhite, P. R.**, Whipping Cream, British Patent 1,125,004, 1968.
182. **Mussellwhite, P. R. and Walker, D. A.**, Frozen Desserts, U.S. Patent 3,535,122, October 20, 1970.
183. **Mutai, M., Aso, K., and Shirota, M.**, Characteristic features of beverage containing live lactobacilli in *Proc. 6th Int. Symp. Conversion and Manufacture of Foodstuffs by Microorganism,* Saikon Publishing, Tokyo, Japan, 1971, 181—189.
184. **National Dairy Council**, Newer Knowledge of Milk, 3rd ed., Rosemont, Ill., 1965.
185. **National Dairy Council**, Composition and nutritive value of dairy foods, *Dairy Counc. Dig.,* 47, 25—30, September-October 1976.
186. **National Dairy Council**, Calcium in bone health, *Dairy Counc. Dig.,* 47(6), 31—35, 1976.
186a. **National Science Foundation**, RANN Division, New Concepts for the Rapid Determination of Protein Quality, Conference at University of Nebraska, Lincoln, 1977.
187. **Neer, K. L., Plimpton, R. F., and Ockerman, H. W.**, Bologna product characteristics as influenced by various sources and levels of cottage cheese whey, *J. Food Sci.,* 39, 993—996, 1974.
188. **Nestlé Products Ltd.**, Process for the Production of Protein Hydrolysates, British Patent 1,107,229, 1968.
189. **Neumann, C. G. and Jelliffe, D. B.**, Eds., in *Symposium on Nutrition in Pediatrics. The Pediatric Clinics of North America,* Vol. 24, W. B. Saunders, February 1977.
190. **Nickerson, T. A.**, Use of milk derivative, lactose, in other foods, *J. Dairy Sci.,* 59, 581—587, 1976.
191. **Nickerson, T. A. and Patel, K. N.**, Crystallization in solutions supersaturated with sucrose and lactose, *J. Food Sci.,* 37, 693—697, 1972.
192. **Neilsen, V. A.**, A 10-year projection for milk production, processing, technology and markets in the United States, *Milk Ind.,* 70(2), 18—21, and 23, 1972.
193. **Nordal, J. and Rossebo, L.**, Enzymatic precipitation in agar gel as a method for the detection of sodium caseinate in raw and heated meat products, *Z. Lebensm. Unters. Forsch.,* 148, 65—69, 1972.
194. **Noyes, R.**, *Protein Food Supplements, Food Process Reviews,* No. 3, Noyes Data Corp., Park Ridge, N.J., 1969.
195. **Oberg, E. B., Nelson, C. E., and Hankinson, C. L.**, Whipping Agent from Casein, U.S. Patent 2,597,136, April 9, 1951.
196. **Olsman, W. J.**, Detection of non-meat proteins in meat products by electrophoresis, *Z. Lebensm. Unters. Forsch.,* 141, 253—259, 1969.
197. **Pallansch, M. J.**, Progress in development of whey-soy drink, in Whey Products Conference, Agricultural Research Service, U.S. Department of Agriculture, Philadelphia, 1974, 48—55.
198. **Pangborn, R. M. and Dunkley, W. L.**, Sensory discrimination of milk salts, lactose, non-dialysable constituents and algin gum in milk, *J. Dairy Sci.,* 49, 1—6, 1968.
199. **Paul, J. K.**, *Fruit and Vegetable Juice Processing. Food Technology Review,* No. 21, Noyes Data Corp., 1975, 259—272.
200. **Petrowski, G. E.**, Emulsion stability and its relation to foods, in *Advances in Food Research,* Vol. 22, Chichester, C. O., Mrak, E. M., and Stewart, G. F., Eds., Academic Press, New York, 1976, 309—359.
201. **Pfaff, W.**, Practical experiences with hydrolyzed milk protein in the manufacture of meat products, *Fleischwirtschaft,* 45, 1427—1437, 1965.
202. **Pfaff, W.**, Hydrolyzed milk protein for pates and cooked sausages, *Fleischwirtschaft,* 54, 661, 1974.
203. *Pharmacopeia of the United States of America,* 18th Revision, Committee of Revision, Board of Trustees, Mack Printing Co., Easton, Pa., 1970, 358.
204. **Phillips, C. M. and Briggs, G. M.**, Milk and its role in the American diet, *J. Dairy Sci.,* 58, 1751—1763, 1975.
205. **Pinkston, P. J. and Claydon, T. J.**, Puffed snacks made from milk curd, *Food Prod. Dev.,* 5(1), 30, 1971.
206. **Pokrovskii, A. A. and Levyant, P. P.**, Protein Preparations from Milk Products, U.S.S.R. Patent 232,747, 1968.
207. **Pomeranz, Y. and Miller, B. S.**, Use of lactase in breadmaking, *Cereal Chem.,* 39, 398, 1962.

208. Pomeranz, Y. and Miller, B. S., Evaluation of lactase preparations for use in breadmaking, *J. Agric. Food Chem.*, 11, 19—22, 1963.

209. Pomeranz, Y., Lactase (beta-galactosidase). II. Possibilities in the food industry, *Food Technol. (Chicago)*, 18, 690—695, 1964.

210. Porter, J. W. G., Nutritional Studies — recent advances, in *Milk Products of the Future,* Rothwell, J., Ed., Society of Dairy Technology, Wembley, England, 1974, 46—50.

211. Porter, J. W. G., *Milk and Dairy Foods,* The Value of Food Ser., Fisher, P. and Bender, A. E., Eds., Oxford University Press, London, 1975.

212. Porter, M. D. and Michaels, A. S., Membrane ultrafiltration, *Chem. Technol.*, 248—254, April 1971.

213. Posati, P. L. and Orr, M. L., Composition of Foods, Dairy and Egg Products, Agriculture Handbook No. 8-1, Agricultural Research Service, U.S. Department of Agriculture, Washington, D.C., 1976.

213a. Protein Advisory Group, United Nations, Low Lactase activity and milk intake, PAG Statement No. 17, in *PAG Compendium,* Halsted Worldmark, New York, 1972, E349-351.

214. Ramshaw, E. H. and Dunstone, E. A., The flavor of milk protein, *J. Dairy Res.*, 36, 203—213, 1969.

215. Ramshaw, E. H. and Dunstone, E. A., Volatile compounds associated with the off-flavour in stored casein, *J. Dairy Res.*, 36, 215—223, 1969.

216. Rash, E., Milk substitutes made from whey for candy provide savings in ingredient, processing costs, *Candy Ind.*, 133(11), 32—34, 1969.

217. Rettger, L. F., Levy, M. N., Weinstein, L., and Weiss, J. E., *Lactobacillus Acidophilus and its Therapeutic Applications,* Yale University Press, New Haven, Conn., 1935.

218. Richert, S. H., Current milk protein manufacturing process, *J. Dairy Sci.*, 58, 985—993, 1975.

219. Rocamora Ruiz, J., Aspectos generales en relación con la incorporation de productos lácteos a otros alimentos, *Via Lactea,* 6(23), 9—13, 1974.

220. Rodier, W. I., III, Wetsel, W. E., Jacobs, H. L., Graeber, R. C., Moskowitz, H. R., Reed, T. J. E., and Waterman, D., The Acceptability of Whey-Soy Mix as a Supplementary Food for Pre-School Children in Developing Countries, Tech. Rep. 74-20 PR, U.S. Army Natick Laboratories, Natick, Mass., 1974.

221. Roeper, J., High-calcium phosphate casein products for use in food systems, *N.Z. J. Dairy Sci. Technol.*, 11, 62—64, 1976.

222. Rosenfield, D., Utilizable protein: quality quantity concepts in assessing food, *Food Prod. Dev.*, 7, 57—62, 1973.

223. Rosenzsweig, N. S., Adult human milk intolerance and intestinal lactase deficiency: a review, *J. Dairy Sci.*, 52, 585—587, 1969.

224. Rothwell, J., Ed., *Milk Products of the Future,* Society of Dairy Technology, Wembleg, England, 1974.

225. Saffle, R. L., Meat emulsions, in *Advances in Food Research,* Vol. 16, Chichester, C. O., Mrak, E. M., and Stewart, G. F., Eds., Academic Press, New York, 1968, 105—160.

226. Sakita, T., Ebisawa, M., and Mimoto, H., Process for Producing Edible Protein Fibre, U.S. Patent 3,749,581, 1973.

227. Sandine, W. E., Muralidhara, K. S., Elliker, P. R., and England, D. C., Lactic acid bacteria in food and health: a review, *J. Milk Food Technol.*, 35, 691—702, 1972.

228. Schoppert, E. F., Sinnamon, H. I., Tally, F. B., Panzer, C. C., and Aceto, N. C., Enrichment of pasta with cottage cheese whey proteins, *J. Food Sci.*, 41, 1297—1300, 1976.

229. Schulz, M. E., Method for the Manufacture of Spreadable Dry Butter, West German Patent 1,201,699, 1966.

230. Schulz, M. E., Problems of combining milk products with other foods, *Milchwissenschaft*, 24, 521—532, 1969.

231. Schulz, W. E. and Voss, E., Preparation of spreadable butter, in *Proc. 17th Int. Dairy Congr.*, Vol. 6, Verlag Th. Mann, Berlin, 1966, 67—69.

232. Schut, J., The effects of fat emulsification and water retention of the consistency of sausages, in *Proc. Kolloquium: Milcheiweiss und die industrielle Lebensmittelherstellung besonders Fleischwaren,* Veghel, Netherlands, 1970, 26—44.

233. Sheffield-Humko Division, Kraft, Inc., A.N.R.C. Reference Protein (brochure), Norwich N.Y., 1960.

234. Shukla, T. P., Beta-galactosidase technology: a solution to the lactose problem, *Crit. Rev. Food Technol.*, 5(3), 325—356, 1975.

235. Singh, M., Use of dairy products in other foods: a market researcher's point of view, *Aust. J. Dairy Technol. Suppl.*, 20—24, September 1971.

236. Singleton, A. D., Whey usage in dairy products, *Dairy Ice Cream Field,* 156(2), 30—32, 1973.

237. Singelton, A. D. and Robertson, R. G., Whey products for the bakery, *Baker's Dig.*, 40(5), 46—48, 1966.

238. Smith, G., Whey protein, *World Rev. Nutr. Diet.,* 24, 88—116, 1976.

239. Smith, J. A. B., Milk and milk products, in *Proteins as Human Food,* Lawrie, R. A., Ed., AVI Publishing, Westport, Conn., 1970, 213—224.

240. Smith, L. M., Symposium: milk lipids, AOCS 46th Annu. Fall Meet., Ottawa, Ontario, Canada, *J. Am. Oil Chem. Soc.,* 50, 175—201, 1973.

241. Southward, C. R., Rennet casein — industrial chemical or food ingredient, *Food Technol. N. Z.,* 9, 11—15, 1974.

242. Speck, M. L., Interaction among lactobacilli and man, *J. Dairy Sci.,* 59, 338—343, 1976.

243. Spurgeon, K. R., Seas, S. W., and Dalaly, B. K., Effects of nonfat milk solids and stabilizers on body, texture, and water retention in low-fat dairy spreads, *Food Prod. Dev.,* 7(3), 34, 36, and 43—44, 1973.

244. Steinitz, W., Freeze-thaw puddings, *Dairy Ice Cream Field,* 152(8), 38, 40, and 46, 1970.

244a. Stephenson, L. S. and Latham, M. C., Lactose intolerance and milk consumption: the relation of tolerance to symptoms, *Am. J. Clin. Nutr.,* 27, 296—303, 1974.

245. Stimpson, E. G., Frozen Concentrated Milk Products, U.S. Patent 2,668,765, 1954.

246. Stimpson, E. G., Conversion of Lactose to Glucose and Galactose, U.S. Patent 2,681,858, 1954.

247. Strange, L. and Singh, M., Australian recombining plants in Southeast Asia, *Aust. J. Dairy Technol. Suppl,* 29—35, September 1971.

248. Strokel, D. R., Bryan, W. G., and Babcock, C. J., Flavors of Milk: A Review of Literature, U.S. Department of Agriculture, Washington, D.C., 1953.

249. Szczesniak, A. S. and Engel, E., U.S. Patent 2,952,543, September 13, 1960.

250. Tomarelli, R. M., Minnick, N., D'Amato, E., and Bernhardt, F. W., Bioassay of the nutritional quality of proteins of human and cow's milk by rat growth procedures, *J. Nutr.,* 68, 265—279, 1959.

251. Tomarelli, R. M. and Bernhardt, F. W., Biological assay of milk and whey protein compositions for infant feeding, *J. Nutr.,* 78, 44—50, 1962.

252. Tumerman, L., Fram, H., and Connelly, K. W., The effect of lactose crystallization in protein stability in frozen concentrated milk, *J. Dairy Sci.,* 37, 830—839, 1954.

253. USDA, Some commercial food and feed products made from or containing whey (appendix 2), in Proc. Whey Utilization Conf., ARS-73-69, Agricultural Research Service, U.S. Department of Agriculture, Washington, D.C., 1970, 132—136.

254. USDA, Proc. Whey Utilization Conf. ARS-73-69, EV Publ. No. 3340, Agricultural Research Service, U.S. Department of Agriculture, Washington, D.C., 1970.

255. USDA, Proc. Whey Products Conf., ERRL Publ. No. 3379, Agricultural Research Service, U.S. Department of Agriculture, Washington, D.C., 1972.

256. USDA, Proc. Whey Products Conf., ERRL Publ. No. 3996, Whey Products Institute, Chicago, Ill., and U.S. Department of Agriculture, Washington, D.C., 1974.

257. USDA, Agricultural Statistics, U.S. Department of Agriculture, Washington, D.C., 1974, 391.

258. USDA, Dairy Situation, Economics Research Service, U.S. Department of Agriculture, Washington, D.C., March 1975, 27.

259. USDA, Dairy Products, U.S. Department of Agriculture, Washington, D.C., January 31, 1977.

260. Voss, E., Beyerlein, V., and Schmanke, E., Problems involved in technical fractionation of butterfat by means of the fat granules filtration process. I. Influence of size and morphology of the fat granules on the filtration ability and yield as well as methods to control the process, *Milchwissenschaft,* 26, 605—613, 1971.

261. Vujinovic, V., Preparation of foods for children with phenylketonuria, *Hrana Ishrana,* 15, 186—189, 1974.

262. Wadsworth, G. R., Milk products of the future — medical aspects, in *Milk Products of the Future,* Rothwell, J., Ed., Society of Dairy Technology, Wembley, England, 1974, 60—65.

263. Wakodo Co. Ltd., Milk-Serum Foodstuff, Japanese Patent 20:537/70, 1970.

264. Walker, N. J., Flavour defects in edible casein and skimmilk powder. I. Malliard reaction, *J. Dairy Res.,* 39, 231—238, 1972.

265. Walker, N. J., Flavour defects in edible casein and skimmilk powders. II. The role of aliphatic monocarboyl compounds, *J. Dairy Res.,* 40, 29—37, 1973.

266. Watts, J. E. and Nelson, J. H., Cheese Flavoring Process, U.S. Patent 3,072,488, January 8, 1963.

267. Webb, B. H., Use of dairy products in bakery goods, *Cereal Sci. Today,* 8, 6—18, 1963.

268. Webb, B. H., Whey — a low cost dairy product for use in candy, *J. Dairy Sci.,* 49, 1310—1313, 1966.

269. Webb, B. H., Utilization of whey in foods and feeds, in Proc. Whey Utilization Conf., ARS-73-69, Agricultural Research Service, U.S. Department of Agriculture, Washington, D. C., 1970, 102—111.

270. Webb, B. H., Recycling whey for profitable uses, *Am. Dairy Rev., Manuf. Milk Prod. Suppl.,* 34(6), 32A-32D, 1972.

270a. *Webster's Third New International Dictionary of the English Language,* Gove, P. B., Editor-in-Chief, GC Merriam, Springfield, Mass., 1966, 62a and 1859.

271. Weisberg, S. M., Recent progress in the manufacture and use of lactose: a review, *J. Dairy Sci.,* 37, 1106—1115, 1954.

272. Weisberg, S. M. and Goldsmith, H. I., Whey for foods and feeds, *Food Technol. (Chicago),* 23, 186—189, 1969.

273. Weisberg, S. M., Food products intended to improve nutrition in the developing world, in *Advances in Food Research,* Vol. 22, Chichester, C. O., Mrack, E. M., and Stewart, G. F., Eds., Academic Press, New York, 1976.

274. Weisberg, S. M., New approaches to marketing milk products, in *New Protein Foods,* Vol. 2, Altschul, A. M., Ed., Academic Press, New York, 1976, 52—59.

275. Wendorff, W. L., Amundson, C. H., and Olson, N. F., The effect of heat treatment of milk upon the hydrolysability of lactose of enzyme lactase, *J. Milk Food Technol.,* 33, 377—379, 1970.

276. Whey Products Institute, U.S. Department of Agriculture/Production of Certain Whey Products, January-December 1974, Whey Products Institute, Chicago, Ill., 1975.

277. Wierzbicki, L. E. and Kosikowski, F. V., Food syrups from acid whey treated with beta-galactosidase of *Aspergillus niger, J. Dairy Sci.,* 56, 1182—1184, 1973.

278. Wingerd, W. H., Lactalbumin Phosphates and a Process of Production, Canadian Patent 790,580, July 23, 1968.

279. Wingerd, W. H., Lactalbumin as a food ingredient, *J. Dairy Sci.,* 54, 1234—1236, 1971.

280. Winkelmann, F., *Imitation Milk and Imitation Milk Products,* Food and Agricultural Organization of the United Nations, Rome, 1974.

281. Wong, N. P. and Parks, O. W., New high-protein from milk, *J. Dairy Sci.,* 53, 978—979, 1970.

282. Woodard, J. C., Short, D. D., Alvarez, M. R., and Reyniers, J., Biological effects of N$^\epsilon$-(DL-2-amino-2-carboxyethyl)-L-lysine, lysinoalanine, in *Protein Nutritional Quality in Foods and Feeds,* Vol. 1, Part 2, Friedman, M., Ed., Marcel Dekker, New York, 1975.

283. Zall, R. R., Goldsmith, R. L., Goldstein, D. J., and Horton, B. S., Membrane Processing of 300,000 Pounds per Day Cottage Cheese Whey for Pollution Abatement, Phase II, Presented at Water Quality Eng. for Industry, 64th Annu. Meet. Am. Inst. Chem. Engineers, San Francisco, Calif., November 28 to December 2, 1971.

# CEREAL BY-PRODUCTS: WHEAT AND RICE

## R. M. Saunders

## INTRODUCTION

Man does not consume cereal grain to any great extent in the form in which it is harvested from the field. Normally the grain is dehulled and then milled further into an endosperm fraction (e.g., wheat flour or white rice) and a bran or by-product fraction. In carrying out this refining process, vast quantities of foodstuffs in the form of by-products are diverted from man's immediate consumption to animal feed, or to fertilizer and fuel. The situation is worsened by the fact that the by-product invariably contains higher percentages of superior quality protein, vitamins, and trace minerals compared to the refined materials traditionally consumed as food. The magnitude of production and potential to be derived from cereal by-products is evident from Table 1.

The purpose of this chapter is to briefly summarize available data underlining the nutritive quality of cereal by-products and of potential food-grade materials obtainable through processing these by-products.

## WHEAT*

When the grain is milled to produce flour, a series of roller mills and sifters are used to separate the flour, which comprises at least 72% of the wheat kernel. The remaining percentage of the kernel is termed "wheat millfeed". Different mill streams may be combined to make a series of products of varying composition as follows:

**Wheat bran** — A mixture of the coarse, outer covering of the wheat kernel, flour, and some fine-ground weed seeds and other nonwheat material. About 50% of total millfeed production is comprised of bran.

**Wheat middlings** — The layer of the wheat kernel just inside the outer bran covering, flour, bran particles, ground weed seeds, and other nonwheat materials. About 45% of total millfeed production is taken off the mill as middlings (or midds), but this can be increased to about 98% by addition of "red dog" and finely ground bran.

**Wheat millrun** — the complete nonflour fraction.

**Wheat shorts** — produced mainly in the Southwest, which confines its millfeeds to a combination of shorts and bran at a 40:60 ratio. Shorts contain more flour than midds.

**Red dog** — Consists of fine particles of wheat bran, germ, and flour, and contains more flour than other millfeeds. About 4% of total millfeed production is red dog.

**Wheat germ meal** — The embryonic plant within the kernel, it can be separated out during the milling process at about 2% of millfeed production. Commercial germ can be obtained by removal of these ingredients.

The composition of millfeed products can be modified by changing the milling and sifting characteristics of the process. However, typical millfeed standards are maintained; these are listed in Table 2.

The Millers National Federation has provided a very comprehensive study of nine different wheats and their milling fractions.[1] These data have been summarized in tabular form (Tables 3 to 6); the mean values for the nine wheats are listed here.

---

* For a more in-depth review of wheat by-products, the reader is referred to References 1, 19, and 20.

Table 1

WORLD PRODUCTION OF CEREAL
GRAINS AND ESTIMATION OF
MILLING BY-PRODUCTS AND THEIR
PROTEIN CONTENT, 1978[21]

Million Metric Tons

| Cereal | Whole grain | Milling by-products[a] | Protein in by-products |
|---|---|---|---|
| Wheat | 439 | 88 | 13 |
| Rice | 385 | 31 | 5 |
| Corn | 383 | NA[a] | NA[a] |
| Barley | 184 | NA | NA |
| Oats | 51 | NA | NA |
| Rye | 30 | NA | NA |
| Sorghum | NA | NA | NA |

*Note:* NA = Not available.

[a]    Excluding hulls.

Table 2

TYPICAL MILLFEED STANDARDS[1]

| Product | Minimum protein (%) | Minimum fat (%) | Maximum fiber (%) |
|---|---|---|---|
| Bran | 13.5 | 2.5 | 12.0 |
| Germ | 25.0 | 7.0 | 4.0 |
| Middlings | 14.0 | 3.0 | 9.5 |
| Millrun | 14.0 | 3.0 | 9.5 |
| Red dog | 15.0 | 2.0 | 4.0 |
| Shorts | 15.0 | 3.5 | 7.0 |

Table 3

PROXIMATE PERCENT ANALYSIS OF WHEAT BY-PRODUCTS[1]

| By-product | Moisture | Protein (N × 6.25) | Crude Fat | Crude fiber | Ash | Starch | Sugars[3] |
|---|---|---|---|---|---|---|---|
| Bran | 11.8 | 15.1 | 3.4 | 10.2 | 6.4 | 9.0 | 15.5 |
| Shorts | 12.2 | 16.7 | 5.0 | 6.4 | 3.8 | 22.2 | 6.7 |
| Red dog | 12.3 | 15.1 | 3.2 | 2.3 | 2.1 | 43.3 | 4.6 |
| Germ | 12.1 | 24.8 | 8.0 | 3.2 | 4.1 | 20.8 | 16.6 |

### Protein

Values for digestibility,[2] protein efficiency ratio (PER),[3] and relative nutritive value[4] measured in rat studies for wheat milling fractions are listed in Table 7. For comparative purposes, the values for flour are included. The amino acid compositions are listed in Table 4.

### Carbohydrates

Excluding the starch and sugar contents listed in Table 2, the balance of the carbo-

Table 4
## AMINO ACID COMPOSITION OF WHEAT BY-PRODUCTS[4]

| Amino acids | By-product (g/16 g N) | | | |
|---|---|---|---|---|
| | Bran | Shorts | Red dog | Germ |
| Lysine | 3.90 | 4.89 | 3.70 | 5.98 |
| Histidine | 2.82 | 2.69 | 2.46 | 2.65 |
| Arginine | 7.10 | 7.33 | 6.23 | 7.54 |
| Aspartic acid | 7.43 | 7.88 | 6.21 | 8.47 |
| Threonine | 3.22 | 3.60 | 3.22 | 3.90 |
| Serine | 4.40 | 4.56 | 4.69 | 4.46 |
| Glutanic acid | 18.59 | 18.50 | 25.86 | 16.21 |
| Proline | 5.72 | 5.80 | 7.82 | 5.04 |
| Glycine | 5.87 | 5.71 | 4.73 | 5.78 |
| Alanine | 5.02 | 5.57 | 4.52 | 6.03 |
| Cystine | 2.43 | 2.26 | 2.45 | 1.91 |
| Valine | 4.56 | 4.90 | 4.54 | 4.62 |
| Methionine | 1.48 | 1.65 | 1.63 | 1.80 |
| Isoleucine | 3.03 | 3.32 | 3.32 | 3.31 |
| Leucine | 6.01 | 6.44 | 6.62 | 6.38 |
| Tyrosine | 2.86 | 2.93 | 2.92 | 2.86 |
| Phenylalanine | 3.80 | 3.97 | 4.25 | 3.78 |

Table 5
## MINERAL COMPOSITION OF WHEAT BY-PRODUCTS[a,1]

| Component | By-product | | | |
|---|---|---|---|---|
| | Bran | Shorts | Red dog | Germ |
| Ash (%) | 6.4 | 3.8 | 2.1 | 4.1 |
| Ca (%) | 0.086 | 0.076 | 0.043 | 0.049 |
| P (%) | 1.3 | 0.79 | 0.47 | 0.86 |
| K (%) | 1.5 | 0.92 | 0.49 | 1.0 |
| Na (%) | 0.021 | 0.016 | 0.012 | 0.021 |
| Mg (%) | 0.50 | 0.25 | 0.13 | 0.23 |
| Zn (ppm) | 111 | 107 | 63 | 116 |
| Fe (ppm) | 86 | 63 | 41 | 46 |
| Mn (ppm) | 105 | 116 | 56 | 117 |
| Cu (ppm) | 12 | 12 | 6.1 | 8.8 |
| Se (ppm) | 0.33 | 0.38 | 0.29 | 0.32 |
| B (ppm) | 4.5 | 3.6 | 2.1 | 4.9 |
| Sr (ppm) | 3.2 | 2.8 | 0.78 | 2.0 |
| Al (ppm) | 5.8 | 5.8 | 5.0 | 5.3 |
| Ba (ppm) | 19.3 | 12.6 | 5.1 | 7.3 |
| Co (ppm) | 0.10 | 0.10 | 0.12 | 0.11 |

[a]   Values reported on 14% moisture basis.

hydrate fraction in wheat milling by-products is comprised of cellulose and hemicellulose (including pentosans), in approximately a 1:1 ratio.[5] Bran sugars include, in descending order of concentration, sucrose, raffinose, neokestose, fructans, fructosylraffinose, stachyose, and monosaccharides (glucose, fructose, xylose, and arabrinose).[6] The sugars in germ in descending concentration are sucrose, raffinose, fructose, glucose, and melibiose.[7]

Table 6

VITAMIN COMPOSITION OF WHEAT
BY-PRODUCTS[a,1]

| | By-product (µg/g) | | | |
|---|---|---|---|---|
| Vitamin | Bran | Shorts | Red dog | Germ |
| Niacin | 298 | 108 | 42 | 75 |
| Pantothenic acid | 32.1 | 23.8 | 13.0 | 21.9 |
| Folic acid | 1.1 | 1.6 | 0.7 | 2.1 |
| Thiamine | 6.1 | 19.7 | 23.2 | 21.8 |
| Riboflavin | 4.9 | 4.8 | 2.5 | 5.8 |
| Pyridoxine | 8.3 | 7.0 | 4.8 | 11.7 |
| Alpha-tocopherol | 24.1 | 59.2 | 31.2 | 132 |
| Betaine | 4810 | 4368 | 3546 | 4827 |
| Choline | 2113 | 2027 | 1603 | 3002 |

[a]   Values reported on 14% moisture basis.

Table 7

RELATIVE NUTRITIVE VALUE,
PROTEIN EFFICIENCY RATIO (PER),
AND DIGESTIBILITY OF WHEAT
BY-PRODUCT PROTEIN[3,4]

| By-product | Relative nutritive value[a] | PER[b] | Protein digestibility (%)[c] |
|---|---|---|---|
| Bran | 49 ± 3 | 1.61 | 73 |
| Shorts | 55 ± 3 | 1.91 | 77 |
| Red dog | 60 ± 3 | 1.95 | 85 |
| Germ | 80 ± 5 | 2.16 | 87 |
| Flour | 23 ± 4 | 0.87 | 93 |

[a]   Relative nutritive value is expressed as percentage of
      the nutritive value of lactalbumin ± the standard er-
      ror.
[b]   Corrected to casein = 2.50.
[c]   Corrected for metabolic N excretion.

## Lipids

The composition and distribution of lipid classes identified in bran and germ are
listed in Table 8. The fatty acid composition of the total lipid and the glycerides from
wheat bran and germ are shown in Table 9.

## Food-Grade Materials from Wheat Milling By-Products

Only small quantities of by-products find direct food application; the bulk of by-
products is customarily used for animal feeds. The recognized exceptions would be
germ and bran in food items such as breakfast cereals. With some success, efforts have
been directed toward recovering food-grade materials from wheat by-products. Dry
milling and classifying wheat bran or shorts has yielded concentrates that are used in
exports to developing countries.[8] The yield and composition of the concentrate can be
varied somewhat; a typical example is shown in Table 10. The PER value of this ma-

Table 8
## LIPIDS DISTRIBUTION IN WHEAT FRACTIONS

| Lipid class | Bran (%) | Germ (%) |
|---|---|---|
| Hydrocarbons, sterylesters | 0.5 | 3.7 |
| Triglycerides | 56.1 | 57.0 |
| Fatty acids, sterols, mono- and diglycerides | 25.1 | 17.8 |
| Phospho- and glycolipids | 22.5 | 16.5 |

From Mecham, D. K., in *Wheat: Chemistry and Technology,* Pomeranz, Y., Ed., American Association of Cereal Chemists, St. Paul, Minn., 1971, 403. With permission.

Table 9
## FATTY ACID COMPOSITION IN WHEAT BY-PRODUCTS

| Fatty acid methyl esters | Total lipid | | Triglyceride | |
|---|---|---|---|---|
| | Bran (%) | Germ (%) | Bran (%) | Germ (%) |
| Myristate | Trace | Trace | Trace | Trace |
| Palmitate | 18.3 | 18.5 | 17.9 | 19.4 |
| Palmitoleate | 0.9 | 0.7 | 0.7 | 0.8 |
| Stearate | 1.1 | 0.4 | 0.8 | 0.5 |
| Oleate | 20.9 | 17.3 | 20.3 | 19.6 |
| Linoleate | 57.7 | 57.0 | 56.2 | 52.5 |
| Linolenate | 1.3 | 5.2 | 2.9 | 4.5 |
| Arachidate | Trace | Trace | 0.7 | 0.5 |
| Others | Trace | 0.8 | 0.8 | 2.4 |

From Mecham, D. K., in *Wheat: Chemistry and Technology,* Pomeranz, Y., Ed., American Association of Cereal Chemists, St. Paul, Minn., 1971, 405. With permission.

Table 10
## YIELD AND COMPOSITION OF FLOUR PRODUCED BY MILLING AND SIFTING WHEAT SHORTS[18]

| Yield (%) | Protein (N × 6.25) (%) | Crude fat (%) | Crude flour (%) | Ash (%) |
|---|---|---|---|---|
| 34.5 | 26.4 | 7.0 | 3.0 | 4.1 |

terial [commercially termed wheat protein concentrate (WPC), or concentrated wheat protein (CWP)] is about 1.9 compared to casein at 2.5, and it is superior to that of regular wheat flour (∼0.8). Compared to the original by-product, the concentrate contains more starch, protein, fat, thiamine, folic acid, and choline but less riboflavin, pantothenic acid, niacin, vitamin $B_6$, and crude fiber.

Table 11
YIELD AND COMPOSITION OF PROTEIN
CONCENTRATES FROM WHEAT MILLING BY-
PRODUCTS BY WET EXTRACTION AT DIFFERENT
pH[9]

| Substrate | pH | Yield (%) | Protein (%) | Fat (%) | Fiber (%) | Ash (%) | Starch (%) |
|---|---|---|---|---|---|---|---|
| Shorts | 8 | 20 | 35 | 7 | 0.4 | 5 | — |
| | 9 | 22 | 35 | 11 | 0.4 | 4 | 36 |
| | 10 | 25 | 41 | 11 | 0.3 | 4 | 38 |
| Millrun | 8 | 18 | 27 | 8 | 0.8 | 5 | 49 |
| | 9 | 20 | 26 | 7 | 0.8 | 4 | 48 |
| | 9 | | | | | | |
| Bran | 9 | 13 | 35 | 10 | 0.8 | 7 | 41 |
| Shorts[a] | 8.6 | 11 | 65 | 18 | 0.5 | 4 | — |
| Shorts (defatted)[a] | — | 10 | 80 | 1 | 0.4 | 4 | — |
| Millrun[a] | 8.6 | 8 | 64 | 19 | 0.4 | 5 | — |

[a]   Starch removed during process.

Table 12
PERCENT COMPOSITION OF RICE MILLING BY-
PRODUCTS[a,3]

| By-products | Protein | Fat | Ash | Fiber | Carbohydrate |
|---|---|---|---|---|---|
| Rice bran | 14.7 | 17.5 | 11.5 | 12.7 | 43.6 |
| Rice polish | 13.4 | 14.2 | 8.4 | 2.7 | 61.3 |
| Rice germ | 21.3 | 21.3 | 9.1 | 13.0 | 35.3 |
| Defatted rice bran[c] | 18.3 | 5.4 | 8.6 | 11.2 | 56.5 |

[a]   Moisture-free basis.
[b]   N × 5.95.
[c]   Commercial product.

Another procedure, though not commercial, can be employed to recover potential food-grade materials from wheat by-products. Mild alkaline extraction followed by precipitation of extracted protein, fat, and other nutrients can provide products with the composition listed in Table 11.[9]

RICE*

In commercial milling of rice, dried paddy is first dehulled to produce brown rice. The hulls have poor nutritive value even for ruminant animals, and it is unlikely that hulls would ever find use as food supplements. Depending on location, the crude bran fraction is disposed for animal feed as is or classified during the milling operation to yield bran, germ, and polish. Germ is sold as a superior-grade animal feed, whereas polish is used in baby foods in the U.S. The actual quantities of germ and polish produced in the world are a meager fraction of the potential quantities. In the U.S., for example, germ is not fractionated from the bran.

Typical compositions for rice milling by-products are listed in Table 12. The amino

* For a more in depth review of rice by-products the reader is referred to References 16 and 17.

Table 13

AMINO ACID COMPOSITION
OF RICE BY-PRODUCTS

| | By-product (g/16 g N) | | |
|---|---|---|---|
| Amino acid | Bran | Polish | Germ |
| Lysine | 4.78 | 4.66 | 4.27 |
| Histidine | 2.73 | 2.70 | 1.48 |
| Arginine | 8.47 | 8.19 | 6.28 |
| Aspartic acid | 8.65 | 8.83 | 9.01 |
| Threonine | 3.77 | 3.52 | 3.50 |
| Serine | 4.71 | 4.50 | 4.96 |
| Glutamic acid | 13.53 | 14.60 | 14.56 |
| Proline | 4.24 | 3.81 | 7.70 |
| Glycine | 5.49 | 5.05 | 4.33 |
| Alanine | 6.24 | 5.87 | 5.27 |
| Cystine | 2.27 | 2.57 | 1.19 |
| Valine | 6.07 | 5.57 | 5.26 |
| Methionine | 2.36 | 2.78 | 2.88 |
| Isoleucine | 3.96 | 3.80 | 3.49 |
| Leucine | 6.97 | 6.97 | 7.70 |
| Tyrosine | 3.17 | 3.39 | 4.70 |
| Phenylala-nine | 4.50 | 4.18 | 4.93 |

Reproduced from *Nutritional Properties of Rice,* pages 13 and 17, With the permission of the National Academy of Sciences, Washington, D.C., 1970.

Table 14

MINERAL CONTENTS OF RICE
BRAN AND POLISH[10]

| | By-product (mg/100 g) | |
|---|---|---|
| Mineral | Bran | Polish |
| Calcium | 25—275 | 9—91 |
| Iron | 13—53 | 10—28 |
| Magnesium | 977—1230 | 568—759 |
| Phosphorus | 1480—2100 | 1770—2440 |
| Potassium | 1365—2270 | 950—1110 |
| Sodium | 23—29 | 6—21 |
| Zinc | 8 | 5—8 |

acid, mineral, vitamin and fatty acid compositions for rice by-products are listed in Tables 13 to 16.

## Protein

Values for digestibility and PER[3] measured in rat feeding studies for rice-milling by-products are listed in Table 17. The quality of rice by-product protein is generally higher than that in other whole cereals or by-products derived from these cereals.

## Carbohydrates

The distribution of cellulose in brown rice is 62% in bran, 4% in germ, 7% in polish,

Table 15

VITAMIN CONTENTS OF RICE BY-
PRODUCTS

| | By-product (mg/100 g) | | |
|---|---|---|---|
| Constituent | Rice bran | Rice polish | Rice germ |
| Thiamine | 2.26 | 1.84 | 6.5 |
| Riboflavin | 0.25 | 0.18 | 0.5 |
| Niacin | 29.8 | 28.2 | 3.3 |
| Pyridoxine | 2.5 | 2.0 | 1.6 |
| Pantothenic acid | 2.8 | 3.3 | 3.0 |
| Folic acid | 0.15 | 0.19 | 0.43 |
| Inositol | 463 | 454 | 373 |
| Choline | 170 | 102 | 300 |
| Biotin | 0.06 | 0.057 | 0.058 |

Reproduced from *Nutritional Properties of Rice,* pages 13 and 17, with the permission of the National Academy of Sciences, Washington, D.C., 1970.

Table 16

FATTY ACID
COMPOSITION OF
BRAN LIPIDS[17]

| Fatty acid | Percent range |
|---|---|
| Myristic | 0.1— 0.3 |
| Palmitic | 12.3—20.5 |
| Palmitoleic | 0.1— 0.2 |
| Stearic | 1.1— 3.0 |
| Oleic | 37.1—52.8 |
| Linoleic | 27.0—40.7 |
| Linolenic | 0.5— 1.4 |
| Arachidic | 0.3— 0.7 |
| Behenic | 0.5— 1.0 |
| Lignoceric | 0.4— 0.9 |

Table 17

PROTEIN EFFICIENCY RATIO (PER)
AND DIGESTIBILITY OF RICE BY-
PRODUCTS[3]

| By-product | PER[a] | Protein digestibility[b] |
|---|---|---|
| Bran | 1.59 | 58 |
| Defatted bran | 2.07 | 71 |
| Polish | — | — |
| Germ | 1.74 | 84 |

[a]   Corrected to casein = 2.50.
[b]   Corrected for metabolic N excretion.

Table 18

YIELD, COMPOSITION, AND PROTEIN EFFICIENCY RATIO (PER) OF
PROTEIN CONCENTRATES DERIVED BY ALKALINE EXTRACTION OF
FULL-FAT AND DEFATTED RICE BRAN[14]

| Source of concentrate | Dry weight basis (%) | | | | | | |
|---|---|---|---|---|---|---|---|
| | Yield | Protein[a] | Fat | Fiber | Ash | Starch | PER[b] |
| Full-fat bran | | | | | | | |
| (1) | ca. 19 | 24 | 33 | 0.7 | 12 | 23 | 1.99 |
| (2)[c] | ca. 12 | 35 | 52 | 0.4 | 5 | — | 2.37 |
| Defatted bran | | | | | | | |
| (1) | ca. 19 | 34 | 8 | 1.6 | 17 | 26 | — |
| (2) | ca. 12 | 72 | 11 | 0.6 | 5 | — | 2.24 |

[a]  N-5.95.
[b]  Corrected to PER 2.50 for casein.
[c]  Starch removed during procedure.

and 27% in dehulled white rice; whereas the distribution of hemicelluloses is 43% in bran, 8% in germ, 7% in polish, and 42% in milled rice.[10] Water-soluble bran hemicelluloses contain mainly arabinose and xylose in the ratio 1.8, with a trace of galactose. The alkali-soluble bran hemicelluloses contain 37% arabinose, 34% xylose, 11% galactose, 9% uronic acid, and a trace of glucose.[10] Commercial rice bran contains about 8% sugars, comprised of sucrose ($\sim$80%), raffinose, and oligosaccharides.[3]

## LIPIDS[11]

Solvent extraction of oil from rice bran is the most important process in recovering food-grade material from rice milling by-products; but it is practiced only limitedly worldwide. The potential world supply is about 4.2 million metric tons, though current production is probably less than 5% of this potential. Processing, properties, composition, and uses are described elsewhere.[11]

### Food-Grade Materials from Rice Milling By-Products*

Oil recovered from rice bran and germ find use as edible food. Small quantities of polish and (reportedly) defatted rice bran are other by-products that find food usage. Consumption of raw bran is limited mainly because of rapid rancidification of the lipid fraction, as well as the presence of hull fragments.

Edible food items could conceivably be prepared from rice by-products by treating the bran to retard lipid deterioration and destroy growth inhibitors.[12] Alternatively, separation of high-protein, low-fiber fractions from raw or heated bran by air-classification[13] or aqueous procedures[14] could potentially yield food-grade materials from bran. Examples of these products ("protein concentrates") that are recoverable from rice bran are listed in Table 18. Conversion of or incorporation of these nutritionally rich materials into foods is not yet documented.

---

*  For a more in-depth review of rice oil, the reader is referred to Reference 11 and other references therein.

# REFERENCES

1. Anon., *Millfeed Manual,* Millers National Federation, Chicago, Ill., 1972.
2. Saunders, R. M. and Kohler, G. O., In vitro determination of protein digestibility in wheat millfeeds for monogastric animals, *Cereal Chem.,* 49, 98-103, 1972.
3. Saunders, R. M., unpublished data, Western Regional Research Center, Albany, Calif., 1970-1976.
4. Miladi, S., Hegsted, D. M., Saunders, R. M., and Kohler, G. O., The relative nutritive value, amino acid content, and digestibility of the proteins of wheat mill fractions, *Cereal Chem.,* 49, 119-127, 1972.
5. Fraser, J. R. and Holmes, D. C., Proximate analysis of wheat flour carbohydrates. IV. Analysis of whole meal flour and some of its fractions, *J. Sci. Food Agric.,* 10, 506-512, 1959.
6. Saunders, R. M. and Walker, H. G., The sugars of wheat bran, *Cereal Chem.,* 46, 85-92, 1969.
7. Linko, P., Cheng, Y., and Milner, M., Changes in the soluble carbohydrates during browning of wheat embryos, *Cereal Chem.,* 37, 548-556, 1960.
8. Fellers, D. A., U.S. Wheat products in world feeding; in *Wheat: Production and Utilization,* Inglett, G. E., Ed., AVI Publishing, Westport, Conn., 1974, 464-483.
9. Saunders, R. M., Connor, M. A., Edwards, R. H., and Kohler, G. O., Preparation of protein concentrates from wheat shorts and wheat millrun by a wet alkaline process, *Cereal Chem.,* 52, 93-101, 1975.
10. Juliano, B. O., The Rice Caryopsis and its composition, in *Rice: Chemistry and Technology,* Houston, D. F., Ed., American Association of Cereal Chemists, St. Paul, Minn., 1972, 16-74.
11. Houston, D. F., Rice bran and polish, in *Rice: Chemistry and Technology,* Houston, D. F., Ed., American Association of Cereal Chemists, St. Paul, Minn., 1972.
12. Barber, S., Bendito de Barber, C., Flores, M. J., and Montes, J. J., Toxic Constituents of Rice Bran. I. Trypsin Inhibitor Activity of Raw and Heat-Treated Bran; and II. Hemagglutinating Activity of Raw and Heat-Treated Bran, 60th Annu. Meet., American Association of Cereal Chemists, St. Louis, Mo., 1975; *Cereal Foods World,* 20(Abstr.), 442, 1975.
13. Houston, D. F. and Mohammad, A., Air-classification and sieving of rice bran and polish, *Rice J.,* 69, 20-21, 1966.
14. Connor, M. A., Saunders, R. M., and Kohler, G. O., Rice bran protein concentrates prepared by wet extraction, *Cereal Chem.,* 53, 488-496, 1976.
15. Mecham, D. K., Lipids, in *Wheat: Chemistry and Technology,* Pomeranz, Y., Ed., American Association of Cereal Chemists, St. Paul, Minn., 1971, 393-405.
16. Houston, D. F., Ed., *Rice: Chemistry and Technology,* American Association of Cereal Chemists, St. Paul, Minn., 1972.
17. Houston, D. F. and Kohler, G. O., *Nutritional Properties of Rice,* National Academy of Sciences, Washington, D.C., 1970.
18. Fellers, D. A., Shephard, A. D., Bellard, N. J., and Mossman, A. P., Protein concentrates by dry milling of wheat millfeeds, *Cereal Chem.,* 43, 715-725, 1966.
19. Pomeranz, Y., Ed., *Wheat: Chemistry and Technology,* American Association of Cereal Chemists, St. Paul, Minn., 1971.
20. Inglett, G. E., Ed., *Wheat: Production and Utilization,* AVI Publishing, Westport, Conn., 1974.
21. USDA, Agricultural Statistics, U.S. Department of Agriculture, Washington, D.C., 1976.

# AQUATIC VASCULAR PLANT FOODS

## B. C. Wolverton and Rebecca C. McDonald

## INTRODUCTION

Research efforts on the nutritional quality of vascular aquatic plants under controlled environmental conditions has been very limited to date. Most of the data in this area have been determined on plants that were collected from natural lakes and ponds. The climate and nutrient content of these aquatic systems were highly variable. In general, the nutritional quality of the plants is a reflection of the conditions under which they were grown. Current research on utilizing vascular aquatic plants to remove nutrients from domestic sewage lagoons has revealed that the crude protein, phosphorus, and other essential elements content of the plants can be improved and consistently maintained at a high level.

In the data following, the nutritional quality of some common vascular aquatic plants has been compiled. A small part on the nutritional value of leaf protein extracts has also been included. All of the information was collected on plants grown on lakes and ponds, unless otherwise noted.

Crude protein was calculated as Kjeldahl nitrogen × 6.25. Carbohydrate was calculated as the difference between 100% and the sum of the percentages of protein, fat, and ash.

# NUTRITIONAL COMPOSITION OF VASCULAR AQUATIC MACROPHYTES

## Table 1
### PROXIMATE COMPOSITION

| Species | Water | Crude protein | Fat | Ash | Carbohydrates | Crude fiber | Cellulose | Tannin | Caloric content (kcal/g) | Ref. |
|---|---|---|---|---|---|---|---|---|---|---|
| Alternanthera philoxerides | 85.5 | 15.6 | 2.68 | 13.9 | 67.82 | — | 21.3 | 1.2 | 3.46 | 2 |
| | — | 19.0 | — | 18.39 | — | — | — | — | — | 3 |
| Aphanizomenon flos-aquae | — | 17.94 | — | 14.72 | — | — | — | — | — | 8 |
| | — | 53.56 | — | 7.21 | — | — | — | — | — | 3 |
| Brasenia schreberi | 89.6 | 12.5 | 4.71 | 8.8 | 73.99 | — | 23.7 | 11.8 | 3.79 | 2 |
| Cabomba caroliniana | 93.0 | 13.1 | 5.42 | 9.6 | 71.88 | — | 26.8 | 15.6 | 3.78 | 2 |
| Ceratophyllum demersum | 94.8 | 21.7 | 5.97 | 20.6 | 51.73 | — | 27.9 | 1.9 | 3.71 | 2 |
| Chara sp. | — | 15.38 | — | 43.41 | — | — | — | — | — | 3 |
| Eichhornia crassipes | 94.0 | 22.85 | 2.12 | 17.75 | 57.28 | 18.3 | — | — | — | 16 |
| | — | 16.31 | — | 15.93 | — | — | — | — | — | 3 |
| | 91.1 | 9.6 | — | — | — | — | — | — | — | 14 |
| | — | 16.50 | — | 18.11 | — | — | — | — | — | 8 |
| | — | 14.94 | — | — | — | — | — | — | — | 9 |
| E. crassipes (leaves) | 84.2 | 10.7 | 2.7 | 14.7 | 71.9 | 17.0 | — | — | — | 14 |
| E. crassipes (leaves)[a] | — | 32.88 | 2.30 | 11.75 | 53.07 | 13.7 | — | — | — | 16 |
| E. crassipes (stalks)[a] | — | 18.88 | 1.79 | 17.85 | 61.48 | 22.4 | — | — | — | 16 |
| E. crassipes (roots)[a] | — | 22.94 | 1.39 | 19.15 | 56.52 | 17.8 | — | — | — | 16 |
| Eleocharis acicularis | 88.9 | 12.5 | 3.59 | 9.9 | 74.01 | — | 27.9 | 2.0 | 3.91 | 2 |
| Elodea canadensis | — | 26.81 | — | 21.87 | — | — | — | — | — | 3 |
| Elodea densa | 90.2 | 20.5 | 3.27 | 22.1 | 54.13 | — | 29.2 | 0.8 | 3.35 | 2 |
| Hydrilla sp. | 92.0 | 18.0 | 3.80 | 28.0 | 50.20 | — | 32.0 | — | 3.40 | 6 |
| Hydrochloa carolinensis | 80.6 | 10.4 | 2.78 | 6.1 | 80.72 | — | 22.0 | 0.8 | 4.10 | 2 |
| Hydrocotyle ranunculoides | 95.8 | 22.4 | 2.19 | 17.4 | 46.21 | 11.8 | — | — | — | 16 |
| Hydrodictyon reticulatum | — | 24.19 | — | 17.94 | — | — | — | — | — | 3 |
| Hydrolea quadrivalvis | 89.0 | 11.1 | 3.85 | 9.3 | 75.75 | — | 22.8 | 2.9 | 4.00 | 2 |
| Hydrotrida caroliniana | 93.6 | 9.7 | 3.85 | 22.7 | 63.75 | — | 29.5 | 2.5 | 3.32 | 2 |

|  |  |  |  |  |  |  |  |  |  | n |
|---|---|---|---|---|---|---|---|---|---|---|
| *Jussiaea decurrens* | 88.2 | 19.1 | 3.93 | 11.7 | 65.27 | — | 29.5 | 4.1 | 3.88 | 2 |
| *J. diffusa* | 86.9 | 10.7 | 3.76 | 11.1 | 74.44 | — | 24.2 | 12.6 | 3.68 | 2 |
| *J. peruviana* | 81.5 | 9.4 | 7.10 | 7.8 | 75.70 | — | 27.5 | 15.6 | 3.89 | 2 |
| *Justicia americana* | 85.0 | 22.9 | 3.40 | 17.4 | 56.30 | — | 25.9 | 1.8 | 3.98 | 8 |
|  |  | 12.63 | — | 16.07 | — | — | — | — | — |  |
| *Lemna minor* | — | 15.94 | — | 18.71 | — | — | — | — | — | 3 |
| *Lemna* sp.[b] | 90.0 | 17.0 | 3.0 | 17.6 | 62.40 | 10.2 | — | — | — | 12 |
| *Microcystis aeruginosa* | — | 50.50 | — | 6.20 | — | — | — | — | — | 3 |
| *Mougeotia* sp. | — | 11.06 | — | 14.54 | — | — | — | — | — | 3 |
| *Myriophyllum brasiliense* | 86.3 | 14.1 | 3.78 | 11.2 | 70.92 | — | 20.6 | 11.9 | 3.69 | 2 |
| *M. heterophyllum* | 90.0 | 8.5 | 2.67 | 15.5 | 73.33 | — | 32.7 | 3.2 | 3.35 | 2 |
| *M. spicatum* | 87.2 | 9.8 | 1.81 | 40.6 | 47.79 | — | 18.8 | 3.2 | 2.47 | 2 |
| *Najas flexilis* | — | 11.63 | — | 19.16 | — | — | — | — | — | 3 |
| *N. guadalupensis* | 92.7 | 22.8 | 3.75 | 18.7 | 54.75 | — | 35.6 | 1.4 | 3.55 | 2 |
| *Nelumbo lutea* | 83.2 | 13.7 | 5.25 | 10.3 | 70.75 | — | 23.6 | 9.2 | 3.74 | 2 |
| *Nuphar advena* | 88.0 | 20.6 | 6.25 | 6.5 | 66.65 | — | 23.9 | 6.5 | 4.30 | 2 |
| *Nymphaea odorata* | 86.3 | 16.6 | 5.38 | 9.2 | 68.82 | — | 20.7 | 15.0 | 3.95 | 2 |
| *Nymphoides aquaticum* | 89.7 | 9.3 | 3.29 | 7.6 | 79.81 | — | 37.4 | 2.9 | 3.95 | 2 |
| *Orontium aguaticum* | 86.8 | 19.8 | 7.85 | 14.1 | 85.90 | — | 23.9 | 3.3 | 3.74 | 2 |
| *Paspalum fluitans* | — | 11.94 | — | 12.71 | — | — | — | — | — | 3 |
| *Phragmites communis* | — | 11.44 | — | 5.90 | — | — | — | — | — | 3 |
| *Pistia stratiotes* | 94.1 | 16.50 | 3.75 | 21.0 | 58.75 | — | 12.0 | — | 3.50 | 5 |
| *Pithophora* sp. | — | 16.06 | — | 27.77 | — | — | — | — | — | 3 |
| *Polygonum hydropiperoides* | 80.8 | 11.9 | 2.39 | 7.8 | 77.91 | — | 26.9 | 6.8 | 4.06 | 2 |
| *P. pensylvanicum* | 76.1 | 10.3 | 2.77 | 7.4 | 79.53 | — | 23.1 | 6.8 | 3.90 | 2 |
| *P. sagittatum* | 85.0 | 11.0 | 2.99 | 8.0 | 78.01 | — | 31.2 | 5.9 | 4.01 | 2 |
| *Potamogeton crispus* | 88.2 | 10.9 | 2.85 | 16.0 | 70.25 | — | 37.2 | 7.2 | 3.61 | 2 |
| *P. diversifolius* | 90.2 | 17.3 | 2.87 | 22.7 | 57.13 | — | 30.9 | 2.0 | 3.40 | 3 |
| *P. illinoensis* | — | 21.44 | — | 26.49 | — | — | — | — | — | 2 |
| *P. nodosus* | 84.2 | 11.2 | 3.62 | 10.9 | 74.28 | — | 21.7 | 3.4 | 3.77 | 3 |
| *Rhizoclonium* sp. | — | 19.75 | — | 17.16 | — | 10.6 | — | — | — | 3 |
| *Ricciocarpus nutans* | 91.0 | 10.6 | 1.1 | 20.6 | 67.7 | — | — | — | — | 12 |
| *Sagittaria latifolia* | 85.0 | 17.1 | 6.71 | 10.3 | 65.89 | — | 27.6 | 2.5 | 4.12 | 2 |
| *Saururus cernuus* | 78.1 | 12.1 | 6.85 | 11.3 | 69.75 | — | 25.3 | 70 | 4.28 | 2 |
| *Sparganium americanum* | 89.1 | 23.7 | 8.11 | 11.4 | 56.79 | — | 20.5 | 3.7 | 4.17 | 2 |
| *Spirodela oligorrhiza*[c] | 87.1 | 28.5 | 5.5 | 17.7 | 48.3 | 11.8 | — | — | — | 12 |
| *S. oligorrhiza*[d] | 91.1 | 37.7 | 4.7 | 11.8 | 45.8 | 7.6 | — | — | — | 12 |
| *S. oligorrhiza* | — | 31.7 | 5.2 | 11.4 | 51.7 | 8.2 | — | — | — | 15 |

# NUTRITIONAL COMPOSITION OF VASCULAR AQUATIC MACROPHYTES

## Table 1 (continued)
## PROXIMATE COMPOSITION

| Species | Water | Crude protein | Fat | Ash | Carbohydrates | Crude fiber | Cellulose | Tannin | Caloric content (kcal/g) | Ref. |
|---|---|---|---|---|---|---|---|---|---|---|
| | | | | | Dry weight (%) | | | | | |
| *S. polyrhiza*[a] | — | 39.53 | 3.40 | 12.5 | 44.57 | 15.6 | — | — | — | 16 |
| *S. polyrhiza*[f] | — | 24.88 | 3.05 | 12.0 | 60.07 | 11.8 | — | — | — | 16 |
| *Spirogyra* sp. | — | 16.88 | — | 13.33 | — | — | — | — | — | 3 |
| *Typha latifolia* | 77.1 | 10.3 | 3.91 | 6.9 | 78.89 | — | 33.2 | 2.1 | 3.69 | 2 |
| | — | 9.94 | — | 9.70 | — | — | — | — | — | 3 |
| | — | 8.56 | — | 6.75 | — | — | — | — | — | 8 |
| *Wolfia arrhiza* | 96.0 | 19.8 | 5.0 | 18.3 | 56.90 | 13.3 | — | — | — | 1 |
| *Wolfia* sp. | — | 21.5 | 5.5 | 14.5 | 58.50 | 10.6 | — | — | — | 12 |

a   Average of the analyses of plants collected from two, heavily loaded, domestic sewage lagoons.
b   Average.
c   Grown in treated waste water effluent.
d   Average of plant samples collected from anaerobic swine waste lagoon.
e   Plants collected from one, heavily loaded, domestic sewage lagoon.
f   Plants collected from natural aquatic system with low nutrient content.

## Table 2
## MINERAL COMPOSITION

| Species | P (%) | K (%) | Na (%) | Ca (%) | S (%) | Mg (%) | Fe (ppm) | Mn (ppm) | Zn (ppm) | Cu (ppm) | B (ppm) | Ref. |
|---|---|---|---|---|---|---|---|---|---|---|---|---|
| *Alternanthera philoxerides* | 0.17 | 4.56 | 0.37 | 1.43 | 0.14 | 0.31 | 720 | 440 | — | — | — | 3 |
| | 0.32 | 5.20 | 0.37 | 0.52 | 0.29 | 0.52 | 720 | 440 | 90 | 15 | — | 8 |
| *Aphanizomenon flos-aquae* | 1.17 | 0.68 | 0.19 | 0.73 | 1.18 | 0.21 | 833 | — | — | — | — | 3 |
| *Brasenia schreberi* | 0.14 | 0.99 | 0.66 | 1.79 | 0.11 | 0.26 | 500 | 265 | 267 | 32 | — | 7 |
| *Cabomba caroliniana* | — | — | — | — | 0.10 | — | — | — | — | — | — | 3 |
| *Ceratophyllum demersum* | 0.26 | 4.01 | 1.16 | 0.77 | 0.18 | 0.42 | 1,053 | 486 | 100 | 30 | — | 3 |
| | — | — | — | — | 0.30 | — | — | — | — | — | — | 7 |
| *Chara* sp. | 0.25 | 2.35 | 0.13 | 9.03 | 0.55 | 0.92 | 2,520 | — | — | — | — | 3 |
| *Eichhornia crassipes* | 0.87 | 3.12 | 1.75 | 0.65 | 0.49 | 0.26 | 1,920 | 189 | 37 | 26 | — | 16 |
| | 0.17 | 4.16 | 0.10 | 1.99 | — | 0.40 | 250 | — | — | — | — | 3 |
| | 0.43 | 4.25 | 0.34 | 1.00 | 0.33 | 1.05 | 250 | 3,940 | 50 | 11 | — | 8 |
| | 0.54 | 4.45 | 0.41 | 1.35 | 0.48 | 0.56 | 3,420 | 270 | 67 | 15 | 20 | 9 |
| *E. crassipes*[a] | 0.91 | 3.60 | 1.83 | 0.53 | 0.45 | 0.85 | 143 | 69 | 21 | 11 | — | 16 |
| *E. crassipes*[a] | 0.95 | 3.02 | 0.94 | 0.64 | 0.34 | 0.21 | 130 | 132 | 24 | 22 | — | 16 |
| *E. crassipes*[a] | 0.56 | 2.92 | 1.79 | 0.61 | 1.62 | 0.23 | 5,790 | 199 | 70 | 63 | — | 16 |
| *Eleocharis acicularis* | 0.24 | 2.86 | 0.54 | 0.53 | 0.18 | 0.33 | 2,920 | 192 | 68 | 42 | — | 3 |
| | — | — | — | — | 0.28 | — | — | — | — | — | — | 7 |
| *Eleocharis quadrangulata* | 0.10 | 1.81 | 0.12 | 0.20 | 0.15 | 0.10 | 560 | 120 | 45 | 20 | — | 7 |
| *Elodea canadensis* | 0.57 | 3.65 | 0.90 | 2.80 | 0.27 | 0.65 | 1,320 | — | — | — | — | 3 |
| *Hydrilla* sp. | 0.28 | 2.80 | — | 4.30 | 0.40 | 0.90 | — | — | — | — | — | 5 |
| *Hydrocotyle ranunculoides* | 0.42 | 3.33 | 1.34 | 0.77 | 0.31 | 0.21 | 7,490 | 357 | 59 | 12 | — | 16 |
| *Hydrodictyon reticulatum* | 0.23 | 4.21 | 0.38 | 0.69 | 1.41 | 0.17 | 1,313 | — | — | — | — | 3 |
| *Juncus effusus* | 0.27 | 0.89 | 0.40 | 0.38 | 0.26 | 0.11 | — | — | — | — | — | 7 |
| *Justicia americana* | 0.12 | 3.28 | 0.17 | 0.90 | 0.18 | 0.41 | 1,085 | 112 | 265 | 26 | — | 8 |
| | — | — | — | — | 0.13 | — | — | — | — | — | 12.1 | 3 |
| *Lemna minor* | 0.63 | 5.20 | 0.30 | 0.70 | 0.30 | 0.51 | 1,690 | 750 | — | — | — | 3 |
| *Lemna* sp. | 0.68 | 2.03 | — | 1.34 | — | 0.30 | 6,500 | 1,500 | 364 | 14 | — | 12 |
| *Microcystis aeruginosa* | 0.68 | 0.79 | 0.04 | 0.53 | 0.27 | 0.17 | 382 | 68 | — | — | — | 3 |
| *Mougeotia* sp. | 0.25 | 1.20 | 0.49 | 1.68 | 0.36 | 0.57 | 1,080 | 2,300 | — | — | — | 3 |
| *Myriophyllum brasiliense* | — | — | — | — | 0.14 | — | — | — | — | — | 23.5 | 3 |
| *M. heterophyllum* | 0.16 | 1.25 | 1.87 | 1.47 | 0.24 | 0.26 | 2,000 | 473 | 54 | 44 | — | 7 |
| *M. spicatum* | 0.42 | 1.87 | 0.75 | 2.77 | 0.43 | 0.74 | 660 | 5,130 | 30 | — | — | 3 |
| *Najas flexilis* | 0.30 | 1.82 | 0.78 | 6.11 | 0.48 | 0.97 | — | — | — | — | — | 3 |
| *N. guadalupensis* | 0.15 | 3.49 | 0.61 | 0.98 | 0.28 | 0.47 | 712 | 201 | 48 | 48 | — | 7 |
| *Nelumbo lutea* | 0.19 | 2.27 | 0.28 | 1.56 | 0.16 | 0.23 | 126 | 607 | 50 | 40 | — | 7 |
| *Nuphar advena* | 0.40 | 1.88 | 1.47 | 1.08 | 0.32 | 0.27 | 740 | 300 | 50 | 35 | — | 7 |
| *Nymphaea odorata* | 0.18 | 1.28 | 1.35 | 1.06 | 0.14 | 0.14 | 600 | 128 | 32 | 36 | — | 7 |
| *Panicum hemitonium* | 0.14 | 1.06 | 0.19 | 0.38 | 0.23 | 0.25 | 133 | 292 | 31 | 26 | — | 7 |
| *Paspalum fluitans* | 0.10 | 2.54 | 0.22 | 0.26 | 0.35 | 0.22 | — | — | — | — | — | 3 |
| *Phragmites communis* | 0.10 | 0.52 | 0.26 | 0.43 | — | 0.27 | — | — | — | — | — | 3 |
| *Pistia stratiotes* | 0.30 | 2.9 | — | 4.40 | 0.39 | 0.90 | — | — | — | — | — | 5 |
| *Pithophora* sp. | 0.30 | 3.06 | 0.07 | 3.82 | 1.42 | 0.20 | 2,836 | 929 | — | — | — | 3 |
| *Pontederia cordata* | 0.24 | 2.58 | 0.83 | 0.96 | 0.22 | 0.15 | 200 | 970 | 67 | 60 | — | 7 |
| *Pontamogeton diversifolius* | 0.27 | 3.08 | 0.44 | 1.14 | 0.50 | 0.19 | 1,240 | 160 | 60 | 36 | — | 7 |
| *Potamogeton illinoensis* | 0.12 | 2.66 | 0.19 | 2.76 | 0.20 | 0.84 | — | — | — | — | — | 3 |
| *Rhizoclonium* sp. | 0.34 | 2.37 | 0.08 | 0.60 | 0.27 | 0.19 | — | — | — | — | — | 3 |
| *Ricciocarpus nutans* | 0.20 | 1.8 | — | 0.79 | — | 0.28 | 26,800 | 9,500 | 82 | 19 | — | 12 |
| *Scirpus americanus* | 0.27 | 0.89 | 0.40 | 0.38 | 0.26 | 0.11 | — | — | — | — | — | 7 |
| *Spirodela oligorrhiza*[b] | 1.0 | 1.57 | — | 1.3 | — | 0.29 | 3,400 | 700 | 420 | 34 | — | 12 |
| *Spirodela oligorrhiza*[c] | 1.71 | 1.82 | — | 0.73 | — | 0.25 | 4,700 | 1,500 | 119 | 13 | — | 12 |
| *Spirodela polyrhiza*[b] | 1.01 | 2.13 | 0.74 | 0.88 | 0.85 | — | — | — | — | — | — | 16 |
| *Spirodela polyrhiza*[d] | 0.36 | 1.22 | 5.54 | 1.34 | 0.45 | — | — | — | — | — | — | 16 |

## Table 2 (continued)
## MINERAL COMPOSITION

| | Dry weight basis | | | | | | | | | | | |
|---|---|---|---|---|---|---|---|---|---|---|---|---|
| Species | P (%) | K (%) | Na (%) | Ca (%) | S (%) | Mg (%) | Fe (ppm) | Mn (ppm) | Zn (ppm) | Cu (ppm) | B (ppm) | Ref. |
| *Spirogyra* sp. | 0.21 | 0.95 | 1.42 | 0.70 | 0.25 | 0.38 | 1,552 | — | — | — | — | 3 |
| *Typha latifolia* | 0.21 | 2.38 | 0.38 | 0.89 | 0.13 | 0.16 | 120 | 412 | 30 | 37 | — | 8 |
| *Utricularia inflata* | 0.12 | 1.98 | 1.52 | 0.67 | 0.26 | 0.21 | 2,112 | 480 | 108 | 47 | — | 7 |
| *Wolfia* sp. | 0.97 | 3.76 | — | 0.77 | — | — | — | — | — | — | — | 12 |

[a] Average of the analyses of plants collected from two, heavily loaded, domestic sewage lagoons.
[b] Grown in treated waste water effluent.
[c] Average of plant samples collected from anaerobic swine waste lagoon.
[d] Plants collected from natural aquatic system with low nutrient content.

## Table 3
## AMINO ACID PROFILE

### Essential Amino Acids

| | | | Dry weight basis (g/100 g protein) | | | | | | | | | |
|---|---|---|---|---|---|---|---|---|---|---|---|---|
| Species | Crude protein | Actual proteins[a] | Ile | Leu | Lys | Met | Phe | Thr | Trp | Val | Ref. |
| FAO reference pattern | — | — | 4.2 | 4.8 | 4.2 | 2.2 | 2.8 | 2.8 | 1.4 | 4.2 | 10 |
| *Eichhornia crassipes*[b] | 25.94 | 19.45 | 5.51 | 9.06 | 6.25 | 1.83 | 5.46 | 4.99 | [c] | 6.00 | 5 |
| *Eichhornia crassipes* | 4.7 | — | 5.6 | 8.7 | 7.6 | 2.3 | 5.2 | 5.0 | [c] | 11.4 | 13 |
| *E. crassipes* (leaves)[d] | 31.3 | 29.81 | 4.89 | 8.68 | 5.96 | 1.47 | 5.70 | 4.56 | 1.04 | 5.83 | 17 |
| *E. crassipes* (stalks)[d] | 18.9 | 16.13 | 3.35 | 5.27 | 3.35 | 0.87 | 3.66 | 3.35 | 1.04 | 3.60 | 16 |
| *Hydrocotyle ranunculoides* | 22.40 | 20.10 | 4.93 | 8.02 | 7.22 | 0.95 | 5.28 | 4.78 | 1.43 | 5.93 | 16 |
| *Justicia americana*[e] | 17.69 | 10.76 | 4.83 | 8.08 | 5.95 | 1.30 | 5.11 | 4.92 | [c] | 5.57 | 4 |
| *J. americana*[f] | 10.19 | 5.93 | 4.55 | 7.42 | 5.90 | 1.69 | 4.89 | 5.40 | [c] | 5.90 | 4 |
| *Pistia stratiotes* | 23.03 | 17.63 | 5.21 | 9.21 | 6.93 | 1.74 | 5.79 | 5.03 | [c] | 6.31 | 5 |
| *Spirodela polyriza*[d,g] | 39.53 | 27.79 | 4.64 | 8.89 | 6.44 | 2.16 | 5.69 | 4.61 | 2.10 | 5.83 | 16 |
| *S. polyriza*[g,h] | 24.88 | 17.74 | 4.51 | 8.35 | 5.53 | 1.86 | 5.13 | 4.46 | 2.36 | 5.47 | 16 |
| *Typha latifolia* | 8.00 | — | 5.0 | 9.2 | 4.6 | 1.5 | 5.6 | 5.3 | [c] | 6.2 | 6 |

| Species | Ala | Asp | Arg | Cys | Glu | Gly | His | Pro | Ser | Tyr | Ref. |
|---|---|---|---|---|---|---|---|---|---|---|---|
| *Eichhornia crassipes*[b] | 6.95 | 14.05 | 6.08 | 0.29 | 12.48 | 6.00 | 2.16 | 4.76 | 4.71 | 3.91 | 5 |
| *E. crassipes* | 7.1 | 10.2 | 5.2 | 0.7 | 9.8 | 6.4 | 2.3 | 4.8 | 4.8 | 3.4 | 13 |
| | 5.59 | 17.37 | 2.98 | 11.60 | 9.29 | 5.14 | 1.90 | 4.73 | 4.32 | 2.98 | 14 |
| *E. crassipes*, (leaves)[d] | 6.50 | 5.49 | 12.63 | 1.37 | 11.56 | 5.39 | 2.31 | 6.30 | 4.29 | 3.55 | 17 |
| *E. crassipes*, (stalks)[d] | 4.15 | 3.10 | 35.40 | 0.76 | 11.97 | 3.66 | 1.43 | 3.84 | 3.10 | 2.29 | 16 |
| *Hdrocotyle uncodes* | 5.88 | 12.40 | 5.18 | 1.54 | 17.28 | 5.18 | 2.34 | 4.43 | 4.58 | 2.74 | 16 |
| *Justicia americana*[e] | 6.13 | 16.44 | 5.76 | 0.09 | 14.03 | 5.95 | 2.69 | 4.74 | 5.02 | 3.44 | 4 |
| *J. americana*[f] | 5.90 | 15.34 | 6.07 | 0.17 | 12.98 | 5.90 | 2.87 | 5.40 | 5.90 | 4.05 | 4 |
| *Pistia stratiotes* | 7.06 | 11.86 | 4.60 | 0.37 | 13.40 | 6.21 | 2.19 | 4.95 | 5.03 | 4.17 | 5 |
| *Spirodela polyriza*[d,g] | 6.88 | 9.68 | 7.99 | 1.66 | 12.67 | 5.94 | 2.05 | 4.61 | 4.68 | 3.53 | 16 |
| *S. polyriza*[g,h] | 7.28 | 14.72 | 6.82 | 1.30 | 13.14 | 5.58 | 1.69 | 4.57 | 4.68 | 2.59 | 16 |
| *Typha latifolia* | 6.2 | 14.5 | 5.0 | 0.1 | 15.4 | 5.8 | 2.0 | 5.2 | 5.1 | 3.3 | 6 |

[a] Sum of amino acids.
[b] Tryptophan analysis not obtained — where tryptophan omitted, author assumed tryptophan to not be present in large quantities and, therefore, the calculated compositional percentages to be reasonably accurate with this omission.
[c] Not analyzed.
[d] Plants grown in domestic sewage.
[e] Maximum protein.
[f] Minimum protein.
[g] Predominant species (small amounts of *Lemna* sp.).
[h] Plants gathered from aquatic system with low nutrient content.

## Table 4
## VITAMINS

Dry weight basis (constituents/100 g)

| Species | Thiamine HCl (B1) (mg) | Riboflavin (B2) (mg) | B$_{12}$ (µg) | Niacin bound (mg) | C (mg) | A (IU) | Pantothenic acid (mg) | Pyroxidine HCl (B6) (mg) | E (IU) | Ref. |
|---|---|---|---|---|---|---|---|---|---|---|
| U.S. RDA | 1.5 | 1.7 | 6.0 | 20.0 | 60 | 5,000 | 10.0 | 2.0 | 30 | 11 |
| *Eichhornia crassipes* | | | | | | | | | | |
| Whole plant[a] | — | — | 23.2 | — | — | — | — | — | — | 17 |
| Leaves[a] | 0.591 | 3.07 | 1.26 | 7.94 | — | 711 | 5.56 | 1.52 | 30 | 17 |
| Stalks[a] | — | — | 1.49 | — | — | — | — | — | — | 17 |
| Roots[a] | — | — | 68.2 | — | — | — | — | — | — | 17 |
| Leaf protein extract | 0.477 | 0.842 | — | 0.28 | 1.30 | — | 0.101 | 0.0613 | 14 | 16 |
| *Hydrocotyle ranunculoides* | 0.563 | 2.32 | 23.0 | 10.4 | 52.3 | 22,500 | 1.64 | — | 32.8 | 16 |
| *Spirodela polyrhiza*[a,b] | 1.38 | — | — | 13.0 | 49.0 | — | | 0.882 | — | 16 |
| *S. polyrhiza*[b,c] | 0.664 | 1.88 | 26.0 | 0.687 | 27.8 | 31,700 | — | 0.876 | — | 16 |

[a] Plants grown in domestic sewage.
[b] Predominant species, small amounts of *Lemna* sp. present.
[c] Plants collected from natural aquatic system with low nutrient content.

## NUTRITIONAL COMPOSITION OF LEAF PROTEIN EXTRACT

### Table 5
### PROXIMATE COMPOSITION OF LEAF PROTEIN EXTRACT

| Species | Crude protein | Fat | Ash | Total carbohydrate | Cellulose | Caloric content (kcal/g) | Ref. |
|---|---|---|---|---|---|---|---|
| *Alternanthera philoxerides* | 31.4 | 7.68 | 12.47 | 48.5 | 5.9 | 4.58 | 2 |
| *Eichhornia crassipes* | 57.8 | 3.94 | 4.77 | 33.5 | — | — | 16 |
| *Justicia americana* | 45.73 | 9.37 | 8.19 | 36.7 | 1.6 | 5.22 | 2 |
| *Nymphaea odorata* | 40.0 | 8.57 | 4.24 | 47.2 | 8.3 | 4.94 | 2 |
| *Orontium aquaticum* | 49. | 14.88 | 7.38 | 28.1 | 2.6 | 5.59 | 2 |
| *Sagittaria latifolia* | 42.8 | 16.62 | 4.23 | 36.4 | — | 5.42 | 2 |

Dry weight basis (%)

Table 6

AMINO ACID PROFILE OF LEAF PROTEIN EXTRACT

Dry weight (%)

| Species | Crude protein | Ala | Asp | Arg | Cys | Glu | Gly | His | Ile | Leu | Lys | Met | Phe | Pro | Ser | Thr | Trp | Tyr | Val | Ref. |
|---|---|---|---|---|---|---|---|---|---|---|---|---|---|---|---|---|---|---|---|---|
| *Alternanthera philoxerides* | 31.4 | — | — | 1.12 | — | — | — | 0.63 | — | 0.94 | 1.61 | 0.20 | Tr[a] | — | — | 0.96 | — | — | 1.37 | 2 |
| *Eichhornia crassipes* | 57.8 | 3.64 | 5.21 | 3.86 | 0.70 | 6.80 | 3.23 | 1.33 | 2.40 | 5.15 | 3.81 | 1.15 | 3.42 | 2.96 | 2.58 | 2.79 | 0.84 | 2.61 | 3.27 | 16 |
| *Justicia americana*[b] | 45.7 | — | — | 2.99 | — | — | — | 1.07 | 2.45 | 4.29 | 2.80 | 0.89 | 2.78 | — | — | 2.27 | — | — | 2.87 | 2 |
| *Nymphaea odorata* | 40.0 | — | — | 2.83 | — | — | — | 1.07 | 1.97 | 3.82 | 3.73 | 0.71 | 2.24 | — | — | 1.91 | — | — | 2.62 | 2 |
| *Orontium aquaticum* | 49.6 | — | — | 3.17 | — | — | — | 1.02 | 2.32 | 4.30 | 2.64 | 0.84 | 2.80 | — | — | 2.26 | — | — | 2.55 | 2 |
| *Sagittaria latifolia* | 42.8 | — | — | 2.14 | — | — | — | 1.14 | 1.46 | 1.87 | 1.52 | 0.56 | Tr | — | — | 1.57 | — | — | 1.80 | 2 |

[a] Tr = trace.
[b] Mean.

# REFERENCES

1. **Bhanthumnavia, K. and McGarry, M. G.**, *Wolffia arrhiza* as a possible source of inexpensive protein, *Nature (London)*, 232, 5311, 495, 1971.
2. **Boyd, C. E.**, Fresh-water plants: a potential source of protein, *Econ. Bot.*, 22(4), 359-368, 1968a.
3. **Boyd, C. E.**, Some Aspects of Aquatic Plant Ecology, in Reservoir Fishery Resources Symp., Athens, Ga., April 5-7, 1967, 114-129, 1968b.
4. **Boyd, C. E.**, Production, mineral nutrient absorption, and biochemical assimilation by *Justica americana* and *Alternanthera philoxerides*, *Arch. Hydrobiol.*, 66(2), 139-160, 1969.
5. **Boyd, C. E.**, The nutritive value of three species of water weeds, *Econ. Bot.*, 23(2), 123-127, 1969.
6. **Boyd, C. E.**, Amino acid, protein, and caloric content of vascular aquatic macrophytes, *Ecology*, 51(5), 902-906, 1970.
7. **Boyd, C. E.**, Chemical analyses of some vascular aquatic plants, *Arch. Hydrobiol.*, 67(1), 73-85, 1970.
8. **Boyd, C. E.**, Vascular aquatic plants for mineral nutrient removal from polluted water, *Econ. Bot.*, 24, 95-103, 1970.
9. **Boyd, C. E.**, Variation in the elemental content of *Eichhornia crassipes, Hydrobiologia*, 38(3-4), 409-414, 1971.
10. **Burton, B. T.**, *Human Nutrition*, 3rd ed., McGraw-Hill, New York, 1976, 162.
11. **Burton, B. T.**, *Human Nutrition*, 3rd ed., McGraw-Hill, New York, 1976, 158.
12. **Culley, D. D. and Epps, E. A.**, Use of duckweed for waste treatment and animal feed, *J. Water Pollut. Control Fed.*, 45, 337-347, 1973.
13. **Taylor, K. G., Bates, R. P., and Robbins, R. C.**, Extraction of protein from water hyacinth, *Hyacinth Control J.*, 9(1), 20-22, 1971.
14. **Taylor, K. G. and Robbins, R. C.**, The amino acid composition of water hyacinth (Eichhornia crassipes) and its value as a protein supplement, *Hyacinth Control J.*, 8, 24-25, 1968.
15. **Truax, T. E., Culley, D. D., Griffith, M., Johnson, W. A., and Wood, J. P.**, Duckweed for chick feed, *La. Agric.*, 16(1), 8-9, 1972.
16. **Wolverton, B. C. and McDonald, R. C.**, National Aeronautics and Space Administrations, National Space Technology Laboratories, unpublished data.
17. **Wolverton, B. C. and McDonald, R. C.**, Nutritional Composition of Water Hyacinths Grown on Domestic Sewage, ERL Rep. No. 173, National Aeronautics and Space Administration, NSTL Station, Mississippi, 1978.

*Foods for Special Uses*

# DIETS FOR THE ELDERLY

## C. L. Justice

## INTRODUCTION

The same foods enjoyed earlier in life should be offered to the aged. The idea that the elderly should be fed a thin gruel concocted in a blender in order to compensate for impaired dentation and diminished powers of digestion, is as wrong as the idea that vitamin and mineral supplements can replace food. Food supplies more than nutrition. The taste, color, form, and texture of foods contribute to the joy of eating. No food should be provided or denied simply because a person is old. Favorite foods shared with family and friends are among the pleasures of life which should be provided to both old and young.

## ADJUSTING DIETS TO INDIVIDUAL REQUIREMENTS

Some dietary adjustments are required for some elderly persons. These adjustments should not be viewed as universal needs of the aged, but rather as adjustments to diseases and disabilities common among the aged. Mechanical and nutritional adjustments, metabolic and digestive limitations, and meal spacing will be examined.

### Mechanical Adjustments

Mechanical adjustments in the diet include adjustments to problems in chewing and swallowing, eating problems of the handicapped and food intolerances. Many but not all elderly require mechanical adjustments in their diets.

#### Chewing and Swallowing

Difficulties in chewing and swallowing sometimes limit food choices, but before resorting to blending or liquifying foods, a sequence should be utilized to determine the maximum capabilities of persons who cannot chew or swallow normally. One should try offering soft foods and food cut into bite-sized pieces before chopping or grinding. A mechanically soft diet is often ordered. A mechanically soft diet is a selection of foods soft in texture. The foods may be cooked or raw (e.g., bananas), as long as they are easily chewed and swallowed. The foods may have mild or strong flavor (e.g., cabbage), as long as the individual can tolerate the food. There is no restriction of salt, sugar, fat, or fiber for a mechanically soft diet, but meats should be chopped or ground unless they are flaky and tender (e.g., fish). Those preparing food for persons who have difficulty chewing and swallowing should blend or liquify foods only as a last resort. Even then, each food should be served separately. Blended foods should never be made into a single-dish meal unless the individual must be tube-fed.

Although it is sometimes necessary to present all food in a liquid form to maintain the patient nutritionally, continued reliance on this mode of feeding may be detrimental to the patient. The muscles exercised in chewing and swallowing are the same as those which make it possible to speak. Speech therapists use a variety of foods mastered in sequence to help persons with oral paralysis, improve breathing, decrease drooling, increase food intake, and regain speech. The Wisconsin Department of Health and Social Services has published such a series that includes four steps: (1) retrains the patient to drink through straw; (2), (3), and (4) advance from foods of gum drop consistency, to foods like melba toast, and finally to foods such as raw carrot. Obviously not every person with oral paralysis can achieve all four steps. The therapist must determine the appropriate step in the suggested sequence and provide preliminary instruction and practice on an individual basis. Mealtime practice with appropriate foods is an important part of the suggested series. For example, the patient at the gum-drop stage should be offered half-inch cubes of cheese, meat, and toasted cheese sandwich; hard cooked egg; dried and fresh fruits and melons; undercooked vegetables; and chewy cookies without nuts. A list of foods to be offered at each of the steps is available from the Wisconsin Department of Health and Social Services, Division of Health, Bureau of Quality Compliance, Facilities Assistance Section, Nutrition Section, Box 309 Madison, Wisconsin 53701. "Supplement for #2 in Series: 'Exercises to Improve the Chewing and Swallowing Ability of an Adult with Oral Paralysis' ''.

### Handicapped

Elderly who are handicapped so severely that they cannot feed themselves often do not get enough to eat. The patient who must be fed frequently loses weight and fails to improve. Every effort should be made to find appropriate knives, forks, spoons, and dishes to enable the handicapped to regain his independence. If a patient must be fed, the person responsible must recognize that feeding takes time. The feeder should seek ways to involve the helpless patient. The patient can often hold his napkin or a piece of bread. A system of signals can be developed to communicate with even the mute patient. Mealtime must be a social time.

### Food Intolerances

Many older persons have a real or fancied intolerance for a number of foods. There is no uniformity among these problems, but these intolerances (whether real or fancied) should be respected. Honoring such attitudes toward specific foods can compromise the nutrient quality of the diet unless someone knowledgeable about the nutrient content of foods offers appropriate substitutes. For example, milk is the food most often omitted. If no milk product is acceptable, a calcium supplement is needed.[1] If the person who refuses milk also consumes less than 5 oz of meat or meat substitutes, protein and riboflavin intake may likewise be marginal when milk is omitted. Fortified milk is the only significant dietary source of vitamin D. No food contains a significant amount of vitamin D unless the vitamin is added in processing.[2] Patients who seldom go out into the sunshine and who refuse to drink milk require another source of vitamin D.

## Nutritional Adjustments

The recommended dietary allowances (RDA, 1980)[3] (Table 1) indicate that the nutrient needs of the aged are so much like those of any other mature adult that the food pattern ensuring an adequate diet for other persons over 21 is appropriate for the elderly. The menu planing check list (Figure 1) developed by the Indiana State Board of Health[4] is a good food guideline.

### Common Nutrient Deficiencies

The U.S. Department of Agriculture (USDA) Food Consumption Survey (1977 to 1978) used 24-hr dietary recalls of the day preceding the interview to calculate nutrient intakes for the various age-sex groups of the population. On the basis of the survey, older Americans seem to have the same patterns of nutrient intakes as other adults. In all adult groups the average individual intakes were below recommended amounts of calcium, magnesium, and vitamin $B_6$ and above the RDA for protein, phosphorus, vitamin A, thiamin, riboflavin, niacin, vitamin $B_{12}$, and vitamin C. Iron was also consumed in recommended amounts by all groups except women in the child-bearing years (Table 2).

Table 1
COMPARISON OF RDA (1980) FOR ADULTS[3]

| Nutrient | Males (years) | | Females (years) | |
|---|---|---|---|---|
| | 23—50 | 51—75 and 75 + | 23—50 | 51—75 and 75 + |
| Protein (g) | 56 | 56 | 44 | 44 |
| Vitamin A ($\mu$g R.E.) | 1000 | 1000 | 800 | 800 |
| Vitamin D ($\mu$g) | 5 | 5 | 5 | 5 |
| Vitamin E (mg$\alpha$—TE) | 10 | 10 | 8 | 8 |
| Vitamin C (mg) | 60 | 60 | 60 | 60 |
| Thiamin (mg) | 1.4 | 1.2 | 1.0 | 1.0 |
| Riboflavin (mg) | 1.6 | 1.4 | 1.2 | 1.2 |
| Niacin (mg NE) | 18 | 16 | 13 | 13 |
| Vitamin $B_6$ (mg) | 2.2 | 2.2 | 2.0 | 2.0 |
| Folacin ($\mu$g) | 400 | 400 | 400 | 400 |
| Vitamin $B_{12}$ | 3.0 | 3.0 | 3.0 | 3.0 |
| Calcium (mg) | 800 | 800 | 800 | 800 |
| Phosphorus (mg) | 800 | 800 | 800 | 800 |
| Magnesium (mg) | 350 | 350 | 300 | 300 |
| Iron (mg | 10 | 10 | 18 | 10 |
| Zinc (mg) | 15 | 15 | 15 | 15 |
| Iodine ($\mu$g) | 150 | 150 | 150 | 150 |

If one examines average nutrient intakes per individual more closely, (Table 2) it is apparent that elderly males consume even less calcium, magnesium, and vitamin $B_6$ than other males, but elderly women have slightly higher calcium, magnesium, and $B_6$ intakes than some younger women. Nevertheless, elderly men had higher, though still less than recommended, intakes of calcium, magnesium, and vitamin $B_6$ than the elderly women surveyed.

Restricted caloric intakes are generally associated with lower intakes of minerals and vitamins. Average caloric intakes reported in the USDA survey peaked at age 5 to 18 in males and age 12 to 14 in females, and declined in each subsequent age group. Although women 75 and over averaged only 1367 kcal/day, these women seem to be selecting foods more wisely than some younger women. The nutrient densities of the foods selected provided more calcium and about the same magnesium and $B_6$ as their daughters got with higher caloric intakes. The limited caloric intake of elderly persons requires more attention to the nutrient densities of foods if recommended amounts of all nutrients are to be included. If caloric restrictions could be eased (as by increasing physical activity for the elderly) nutrient density would be less critical. Increased caloric intakes tend to be associated with better mineral and vitamin intakes.

The nutrient density of foods eaten at breakfast tends to be high. This quality suggests a useful strategy to improve the diets of the elderly since older persons generally eat better at breakfast than at other meals. The elderly, even more than younger persons, should be encouraged to eat a complete beakfast and to avoid omitting breakfast or having only a continental breafast — a cup of coffee and a roll. A good breakfast should provide not less than one fourth of the day's calories and can easily supply more than one fourth of the daily allowancs for several minerals and vitamins if the pattern includes fruit, milk, a grain food, and a good quality protein food.

What kinds of foods should be added to diets to increase calcium, magnesium, and vitamin $B_6$ intakes? It is almost impossible to supply adequate dietary calcium unless milk products are included in the diet. No one food group can guarantee recommended amounts of magnesium or $B_6$, however. There is little magnesium in meats but nuts and legumes are good sources. Whole grain cereals are higher in magnesium and vita-

Indiana State Board of Health
1330 West Michigan Street
Indianapolis, Indiana 46206

SBM25-007
1974

INSTITUTION _____

DATE OF MENUS _____

DATE CHECKED _____

CHECKED BY _____

| FOOD GROUP | M | T | W | T | F | S | S | Total |
|---|---|---|---|---|---|---|---|---|
| **VEGETABLES AND FRUITS** | | | | | | | | |
| Dark green or deep yellow vegetable or fruit or equivalent sources of Vitamin A — 4 or more servings per week. | | | | | | | | |
| 1 serving is equivalent to ½ cup broccoli, collards, kale, spinach, turnip greens, or other dark green leaves, carrots, pumpkins, sweet potato, winter squash or five apricot halves or ¼ medium cantaloupe. | | | | | | | | |
| Note: One two ounce serving of cooked liver can be used as an alternate for four servings of Vitamin A rich fruits and vegetables. | | | | | | | | |
| Citrus fruit or equivalent sources of Vitamin C — 1 serving per day. | | | | | | | | |
| 1 serving is equivalent to ½ grapefruit, 1 medium orange, ½ cantaloupe, ½ cup strawberries, ½ cup orange or grapefruit juice, ½ cup broccoli, brussels sprouts, or mustard greens. | | | | | | | | |
| ½ serving is equivalent to 1 wedge honeydew, 1 tangerine or ½ cup tangerine juice, ½ cup tomato juice or cooked tomato, 1 medium raw tomato, 1 medium baked potato, ½ green pepper, ½ cup cauliflower, rutabaga, raw cabbage, collards, kale or turnip greens. | | | | | | | | |
| Other vegetables and fruits — 4 servings daily (include Vitamin A & C sources in total) | | | | | | | | |
| 1 serving is equivalent to ½ cup of fruit or vegetable, or a usual serving such as one medium apple, banana, peach or potato. | | | | | | | | |
| **MILK** | | | | | | | | |
| Milk, fluid whole, 2%, skim, buttermilk or equivalent — 2 cups daily for adults, 4 cups daily for children. | | | | | | | | |
| ½ cup milk is equivalent to *1 ounce processed cheese, ½ cup custard or milk pudding, or 1 serving cream soup made with milk. | | | | | | | | |
| ¼ cup milk is equivalent to ½ cup ice cream, *½ ounce processed cheese, *½ cup cottage cheese. | | | | | | | | |
| **MEAT AND OTHER PROTEIN FOODS** | | | | | | | | |
| Meat, poultry, fish or protein equivalent — 5 ounces per day. | | | | | | | | |
| 1 ounce is equivalent to 1 ounce of cooked, edible lean beef, veal, lamb, pork, poultry, fish, sea food or variety meats such 1 frankfurter, 1 ounce slice luncheon meat. *1 ounce processed cheese, *¼ cup cottage cheese, 1 egg, ½ cup cooked dried beans or peas, 2 tablespoons peanut butter, 4 strips bacon, 3 links pork sausage. | | | | | | | | |
| **BREAD AND CEREALS** | | | | | | | | |
| Bread and cereals, whole grain or enriched — 4 or more servings per day. | | | | | | | | |
| 1 serving is equivalent to 1 slice of bread, 1 roll, muffin or biscuit, 2 squares graham crackers, 5 squares saltines, 1 ounce ready to eat cereal, ½ to ¾ cup cooked cereal, cornmeal, grits, rice, macaroni, noodles or spaghetti. | | | | | | | | |
| **OTHER FOODS** | | | | | | | | |
| Butter or fortified margarine — 3 or more teaspoons per day used as a spread or in cooking. | | | | | | | | |
| IS there meat or another protein food (above) in each dinner and supper? | | | | | | | | |
| IS there at least one serving of a fruit and/or vegetable in each meal? | | | | | | | | |

*If serving of chedder or cottage cheese is being counted as a milk equivalent, it should not also be counted as a meat equivalent.

FIGURE 1.   Menu planning check list.

min $B_6$ than white bread and refined cereals, but unless a variety of foods is included recommended allowances for these two nutrients can hardly be attained. A variety of foods is the secret of an adequate diet which will supply not only magnesium and

Table 2
## 1977-1978 U.S. DEPARTMENT OF AGRICULTURE FOOD CONSUMPTION SURVEY (AVERAGE INTAKE PER INDIVIDUAL)

| | | | | Age and sex | | | | |
|---|---|---|---|---|---|---|---|---|
| | 35—50 | | 51—64 | | 65—74 | | 75 + | |
| RDAs | ♂ | ♀ | ♂ | ♀ | ♂ | ♀ | ♂ | ♀ |
| kcal | 2314 | 1514 | 2148 | 1522 | 1970 | 1444 | 1808 | 1367 |
| Protein (g) ♂ 56 ♀ 44 | 95.6 | 63.9 | 90.1 | 65.2 | 81.0 | 60.4 | 74.6 | 54.1 |
| Fat (g) | 109.3 | 70.8 | 101.6 | 71.2 | 92.8 | 65.8 | 86.2 | 59.0 |
| CHO (g) | 220.8 | 151.2 | 208.8 | 153.8 | 205.3 | 155.4 | 184.3 | 157.4 |
| Calcium (mg) all 800 | 764[a] | 515[a] | 702[a] | 532[a] | 729[a] | 566[a] | 679[a] | 591[a] |
| Iron (mg) ♂ 10 — ♀ 10 ♀ under 50 −18 | 15.8 | 10.7[a] | 15.5 | 11.4 | 14.5 | 10.6 | 13.4 | 10.1 |
| Magnesium (mg) ♂ 350 ♀ 300 | 310[a] | 222[a] | 304[a] | 235[a] | 287[a] | 227[a] | 267[a] | 214[a] |
| Phophorous (mg) | 1397 | 922 | 1289 | 948 | 1246 | 930 | 1137 | 880 |
| Vitamin A (IU) | 5690 | 4264 | 6945 | 6044 | 6834 | 6218 | 6693 | 5931 |
| Thiamin (mg) ♂ 1.4—1.2 ♀ 1.0 | 1.45 | 1.01 | 1.47 | 1.05 | 1.40 | 1.07 | 1.41 | 1.01 |
| Riboflavin (mg) ♂ 1.6—1.4 ♀ 1.2 | 1.88 | 1.27 | 1.88 | 1.40 | 1.85 | 1.41 | 1.73 | 1.40 |
| Preformed niacin (mg) | 23.8 | 16.2 | 23.1 | 17.2 | 20.9 | 15.6 | 18.7 | 13.8 |
| Vitamin B$_6$ (mg) ♂ 2.2 ♀ 2.0 | 1.73[a] | 1.19[a] | 1.75[a] | 1.29[a] | 1.58[a] | 1.24[a] | 1.51[a] | 1.15[a] |
| Vitamin B$_{12}$ (μg) | 5.55 | 3.78 | 7.18 | 5.27 | 5.82 | 4.21 | 4.95 | 4.07 |
| Vitamin C (mg) | 86 | 79 | 98 | 93 | 100 | 92 | 96 | 90 |

[a]   Less than Recommended Daily Dietary Allowance.

vitamin B$_6$ but all of the vitamins and minerals even those for which no allowance has been identified. Any practice which restricts variety — a limited caloric allowance, limited funds to purchase food, problems of chewing and swallowing and feeding independently — tends to diminish the nutritional adequacy of one's diet.

## Calories

The suggested caloric allowance (RDA, 1980) for adults over 75 years of age is 1600 cal (1200 to 2000) for the average woman and 2050 cal (1650 to 2450) for the average man engaged in very light activity. Durnin and Passmore[6] state that during adult life there is a decline in the rate of resting metabolism of just over 2% per decade. Hence, by age 80 one's resting metabolism is 85% of its caloric cost at age 25. This decline in resting metabolism is thought to be one of the essential features of aging. However, the total differences between resting metabolism at age 25 and age 80 years is small — approximately 200 cal/day. Differences in activity may obliterate this difference in resting metabolism. In a study of elderly and middle-aged housewives, Durnin and Passmore[6] found a range of caloric expenditure in the elderly of 1490 to 2410 cal/day, while the expenditure range for middle-aged housewives (1750 to 2320 cal/day) fell within the range required by the elderly housewife.

The inactivity of most institutionalized aged seems to reduce their total caloric needs. In one study[7] of a nursing home population, the daily caloric intake of this population was calculated to be approximately 1400 cal for the women and 1600 cal for the men. The women consuming more than 1600 cal were considered obese by their physicians.

No caloric guideline alone can indicate what is a satisfactory caloric intake for an individual whether young or old. The adequacy of the caloric intake is best measured by a weight record of the individual. Weights should be taken and recorded in patients' charts at least once a month. A gain or loss of more than 2 lb is indicative of more than normal diurnal fluctuation. Illness and trauma are not uncommon among the elderly. Although decreases in both resting metabolism and activity are typical of the aging process, major surgery, multiple fractures, severe burns, and other traumas increase caloric needs dramatically.[8]

*Protein*

The protein needs of the elderly may be slightly less than the protein requirements of other mature adults, but a standard of 1.0 g/kgram of body weight is generally accepted in menu planning.[9] As the RDA reference female weighs 58 kg and the reference male 70 kg, menus should provide approximately 60 to 70 g protein per day. Impaired renal function may require severe restriction of total protein and selection of only the best quality protein. However, if the patient is on dialysis, dietary protein is usually approximately the same as for other persons of similar size.[4] Major trauma not only causes an increase in caloric requirements, but also causes the body to waste protein.[10] The patient may benefit from a high-protein diet during convalescence. Walker and Linkswiler[11] have suggested that high-protein diets can cause abnormal losses of calcium from the body. They have associated negative calcium balances with excessive intakes of protein (more than 100 g of protein for young women and more than 140 g in the diets of young men). Possibly, dietary protein should not be allowed to exceed 2 g of protein per kilogram, even on high-protein diets.

Four to five ounces of cooked, lean meat and 2 cups of milk will supply approximately 50 g of protein and another 12 g is obtained from the minimal four servings of breads and/or cereals and, two vegetables. Meat substitutes may replace all or part of the meat, but meat substitutes generally do not seem to supply trace minerals as well as animal products. The vegetarian who avoids all animal products should also have a supplement of vitamin $B_{12}$.

*Fat*

The epidemiological association of high-fat diets with heart disease and some forms of cancer are the rationale for a generally accepted guideline that not more than 28%—35% of the total calories come from fat. By this guideline, an individual who requires 2000 calories would be allowed less than 80 g of fat per day. It is difficult to fit fried foods into the framework of this caloric limitation even if the person can digest and absorb fat well.

*Carbohydrate*

Dietary carbohydrates should provide more calories than either protein or fat. Table sugar is not forbidden unless the individual is diabetic, but the carbohydrates in fruits and vegetables, nuts and legumes, and whole-grain breads and cereals are better because they provide minerals and vitamins as well as carbohydrates. These foods are also significant sources of dietary fiber, which helps ensure normal bowel action. Whole-grain cereals, legumes and nuts, and fruits and vegetables are good sources of fiber. The 1976 Symposium on Food and Fiber[12] recommended a variety of foods to assure the consumption of good mixtures of plant fibers, but stated that the fortification of foods with specific polysaccharides (such as cellulose) is not justified by the present state of knowledge.

The minimum dietary intake of carbohydrate foods is four servings of fruits and vegetables and four servings (slices) of breads and cereals, however, if the individual requires more than 1200 cal/day he will require more than four servings of each of these carbohydrate food groups. Between 40 and 60% of the total calories must be supplied by carbohydrate foods if dietary fat is not to exceed 35% of the total calories protein intake is to be between 1 and 2 g/kg.

## Metabolic and Digestive Limitations

Modified diets appear to be prescribed for a larger proportion of aged than younger persons. Many aged are institutionalized because they cannot follow their diet prescriptions. The physician who prescribes a highly restrictive diet for an elderly person may be denying his patient one of the few remaining pleasures of living. Nevertheless, diets restricting carbohydrate, protein, and fat and diets limiting sodium intake are often necessary to control disease states common among the elderly. The dietitian is the professional who should fit the diet to the patient. It is difficult to change long established food habits. Dietary restrictions should be supported by laboratory or clinical evidence of their necessity. Physicians who prescribe modified diets have a responsibility for ordering laboratory tests to support the necessity of the diet prescription and to monitor its effectiveness.

There are few guidelines to the nutrient needs of the aged who are ill, but clinical malnutrition is more apt to develop among those whose nutritional status was already marginal due to a lifetime of poor diet habits. The treatment of clinical malnutrition, e.g., the various forms of anemia, is a medical rather than dietary problem. For example, dietary iron is not sufficient to treat iron deficiency anemia. The patient must follow a regimen of medicinal iron for several months to cure his anemia. This is not to belittle the importance of helping him improve his dietary practices, but good dietary habits prevent rather than cure disease.

Food for the elderly should be seasoned with the same care appropriate for younger persons. One of the changes characteristic of aging appears to be a decrease in the number of taste buds. Unless the individual is on a sodium restriction so strict that he must use "salt free" bread, his food should be cooked with salt. Sweet, sour, and bitter, as well as salt, are needed to povide a variety of flavors. Current diet theory advises ulcer patients to avoid pepper and caffeine, but such restrictions are not appropriate for the elderly as a group.

## Sodium Restrictions and High-Potassium Foods

Sodium restrictions are appropriate for persons with hypertension.[13] Although attempts to control hypertension by diet alone are not advisable, a smaller dose of medication is required if the person with hypertension adheres to a sodium restricted diet. The amount of sodium allowed should be specified when the dosage of the diuretic is determined.

Hypertension is common. Guyton[14] points out that 20% of the entire population will develop hypertension at some time during life and that 12% of all deaths are due to hypertension. Restrictions of dietary sodium are helpful in the control of hypertension, but the use of coffee or tea in moderation is probably harmless to most patients who have essential hypertension.[15]

Potassium may also be a dietary consideration for the person with hypertension. One fourth to one third of the hypertensives controlled with thiazide diuretics become potassium deficient.[16] Potassium occurs in almost all foods; thus, too severe a restriction in caloric intake may be the critical factor in the development of a potassium deficiency. Potassium is often leached out of foods during cooking, as it is highly water soluble. Hence, a baked potato is a better source of potassium than one which is peeled and boiled. Persons taking thiazide diuretics to control hypertension require foods which are high in potassium and low in sodium. They should not add salt to the baked potato. Raw fruits (especially banana, avocado, and melons) are reliable sources of dietary potassium which contain almost no sodium. Dried fruits are not better than other fruits in potassium content unless eaten in much larger amounts than individuals would normally consume. However, a cup of prune juice provides more potassium (470 mg) than a cup of orange juice (372 mg). A small baked potato (2 in in diameter) provides more potassium than any fruit except the avocado.[17]

### Cholesterol Control

High blood pressure is often observed in atherosclerosis, but weakened heart pumping action and elongation of blood vessels may produce lowered blood pressure even though the vessels have lost much of their elasticity. In aged persons a "normal" blood pressure reading does not necessarily mean a healthy cardiovascular system. The National Academy of Science and the American Association recommend the following:

> Routine medical examinations should include measurement of the plasma lipid profile. If the plasma lipid values indicate that one is in a high risk group, he should be given dietary advice designed to correct his abnormal blood lipid picture . . . it will usually entail a reduced intake of cholesterol and saturated fats . . . [18]

Diets to alter the blood lipid profile are often necessary, but a cholesterol lowering diet is not appropriate for all aged persons. On the average, plasma cholesterol concentrations appear to peak at approximately age 50 in men and 65 in women. Gillum et al.[19] also observed a sharp fall of cholesterol concentrations in both their male and female subjects after age 75 It is generally recommended that the total fat (both saturated and unsaturated) in diets not exceed 35% of the total calories and that cholesterol lowering diets be required of those considered to have a high risk of coronary or vascular disease.

### Additional Modifications and Drug-Food Adjustments

Other problems which require dietary modification in diets for the elderly are lactase insufficiency, celiac disease, fat malabsorption, and dumping syndrome. Diabetes and renal impairment are also common and require diet modification for their control.

The medication an older person must use may also require some adjustent in his food intake or in the timing associated with medicine and meals.[20] Monoamine oxidase (MAO) inhibitors, anticoagulant, isoniazid (INH), dilantin or phenobarbitol, tetracyclines, and penicillin are among the widely used drugs which have some drug nutrient interaction. Some drugs are absorbed better when taken 1 hr before meals or 2 hr after, while others are irritating to the digestive tract if not taken with food.

### Meal Spacing

A regular meal schedule should be followed. It has been suggested, on one hand, that five or six meals a day are better than three meals a day and, on the other hand, that one hot meal a day in a congregate setting can alleviate many social and nutritional problems of the aged. Whatever meal schedule is followed it should be remembered that not more than 50% and not less than 20% of the day's calories should be consumed in any 5-hr period between 7:00 a.m. and 10:00 p.m.[21] In addition, no more than 14 hr should elapse between the last "substantial meal" in the evening and break-

| | Breakfast | Noon | Evening |
|---|---|---|---|
| **Monday** | Orange juice<br>Corn Flakes<br>or<br>Poached eggs<br>Buttered toast<br>Jelly<br>Coffee, tea, milk | Meat loaf with tomato sauce<br>Buttered green limas<br>Pear half<br>Bread and butter<br>Chocolate pudding<br>Milk, coffee, tea | Chicken livers — bacon<br>Hash brown potatoes<br>Creamed peas<br>Fruit cocktail in jello<br>Bread and butter<br>Milk, coffee, tea |
| **Tuesday** | Orange juice<br>Cream of Rice<br>or<br>Scrambled eggs<br>Buttered toast<br>Jelly<br>Milk, coffee, tea | Chop suey (pork)<br>Rice<br>Apricot with cottage cheese<br>Salad<br>Sherbet — Cookie<br>Bread and butter<br>Milk, coffee, tea | Smoked sausage<br>Buttered parsnips<br>Hot apple slices<br>Russian cream with<br>  red raspberries<br>Bread and butter<br>Milk, coffee, tea |
| **Wednesday** | Orange juice<br>Wheaties<br>or<br>Pancakes<br>Sausage link<br>Butter — Syrup<br>Milk, coffee, tea | Baked haddock fillets in<br>  tomato sauce<br>Macaroni and cheese<br>Buttered spinach<br>Bread and butter<br>Strawberry shortcake<br>Milk, coffee, tea | Sloppy joe on bun<br>Escalloped corn<br>Lettuce and Old Dutch<br>  dressing<br>Chilled plums<br>Plain cookie<br>Milk, coffee, tea |
| **Thursday** | Orange juice<br>Cream of Wheat<br>or<br>Poached eggs<br>Buttered toast<br>Jelly<br>Milk, coffee, tea | Oven fried steak<br>Mashed potatoes<br>Zucchini and tomatoes<br>Three-bean salad<br>Bread and butter<br>Pumpkin pie<br>Milk, coffee, tea | Chicken noodle soup<br>Crackers<br>Ham and cheese sandwich<br>Cabbage apple salad<br>Cherry delight<br>Milk, coffee, tea |
| **Friday** | Orange juice<br>Grapenut Flakes<br>or<br>Scrambled eggs<br>Buttered toast<br>Jelly<br>Milk, coffee, tea | Weiners and kraut<br>Glazed carrots<br>Mashed potatoes<br>Bread and butter<br>Baked apple<br>Milk, coffee, tea | Sliced turkey roll<br>  sandwich<br>Beef vegetable soup<br>Crackers<br>Pickle chip<br>Peach shortcake<br>Milk, coffee, tea |
| **Saturday** | Orange juice<br>Oatmeal<br>or<br>Fried eggs<br>Buttered toast<br>Jelly<br>Milk, coffee, tea | Chicken and noodles<br>Harvard beets<br>Pineapple and cottage<br>  cheese salad<br>Bread and butter<br>Lime sherbet<br>Milk, coffee, tea | Japanese meat balls<br>Buttered broccoli<br>Rice<br>Mandarin oranges in<br>  orange gelatine<br>Square of spice (apple) cake<br>Bread and butter<br>Milk, coffee, tea |
| **Sunday** | Grapefruit sections<br>Cream of Rice<br>Sweet roll<br>Butter<br>Milk, coffee, tea | Baked ham<br>Sweet potatoes<br>Green beans in mushroom sauce<br>Perfection salad<br>Sugar cream pie<br>Dinner rolls | Mush and milk<br>Salad plate — two squares jello,<br>  cottage cheese, and<br>  sliced cling peaches<br>Bread and butter<br>Fresh fruit (apple, banana,<br>  or grapes) |

FIGURE 2. Sample menus for the aged.

fast.[22] Health authorities define a "substantial meal" as one which contains at least three different menu items, one of which is a good source of protein, and at least 20% of the day's calories. Most would also require that one of the menu items be a fruit or vegetable.

## SUMMARY

Good diets for the elderly are like good diets for other adults. A wide variety of foods is needed — milk and milk products, meats and meat substitutes, fruits and vegetables, and enriched or whole-grain breads and cereals. (Some sample menus for the aged are shown in Figure 2.) Restrictions and modifications should be imposed solely on the basis of food and nutrition problems experienced by the individual. Elderly persons more often require dietary modifications and restrictions than do other adults, but this is because they are ill or handicapped and not because they are elderly. Diabetes and hypertension occur frequently in aged populations. Because each of these conditions requires diet modification, persons preparing foods for groups of elderly persons should try to provide menu choices to simplify adherence to these two types of diets. In addition, each menu should include some soft foods for those who have difficulty in chewing and swallowing. However, menus made up only of soft foods should be offered only to those who cannot chew.

Meals should be planned to stimulate the appetite and please the diner. A desirable weight should be established for each person and excessive loss or gain avoided. Serving good food may be almost all that can be done for many of the elderly who are ill. Attractive meals reassure the diner that he is appreciated. Neither seasoning nor socialization should be neglected in planning meals for the elderly.

# REFERENCES

1. Watkin, D. M., Nutrition for the aging and the aged, in *Nutrition in Health and Diseases,* Goodhardt, R. S. and Shils, M. E., Eds., Lea Febiger, Philadelphia, 1974, 681-710.
2. Scott, H. T., Vitamin D group, in *The Vitamins,* Sebrell, W. H., Jr. and Harris, R. S., Eds., Academic Press, New York, 1971, 209-211.
3. Food and Nutrition Board, Recommended Dietary Allowances, 9th ed., National Academy of Sciences—National Research Council, Washington, D.C., 1980.
4. Indiana State Board of Health Menu Planning Check List, in *Indiana Diet Manual,* 1981. May be ordered from Louis Gumpper, 809-G Lincolnwood Lane, Indianapolis, Ind. 46260.
5. Science and Education Administration, Food and Nutrient Intake of Individuals in 1 Day in the United States, Spring 1977, U.S. Department of Agriculture, Washington, D.C., 1980.
6. Durnin, J. V. G. A. and Pasmore, R., *Energy, Work and Leisure,* Heinemann, London, 1967, 104 and 116.
7. Justice, C. L., Howe, J. M., and Clark, H. E., Dietary intakes and nutritional status of elderly patients, *J. Am. Diet. Assoc.,* 65, 639-646, 1974.
8. Caldwell, F. T., Changes in energy metabolism during recovery from injury, in Ciba Foundation Symposium, *Energy Metabolism in Trauma,* Porter, R. and Knight, J., Eds., J A. Churchill, London, 1970.
9. Young, V. R., Perera, W. D., Winterer, J. C., and Scrimshaw, N. S., Protein and amino acid requirements of the elderly, in *Nutrition and Aging,* Winick, M., Ed., John Wiley Sons, New York, 1976, 77-112.
10. Kinney, J. M., Long, C. L., and Duke, D. H., Jr., Energy demands in the surgical patient, in *Body Fluid Replacement in the Sugical Patient,* Nahas, G. G. and Fox, C. L., Eds., Grune Stratton, New York, 1970, 296-300.
11. Walker, R. M. and Linkswiler, H. M., Calcium retention in adult human males as affected by protein intake, *J. Nutr.,* 102, 1237-1302, 1972.
12. Maraboce Symposium on Food and fibre, *Nutr. Rev.,* 35, 72, 1977.
13. Freis, E. D., The Modern Management of Hypertension, Veterans Administration, Washington, D.C., 1973.
14. Guyton, A. C., *Textbook of Medical Physiology,* W. B. Saunders, Philadelphia, 1971, 304.
15. Kark, R. M. and Oyama, J. H., Nutrition and cardiovascular-renal diseases, in *Modern Nutrition in Health and Disease,* Goodhart, R. S. and Shils, M. E., Eds., Lea Febiger, Philadelphia, 1974, 863-869.
16. Veterans Administration Cooperative Study Group of Antihypertensive Agents, Effects of treatment on morbidity in hypertension, *Circulation,* 45, 991-1004, 1972.
17. Agriculture Research Service, Composition of Foods, in Agriculture Handbook No. 8, U.S. Department of Agriculture, Washington, D.C., 1963.
18. A joint statement of the Foods and Nutrition Board of the National Academy of Sciences-National Research Council and the Council on Foods and Nutrition, American Medical Association, Diet and coronary disease, *Nutr. Rev.,* 30, 223-225, 1972.
19. Gillum, H. L., Morgan, A. F., and Jerome, D., Nutritional status of the aging. IV. Serum cholesterol and diet, *J. Nutr.,* 55, 449-468, 1955.
20. Cooper, J. W., Food-drug interactions, U.S. Pharmacist, pp. 17-28, November - December 1976.
21. Nutrition Section, Wisconsin Division of Health, Nutritional Guidelines for Alternate Menu Patterns, Issue 2-74, April-May-June 1974.
22. Interpretive Guidelines and Survey Procedures for the Application of the Conditions of Participation for Skilled Nursing Facilities, 1974, 405.1125, p. 43.

# THERAPEUTIC DIETS FOR MAN

## Wanda Chenoweth

## INTRODUCTION

A therapeutic diet is basically a normal diet which is modified because of the changes during disease or illness that occur in a person's ability to tolerate or utilize food and nutrients. Most therapeutic diets involve modifications in consistency or bulk, energy content, or kinds and amounts of one or more nutrients. Although little is known about changes in nutrient requirements in illness, it is important that the food restrictions used in a therapeutic diet do not lead to an inadequate intake of nutrients. The nutritional adequacy of the diet must be carefully evaluated, especially if the diet is to be used for a long period of time.

It also is important that therapeutic diets be adapted to meet the needs of the individual patient. All patients with renal disease may not need restriction of dietary protein or sodium, nor is there one diet which is appropriate for all persons with diabetes. Because strong experimental data are often lacking to support the rigid diet regimens traditionally prescribed for patients with gastrointestinal diseases, there has been a trend toward using such diets only as guides to foods which may cause problems and to eliminate "restricted" foods only if they are not tolerated. Therapeutic diets should also be planned as much as possible to fit the patient's food habits and preferences, economic status, religious practices, and other factors influencing food intake such as place where meals are eaten or facilities available for preparation and storage of food.

In the following discussion of therapeutic diets, an attempt has been made to describe diets on the basis of the diet modifications rather than the disease conditions in which they are used. Because agreement is often lacking regarding individual foods which should be included in specific diets, it seems appropriate to describe the characteristics of the diet rather than to include detailed lists of foods allowed and restricted. However, sample diets have been included for the most common therapeutic diets; for the other diets, references where detailed information can be found are given.

## DIETS MODIFIED IN TEXTURE AND CONSISTENCY

### Routine Hospital Diets

**Light or simple general diet** — This diet is often included as one of the basic or routine hospital diets (Table 1). Fried foods, rich pastries, highly seasoned foods, and coarse foods such as whole-grain cereals, nuts, and fruits and vegetables with coarse skins or seeds are omitted. It is sometimes considered as a transitional diet during convalescence from surgery or acute illness; however, it is also appropriate for individuals who habitually cannot tolerate rich or highly seasoned foods.[1,2]

**Soft diet** — The diet consists of foods that are soft in texture and moderately low in indigestible carbohydrates and connective tissue found in meat (Table 1). Fried foods and highly seasoned foods are omitted. The diet may be used as a progression step from a liquid diet to a regular diet after acute illness or surgery. The **mechanical** or **dental soft** diet is similar, except that all foods must be in a form which can be swallowed with little or no chewing. Foods are finely ground, mashed, or pureed. The diet may be prescribed for patients with very poor teeth, oral or esophageal lesions, or after oral or eye surgery.[2-4]

**Full liquid** — Foods that are liquids or become liquid at body temperature are included in a full liquid diet (Table 1). Strained cereal gruels, strained cream soups, soft

Table 1
## DIETS MODIFIED IN CONSISTENCY

| Food Groups | Clear liquid | Full liquid | Soft | Light or simple, general |
|---|---|---|---|---|
| Soup | Broth, bouillon | Same, plus strained soups | Same | All |
| Cereal | | | Refined cooked cereals, cornflakes, rice, noodles, macaroni, spaghetti | Same |
| Bread | | | White bread, crackers, melba, zwieback | Same, plus graham and rye bread |
| Protein foods | | Milk, cream, milk drinks | Same, plus eggs (not fried), mild cheese, fowl, fish, sweet-breads, tender beef, veal, lamb, liver, bacon, gravy | Same |
| Vegetables | | | Potatoes — baked, mashed, creamed, steamed, escalloped; tender, cooked-whole, bland vegetables (may be strained or pureed) | Same, cooked-whole bland; lettuce |
| Fruit and fruit juices | Apple juice | All fruit juices | Same, plus cooked fruit — peaches, pears, applesauce, peeled apricots, white cherries, bananas, orange and grapefruit sections without membrane | All |
| Desserts, gelatin | Plain gelatin, water ice | Same, plus sherbet, ice cream, puddings, custard | Same, plus plain sponge cakes, plain cookies, plain cake, simple puddings | Same |
| Miscellaneous | Ginger ale, carbonated water, coffee, tea | Same | Same, plus butter, salt, pepper | Same |

Adapted from Williams, S. R., *Nutrition and Diet Therapy,* 4th ed., C. V. Mosby, St. Louis, 1981, 498. With permission.

custard or puddings, and plain ice cream and sherbet may be used in addition to fruit juices, milk beverages, broth soup, tea, coffee, and carbonated beverages. Six or more feedings per day are recommended. The diet may be used in the acute stage of numerous diseases, for patients with fractured jaws, after oral or other types of surgery, or for patients who are too ill to eat solid foods.[5]

**Clear liquid** — This diet provides minimal residue and may be used after surgery, in acute infections, in acute inflammatory conditions of the gastrointestinal tract, or to minimize fecal material.[5] The purpose of the diet is to relieve thirst, prevent dehydration, and promote a gradual return to normal intake of food. Since an adequate intake of nutrients is not possible with this diet, it should not be continued for more than a few days. In addition to the foods shown in Table 1, some hospitals include all strained fruit juices and plain sugar candy.

**Low or minimal residue diet** — This diet is poorly defined and foods included in the diet may vary appreciably. In general, the diet is designed to leave a minimum of residue in the colon in the form of indigestible carbohydrate, connective tissue from meat, or insoluble salts. Milk may be eliminated or restricted in amount. Whole-grain cereals, nuts, tough cuts of meat, and fish or poultry with skin are eliminated. Nonfibrous cooked or strained fruits and vegetables may be allowed, although in some diets all fruits and vegetables are eliminated. The diet may be used prior to and following surgery of the colon or rectum or during acute stages of diarrhea and other gastrointestinal disturbances. It may also be used for patients with partial intestinal obstruction or those receiving radiation therapy of the pelvic area.[6,7] Commercial low-residue liquid products have tended to replace the use of this diet in many of these conditions.

**Bland diet** — The bland diet consists of foods that are considered bland or mild flavored. Foods which have traditionally been believed to cause chemical, mechanical, or thermal irritation to the gastrointestinal tract or to stimulate gastric acid secretion are eliminated. The diet has been used most frequently in the treatment of patients with gastric or duodenal ulcers, but may also be prescribed for patients with hiatal hernia or various conditions involving inflammation of the gastrointestinal tract. Alcohol and caffeine-containing beverages and meat broth soups are eliminated because they contain substances which stimulate gastric secretion. Recent evidence suggests that decaffeinaed coffee may nearly be as strong a stimulus to gastric acid secretion as regular coffee.[8] All spices, herbs, and condiments are usually excluded, although only a few (black pepper, chili powder, cayenne pepper, and possibly nutmeg) have been demonstrated to cause gastric irritation.[9] Fried foods, legumes, and vegetables such as cabbage, onions, and cauliflower are eliminated because they are considered to be difficult to digest. Coarse, raw, or hard foods are frequently omitted; however, there is little evidence that these foods irritate the gastric mucosa if a person is able to chew properly.[10] Small, frequent meals are recommended to help buffer gastric acid and avoid the distention stimulus to acid secretion.[11] After the initial neutralizing effect of ingested food, almost all foods will stimulate acid secretion; consequently, bedtime snacks should be avoided to prevent occurrence of hyperacidity during sleep.[12] A typical bland diet is described in Table 2.

Dietary treatment of patients with gastric or duodenal ulcer may consist of a series of bland diets sometimes referred to as "progressive" bland diets. Diets may be defined in terms of stages or degree of restriction (strict, moderate, or liberal). Foods allowed in the first stages may be limited to milk and cream, soft eggs, refined cooked cereals, white bread, potatoes, cottage cheese, strained cream soups, ice cream, plain puddings, and gelatin desserts. Tender meat, cooked or canned fruits and vegetables (sometimes pureed), and other foods are gradually introduced into the diet until it is similar to the one described in Table 2.

Because of the lack of evidence that strict bland diets are beneficial, dietary management of patients with nonbleeding ulcers has become much more liberal in recent years.[12-15] Patients are generally encouraged to eat a regular diet eliminating only alcohol, caffeine-containing beverages, and occasional foods or condiments that exacerbate ulcer pain.

### Tube Feedings

Various types of liquid diets may be administered by nasogastric, gastric, or jejunal tube whenever a patient is unable to consume food orally. This form of feeding may be used following surgery or injury, if a patient is comatose, when there is an obstruction of the gastrointestinal tract, or in treatment of certain mental disturbances.[16] Occasionally, nasogastric feeding may be used to supplement what would otherwise be an inadequate oral intake of food.

There are four basic types of tube feeding: milk-base formulas, low-residue formulas, homogenized food formulas, and elemental diets. Commercial preparations of all

Table 2
BLAND DIET

| Foods allowed | Foods to avoid |
|---|---|
| Beverages | |
| Cereal beverages; decaffeinated coffee | Alcoholic and carbonated beverages; coffee or tea (unless tolerated) |
| Milk | |
| Milk, cream, buttermilk | |
| Meat, eggs, cheese | |
| Tender meat, fish or fowl; liver; eggs boiled, poached, or scrambled in double boiler; cream, cottage, and other soft, mild cheeses | Fried, smoked, and preserved meat, fish, or fowl |
| Breads, cereals, macaroni products | |
| White bread and rolls, crackers; all refined cereals; macaroni, spaghetti, noodles | Breads or cereals made from whole grains or bran; dried legumes |
| Vegetables | |
| Potatoes, peas, squash, asparagus tips, carrots, tender string beans, beets, spinach | All raw; all cooked except those listed as allowed |
| Fruits | |
| Fruit juices (if tolerated); banana; avocados; baked apple (no skin), applesauce; canned peaches; pears; apricots; white cherries | All except those listed as allowed |
| Soups | |
| Cream soups made with "allowed" foods | Bouillon; broth-based soups |
| Desserts | |
| Custard; ice cream; simple puddings; gelatin desserts; sponge cake; plain cookies and cakes | Pastries; desserts made with coconut, raisins, nuts |
| Fats | |
| Butter, margarine; plain salad dressing | Fried and fatty foods; nuts; olives; highly seasoned salad dressing |
| Sweets and miscellaneous | |
| Sugar, jelly, salt, cocoa | Preserves; candy made with coconut, nuts, or other foods not allowed; pepper; other spices; mustard; ketchup; relishes; meat gravies |

*Note:* Principles — (1) low in fiber and connective tissue; (2) little or no condiments or spices; and (3) foods simply prepared.

Adapted from Mitchell, H. S., Rynbergen, H. J., Anderson, L., and Dibble, M. V., *Nutrition in Health and Disease*, 16th ed., J. B., Lippincott, New York, 1976, 348. With permission.

types are available, and most hospitals use these products rather than prepare their own.

Diarrhea has been associated with many types of tube feedings and may be related to bacterial contamination, a formula too high in osmolality, too rapid administration of the feeding, improper insertion of the tube, and use of excessively cold feedings.[17]

**Milk-base formulas** — These were the most common form of tube feeding for many years because of ease of preparation. Frequent problems with diarrhea probably occurred because of the high lactose content and osmolality of these formulas. Certain commercial products made from skim milk without added fat may have an excessively low-fat content, whereas the protein and lactose are undesirably high.

**Low-residue, low-lactose formulas** — Common ingredients in these products include intact proteins such as casein, egg whites or soy isolate, vegetable oils, and corn syrup solids or sugars. Their low osmolality, residue, and lactose content make them more suitable for treating some conditions than milk-based formulas, but the palatibility of some products tends to be lower.

**Homogenized-food formulas** — These diets are composed of a blended mixture of meat, vegetables, fruits, some form of complex carbohydrate, eggs, fats, milk, and sometimes added carbohydrate. In some instances, the formula is administered by a food pump, which allows use of a more viscous mixture and administration at a slow, constant speed. These diets have a distribution of energy sources more similar to that of a normal diet and are generally better tolerated than milk-base formulas.

**Elemental diets (or chemically defined diets)** — These commercial liquid formulas are often a mixture of synthetic amino acids or hydrolyzed protein, sugars, vitamins, and minerals. Carbohydrate in such products may provide more than 80% of the calories, with protein supplying most of the remaining calories. However, some products, may also contain fat, frequently in the form of medium chain triglycerides, which provides 30 to 35% of the total calories. The diets are free of indigestible matter thereby reducing residue in the intestines to the endogenous minimum. The formulas require minimal digestion and are generally absorbed rapidly in the upper portion of the small intestine. Numerous uses for elemental diets have been described, including pancreatic and biliary dysfunctions, inflammatory bowel disease, preoperative bowel preparations, fistulas of the alimentary tract, postoperative clear liquid, and after oral surgery. A special branch-chain amino-acid enriched elemental diet has recently been shown to be valuable in the treatment of chronic hepatic encephalopathy (18). Because the products tend to be expensive and some are also relatively low in protein, nearly fat free, and high in sodium, their use is best restricted to those conditions in which minimal residue and ease of digestion are of primary importance.[19]

An example of a blenderized food formula which can be prepared in the hospital or at home is given in Table 3. Tables 4 and 5 show the ingredients and nutrient composition found in various commercially available products for tube feeding. Most of these formulas also can be used as oral supplements to provide extra calories and protein, and several of the commercial products are available in different flavors.

**Total parenteral nutrition (hyperalimentation)** — Total parenteral nutrition is a means of feeding patients by the intravenous route using solutions which provide calories and other essential nutrients in amounts greater than those found in standard intravenous fluids. Proteins may be provided as crystalline amino acids or as hydrolyzates of proteins such as fibrin. Glucose is the major energy source. Vitamins and minerals may be added to the solution daily or at appropriate intervals. Fat preparations (Intralipid®, Cutter Laboratories, Inc. and Liposyn®, Abbott Laboratories) have recently been approved for intravenous use. Hyperalimentation solutions must be prepared under sterile conditions and their composition altered as indicated by the patient's condition.[20-23] Total parenteral nutrition has been of particular value in the management of the cancer patient.[24]

## DIETS MODIFIED IN SPECIFIC NUTRIENTS AND ENERGY CONTENT

### Modification in Protein

**Protein-free (0 to 5 g) diet** — Complete elimination of dietary protein is usually indicated for the patient with hepatic encephalopathy who is comatose or semicomatose.[25] The only foods allowed are sugar, hard candies, fat, and carbonated beverages. If restriction of sodium is indicated, the sodium content of these foods must be taken

Table 3
BLENDERIZED TUBE FEEDING

| Ingredients[a] | Weight (g) | Household measure |
|---|---|---|
| Milk (whole) | 244 | 1 cup |
| Milk (dry skim) | 16 | 2 tbsp |
| Cream (20% fat) | 100 | ½ cup |
| Egg (pasteurized powder) | 30 | 4 tbsp |
| Corn syrup | 70 | ½ cup |
| Strained pears | 70 | ½ jar |
| Strained peas | 70 | ½ jar |
| Strained beef | 100 | 6 tbsp |
| Orange juice | 100 | ½ cup |
| Water (add to make 1000 m$l$) | | |

| Composition (per 1000 m$l$) | |
|---|---|
| Energy (kcal) | 1022 |
| Protein (g) | 49.5 |
| Fat (g) | 45.5 |
| Carbohydrate (g) | 106.3 |
| Calcium (mg) | 711 |
| Iron (mg) | 8.5 |
| Vitamin A (IU) | 2946 |
| Vitamin C (mg) | 57 |

[a]   Place all ingredients in a mechanical blender and mix 10 min. Refrigerate immediately. Shake well before using.

[b]   Pasteurized powdered egg used to avoid *Salmonella;* 15 g powdered egg is equivalent to one egg.

Adapted from Mitchell, H. S. Rynbergen, H. J., Anderson, L., and Dibble, M. V., *Nutrition in Health and Disease,* 16th ed., J. B. Lippincott, New York, 1976, 367. With permission.

into consideration. Recipes are available for butter soup, butter pudding, and butter-sugar balls.[26,27] Appropriate commercial diet supplements or formulas may also be available for use.[18] The Borst diet, a zero-protein, low-potassium diet, was proposed by Borst[28] for patients in acute renal failure; however, the diet is generally considered drastic and is seldom used.[27]

Minimal or low-protein diets (20 to 40 g) — Sample diet patterns providing approximately 20, 30, and 40 g protein are presented in Table 6. Other patterns have been described.[29,30] Because of the higher content of essential amino acids in eggs and milk as compared to meat, fish, and poultry, these foods are usually used as the major source of protein in the very low-protein diets. If special low-protein bread is substituted for the regular bread, additional milk or egg may be included in the diet. Extra calories are provided by liberal use of sugars and protein-free fats and starches. Diets with varying degrees of protein restriction may be used in the treatment of patients with hepatic encephalopathy and acute or chronic uremia.[31,32] Protein restriction in the treatment of acute glomerulonephritis is controversial, but is generally used only if oliguria or anuria develops.[33] Because the control of sodium and/or potassium intake may also be indicated in many of these conditions, additional foods may need to be restricted because of their mineral content (see section on diets for treatment of chronic renal failure).

## Table 4
## INGREDIENTS IN COMMERCIALLY AVAILABLE PRODUCTS FOR TUBE FEEDING

| Product | Major ingredients |
| --- | --- |
| **Milk-based products** | |
| Nutri-1000®, Cutter Laboratories, Inc. | Skim milk, corn oil, corn syrup solids sodium caseinate vitamins, and minerals |
| Meritene® liquid, Doyle Pharmaceutical Company | Concentrated sweet skim milk, corn syrup solids, vegetable oil, sodium caseinate, sucrose |
| Sustacal® liquid, Mead Johnson Laboratories | Sucrose, concentrated sweet skim milk, corn syrup solids, partially hydrogenated soy oil, sodium and calcium caseinate, soy protein isolate |
| **Low-residue, lactose-free products (intact protein)** | |
| Ensure®, Ross Laboratories | Corn syrup solids, sucrose, sodium and calcium caseinates, corn oil, soy protein isolates |
| Isocal® Tube Feeding, Mead Johnson Laboratories | Corn syrup solids, soy oil, calcium and sodium caseinate, MCT oil, soy protein isolate |
| Portagen®, Mead Johnson Laboratories | Corn syrup solids, sugar, MCT oil, sodium caseinate, corn oil |
| Precision® Low-Residue Diet, Doyle Pharmaceutical Co., | Maltodextrin, pasteurized egg white solids, sugar, vegetable oil |
| Precision® High Nitrogen Diet, Doyle Pharmaceutical Co., | Maltodextrin, pasteurized egg white solids, sugar, calcium glycerophosphate, vegetable oil |
| Precision® Isotonic Diet, Doyle Pharmaceutical Co. | Glucose oligosaccharides, pasteurized egg white solids, sugar, vegetable oil |
| **Elemental diets (hydrolyzed protein or amino acids)** | |
| Flexical®, Mead Johnson Laboratories | Sucrose, dextrin, enzymatically hydrolyzed casein, soy oil, MCT, citric acid, mono- and diglyceride, lecithin, L-amino acids (L-methionine, L-tyrosine, L-tryptophan) |
| Vivonex® Standard, Eaton Laboratories, Inc. | Glucose oligosaccharides, purified L-amino acids, safflower oil |
| Vivonex® High Nitrogen, Eaton Laboratories, Inc. | Glucose oligosaccharides, purified L-amino acids, safflower oil |
| **Blenderized tube feedings** | |
| Formula 2®, Cutter Laboratories, Inc. | Nonfat dry milk, beef, sucrose, carrots, corn oil, orange juice concentrate, egg yolks, green beans, farina, cellulose gum |
| Compleat-B®, Doyle Pharmaceutical Co. | Beef puree, maltodextrin, green bean puree, pea puree, nonfat dry milk, corn oil, sucrose, peach puree, orange juice |
| Vitaneed®, Organon, Inc. | Corn syrup solids, puree beef, soy oil, calcium caseinate, maltodextrin, puree green beans, peaches, carrots |

**Gluten-restricted or gliadin-free diet** — This diet eliminates wheat, rye, oats, barley, buckwheat, and products containing these cereal grains. Food restrictions are usually based on those originally described by Sleisenger et al.[34] Special recipes are available for baked products using gluten-free wheat starch and flour from nonrestricted cereals.[34,35] The diet is used primarily in the treatment of celiac disease or gluten-induced enteropathy,[36] but has recently been shown to be of value in patients with dermatitis herpetiformis.[37,38]

**Purine-restricted diet** — A diet low in purines may occasionally be used to aid in

## Table 5
## COMPARISON OF NUTRIENT COMPOSITION OF 2000 ml OF VARIOUS COMMERCIALLY AVAILABLE TUBE FEEDINGS[a,b]

| Energy and nutrients | Milk-base products | | Low-residue, low-lactose products (intact protein) | | | | Elemental diets | | Blenderized tube feeding | | |
|---|---|---|---|---|---|---|---|---|---|---|---|
| | I | II | III | IV | V | VI | VII | VIII | IX | X | XI |
| Energy (kcal) | 2000 | 2000 | 2120 | 2120 | 2220 | 2100 | 2000 | 2000 | 2000 | 2000 | 2040 |
| Protein (g) | 120 | 120 | 74 | 68 | 52 | 88 | 45 | 84 | 80 | 76 | 75 |
| Fat (g) | 46 | 67 | 74 | 88 | 2 | 1 | 68 | 2 | 80 | 80 | 80 |
| CHO (g) | 279 | 230 | 290 | 260 | 498 | 436 | 305 | 420 | 240 | 246 | 260 |
| Calcium (mg) | 2000 | 2500 | 1060 | 1260 | 1160 | 800 | 1200 | 666 | 1260 | 1440 | 1150 |
| Phosphorus (mg) | 1840 | 2500 | 1060 | 1060 | 1160 | 800 | 1000 | 666 | 3400 | 1120 | 1050 |
| Magnesium (mg) | 760 | 667 | 420 | 420 | 468 | 280 | 400 | 266 | 500 | 200 | 500 |
| Iron (mg) | 34 | 30 | 19 | 19 | 21 | 13 | 18 | 12 | 23 | 25 | 24 |
| Sodium (mg) | 1840 | 1833 | 1480 | 1060 | 1400 | 2000 | 700 | 1542 | 3120 | 1200 | 1100 |
| Potassium (mg) | 4120 | 3333 | 2540 | 2640 | 1740 | 1800 | 2500 | 1400 | 2620 | 3520 | 2500 |
| Vitamin A (IU) | 9280 | 8333 | 5284 | 5280 | 5840 | 3520 | 5000 | 3332 | 6250 | 5000 | 7000 |
| Thiamin (mg) | 2.8 | 3.8 | 3.2 | 4.0 | 2.6 | 1.6 | 3.8 | 1.0 | 2.8 | 1.6 | 2.6 |
| Riboflavin (mg) | 3.4 | 3.8 | 3.6 | 4.6 | 3.0 | 1.8 | 4.4 | 1.0 | 2.8 | 1.8 | 3.0 |
| Niacin (mg) | 38 | 33 | 42 | 52 | 23 | 14 | 50 | 13 | 25 | 20 | 36 |
| Ascorbic acid (mg) | 112 | 150 | 320 | 316 | 106 | 64 | 300 | 40 | 113 | 78 | 120 |

[a] Since manufacturers may modify composition periodically, accuracy of values should be checked carefully with product labels.

[b] I, Sustacal®, Mead Johnson Laboratories; II, Meritene,® Doyle Pharmaceutical Co.; III, Ensure®, Ross Laboratories; IV, Isocal®, Mead Johnson Laboratories; V, Precision® Low-Residue, Doyle Pharmaceutical Co.; VI, Precision® High Nitrogen, Doyle Pharmaceutical Co.; VII, Flexical®, Mead Johnson Laboratories; VIII, Vivonex® High Nitrogen, Eaton Laboratories, Inc.; IX, Compleat B®, Doyle Pharmaceutical Co.; X, Formula 2®, Cutter Laboratories, Inc.; and XI, Vitaneed®, Organon, Inc.

Table 6
MINIMAL OR LOW-PROTEIN DIETS

| | Approximate protein intake (g) | | |
| --- | --- | --- | --- |
| Food group | 20 | 30 | 40 |
| Milk | 4 oz | 4 oz | 8 oz |
| Egg | 1 | 1 | 1 |
| Meat, fish, or poultry | — | 1 oz | 2 oz |
| Fruit | 3 servings | 3 servings | 3 servings |
| Bread, cereals, legumes[a] | 3 servings | 3 servings | 3 servings |
| Vegetables | 2 servings[b] | 2 servings | 2 servings |

[a]  Size of serving adjusted to provide 2 g protein/serving.
[b]  For this diet the kind and amount of vegetable is adjusted to provide
    ≤ 1 g protein/serving; in the other diets vegetables provide 2 to 5 g
    protein.

lowering elevated blood uric acid or maintaining normal concentrations in patients with gout or uric acid renal calculi. Foods commonly eliminated or restricted include organ meats, sardines, anchovies, meat extracts, broth soups, gravy, dried legumes, wheat germ and bran, and oatmeal. Diets containing approximately 35 or 100 mg[39] and 125 mg purines[40] have been described.

Low phenylalanine diet — Restriction of dietary phenylalanine forms the basis of treatment for infants and children with the hereditary metabolic disease phenylketonuria.[41] Since phenylalanine is an essential amino acid required for growth, it cannot be completely eliminated from the diet. However, dietary intake is adjusted to an amount (approximately 15 to 25 mg/kg body weight) which will reduce elevated serum phenylalanine and maintain concentrations within acceptable ranges. Frequent determinations of blood phenylalanine levels are required, followed by appropriate adjustments in dietary intake. The diet for the young infant is based on a proprietary formula low in phenylalanine such as Lofenalac® (Mead Johnson). Solid foods are introduced into the diet as the child grows. These foods are selected from lists of phenylalanine food exchange groups or equivalents.[42,43]

Other diet modifications involving amino acids — Diets or infant formulas modified in amino acids have been tried in the treatment of a number of hereditary metabolic disorders. Tyrosinemia may be treated by restriction of dietary tyrosine and phenylalanine[41,44] and methionine.[45] Artificial formula and diets low in branched chain amino acids (valine, leucine, and isoleucine) have been described for treatment of maple syrup urine disease.[46-48] Low-methionine or low-methionine, high-cystine diets have been proposed for treatment of homocystinuria[49,50] and cystinuria.[51] Dietary restriction of leucine may be beneficial for infants with leucine-induced hypoglycemia.[52]

Modification in Fat

Fat-restricted diets (30 and 50 g) — Approximately 50 g fat will be provided by a diet containing the following foods: 5 oz cooked meat, fish or poultry (moderate fat, 5 g/oz meat), 1 egg, and 4 tsp fat (butter, margarine, or oil). Fruits, vegetables cereals, plain bread, skim milk, sugars, and fat-free sweets may be used to provide additional calories and protein. The amount of fat can be reduced to approximately 30 g by omitting 3 tsp fat and 1 oz meat (or 1 egg) from the diet pattern described above. Fat-restricted diets may be used in the management of patients with steatorrhea or serious diseases of the biliary tract or pancreas.[53]

Diets modified in type and amount of fat — Modifications in the type and amount of dietary fat have been recommended to lower and control serum cholesterol and total circulating lipids.[54] The total amount of fat in the diet is restricted to approximately 30 to 35% of the total calories. The amount of polyunsaturated (P) fat is increased and the saturated (S) fat decreased to give P:S ratios ranging from approximately 1:1 to 2.8:1 in contrast to the 0.5:1 ratio found in the average American diet. Dietary cholesterol is restricted to less than 300 mg a day. Many different diet plans have been described following these general principles. The American Heart Association has prepared pamphlets listing amounts and kinds of foods to be used in fat-modified diets at several levels of caloric intake.[55] Recommendations for a modified fat diet unrestricted in calories are summarized in Table 7.

Diets for specific types of hyperlipoproteinemia will be described later.

## Modification in Carbohydrate

**Lactose-restricted diet** — This diet excludes lactose in the form of milk, most milk products, and processed foods with added lactose or whey. The diet may be prescribed for persons with lactose intolerance related to decreased activity of intestinal lactase. The degree of restriction necessary to control symptoms varies among individuals. Many adults tolerate the small amount of lactose present in such foods as butter, margarine, bread, and hard cheeses. Typical uses of lactose in foods and medications were listed by Koch et al.[56]

**Galactose-free diet** — All foods containing lactose and galactose are eliminated in the treatment of infants and children with galactosemia. In addition to milk, milk products, and all processed foods containing lactose, galactose-storing organ meats such as liver, pancreas, and brain are eliminated. Legumes are sometimes omitted on the basis that they contain oligosaccharides which may yield galactose on hydrolysis.[56] A protein hydrolysate or meat-base formula may be used as a milk substitute for infant feeding. Use of soy formulas has been controversial; however, the oligosaccharides do not seem to be broken down in the intestine and appear to be satisfactory.[57]

**Fructose-restricted diet** — Dietary restriction of fructose from fruits and foods high in sucrose may be used in the treatment of hereditary fructose intolerance or abnormalities in fructose absorption.[58] Table sugar, syrups, sweets, and processed foods containing sugar are eliminated. Vegetables which are permitted include asparagus, cabbage, cauliflower, celery, green beans, green peppers, lettuce, spinach, wax beans, and white potatoes. All other vegetables, sweet potatoes, and all fruits are omitted.[58]

## Other Diets with Controlled Intake of Protein, Fat, and Carbohydrate

**Diabetic diets** — The single most important objective in dietary treatment of diabetic patients is control of caloric intake to achieve and maintain ideal body weight. Although opinions differ regarding the need for additional modifications, most diets used to treat diabetics have the following characteristics: (1) elimination of sucrose and most foods with added sucrose and (2) regularity of meals, with a similar intake of calories at the same time each day.[59] For the insulin-dependent patient, the distribution of meals will be influenced by the type of insulin he is receiving and his response to it.

In 1950 a committee representing the American Diabetes Association, U.S. Public Health Service, and The American Dietetic Association published a widely used method of calculating diabetic diets. Commonly used foods were grouped according to similar nutrient composition into six groups called "Exchange Lists".[60] Ideally, a daily diet plan, giving the number of exchanges permitted at each meal was calculated for each individual diabetic patient. However, for the convenience of physicians a series of diet plans ranging in caloric value from 1200 to 3000 cal was outlined by the American Diabetes Association.[61] A similar series of diet plans with modifications in the type and amount of fat was published in 1967.[62] In 1976 an expanded and revised version of the original Exchange Lists was presented in the booklet, "Exchange Lists for Meal Planning".[63] These Exchange Lists are shown in Table 8. The major revisions

Table 7

MODIFIED FAT DIET WITH UNRESTRICTED CALORIES[a]

| Food Group | Amount | Recommended | Avoid or use sparingly |
|---|---|---|---|
| Meat, fish, poultry, dried beans and peas | 6—8 oz (cooked) | Limit use of lean beef, lamb, pork, and ham to 9 oz./week; use chicken, turkey, veal, legumes for remaining meals; cottage cheese (preferably uncreamed) or low-fat yogurt also may be used as meat substitutes | Duck, goose; heavily marbled and fatty meats; organ meats; shellfish |
| Eggs | | Limit egg yolk to 3 per week including eggs used in cooking | |
| Milk products | 2—3 cups | Use skim milk, nonfat dry milk; buttermilk and yogurt from skimmed milk; 1 oz cheese made from skimmed or partially skimmed milk can be substituted for 1 cup milk | Whole milk and whole milk products: ice cream, whipped cream; nondairy cream substitute; cheese made from cream or whole milk |
| Fats and oils | 4 or more Tbsp | Use polyunsaturated vegetable oils: corn, cottonseed, safflower, sesame, soybean; 1—2 tbsp special polyunsaturated margarine may be substituted for the oil; salad dressings and mayonnaise containing these oils | Solid fats and shortenings: butter, lard, salt pork, hydrogenated shortening, coconut oil, bacon fat |
| Breads and cereals | As desired (8—10 servings) | Breads made with a minimum of saturated fat | Commercial or homemade products or mixes containing egg yolk or saturated fat |
| Vegetables and fruits Desserts, beverages, sweets, sugars | As desired As desired | | Commercial or homemade products or mixes containing egg yolk or saturated fat |

[a]  This diet would provide approximately 30% of the calories from fat, with 4% from saturated fatty acids, and 11% from linoleic fatty acid. Cholesterol intake would be 250-300 mg.

Adapted from *Planning Fat-Controlled Meals for Approximately 2000-2600 Calories* (revised), American Heart Association, New York, 1967. With permission.

## Table 8
## EXCHANGE LISTS FOR MEAL PLANNING

### List 1. Milk Exchanges

One exchange contains 12 g carbohydrate, 8 g protein, a trace of fat, and 80 kcal; this list shows the kinds and amounts of milk or milk products to use for one milk exchange; Foods listed in bold type are nonfat

| | |
|---|---|
| **Nonfat fortified milk** | |
| **Skim or nonfat milk** | 1 cup |
| **Powdered (nonfat dry, before adding liquid)** | ⅓ cup |
| **Canned, evaporated skim milk** | ½ cup |
| **Buttermilk made from skim milk** | 1 cup |
| **Yogurt made from skim milk (plain, unflavored)** | 1 cup |
| Low-fat fortified milk | |
| 1% Fat fortified milk (omit ½ fat exchange) | 1 cup |
| 2% Fat fortified milk (omit 1 fat exchange) | 1 cup |
| Yogurt made from 2% fortified milk (plain, unflavored) (omit 1 fat exchange) | 1 cup |
| Whole milk (omit 2 fat exchanges) | |
| Whole milk | 1 cup |
| Canned, evaporated whole milk | ½ cup |
| Buttermilk made from whole milk | 1 cup |
| Yogurt made from whole milk (plain, unflavored) | 1 cup |

### List 2. Vegetable Exchanges

One exchange contains about 5 g carbohydrates, 2 g protein, and 25 kcal; this list shows the kinds of vegetables to use for one vegetable exchange; one exchange is ½ cup

| | |
|---|---|
| Asparagas | **Greens** |
| Bean sprouts | Mustard |
| Beets | Spinach |
| Broccoli | Turnip |
| Brussel sprouts | **Mushrooms** |
| Cabbage | Okra |
| Carrots | Onions |
| Cauliflower | Rhubarb |
| Celery | Rutabaga |
| Cucumbers | Sauerkraut |
| Eggplant | **String beans (green or yellow)** |
| Green pepper | **Summer squash** |
| Greens | Tomatoes |
| Beet | Tomato juice |
| Chards | Turnips |
| Collards | **Vegetable juice cocktail** |
| Dandelion | Zucchini |
| Kale | |

The following raw vegetables may be used as desired

| | |
|---|---|
| Chicory | Lettuce |
| Chinese cabbage | Parsley |
| Endive | Radishes |
| Escarole | Watercress |

### List 3. Fruit Exchanges

One exchange of fruit contains 10 g carbohydrate and 40 kcal; fruit may be used fresh, dried, canned or frozen, cooked or raw, as long as no sugar is added; this list shows the kinds and amounts of fruit to use for one fruit exchange

Table 8 (continued)
## EXCHANGE LISTS FOR MEAL PLANNING
### List 3. Fruit Exchanges

| | | | |
|---|---|---|---|
| Apple | 1 small | Mango | ½ small |
| Apple juice | ⅓ cup | Melon | |
| Applesauce (unsweetened) | ½ cup | Cantaloupe | ¼ small |
| Apricots (fresh) | 2 medium | Honeydew | 1/8 medium |
| Apricots (dried) | 4 halves | Watermelon | 1 cup |
| Banana | ½ small | Nectarine | 1 small |
| Berries | | Orange | 1 small |
| Blackberries | ½ cup | Orange juice | ½ cup |
| Blueberries | ½ cup | Papaya | ¾ cup |
| Raspberries | ½ cup | Peach | 1 medium |
| Strawberries | ¾ cup | Pear | 1 small |
| Cherries | 10 large | Persimmon, native | 1 medium |
| Cider | ⅓ cup | Pineapple | ½ cup |
| Dates | 2 | Pineapple juice | ⅓ cup |
| Figs, fresh | 1 | Plums | 2 medium |
| Figs, dried | 1 | Prunes | 2 medium |
| Grapefruit | ½ | Prune juice | ¼ cup |
| Grapefruit juice | ½ cup | Raisins | 2 Tbsp |
| Grapes | 12 | Tangerine | 1 medium |
| Grape juice | ¼ cup | | |

Cranberries may be used as desired if no sugar is added

### List 4. Bread Exchanges (Includes Cereals and Starchy Vegetables)

One exchange contains 15 g carbohydrate, 2 g protein, and 70 kcal; this list shows the kinds and amounts of breads, cereals, starchy vegetables, and prepared fruit to use for one bread exchange; those which appear in Bold type are low fat

| | | | |
|---|---|---|---|
| **Bread** | | Oyster | 20 |
| **White (including French and Italian)** | 1 slice | Pretzels, 3 1/8 long × 1/8 in. diam. | 25 |
| **Whole wheat** | 1 slice | Rye wafers, 2 × 3½ in. | 3 |
| **Rye or pumpernickel** | 1 slice | **Saltines** | 6 |
| **Raisin** | 1 slice | Soda, 2½ in.² | 4 |
| **Bagel, small** | ½ | **Dried beans, peas, and lentils** | |
| **English muffin, small** | ½ | **Beans, peas, lentils (dried and cooked)** | ½ cup |
| **Plain roll, bread** | 1 | **Baked beans, no pork (canned)** | ¼ cup |
| **Frankfurter roll** | ½ | Starchy vegetables | |
| **Hamburger bun** | ½ | **Corn** | ⅓ cup |
| **Dried bread crumbs** | 3 Tbsp | **Corn on cob** | 1 small |
| **Tortilla, 6 in.** | 1 | **Lima beans** | ½ cup |
| **Cereal** | | **Parsnips** | ⅔ cup |
| **Bran flakes** | ½ cup | **Peas, green (canned or frozen)** | ½ cup |
| **Other ready-to-eat unsweetened cereal** | ¾ cup | **Potato, white** | 1 small |
| **Puffed cereal (unfrosted)** | 1 cup | **Potato (mashed)** | ½ cup |
| **Cereal (cooked)** | ½ cup | **Pumpkin** | ¾ cup |
| **Grits (cooked)** | ½ cup | **Winter squash, acorn or butternut** | ½ cup |
| **Rice or barley (cooked)** | ½ cup | **Yam or sweet potato** | ¼ cup |
| **Pasta (cooked), spaghetti, noodles, macaroni** | ½ cup | | |
| **Popcorn (popped, no fat added)** | 3 cups | Prepared Foods | |
| **Cornmeal (dry)** | 2 Tbsp | Biscuit 2 in. diam. (omit 1 fat exchange) | 1 |
| **Flour** | 2½ Tbsp | Corn bread, 2 × 2 × 1 in. (omit 1 fat exchange) | 1 |
| **Wheat germ** | ¼ cup | Corn muffin, 2 in. diam. (omit 1 fat exchange) | 1 |
| **Crackers** | | Crackers, round butter type (omit 1 fat exchange) | 5 |
| **Arrowroot** | 3 | | |
| **Graham, 2½ in.²** | 2 | | |
| **Matzoth, 4 × 6 in.** | ½ | | |

## Table 8 (continued)
## EXCHANGE LISTS FOR MEAL PLANNING

### List 4. Bread Exchanges (Includes Cereals and Starchy Vegetables)

| | | | |
|---|---|---|---|
| Muffin, plain small (omit 1 fat exchange) | 1 | Pancake, 5 × ½ in. (omit 1 fat exchange) | 1 |
| Potatoes, french fried, length 2—3½ in. (omit 1 fat exchange) | 8 | Waffle, 5 × ½ in. (omit 1 fat exchange) | 1 |
| Potato or corn chips (omit 2 fat exchanges) | 15 | | |

### List 5. Meat Exchanges

*Lean Meat* — One exchange of lean meat (1 oz) contains 7 g protein, 3 g fat, and 55 kcal; this list shows the kinds and amounts of lean meat and other protein-rich foods to use for one low-fat meat exchange

| | |
|---|---|
| Beef | 1 oz |
| Baby beef (very lean), chipped beef, chuck, flank steak, tenderloin, plate ribs, plate skirt steak, round (bottom, top), all cuts rump, spare ribs, tripe | |
| Lamb | |
| Leg, rib, sirloin, loin (roast and chops), shank, shoulder | 1 oz |
| Pork | |
| Leg (whole rump, center shank), ham, smoked (center slices) | 1 oz |
| Veal | |
| Leg, loin, rib, shank, shoulder cutlets | 1 oz |
| Poultry | |
| Meat without skin of chicken turkey, cornish hen, guinea hen, pheasant | 1 oz |
| Fish | |
| Any fresh or frozen | 1 oz |
| canned salmon, tuna, mackerel, crab and lobster, | ¼ cup |
| clams, clams, oysters, scallops, shrimp | 5 or 1 oz |
| sardines, drained | 3 |
| Cheeses containing less than 5% butterfat | 1 oz |
| Cottage cheese, dry and 2% butterfat | ¼ cup |
| Dried beans and peas (omit 1 bread exchange) | ½ cup |

*Medium-Fat meat* — For each exchange of medium fat meat omit ½ fat exchange; this list shows the kinds and amounts of medium-fat meat and other protein-rich foods to use for one medium-fat meat exchange

| | |
|---|---|
| Beef | |
| Ground (15% fat), corned (canned), rib eye, round (ground commercial) | 1 oz |
| Pork | |
| Loin (all cuts tenderloin), shoulder arm (picnic), shoulder blade, Boston butt, Canadian bacon, boiled ham | 1 oz |
| Liver, heart, kidney and sweetbreads (these are high in cholesterol) | 1 oz |
| Cottage cheese, creamed | ¼ cup |
| Cheese | |
| Mozzarella, ricotta, farmer's cheese, neufchatel, | 1 oz |
| Parmesan | 3 Tbsp |
| Egg (high in cholesterol) | 1 |
| Peanut butter (omit 2 additional fat exchanges) | 2 Tbsp |

*High-Fat Meat Exchanges* — For each exchange of high-fat meat omit 1 fat exchange; this list shows the kinds and amounts of high-fat meat and other protein-rich foods to use for one high-fat meat exchange

| | |
|---|---|
| Beef | |
| Brisket, corned beef (brisket), ground beef (more than 20% fat), hamburger (commercial), chuck (ground commercial), roasts (rib), steaks (club and rib) | 1 oz |

**Table 8 (continued)**
**EXCHANGE LISTS FOR MEAL PLANNING**

### List 5. Meat Exchanges

| | |
|---|---|
| Lamb | |
|   Breast | 1 oz |
| Pork | |
|   Spare ribs, loin (back ribs), pork (ground), country style ham, deviled ham | 1 oz |
| Veal | |
|   Breast | 1 oz |
| Poultry | |
|   Capon, duck (domestic), goose | 1 oz |
| Cheese | |
|   Cheddar types | 1 oz |
| Cold cuts | 4½ × 1/8 in. slice |
| Frankfurters | 1 small |

### List 6. Fat Exchanges

One exchange of fat contains 5 g fat and 45 kcal; this list shows the kinds and amounts of fat-containing foods to use for one fat exchange; to plan a diet low in saturated fat, select only those exchanges which appear in **bold type** — they are polyunsaturated

| | | | |
|---|---|---|---|
| Margarine, soft, tub or stick[a] | 1 tsp | Margarine, regular stick | 1 tsp |
| Avocado, (4 in. in diam.)[b] | 1/8 | Butter | 1 tsp |
| Oil, corn, cottonseed, safflower, soy, sunflower | 1 tsp | Bacon fat | 1 tsp |
| | | Bacon, crisp | 1 strip |
| Oil, olive[b] | 1 tsp | Cream, light | 2 Tbsp |
| Oil, peanut[b] | 1 tsp | Cream, sour | 2 Tbsp |
| Olives[b] | 5 small | Cream, heavy | 1 Tbsp |
| Almonds[b] | 10 whole | Cream cheese | 1 Tbsp |
| Pecans[b] | 2 whole large | French dressing[c] | 1 Tbsp |
| Peanuts[b] | | Italian dressing[c] | 1 Tbsp |
|   Spanish | 20 whole | Lard | 1 tsp |
|   Virginia | 10 whole | Mayonnaise[c] | 1 tsp |
| Walnuts | 6 small | Salad dressing, mayonnaise type[c] | 2 tsp |
| Nuts, other[b] | 6 small | Salt pork | ¾ in.³ |

[a]  Made with corn, cottonseed, safflower, soy, or sunflower oil only.
[b]  Fat content is primarily monounsaturated.
[c]  Can be used on fat modified diet if made with corn, cottonseed, safflower, soy, or sunflower oil.

Adapted from *Exchange Lists for Meal Planning*, American Diabetes Association, Inc., and the American Dietetic Association, New York, 1976. With permission.

were in the milk and meat exchanges, with skim milk and lean meat being the basis for the respective exchanges, rather than whole milk and medium-fat meat. Other changes were also designed to assist the diabetic in selecting foods with a low-cholesterol, high-polyunsaturated fat content.

The intent of the revised booklet is to promote individualization of diabetic diets. The diet for each patient is calculated by the dietitian in consultation with the physician.[64] The diet prescription is formulated to meet the needs of the individual patient. Energy intake is adjusted to achieve and maintain desirable body weight. Intake of protein, fat, and carbohydrate is controlled, but does not differ significantly from amounts found in desirable diets for normal persons. Many diabetic diets tend to be generous in protein, with at least 15 to 20% of the calories supplied by protein. For

Table 9

SAMPLE DIET PLAN FOR A 2200 CALORIE
DIABETIC DIET[a]

| | Number of food exchanges[b] | | Number of food exchanges |
|---|---|---|---|
| Breakfast | | Lunch | |
| Fruit | 2 | Meat | 3 |
| Meat | 1 | Bread | 2 |
| Bread | 3 | Vegetable | 1 |
| Fat | 4 | Fruit | 2 |
| Milk | 1 | Fat | 3 |
| | | Milk | 1 |
| Dinner | | Bedtime | |
| Meat | 3 | Milk | 1 |
| Bread | 3 | Bread | 1 |
| Vegetable | 1 | Meat | 2 |
| Fruit | 2 | Fat | 2 |
| Fat | 3 | | |

[a]  Diet provides approximately 110 g protein, 90 g fat (37% of calories), and 240 g carbohydrates; fraction of total calories at each meal is approximately 2/7, 2/7, 2/7, and 1/7.

[b]  Exchange lists are given in Table 8.

many years, diabetic diets were restricted in total carbohydrate; however, results of recent investigations indicate that high-carbohydrate diets do not have an adverse effect on diabetic control or insulin requirements.[65] There is some evidence that high-fiber diets or supplementation with fiber sources such as guar gum may improve glucose tolerance and reduce insulin requirements.[66,67] Because of the increased susceptibility of the diabetic to cardiovascular disease, many diets currently being recommended are moderately restricted in total fat (approximately 35% of calories), with an emphasis on decreased saturated fat and cholesterol intake. Factors such as food preferences, life style, and economic status are taken into consideration in planning the number and kinds of exchanges and their distribution into meals. A sample diet plan for a 2200 kcal diabetic diet is shown in Table 9.

Probably the majority of diabetic patients are placed on diets using Exchange Lists with amounts of food given in household measures. However, some physicians instruct patients to weigh all food. At the other extreme, some diabetic patients are advised only to eat regular meals and omit foods containing sugar.

**Low-carbohydrate, high-protein diet** — Diets designed to provide a minimum stimulation for insulin secretion may be prescribed for persons experiencing alimentary or reactive hypoglycemia. The diet usually emphasizes high-protein foods with limited amounts of carbohydrates as milk, cereals, frutis, and vegetables.[68] Sugars and foods with added sugar are eliminated. Foods should be distributed in six or more balanced feedings per day. The following pattern of food exchanges would provide approximately 120 g carbohydrate, 130 g protein, and 2000 kcal: 2 milk (regular), 3 vegetable, 2 fruit, 4 bread, 14 meat, and 10 fat. Additional calories can be supplied by increasing the number of meat and fat exchanges. Recently, diets low in simple sugar, but unrestricted in complex carbohydrate and dietary fiber, have been advocated in the treatment of alimentary hypoglycemia.[69]

**Low-carbohydrate, high-protein, restricted fluid diet** — This diet may be used in treating patients with the dumping or postgastrectomy syndrome.[70] General characteristics of the diet and a suggested meal pattern are given in Table 10.

## Table 10
## LOW-CARBOHYDRATE, HIGH-PROTEIN, RESTRICTED FLUID DIET[a]

### General description[b]

1. Five or six small meals daily
2. Relatively high-fat content to retard passage of food
3. High-protein content to rebuild tissue
4. Relatively low-carbohydrate content to prevent rapid passage of quickly utilized foods
5. No milk; no sugar, sweets, or desserts; no alcohol or sweet carbonated beverages
6. Liquids between meals only; avoid fluids for at least 1 hr before and after meals
7. Relatively low roughage foods; raw foods as tolerated

### Patterns of food exchanges[c]

| Breakfast | | a.m. Snack | |
|---|---|---|---|
| Fruit | 1 | Meat | 2 |
| Bread | 1 | Bread | 1 |
| Meat | 2 | Fat | 1 |
| Fat | 2 | | |
| | | | |
| Lunch | | p.m. Snack | |
| Meat | 3 | Meat | 2 |
| Bread | 1 | Bread | 1 |
| Vegetable | 1 | Fat | 1 |
| Fruit | 1 | | |
| Fat | 2 | | |
| | | | |
| Dinner | | Bedtime snack | |
| Meat | 4 | Meat | 2 |
| Vegetable | 1 | Bread | 1 |
| Fruit | 1 | Fat | 1 |
| Fat | 2 | | |

[a]  Diet provides approximately 120 g protein, 115 g carbohydrate, and 2000 kcal.
[b]  Adapted from Williams, S. R., *Nutrition and Diet Therapy,* 4th ed., C. V. Mosby, St. Louis, 1981, 675.
[c]  Food Exchange lists given in Table 8. Calories calculated on the basis of medium-fat meat.

**Ketogenic diet** — A ketogenic diet may be used in the treatment of some types of epilepsy and convulsive disorders in children. The diet is high in fat and severely restricted in carbohydrate. Protein and energy intake should be sufficient to allow normal growth. Foods must be carefully measured or weighed. To produce ketosis, the ketogenic-antiketogenic (K-AK) ratio of the diet must usually be 3:1 or 4:1. In computing the K-AK ration, 90% of fat and 50% of protein are calculated as ketogenic; 100% of carbohydrate, 10% of fat, and 50% of protein are considered antiketogenic. Details regarding diet calculations and foods allowed in the diet have been described by Mike[71] and Lasser and Brush.[72] Medium-chain triglycerides (MCT) appear to induce ketosis more readily than regular dietary fats, and a ketogenic diet using MCT has recently been described.[73]

**Fat and carbohydrate modifications for specific types of hyperlipoproteinemias** — A system for classifying blood lipid abnormalities based on measurements of lipoproteins has been described by Frederickson et al.[74] and Levy.[75] Five types of hyperlipoproteinemia were originally described. Type II was later modified to Type IIa and IIb.[76] Table 11 lists the changes in blood lipids characteristic of each type of hyperlipoproteinemia and the diet modifications recommended to correct the abnormalities. Detailed dietary plans for each of the types of hyperlipoproteinemia are available, including food lists, guidelines for purchase and preparation of food, and suggestions for eating out.[77] Food allowances for an 1800 kcal diet are shown in Table 12.

# Table 11
## BLOOD LIPID CHARACTERISTICS AND DIET MODIFICATIONS FOR SPECIFIC TYPES OF HYPERLIPOPROTEINEMIAS

| | Type I | Type IIa | Type IIb and Type III | Type IV | Type V |
|---|---|---|---|---|---|
| | | | **Characteristics of Blood Lipid Patterns** | | |
| Serum cholesterol | Normal or elevated | Elevated | Elevated | Normal or elevated | Elevated or normal |
| Serum triglyceride | Markedly elevated | Normal or slightly elevated | Usually elevated | Elevated | Elevated to markedly elevated |
| Lipoprotein[a] profile | Elevated chylomicrons | Increased LDL | Type IIb, increased LDL and VLDL; Type III, increased ILDL | Increased VLDL | Increased VLDL and chylomicrons |
| | | | **Diets Modifications** | | |
| General prescription | Low fat (25—35 g) | Low cholesterol, increased polyunsaturated fat | Low cholesterol, approximately 20% kcal protein, 40% kcal fat, and 40% kcal CHO | Controlled carbohydrate, moderately restricted cholesterol | Restricted fat, controlled carbohydrate, moderate cholesterol |
| Energy | Calories not restricted | Calories not restricted | Achieve and maintain "ideal" body weight | Achieve and maintain "ideal" body weight | Achieve and maintain "ideal" body weight |
| Protein | Amount not limited | Amount not limited | 18—21% total calories; 1½—2 g/kg body weight | Amount not limited | 21—24% total calories; 1½—2 g/kg body weight |
| Fat | Restrict amount 25—35 g; type not important | Increased polyunsaturated; limited saturated | 40% of total calories; emphasis on polyunsaturated | Not limited unless calorie restriction is indicated; emphasis on polyunsaturated fat | 0.9—1.3 g/kg body weight; polyunsaturated fat in preference to saturated |

| Cholesterol | Not restricted | Less than 300 mg/day; 100—200 mg preferred | Less than 300 mg/day | 300—500 mg/day | 300—500 mg/day |
|---|---|---|---|---|---|
| Carbohydrates | Not limited | Not limited | Controlled, restriction of sucrose and concentrated sweets | Limited to 4—5 g/kg body weight, restriction of concentrated sweets | Limited to 5 g/kg body weight, limited sucrose and concentrated sweets |
| Alcohol | Not recommended | Use with discretion | Limited use[b] | Limited use[b] | Not recommended |

[a] LDL = low-density lipoprotein; VLDV = very low-density lipoprotein; and ILDL = intermediate low-density lipoprotein.

[b] Limit to two servings per day. One serving equivalent to 1 oz gin, rum, vodka, or whiskey, 1½ oz sweet wine, 2½ oz dry wine, or 5 oz beer.

Adapted from Frederickson, D. S., Levy, R. I., Bonnell, M., and Ernst, N., The Dietary Management of Hyperlipoproteinemia, A Handbook for Physicians and Dietitians, Publ. No. (NIH) 76-110, U.S. Department of Health, Education and Welfare, Washington, D.C., 1974.

Table 12
## FOOD ALLOWANCES FOR 1700-2000 CALORIE DIETS FOR HYPERLIPOPROTEINEMIA

|  | Type I | Type II | Type IIb and Type III | Type IV | Type V |
|---|---|---|---|---|---|
| Skim milk (cups) | 4 | 2 | 2 | 2 | 4 |
| Lean meat, poultry, fish, (oz) | 5 | 6—9[a] | 6 | Ad lib | 6 |
| Egg yolks as substitute for 1 oz meat | 3 per week | None | None | 3 per week | 3 per week |
| Breads, cereals | 6+ | 7+ | 7 | 7 | 9 |
| Potato or other starchy vegetable | 1+ | 1+ | 1 | 1 | 1 |
| Vegetables and fruits | 5 | 5 | Ad lib 3 | Ad lib 6 | Ad lib 3 |
| Fats (tsp) | None | 6—9[b] | 12 | Ad lib | 6 |
| Sugars, sweets | Ad lib | Ad lib | None | None | None |
| Low-fat desserts | Ad lib | Ad lib | None | None | None |
| Alcohol | None | With discretion | Limit use[c] | Limit use[c] | None |

[a]   Limit lean beef, lamb, ham, or pork to 3 oz three times per week; use fish, shellfish, chicken, turkey, veal, and dried or chipped beef for remaining meat.
[b]   For each ounce of meat eaten use at least 1 tsp of one of the following: corn oil, safflower oil, soft safflower margarine, or commercial mayonnaise.
[c]   Limit alcohol to two servings per day. One serving is equivalent to the following: 1 oz gin, rum, vodka, or whiskey, 1½ oz sweet wine, 2½ oz dry wine, 5 oz beer.

Adapted from Frederickson, D. S., Levy, R. I., Bonnell, M., and Ernst, N., The Dietary Management of Hyperlipoproteinemia, A Handbook for Physicians and Dietitians, Publ. No. (NIH) 76-110, U.S. Department of Health Education and Welfare, Washington, D.C., 1974.

## Calorie-Restricted Diets
Diets based on the diabetic Exchange Lists (Table 8) are often used for persons who must restrict their caloric intake to lose weight. Such diets eliminate the need for constant calorie counting and allow flexibility in food intake with a minimum of planning. Diet patterns should be adjusted to the needs and preferences of the individual. Sample diet patterns for diets providing 1000, 1200, and 1500 kcal are presented in Table 13.

## Diet Modifications to Control Mineral Intake
Sodium-restricted diets — Diets restricted in sodium are used primarily to prevent, control, or eliminate edema associated with cardiovascular disease, various types or stages of renal disease, cirrhosis of the liver, and certain types of hormone therapy. Sodium restriction may also be beneficial in treatment of some patients with hypertension and Meniere's disease.[78] The average American diet contains approximately 4 to 6 g sodium, although some persons may ingest as much as 10 to 12 g.[79] The two principal sources of dietary sodium are sodium chloride added to food during cooking or processing and sodium occurring in foods as a natural mineral. Small amounts of sodium may be contributed by other sodium compounds such as baking soda, baking powder, or sodium benzoate. Four levels of dietary sodium restriction have been described by the American Heart Association.[80] Restrictions for a mild sodium-restricted diet are listed in Table 14. Food allowances and restrictions for a 500 mg sodium diet are summarized in Table 15, with suggested modifications for 250 or 1000 mg sodium diets listed in Table 16.

Table 13
## SAMPLE DIET PLANS FOR CALORIE-RESTRICTED DIETS

Number of exchanges[a]

| | Calories | | |
|---|---|---|---|
| | 1000 | 1200 | 1500 |
| Breakfast | | | |
| Fruit | 1 | 1 | 1 |
| Meat (lean) | 1 | 1 | 1 |
| Bread | 1 | 1 | 1 |
| Fat | 1 | 1 | 2 |
| Milk (skim) | 1 | 1 | 1 |
| Lunch | | | |
| Meat (lean) | 2 | 2 | 3 |
| Bread | 1 | 2 | 2 |
| Vegetable | 1 | 1 | 1 |
| Fruit | 1 | 1 | 2 |
| Fat | 1 | 2 | 3 |
| Milk (skim) | 1 | 1 | 1 |
| Dinner | | | |
| Meat (lean) | 2 | 3 | 3 |
| Bread | 1 | 1 | 2 |
| Vegetable | 1 | 1 | 1 |
| Fruit | 1 | 1 | 2 |
| Fat | 2 | 3 | 3 |
| Milk (skim) | — | — | — |

[a] Food Exchange Lists are described in Table 8.

Table 14
## MILD SODIUM-RESTRICTED DIET (2 to 3 g SODIUM)

Light salting of food during cooking is permitted;
  do not add salt to cooked or processed foods
Do not use
  Salty or smoked meat
    Bacon, bacon fat, bologna, chipped or corn beef, frankfurters,
    ham, kosher meats, luncheon meats, salt pork, sausage
  Salt or smoked fish
    Anchovies, caviar, salted and dried cod, herring, sardines, etc.
  Processed cheese,[a] cheese spreads or any cheese such as
   Roquefort, Camembert, or Gorgonzola
  Peanut butter[a]
  Sauerkraut, pickles, olives
  Heavily salted foods
    Potato chips, pretzels, salted crackers, salted nuts,
    salted popcorn, other salted snack foods
  Spices and condiments
    Bouillon,[a] meat sauces, meat tenderizers, catsup,[a] chili sauce,
    prepared mustard, relishes, worcestershire sauce, soy sauce,
    seasoned salts, monosodium glutamate, cooking wine

[a] Low-sodium dietetic products may be used.

Adapted from *Your Mild Sodium-Restricted Diet* (revised), American Heart Association, New York, 1969. With permission.

Table 15
500 MG SODIUM DIET (STRICT LOW-SODIUM DIET)

| Food | Daily intake | Sodium content[a] | Foods to Use | Foods to Avoid |
|---|---|---|---|---|
| Milk | 16 oz | 120 mg/8 oz | Regular (whole) milk; evaporated, skim, or powdered milk; buttermilk; substitute: 6 oz plain yogurt | |
| Meat, poultry fish | 6 oz | 25 mg/oz | Use fresh, frozen, or dietetic canned | Brains or kidneys; canned, salted, or smoked meat (bacon, ham, luncheon meats, sausages, etc.) |
| Substitutes for 1 oz meat | | | | |
| Egg | 1 | 70 mg/1 egg | Limit to 1 egg/day | Frozen fish fillets; canned, salted, or smoked fish (anchovies, sardines, etc); canned tuna or salmon unless low-sodium; shellfish; regular cheese, cottage cheese, and peanut butter |
| Cheese | 1 oz | | Low-sodium dietetic cheese | |
| Cottage cheese | ¼ cup | | Unsalted cottage cheese | |
| Peanut butter | 2 tbsp | | Low-sodium peanut butter | |
| Potatoes, bread, cereal, cereal product | 6—9 servings | 5 mg/serving (1 serving = 1 slice bread, ½ cup cooked cereal ¾ cup dry cereal ½ cup cooked rice, noodles, etc.) | Low sodium breads, rolls and crackers, unsalted cooked cereals, puffed wheat, shredded wheat, unsalted macaroni, noodles, spaghetti, rice, popcorn; flour | Regular bread, crackers, etc., cooked cereals containing a sodium compound; dry cereals except those listed; potato chips, pretzels, salted popcorn. |
| Vegetables | 2—4 servings | 5—9 mg/serving (about ½ cup) | Any fresh, frozen, or dietetic canned vegetables except those listed to avoid | Canned vegetables or vegetable juice unless low-sodium dietetic; frozen peas, limas, mixed vegetables; artichokes, beets, carrots, celery, chard, greens, spinach, sauerkraut, turnips |
| Fruits | 3—4 servings | 2 mg/average serving | Any fresh, frozen, canned, or dried | Dried fruit if processed with sodium sulfite; frozen melon balls if salt added |

| | | |
|---|---|---|
| Fats | 2 or more Little or no sodium | Unsalted butter, margarine, cooking fat, or oil; unsalted salad dressing, mayonnaise, unsalted nuts; limit cream to 2 tbsp/day | Regular butter or margarine, commercial salad dressings unless low-sodium dietic; bacon fat, salt pork; olives salted nuts; gravies |
| Miscellaneous | As calories permit | Homemade soup with foods allowed; jelly, jam, sugar, honey, calcium saccharin; gelatin dessert made with plain gelatin; puddings made without milk; pies, cakes, cookies made with sodium-free baking powder; coffee, tea, coffee substitute, lemon | Instant cocoa mix, malted milk, soft drinks, bouillon, meat extract; commercial candies, gelatin desserts, regular baking powder or soda; rennet tablets, seasoned salts, prepared mustard, ketchup, chili sauce, horseradish, meat tenderizer, soy sauce, Worcestershire sauce, olives, pickles, relishes |

<sup>a</sup>  Approximate sodium content.

Adapted from *Your 500 Milligram Sodium Diet*(revised), American Heart Association, New York, 1968. With permission.

## Table 16
## MODIFICATIONS OF THE LOW-SODIUM DIET

### Modifications for a 250-mg Sodium Diet

The 250-mg sodium diet is basically the same as the 500-mg sodium diet except
1. Substitute low-sodium milk (2 or more cups) for the regular milk
2. Reduce the amount of meat to 5 oz

### Modifications for a 1000-mg Sodium Diet

The sodium content of the 500-mg sodium diet can be increased to 1000 mg by using *one* of the following modifications
Modification I
1. Two slices regular bread and 2 tsp salted butter or margarine may be used to replace the same amount of the unsalted foods
2. One serving (½ cup) is allowed daily of high-sodium vegetables: spinach, celery, carrots, beets, artichokes, white turnips.
Modification II (high protein)
1. 10 oz meat are allowed instead of 6 oz
2. One serving of prepared or milk dessert such as ice cream, custard, gelatin or 1 cup milk
3. Two eggs instead of one
4. One serving of high-sodium vegetables
Modification III
1. Three slices regular bread may be substituted for low-sodium bread (if additional bread is desired, unsalted bread must be used)

Adapted from Williams, S. R., *Nutrition and Diet Therapy,* 4th ed., C. V. Mosby, St. Louis, 1981, 624. With permission.

**Diets with decreased or increased amounts of potassium** — Dietary restriction of potassium may be used in the treatment of patients who have elevated serum potassium as a consequence of renal disease or certain endocrine disorders. In renal disease, diet modifications are seldom limited to potassium and often include restriction of protein, sodium, and fluid. These diets are discussed in the following section. Potassium is widely distributed in foods. Rich sources include milk, meat, legumes, whole-grain cereals, potatoes, leafy vegetables, tomatoes, and certain fruits (bananas, prunes, melons, and citrus fruits). Long-term use of certain diuretics may lead to hypokalemia. Increased intake of high-potassium foods may be recommended; however, dietary intake alone is seldom sufficient to provide the necessary potassium and supplements such as potassium chloride are usually prescribed.[82,83]

**Controlled-protein, -sodium, and -potassium diets for treatment of chronic renal failure** — Diet management of patients with renal disease varies from patient to patient. Diet restrictions involve primarily protein, sodium, potassium, and water. Levels of nutrient intake depend on the individual patient's degree of renal impairment, the type of treatment being used, and the patient's response to that treatment. The Giordano-Giovannetti diet is a highly restricted, very low-protein diet used to treat patients with severe chronic uremia.[84] A British adaption of the diet provides approximately 2000 kcal and 18 to 20 g protein.[85] Approximately 12 g of protein are supplied by 6½ oz milk and 1 egg with the remainder of the protein coming from fruits, vegetables, and cereals. Food exchange lists and recipes for a modified Giovanetti diet (20 g protein, 1500 mg potassium) have been described by Williams.[86] Less rigid dietary control is possible for many patients with chronic renal disease, especially those being managed on dialysis programs. Diets appropriate for the individual patient are planned using food exchange lists based on the protein, sodium, and potassium content of foods. Numerous exchange lists and diet plans have been described.[87-93]

Table 17
## ROWE ELIMINATION DIETS[1]

| Cereal free elimination diet | Fruit-free, cereal-free elimination diet | Minimal elimination diets |
|---|---|---|
| Tapioca | Tapioca (pearl only) | 1. Lamb, white potatoes, pearl tapioca, carrots, peas, cottonseed or sesame oil (not Chinese), salt, water, and soy milk[a] may be tried; this eliminates beef, all cereals and fruits, soy and lima beans, and most vegetables which are in one or both of the preceding diets |
| White potatoes | White potatoes | |
| Sweet potatoes or yams | Potato starch | |
| Soybean-potato bread | Sweet potatoes or yams | |
| Lima bean-potato bread | Soybean-potato bread | |
| Soy milk[a] | Lima bean-potato bread | |
| Lamb | Soy milk[a] | |
| Chicken fryers, roosters and capon (no hens) | Cooked carrots | |
| Bacon | Squash | |
| Liver (lamb) | Artichokes | 2. Chicken, turkey, rice, pearl tapioca, cottonseed or sesame oil, salt, sugar, water, and soy milk[a] or a similar diet may be used; this eliminates all cereals, legumes, meat, vegetables, and fruits |
| Artichokes | Peas | |
| Asparagus | Lima beans | |
| Carrots | String beans | |
| Lettuce | Lamb | |
| Lima beans | Bacon | |
| Peas | Chicken (no hens) | |
| Spinach | Cane or beet sugar | 3. Fin fish, crab, eggs, pearl tapioca, soy-tapioca bread, cake and cookies, margarine,[b] sugar, salt, water, and soy milk |
| Squash | Margarine[b] | |
| String beans | Soybean oil | |
| Tomatoes | Gelatin, plain | |
| Apricots[c] | Salt | |
| | Syrup made with cane sugar (no maple syrup) | |
| Grapefruit | Corn-free tartaric acid-free baking powder | |
| Lemon | | |
| Peaches | | |
| Pineapples | | |
| Prunes | | |
| Pears | | |
| Cane or beet sugar | | |
| Salt | | |
| Sesame oil (not Chinese) | | |
| Soybean oil | | |
| Margarine[b] | | |
| Gelatin, plain, flavored with allowed fruit juices | | |
| White vinegar | | |
| Vanilla extract | | |
| Lemon extract | | |
| Corn starch-free baking powder | | |
| Baking soda | | |
| Cream of tartar | | |
| Maple syrup or syrup made with cane sugar flavored with maple | | |

[a]  Free of corn syrup solids and corn oil.
[b]  Free of milk solids and corn oil.
[c]  Fruits, fresh or canned in cane sugar (not corn syrup).

Adapted from Rowe, A. H., *Food Allergy*, Charles C Thomas, Springfield, Ill., 1972, 41—75. With permission.

Diets restricted in calcium and/or phosphorus — A diet providing 400 mg calcium has been described by Williams.[94] Foods eliminated from the diet include milk and all foods made from or containing milk (except bread), oatmeal and whole-grain cereals, dried fruit, rhubarb, clams, oysters, shrimp, legumes, broccoli, green cabbage, celery, green leafy vegetables, nuts, olives, and chocolate. Phosphorus is widely distributed in foods. Rich sources include milk and milk products, legumes, fish, meat, green leafy vegetables, and whole-grain cereals. A low phosphorus diet (approximately 1000 mg) has been described by Williams.[95] Low calcium and/or low phosphorus diets may be used to prevent or control renal calculi composed largely of calcium phosphate. Mitchell et al.[96] have outlined a diet containing 500 to 700 mg calcium and 1000 to 1200 mg phosphorus based on the diet originally recommended by Shorr[97] for management of calcium phosphate stones. Restriction of dietary phosphorus may become necessary in certain patients with chronic renal failure.[98]

Copper-restricted diets — Restriction or control of the dietary intake of copper may be included in the treatment of patients with Wilson's disease.[99,100] Foods restricted or eliminated include organ meats, shellfish, whole-grain cereals, legumes, mushrooms, nuts, and chocolate.

## OTHER THERAPEUTIC DIETS

Acid-ash diet — This diet contains foods having a total anion-forming metabolic ash or residue content in excess of the total cation-forming ash.[101] Foods having an acid ash include meat, whole-grain cereal, eggs, cheese, cranberries, prunes, and plums. These foods have a high content of chloride, and phosphate. Foods with a high alkaline ash (milk, vegetables, and fruits, except those listed above) are restricted. Only 1 pt milk, one to two servings of fruit, and two servings of vegetables are usually permitted. An acid-ash diet may be used to prevent or control kidney stones composed of calcium, magnesium, phosphates, or carbonates.[102]

Alkaline-ash diet — This diet emphasizes liberal use of milk, fruits, and vegetables to provide a metabolic ash with an excess of cation-forming elements such as sodium, potassium, calcium, and magnesium. Foods having a high acid ash are restricted. An alkaline-ash diet may be used to prevent or treat kidney stones with a high content of uric acid or cystine.[101]

Diets used in treatment of food allergy — Various diets have been used in the diagnosis and treatment of food allergy. The best known of these are the Rowe elimination diets (Table 17).[103] The cereal-free diet is usually used first and if improvement does not occur, the fruit-free, cereal-free diet is tried. If these two diets do not relieve symptoms and symptoms continue to appear to be related to food, one of the "minimal elimination diets" may be used. The length of time during which the initial elimination diet should be used varies with the frequency of occurrence of symptoms. If use of the diet for 2 weeks leads to disappearance of symptoms which previously occurred almost daily, it can be assumed that the allergenic foods have been eliminated. If symptoms ordinarily occur every 2 to 6 weeks, a trial period as long as several months may be required. When relief is apparent, other foods are added one at a time for 2 to 4 days to test the patient's response. Other diets used to diagnose food allergies may eliminate all common irritants[104] or all vegetable- or animal-protein foods.[105] Diets eliminating specific foods such as eggs, wheat, milk, seafood, or nuts have been described[106] and may be used for diagnosis or treatment of allergic conditions. Because most of these diets involve elimination of numerous common foods, it is essential that the nutritional adequacy of the diet be carefully evaluated and appropriate supplements provided if necessary.

# REFERENCES

1. Krause, M. V. and Mahan, L. K., *Food, Nutrition and Diet Therapy*, 6th ed., W. B. Saunders, Philadelphia, 1979, 445-446.
2. Mitchell, H. S., Rynbergen, H. J., Anderson, L., and Dibble, M. V., *Nutrition in Health and Disease*, 16th ed., J. B. Lippincott, New York, 1976, 321-322.
3. Committee on Dietetics of The Mayo Clinic, *Mayo Clinic Diet Manual*, 5th ed., W. B. Saunders, Philadelphia, 1981, 14.
4. Nutrition Service of Iowa State Department of Health, *Simplified Diet Manual*, 4th ed., Iowa State University Press, Ames, 1975, 27.
5. American Dietetic Association, *Handbook of Clinical Dietetics*, Yale University Press, New Haven, 1981, B3-B7.
6. Robinson, C. H. and Lawler, M. R., *Normal and Therapeutic Nutrition*, 15th ed., Macmillan, New York, 1977, 445-447.
7. Committee on Dietetics of The Mayo Clinic, *Mayo Clinic Diet Manual*, 5th ed., W. B. Saunders, Philadelphia, 1981, 143.
8. Cohen, S. and Booth, G. H., Gastric acid secretion and lower-esophageal-sphincter pressure in response to coffee and caffeine, *N. Engl. J. Med.*, 293, 897-899, 1975.
9. Schneider, M. A., DeLuca, V., and Gray, S. J., The effect of spice ingestion upon the stomach, *Am. J. Gastroenterol.*, 26, 722-731, 1956.
10. Shull, H. J., Diet in the management of peptic ulcer, *JAMA*, 170, 1068-1071, 1959.
11. Fein, H. D., Nutrition in diseases of the stomach, including related areas in the esophagus and duodenum, in *Modern Nutrition in Health and Disease*, 6th ed., Goodhart, R. S. and Shils, M. E., Eds., Lea & Febiger, Philadelphia, 1980, 903.
12. Richardson, C. T., Gastric acid, in *Gastrointestinal Disease*, Sleisenger, M. H. and Fordtran, J. S., Eds., W. B. Saunders, Philadelphia, 1978, 882.
13. American Dietetic Association Position Paper on Bland Diet in the Treatment of Chronic Duodenal Ulcer Disease, *J. Am. Diet. Assoc.*, 59, 244-245, 1971.
14. Dunkerley, R. C., Dunn, G. D., and Wilson, F. A., Gastrointestinal disorders: the role of diet in cause and management, *Postgrad. Med.*, 59, 182-187, 1976.
15. Weser, E. and Kim, Y., Nutrition and the gastrointestinal tract, in *Gastrointestinal Disease*, Sleisenger, M. H. and Fordtran, J. S., Eds., W. B. Saunders, Philadelphia, 1978, 43-44.
16. Bennion, M., *Clinical Nutrition*, Harper & Row, New York, 1979, 185-191.
17. Gormican, A. and Liddy, E., Nasogastric tube feedings, *Postgrad. Med.*, 53, 71-76, 1973.
18. Freund, H., Yoshimura, N., and Fischer, J. E., Chronic hepatic encephalopathy: long-term therapy with a branched-chain amino-acid-enriched elemental diet, *JAMA*, 242, 347-349, 1979.
19. Kark, R. M., Liquid formula and chemically defined diets, *J. Am. Diet. Assoc.*, 64, 477-479, 1974.
20. Dudrick, S. J. and Rhoads, J. E., New horizons for intravenous feeding, *JAMA*, 215, 939-949, 1971.
21. Paradis, C., Spanier, A. H., Calder, M., and Shizgal, H. M., Total parenteral nutrition with lipid, *Am. J. Surg.*, 135, 164-171, 1978.
22. Wretlind, A., Parenteral nutrition, *Surg. Clin. North Am.*, 58, 1055-1070, 1978.
23. Harries, J. T., Aspects of intravenous feeding in childhood, in *Advances in Parenteral Nutrition*, Johnson, I. D. A., Ed., University Park Press, Baltimore, 267-280, 1978.
24. Brennan, M. F., Total parenteral nutrition in the management of the cancer patient, *Ann. Rev. Med.*, 32, 233-243, 1981.
25. Jeffries, G. H., Diseases of the liver, in *Textbook of Medicine*, 15th ed., Beeson, P. B., McDermott, W., and Wyngaarden, J. B., Eds., W. B. Saunders, Philadelphia, 1979, 1666.
26. Ohlson, M. A., *Experimental and Therapeutic Dietetics*, 2nd ed., Burgess Publishing, Minneapolis, 1972, 143.
27. Williams, S. R., *Nutrition and Diet Therapy*, 4th ed., C. V. Mosby, St. Louis, 1981, 638-639.
28. Borst, J. C. G., Protein katabolism in uraemia: effects of protein-free diets, infections, and blood transfusions, *Lancet*, 1, 824-828, 1948.
29. Grills, N. J. and Bosscher, M. V., Eds., *Manual of Nutrition and Diet Therapy*, Macmillan, New York, 1981, 163-168.
30. Williams, S. R., *Nutrition and Diet Therapy*, 4th ed., C. V. Mosby, St. Louis, 1981, 599.
31. Thiele, V. F., *Clinical Nutrition*, 2nd ed., C. V. Mosby, St. Louis, 1980, 100-102.
32. Burton, B. T., Current concepts of nutrition and diet in diseases of the kidney. I. General principles of dietary management. II. Dietary regimen in specific kidney disorders, *J. Am. Diet Assoc.*, 65, 623-626, 627-633, 1974.
33. Kark, R. M. and Oyama, J. H., Nutrition, hypertension and kidney disease, in *Modern Nutrition in Health and Disease*, 6th ed., Goodhart, R. S., and Shils, M. E., Eds., Lea & Febiger, Philadelphia, 1980, 1022.

34. Sleisenger, M. H., Rynbergen, H. J., Pert, J. H., and Almy, T. P., A wheat- , rye- , and oat-free diet, *J. Am. Diet. Assoc.,* 33, 1137-1140, 1957.
35. Hjortland, M., *Low Gluten Diet with Tested Recipes,* Clinical Research Unit, University of Michigan, Ann Arbor, 1973.
36. Trier, J. S., Celiac sprue disease, in *Gastrointestinal Disease,* Sleisenger, M. H. and Fordtran, J. S., Eds., W. B. Saunders, Philadelphia, 1978, 1046-1048.
37. Cooper, B. T., Mallas, E., Trotter, M. D., and Cooke, W. T., Response of the skin in dermatitis herpetiformis to a gluten free diet, with reference to jejunal morphology, *Gut,* 19, 754-758, 1978.
38. Moorthy, A. V., Zimmerman, S. W., and Maxim, P. E., Dermatitis herpetiformis and celiac disease, *JAMA,* 239, 2019, 1978.
39. Ohlson, M. A., *Experimental and Therapeutic Dietetics,* 2nd ed., Burgess Publishing, Minneapolis, 1972, 90-91.
40. Williams, S. R., *Nutrition and Diet Therapy,* 4th ed., C. V. Mosby, St. Louis, 1981, 656-657.
41. Berry, H. K., Hyperphenylalanemias, *Clin. Perinatol.,* 3, 15-40, 1976.
42. Acosta, P. B. and Centerwall, W. R., Phenylketonuria: dietary management, *J. Am. Diet. Assoc.,* 36, 206-211, 1960.
43. Bureau of Public Health Nutrition of the California State Department of Public Health, PKU, a diet guide for parents of children with phenylketonuria, 1969, in *Nutrition and Diet Therapy,* 4th ed., Williams, S. R., Ed., C. V. Mosby, St. Louis, 1981, 440-445.
44. Hill, A., Nordin, P. M., and Zaleski, W. A., Dietary treatment of tyrosinosis, *J. Am. Diet. Assoc.,* 56, 308-312, 1970.
45. Michals, K., Matalon, R., and Wong, P. W. K., Dietary treatment of tyrosinemia type I, *J. Am. Diet. Assoc.,* 73, 507-514, 1978.
46. Smith, B. A. and Waisman, H. A., Leucine equivalency system in managing branched chain ketoaciduria, *J. Am. Diet. Assoc.,* 59, 342-346, 1971.
47. Noel, M. B., Stanley, P. B., Girz, J. C., and Allen, R. J., Dietary treatment of maple sirup urine disease (branched-chain ketoaciduria), *J. Am. Diet. Assoc.,* 69, 62-68, 1976.
48. Bell, L., Chao, E., and Milne, J., Dietary management of maple-sirup-urine disease: extension of equivalency systems, *J. Am. Diet. Assoc.,* 74, 357-361, 1979.
49. Sardharwalla, I. B., Jackson, S. H., Hawke, H. D., and Sass-Kortsak, A., Homocystinuria: a study with low-methionine diet in three patients, *Can. Med. Assoc. J.,* 99, 731-740, 1968.
50. Committee on Nutrition, American Academy of Pediatrics, Special diets for infants with inborn errors of amino acid metabolism, *Pediatrics,* 57, 783-790, 1976.
51. Smith, D. R., Kolb, F. O., and Harper, H. A., The management of cystinuria and cystine-stone disease, *J. Urol.,* 81, 61-71, 1959.
52. Roth, H. and Segal, S., The dietary management of leucine sensitive hypoglycemia, with report of a case, *Pediatrics,* 34, 831-838, 1964.
53. Arvanitakis, C., Diet therapy in gastrointestinal disease: a commentary, *J. Am. Diet. Assoc.,* 75, 449-452, 1979.
54. American Heart Association Committee on Nutrition, Diet and coronary heart disease, *Circulation,* 58, 762A-765A, 1978.
55. *Planning Fat-Controlled Meals for 1200 and 1800 Calories* (revised): *Planning Fat-Controlled Meals for Approximately 2000-2600 Calories* (revised), American Heart Association, New York, 1966 and 1967.
56. Koch, R., Acosta, P., Ragsdale, N., and Donnell, G. N., Nutrition in the treatment of galactosemia, *J. Am. Diet. Assoc.,* 43, 216-222, 1963.
57. Donnell, G. N., Koch, R., and Bergren, W. R., Observations on results of management of galactosemic patients, in *Galactosemia,* Hsia, D. Y.-Y., Ed., Charles C Thomas, Springfield, Ill., 1969, 247.
58. Cornblath, M. and Schwartz, R., *Disorders of Carbohydrate Metabolism in Infancy,* 2nd ed., W. B. Saunders, Philadelphia, 1976, 322-339, 472.
59. Nuttall, F. Q. and Brunzell, J. D., Principles of nutrition and dietary recommendations for individuals with diabetes mellitus: 1979, *J. Am. Diet. Assoc.,* 75, 527-531, 1979.
60. *Meal Planning with Exchange Lists,* American Dietetic Association, Chicago, and American Diabetes Association, New York, 1950.
61. *ADA Meal Plans Nos. 1-9,* The American Diabetes Association, New York, and the American Dietetic Association, Chicago, 1956.
62. *Diabetic Diet Card for Physicians and Dietitians for Use with Fat-Controlled Diets,* American Diabetes Association, New York, and the American Dietetic Association, Chicago, 1967.
63. *Exchange Lists for Meal Planning,* American Diabetes Association, New York, and the American Dietetic Association, Chicago, 1976.
64. ADA, *A Guide for Professionals: The Effective Application of "Exchange Lists for Meal Planning,"* American Diabetes Association, New York, 1977.

65. Reaven, G. M., How high the carbohydrate, *Diabetologia,* 19, 409-413, 1980.
66. Kay, R. M., Grobin, W., and Track, N. S., Diets rich in natural fiber improve carbohydrate tolerance in maturity-onset, non-insulin dependent diabetics, *Diabetologia,* 20, 18-21, 1981.
67. Jenkins, D. J. A., Dietary fiber, diabetes, and hyperlipidaemia, *Lancet,* 2, 1287-1289, 1979.
68. Leggett, J. and Favazza, A. R., Hypoglycemia: an overview, *J. Clin. Psychiatry,* 39, 51-57, 1978.
69. Leichter, S. B., Alimentary hypoglycemia: a new appraisal, *Am. J. Clin. Nutr.,* 32, 2104-2114, 1979.
70. American Dietetic Association, *Handbook of Clinical Dietetics,* Yale University Press, New Haven, 1981, D3-D5.
71. Mike, E. M., Practical guide and dietary management of children with seizures using the ketogenic diet, *Am. J. Clin. Nutr.,* 17, 399-409, 1965.
72. Lasser, J. L. and Brush, M. K., An improved ketogenic diet for treatment of epilepsy, *J. Am. Diet. Assoc.,* 62, 281-285, 1973.
73. Signore, J. M., Ketogenic diet containing medium-chain triglycerides, *J. Am. Diet. Assoc.,* 62, 285-290, 1973.
74. Frederickson, D. S., Levy, R. I., and Lees, R. S., Fat transport in lipoproteins — an integrated approach to mechanisms and disorders, *N. Engl. J. Med.,* 276, 34-44, 94-103, 148-156, 215-225, and 273-281, 1967.
75. Levy, R. I., Classification and etiology of hyperlipoproteinemias, *Fed. Proc. Fed. Am. Soc. Exp. Biol.,* 30, 829-834, 1971.
76. Levy, R. I., Morganroth, J., and Rifkind, B. M., Treatment of hyperlipidemia, *N. Engl. J. Med.,* 209, 1295-1301, 1974.
77. Frederickson, D. S., Levy, R. I., Bonnell, M., and Ernst, N., The Dietary Management of Hyperlipoproteinemia, A Handbook for Physicians and Dietitians, Publ. No. (NIH) 76-110, U.S. Department of Health, Education and Welfare, Washington, D.C., 1974.
78. American Dietetic Association, *Handbook of Clinical Dietetics,* Yale University Press, New Haven, 1981, G3-G6.
79. Institute of Food Technologist's Expert Panel on Food Safety and Nutrition, Dietary salt, *Food Technol. (Chicago),* 34, 85-91, 1980.
80. *Your Mild Sodium-Restricted Diet* (revised); *Your 1000 milligram Sodium Diet* (revised); and *Your 500 milligram Sodium Diet* (revised), American Heart Association, New York, 1968 and 1969.
81. Williams, S. R., *Nutrition and Diet Therapy,* 4th ed., C. V. Mosby, St. Louis, 1981, 624.
82. Kosman, M. E., Management of potassium problems during long-term diuretic therapy, *JAMA,* 230, 743-748, 1974.
83. Davies, D. L. and Wilson, G. M., Diuretics: mechanisms of action and clinical application, *Drugs,* 9, 178-226, 1975.
84. Giovannetti, S. and Maggiore, Q., A low nitrogen diet with proteins of high biological value for severe chronic uraemia, *Lancet,* 1, 1000-1003, 1964.
85. Shaw, A. B., Bazzard, F. J., Booth, E. M., Nilwarangkur, S., and Berlyne, G. M., The treatment of chronic renal failure by a modified Giovannetti diet, *Q. J. Med.,* 34, 237-253, 1965.
86. Williams, S. R., *Nutrition and Diet Therapy,* 4th ed., C. V. Mosby, St. Louis, 1981, 645-649.
87. Jordan, W. L., Cimino, J. E., Grist, A. C., McMahon, G. E., and Doyle, M. M., Basic pattern for a controlled protein, sodium and potassium diet, *J. Am. Diet. Assoc.,* 50, 137-141, 1967.
88. Association of Michigan Nephrology Dietitians, *Diet Instruction Manual,* Kidney Foundation of Michigan, Ann Arbor, 1975.
89. Jones, W. O., Diet Guide for Patients on Chronic Dialysis, Publ. No. (NIH) 76-685, U.S. Department of Health, Education and Welfare, Washington, D.C., 1976.
90. Kopple, J. D., Nutritional management of chronic renal failure, *Postgrad. Med.,* 64(5), 135-144, 1978.
91. Berger, M., Dietary management of children with uremia, *J. Am. Diet. Assoc.,* 70, 498-505, 1977.
92. Davis, M., Comty, C., and Shapiro, F., Dietary management of patients with diabetes treated by hemodialysis, *J. Am. Diet. Assoc.,* 75, 265-269, 1979.
93. Furst, P., Allberg, M., Alvestrand, A., and Bergstrom, J., Principles of essential amino acid therapy in uremia, *Am. J. Clin. Nutr.,* 31, 1744-1755, 1978.
94. Williams, S. R., *Nutrition and Diet Therapy,* 4th ed., C. V. Mosby, St. Louis, 1981, 652.
95. Williams, S. R., *Nutrition and Diet Therapy,* 4th ed., C. V. Mosby, St. Louis, 1981, 653.
96. Mitchell, H. S., Rynbergen, H. J., Anderson, L., and Dibble, M. V., *Nutrition in Health and Disease,* 16th ed., J. B. Lippincott, New York, 1976, 455.
97. Shorr, E., Aluminum hydroxide gels in the management of renal stones, *J. Urol.,* 53, 507-520, 1945.
98. Schoolwerth, A. C. and Engle, J. E., Calcium and phosphorus in diet therapy of uremia, *J. Am. Diet. Assoc.,* 66, 460-464, 1975.
99. Sternlieb, I. and Scheinberg, I. H., Penicillamine therapy for hepatolenticular degeneration, *JAMA,* 189, 748-754, 1964.

100. Sass-Kortsak, A. and Bearn, A. G., Hereditary disorders of copper metabolism, in *The Metabolic Basis of Inherited Disease,* 4th ed., Stanbury, J. B., Wyngaarden, J. B., and Frederickson, D. S., Eds., McGraw-Hill, New York, 1978, 1115.
101. Krause, M. V. and Mahan, L. K., *Food Nutrition and Diet Therapy,* 6th ed., W. B. Saunders, Philadelphia, 1979, 644.
102. Robinson, C. H., *Normal and Therapeutic Nutrition,* 15th ed., Macmillan, New York, 1977, 564.
103. Rowe, A. H., *Food Allergy,* Charles C Thomas, Springfield, Ill., 1972, 41-75.
104. Committee on Dietetics of The Mayo Clinic, *Mayo Clinic Diet Manual,* 5th ed., W. B. Saunders, Philadelphia, 1981, 159-160.
105. Ohlson, M. A., *Experimental and Therapeutic Dietetics,* 2nd ed., Burgess Publishing, Minneapolis, 1972, 92-94.
106. Goodhart, R. S. and Shils, M. E., Eds., *Modern Nutrition in Health and Disease,* 6th ed., Lea & Febiger, Philadelphia, 1980, 1306-1307.

# PARENTERAL NUTRITION

Paul Starker, Arvid Wretlind, and John M. Kinney

Parenteral nutrition refers to the administration of nutrients by the intravenous route. This method of nutrition is used in order to prevent or treat starvation and its complications when feedings via the enteral route are not possible. Determination of which patients require nutritional support is best accomplished by a careful history and physical examination. Many biochemical and anthropometric parameters are used in nutritional assessment, but a weight loss of greater than 10% of the total body weight in a nonobese patient remains the major factor in determining necessity for nutritional support. There are many conditions where there are indications for the use of the parenteral (as opposed to the enteral) route for delivery of nutrients. Some of the more important ones are listed in Table 1.*

The essential nutrients which must be delivered during parenteral nutrition are listed in Table 2. There are a number of commercially available solutions which allow delivery of these nutrients. The amino acid solutions are listed and compared to egg protein in Table 3.

There are specific mixtures of amino acids which are to be used for patients with renal disease (Aminess®, Aminosyn RF®, and Nephramine®) (Table 4). These solutions mainly provide essential amino acids. The assumption is that nitrogen will be recycled into synthesis of nonessential amino acids instead of urea formation. The amino acid imbalance seen in liver failure is characterized by low levels of branched-chain amino acids and high levels of aromatic amino acids. This is thought to contribute to the synthesis of false neurotransmitters and exacerbate the encephalopathy of hepatic failure. The amino acid solutions commercially available today add to this imbalance and therefore are not recommended for patients with liver dysfunction. As yet, there is no commercially available amino acid solution for patients with liver failure.

The various carbohydrates and glucose substitutes used in parenteral nutrition are listed in Table 5. Of these, glucose is the carbohydrate of choice and is also the most commonly used.

The composition of the fat emulsions available for parenteral nutrition are listed in Table 6. The fatty acid breakdown of the various oils used in these emulsions are given in Table 7.

Table 8 shows the energy conversion factors for amino acids, fat, carbohydrates, and some other nutrients. The energy content of the infusion solutions becomes important not only when considering the total energy requirement of the patient but also when determining the fat to carbohydrate calorie ratio. The debate as to whether fat should be used as a calorie source or only to prevent essential fatty acid deficiency continues. However, it is becoming more widely accepted that the nonprotein calories should be given in a fat to carbohydrate ratio of 1:1.

The daily energy allowances and clinical conditions which may cause an increase or decrease in these allowances are listed in Table 9. The allowances for water, protein, fat, carbohydrate, vitamins, and minerals are detailed in Tables 10-14.

The decision to administer the needed amount of parenteral nutrition via a peripheral or a central vein is generally dictated by the osmotic activity of the nutritional solutions (Table 15). Peripheral veins will rapidly develop thrombophlebitis if a solu-

---

* All tables appear at end of text.

tion with an osmolality of greater than 600 to 800 mOsm is infused. Therefore, when the amount of nutrients required exceeds the amount which can be delivered (in a clinically acceptable fluid volume) by peripheral vein, central venous access must be obtained for parenteral nutrition.

Examples of some regimens for parenteral nutrition via a central vein are given in Table 16. Once central vein parenteral nutrition has been undertaken, the complications of such therapy must be prevented whenever possible. Complications fall into three categories. The first is mechanical and has to do with the actual insertion of the central venous catheter and its interaction with the structures it encounters. Among the major complications in this group are pneumothorax and subclavian or jugular vein thrombosis. The second category of complications is infectious. "Catheter sepsis" is defined as an increase in body temperature with no other apparent source which disappears when the catheter is removed. The offending organisms are usually skin flora such as *Staphylococcus epidermidis, Staphylococcus aureus* and *Klebsiella.* However, *Candida albicans* is also a common organism and is found in association with contamination of the intravenous system. The third category of complications is metabolic and these are detailed in Table 17.

Parenteral nutrition should always be monitored carefully. A summary of monitoring is given in Table 18.

With an awareness of the indications, requirements, limitations, methods of administration, and complications of parenteral nutrition, patients can safely and effectively be treated for their nutritional problems using this route.

Several review articles on parenteral nutrition,[1-8] as well as several journals on parenteral nutrition or related subjects[9-16] are listed for further reference.

Table 1
## CONDITIONS WHERE PARENTERAL NUTRITION MAY BE INDICATED

The general indications for use of the parenteral route to deliver nutrients are when the patients cannot eat, must not eat, will not eat, do not eat enough; and when tube feeding cannot be used.

Indications for parenteral nutrition may occur in the following situations or diseases
Preoperatively
Postoperatively
Gastrointestinal obstruction
Ileus
Short-gut syndrome
Malabsorption
Pancreatitis
Inflammatory bowel disease
Gastrointestinal fistula
Ulcers
Renal failure
Cachexia

Table 2
## ESSENTIAL NUTRIENTS IN PARENTERAL NUTRITION

| Fluid | Water | Major electrolytes | Trace elements |
|---|---|---|---|
| Sources for synthesis of body proteins and energy | Amino acids<br>Glucose<br>Fat | Sodium<br>Potassium<br>Calcium<br>Magnesium<br>Chloride<br>Phosphorus | Iron<br>Zinc<br>Copper<br>Cobalt<br>Chromium<br>Manganese<br>Selenium<br>Molybdenum<br>Fluoride<br>Iodide |
| Water-soluble vitamins | Thiamin<br>Riboflavin<br>Niacin<br>Vitamin $B_6$<br>Folacin<br>Vitamin $B_{12}$<br>Pantothenic acid<br>Biotin<br>Ascorbic acid | | |
| Fat-soluble vitamins | Vitamin A<br>Vitamin D<br>Vitamin E<br>Vitamin K | | |

Table 3
COMPOSITION OF SOME AMINO ACID MIXTURES FOR PARENTERAL NUTRITION

g of Amino Acid/16 g of Total Amino Acid Mixture

| | Aminoplex®[a] | Aminosteril®[b] | Aminosyn®[c] | Freamine®[d] | Travasol®[e] | Totamine®[f] | Vamin®[g] | Egg protein |
|---|---|---|---|---|---|---|---|---|
| Isoleucine | 3.8 | 2.5 | 7.4 | 7.6 | 4.6 | 5.5 | 6.6 | 6.6 |
| Leucine | 5.2 | 3.7 | 9.6 | 9.9 | 6.0 | 8.6 | 9.0 | 8.8 |
| Lysine | 8.1 | 3.3 | 7.4 | 7.9 | 5.5 | 6.2 | 6.6 | 6.4 |
| Phenylalanine | 5.2 | 2.55 | 4.5 | 6.0 | 6.0 | 8.6 | 9.4 | 5.8 |
| Methionine | 7.6 | 2.15 | 4.1 | 5.8 | 5.5 | 8.6 | 3.2 | 3.1 |
| Threonine | 3.8 | 2.2 | 5.4 | 4.4 | 4.1 | 3.8 | 5.1 | 5.1 |
| Tryptophan | 1.9 | 1.0 | 1.7 | 1.7 | 1.7 | 1.9 | 1.7 | 1.6 |
| Valine | 6.2 | 3.1 | 8.1 | 7.2 | 4.4 | 6.2 | 7.3 | 7.3 |
| Essential AA | 41.9 | 20.5 | 48.2 | 55.8 | 37.8 | 49.5 | 52.1 | 51.3 |
| Alanine | 17.6 | 7.5 | 13.0 | 7.7 | 19.9 | 6.9 | 5.1 | 7.4 |
| Arginine | 11.0 | 6.0 | 10.0 | 4.0 | 9.9 | 10.3 | 5.6 | 6.1 |
| Aspartic acid | — | — | — | — | — | 3.4 | 7.0 | 9.0 |
| Cysteine/cystine | — | — | — | — | — | 1.7 | 2.4 | 2.4 |
| Glutamic acid | — | — | — | — | — | 3.5 | 15.3 | 16.0 |
| Glycine | 14.3 | 7.0 | 13.0 | 23.0 | 19.9 | 12.1 | 3.6 | 3.6 |
| Histidine | 3.3 | 1.5 | 3.0 | 3.1 | — | 3.2 | 4.1 | 2.4 |
| Ornithine-aspartate | 2.4 | — | — | — | — | 2.4 | — | — |
| Proline | 4.8 | 7.5 | 8.8 | 12.2 | 4.1 | 6.9 | 13.8 | 8.1 |
| Serine | — | — | 4.4 | 6.4 | — | 3.4 | 12.8 | 8.5 |
| Tyrosine | — | — | 0.6 | — | 0.3 | 0.5 | 0.8 | 4.2 |
| Total AA | 95.3 | 50.0 | 101.0 | 112.2 | 91.9 | 104.4 | 121.0 | 119.0 |

[a]    Geistlich Sons Ltd., Chester, England.
[b]    Fresenius, Bad Homburg, West Germany.
[c]    Abbott, North Chicago, Ill.
[d]    McGaw, Glendale, Calif.
[e]    Travenol, Deerfield, Ill.
[f]    Egic, Loiret, France.
[g]    Vitrum, Stockholm, Sweden.

## Table 4
## COMPOSITION OF SOME AMINO ACID MIXTURES FOR PARENTERAL NUTRITION IN RENAL FAILURE

g of Amino Acid/16 g of Total Amino Acid Mixture

| | Aminess®[a] | Aminosyn RF®[b] | Nephramine®[c] |
|---|---|---|---|
| Isoleucine | 12.7 | 12.9 | 15.4 |
| Leucine | 20.0 | 20.4 | 24.2 |
| Lysine | 14.5 | 14.8 | 17.6 |
| Phenylalanine | 20.0 | 20.4 | 24.2 |
| Methionine | 20.0 | 20.4 | 24.2 |
| Threonine | 9.1 | 9.2 | 11.0 |
| Tryptophan | 4.5 | 4.5 | 5.5 |
| Valine | 14.5 | 14.8 | 17.9 |
| Essential AA | 115.3 | 117.4 | 140.0 |
| Alanine | | | |
| Arginine | | 16.8 | |
| Aspartic acid | | | |
| Cysteine/cystine | | | |
| Glutamic acid | | | |
| Glycine | | | |
| Histidine | 10.0 | 12.0 | |
| Ornithine-aspartate | | | |
| Proline | | | |
| Serine | | | |
| Tyrosine | | | |
| Total AA | 125.3 | 146.2 | 140.0 |

[a] Vitrum, Stockholm, Sweden.
[b] Abbott, Chicago, Ill.
[c] McGaw, Irvine, Calif.

## Table 5
## METABOLIC PROPERTIES OF CARBOHYDRATES AND POLYOLS FOR PARENTERAL NUTRITION

| | Carbohydrates | | Polyols | |
|---|---|---|---|---|
| | Glucose | Fructose | Sorbitol | Xylitol |
| Normal metabolite | + | | | |
| Metabolized by cells in all tissues | + | | | |
| Increases nitrogen utilization | + | + | + | + |
| Anitketogenic | + | + | + | + |
| "Partial insulin independency" | | + | + | + |

| | Carbohydrate | Polyols | |
|---|---|---|---|
| | Fructose | Sorbitol | Xylitol |
| Some adverse reactions of fructose, sorbitol, and xylitol | | | |
| Metabolic acidosis | + | + | + |
| Hyperuricemia | + | + | + |
| Decrease of adenine nucleotide in the liver and phosphate in the blood | + | + | + |
| Osmotic diuresis with electrolyte losses | | + | + |
| Crystal deposition in kidney and brain | | | + |

Reprinted with permission from Wretlind, A., *Nutr. Metab.*, 18(Suppl. 1), 242-255, 1975. S. Karger AG, Basel, Switzerland.

Table 6
COMPOSITION OF INTRAVENOUS EMULSIONS (g/$l$)[a]

| | Intralipid®[b] | Lipiphysan®[c] | Lipofundin S®[d] | Intrafat®[e] | Liposyn®[f] |
|---|---|---|---|---|---|
| Oils | | | | | |
| Soybean | 100 or 200 | | 100 or 200 | 100 | |
| Cottonseed | | 150 | | | |
| Safflower | | | | | 100 |
| Egg yolk phospholipids | 12 | | | 12 | 12 |
| Soybean lecithin | | 20 | | | |
| Soybean phospholipids | | | 7.5 or 15 | | |
| Glycerol | 25 | | 25[g] | 25 | 25 |
| Sorbitol | | 50 | | | |
| DL-Tocopherol | | 0.5 | | | |

[a]    All amounts listed are for water added to make 1 $l$
[b]    Vitrum AB, Stockholm, Sweden.
[c]    Egic, Loiret, France.
[d]    Braun, Melsungen, Germany.
[e]    Diago, Osaka, Japan.
[f]    Abbott, North Chicago, Ill.
[g]    Or 50 g of xylitol instead of glycerol.

Table 7
FATTY ACID PATTERNS OF OILS AND PHOSPHOLIPIDS USED
IN INTRAVENOUS FAT EMULSIONS

| | Oils (%) | | | Phospholipids (%) | |
|---|---|---|---|---|---|
| | Cottonseed | Safflower | Soybean | Egg yolk | Soybean lecithin |
| Myristic acid ($C_{14}$) | 1.4 | | 0.04 | 0.09 | |
| Myristoleic acid ($C_{14:1}$) | 0.1 | | | | |
| Palmitic acid ($C_{16}$) | 23.4 | 7 | 9 | 33 | 15.8 |
| Palmitoleic acid ($C_{16:1}$) | 2.0 | | 0.03 | 0.4 | |
| Stearic acid ($C_{18}$) | 1.1 | 2.5 | 3 | 16 | 6.3 |
| Oleic acid ($C_{18:1}$) | 22.9 | 13 | 26 | 32 | 62.9 |
| Linoleic acid ($C_{18:2}$) | 47.8 | 77 | 54 | 11 | 2.0 |
| Linolenic acid ($C_{18:3}$) | | 0.1 | 8 | 0.3 | |
| Arachidic acid ($C_{20}$) | 1.3 | | 0.1 | 0.1 | 13.0 |
| Arachidonic acid ($C_{20:4}$) | | | | 0.2 | |
| Behenic acid ($C_{22}$) | | | 0.06 | 3 | |
| Unidentified acids | | | | 0.2 | |

Table 8
ENERGY CONVERSION
FACTORS USED IN
PARENTERAL NUTRITION

| Nutrient | kcal/g | kJ/g |
|---|---|---|
| Amino acids[a] | 4.1 | 17.2 |
| Fat (soybean oil) | 9.4 | 39.3 |
| Phospholipids (egg) | 8 | 33.5 |
| Glucose | 3.75 | 16 |
| Fructose | 3.75 | 16 |
| Glycerol | 4.3 | 18 |
| Sorbitol | 4 | 17 |
| Xylitol | 4 | 17 |

[a] Amino acid pattern according to Vamin®.

Table 9
RECOMMENDED ENERGY ALLOWANCES
FOR TPN TO COVER RESTING METABOLISM,
SPECIFIC DYNAMIC EFFECT,[a] SOME
PHYSICAL ACTIVITY,[b] AND GROWTH (IN
CHILDREN)

| Age (years) | kcal/kg | MJ/kg | kcal/day | MJ/day |
|---|---|---|---|---|
| 0—1 | 90—120 | 0.38—0.50 | 500—1000 | 2.1—4.2 |
| 1—7 | 75—90 | 0.31—0.38 | 1000—1500 | 4.2—6.3 |
| 7—12 | 60—75 | 0.25—0.31 | 1500—2000 | 6.3—8.4 |
| 12—18 | 30—60 | 0.13—0.25 | 2000 | 8.4 |
| 18—35 | | | | |
| Men | 26—31 | 0.11—0.13 | 1700—2000 | 7.1—8.4 |
| Women | 25—31 | 0.10—0.13 | 1400—1675 | 5.8—7.9 |
| 35—75 | | | | |
| Men | 25—29 | 0.10—0.12 | 1600—1900 | 6.7—7.9 |
| Women | 24—30 | 0.10—0.13 | 1300—1575 | 5.3—6.6 |
| 75 | | | | |
| Men | 23—28 | 0.09—0.12 | 1450—1750 | 6.0—7.2 |
| Women | 22—28 | 0.09—0.12 | 1200—1450 | 4.9—6.1 |

[a] Specific dynamic effect = 6% of ingested energy.
[b] Sitting requires an additional 0.4 kcal/min (0.0017 MJ/min). Walking requires an additional 1.4 kcal/min (0.006 MJ/min).

## CLINICAL CONDITIONS THAT ALTER ENERGY EXPENDITURE

### Increased energy expenditure

| | |
|---|---|
| Postoperatively | ↑0—10% |
| Multiple fractures | ↑10—30% |
| Sepsis | ↑25—60% |
| 3° burn >20% of body | ↑50—100% |

### Decreased energy expenditure

| | |
|---|---|
| Reduced body weight and starvation | ↓0—30% |

## Table 10
### DAILY ALLOWANCES OF WATER, ENERGY, AMINO ACIDS, CARBOHYDRATES, AND FAT FOR PATIENTS ON TOTAL PARENTERAL NUTRITION (TPN) (PER kg OF BODY WEIGHT PER DAY)[2,3]

### Adults

| Nutrients energy | Basal[a] | Moderate[b] | High[c] |
|---|---|---|---|
| Water (ml) | 30 | 50 | 100—150 |
| Energy | | | |
| kcal | 30 | 35—40 | 50—60 |
| MJ | 0.13 | 0.15—0.17 | 0.21—0.25 |
| Amino acid N | | | |
| g | 0.09 | 0.2—0.3 | 0.4—0.5 |
| | 0.7 | 1.5—2 | 3—3.5 |
| Glucose (g) | 2 | 5 | 7 |
| Fat (g) | 2 | 3 | 3—4 |

### Children (Years)

| Nutrients energy | Basal[a] | | | Moderate[b] | | | High[c] | | |
|---|---|---|---|---|---|---|---|---|---|
| | 0-1 | 1-8 | 8-15 | 0-1 | 1-8 | 8-15 | 0-1 | 1-8 | 8-15 |
| Water (ml) | 100 | 70—100 | 30—70 | 125 | 100—125 | 50—100 | 125—200 | 100—150 | 100—125 |
| Energy | | | | | | | | | |
| kcal | 90—100 | 60—80 | 40—60 | 125 | 100 | 50—70 | 150 | 125 | 60—100 |
| MJ | 0.4—0.5 | 0.2—0.3 | 0.17—0.25 | 0.52 | 0.42 | 0.32 | 0.63 | 0.52 | 0.25—0.42 |
| Amino acid N | | | | | | | | | |
| g | 0.3 | 0.2 | 0.15 | 0.45 | 0.3 | 0.25 | 0.5 | 0.45 | 0.3—0.4 |
| | 2.5 | 1.5—2.0 | 1—1.5 | 3.5 | 2.5 | 2.1 | 4 | 3.5 | 2.5—3.0 |
| Glucose (g) | 12 | 10—15 | 10 | 15—20 | 12—15 | 12 | 20—25 | 18—20 | 12—15 |
| Fat (g) | 1—4 | 2.4 | 4 | 4 | 4 | 3—4 | 6 | 5 | 4 |

[a] Resting metabolism, specific dynamic effect, and some physical activity.
[b] Postoperative state or depletion.
[c] Burns, sepsis, or major trauma.

Table 11
## DAILY ALLOWANCES OF ELECTROLYTES AND TRACE ELEMENTS FOR PATIENTS ON TPN (PER KG OF BODY WEIGHT PER DAY)[2,3]

Adults

| Electrolytes and trace elements | Basal[a] | Moderate[b] | High[c] |
|---|---|---|---|
| Sodium, mmol (mg) | 1—1.4 (23—32) | 2—3 (46—69) | 3—4 (69—92) |
| Potassium, mmol (mg) | 0.7—0.9 (27—35) | 2 (78) | 3—4 (117— 156) |
| Calcium, mmol (mg) | 0.11 (4.4) | 0.15 (6) | 0.2 (8) |
| Magnesium, mmol (mg) | 0.04 (1) | 0.15—0.20 (3.6—4.8) | 0.3—0.4 (7.2—9.6) |
| Iron, $\mu$mol ($\mu$g) | 0.25—1.0 (14—56) | 1.0 (56) | 1.0 (56) |
| Manganese, $\mu$mol ($\mu$g) | 0.1 (5.5) | 0.3 (16.5) | 0.6 (33) |
| Zinc, $\mu$mol ($\mu$g) | 0.7 (46) | 0.7—15 (46—89) | 1.5—3.0 (89—195) |
| Copper, $\mu$mol ($\mu$g) | 0.07 (4.5) | 0.3—0.4 (19—26) | 0.4—1 (26-69) |
| Chromium, $\mu$mol ($\mu$g) | 0.015 (0.8) | | 0.8 (4) |
| Selenium, $\mu$mol ($\mu$g) | 0.006 (0.5) | | |
| Molybdenum, $\mu$mol ($\mu$g) | 0.003 (0.3) | | |
| Chloride, mmol (mg) | 1.3—1.9 (46—67) | 2—3 (71—107) | |
| Phosphorus, mmol (mg) | 0.15 (4.7) | 0.4 (12) | 0.6—1.0 (19—31) |
| Fluoride, $\mu$mol ($\mu$g) | 0.7 (13) | 0.7—1.5 (13—29) | |
| Iodide, $\mu$mol ($\mu$g) | 0.015 (69) | | |

[a]   Resting metabolism, specific dynamic effect and some physical activity.
[b]   Postoperative state or depletion.
[c]   Burns, sepsis, or major trauma.

Table 12

DAILY ALLOWANCES OF ELECTROLYTES AND TRACE ELEMENTS FOR PATIENTS ON TPN (PER kg OF BODY WEIGHT PER DAY)[2,3]

Children (Years)

| Electrolytes and trace elements | Basal[a] | | Moderate[b] | | High[c] | |
|---|---|---|---|---|---|---|
| | 0—1 | 1—5 | 0—1 | 1—15 | 0—1 | 1—15 |
| Sodium, mmol (mg) | 2 (46) | 1—2 (23—46) | 2.5—3.5 (58—81) | 2—3 (46—69) | 4—5 (92—115) | 3—4 (69—92) |
| Potassium, mmol (mg) | 2 (78) | 1—2 (39—78) | 2—3 (78—117) | 2—2.5 (78—98) | 3—4 (117—156) | 3 (117) |
| Calcium, mg | 0.5—1 (20—40) | 0.5—1 (20—40) | 1—1.5 (40—60) | 1 (40) | 1.5—2 (60—80) | 1.5 (60) |
| Magnesium, mmol (mg) | 0.15 (3.6) | 0.1 (2.4) | 0.3 (7.2) | 0.15 (3.6) | 0.5 (12) | 0.2—0.3 (4.8—7.2) |
| Iron, µmol (µg) | 2 (112) | 1.5 (84) | 3 (168) | 2 (112) | 4 (224) | 3 (168) |
| Manganese, µmol (µg) | 0.3 (17) | 0.2 (11) | 0.1 (5) | 0.3 (17) | | 0.6 (33) |
| Zinc, µmol (µg) | 1 (65) | 1 (65) | 1.5 (98) | 1 (65) | 3 (195) | 1.5 (98) |
| Copper, µmol (µg) | 0.3 (19) | 0.2 (13) | 0.3—0.4 (19—26) | | | |
| Chromium, µmol (µg) | 0.01 (0.5) | 0.01 (0.5) | | | | |
| Selenium, µmol (µg) | 0.04 (3) | 0.003 (2.4) | | | | |
| Molybdenum, µmol (µg) | 0.12 (12) | 0.003—0.12 (0.3—12) | | | | |
| Chloride, mmol (mg) | 3 (107) | 2 (71) | 1—3 (36—107) | 2—3 (71—107) | 4—15 (142—178) | 3—44 (7—142) |
| Phosphorus, mmol (mg) | 1 (31) | 0.3 (9) | 1.5 (47) | 0.5 (16) | 2—2.5 (69—78) | 1 (31) |
| Fluoride, µmol (µg) | 3 (57) | 1 (19) | | | | |
| Iodide, µmol (µg) | 0.04 (5) | 0.02 (2.5) | | | | |

[a]   Resting metabolism, specific dynamic effect, and some physical activity.
[b]   Postoperative state or depletion.
[c]   Burns, sepsis, or major trauma.

## Table 13
### DAILY ALLOWANCES OF VITAMINS FOR PATIENTS ON TPN (PER KG BODY WEIGHT PER DAY)[2,3]

### Adults

| Vitamins | Basal[a] | Moderate[b] | High[c] |
|---|---|---|---|
| Thiamine, mg | 0.02 | 0.04 | 0.3 |
| Riboflavin, mg | 0.03 | 0.06 | 0.3 |
| Niacin, mg | 0.2 | 0.4 | 2 |
| Pyridoxine, mg | 0.03 | 0.06 | 0.4 |
| Folic acid, $\mu$g | 3 | 6 | 6—9 |
| Vitamin $B_{12}$, $\mu$g | 0.03 | 0.06 | 0.06 |
| Pantothenic acid, mg | 0.2 | 0.4 | 0.4 |
| Biotin, $\mu$g | 5 | 10 | 10 |
| Ascorbic acid, mg | 0.5 | 2 | 25 |
| Retinol, $\mu$g (IU) | 10 (33) | 10 (33) | 20 (67) |
| Vitamin D, $\mu$g (IU) | 0.04 (2) | 0.04 (2) | 0.1 (4) |
| Vitamin K, $\mu$g | 2 | 2 | 2 |
| Tocopherol, IU | 0.5 | 0.75 | 1 |

[a]   Resting Metabolism, specific dynamic effect, and some physical activity.
[b]   Postoperative state or depletion.
[c]   Burns, sepsis, or major trauma.

## Table 14
### DAILY ALLOWANCES OF VITAMINS FOR PATIENTS ON TPN (PER KG BODY WEIGHT PER DAY[2,3]

### Children (Years)

| Vitamins | Basal[a] | | Moderate[b] | | High[c] | |
|---|---|---|---|---|---|---|
| | 0-1 | 1-15 | 0-1 | 1-15 | 0-1 | 1-15 |
| Thiamine, mg | 0.05 | 0.05—0.02 | 0.1 | 0.04—0.1 | 2 | 0.3—2 |
| Riboflavin, mg | 0.1 | 0.1—0.03 | 0.2 | 0.06—0.2 | 0.4 | 0.3—0.4 |
| Niacin, mg | 1 | 1—0.2 | 2 | 0.4—2 | 4 | 2—4 |
| Pyridoxine, mg | 0.1 | 0.1—0.03 | 0.2 | 0.06—0.2 | 0.6 | 0.4—0.6 |
| Folic acid, $\mu$g | 20 | 3—20 | 40 | 6—40 | 50 | 9—50 |
| Vitamin $B_{12}$, $\mu$g | 0.2 | 0.2—0.03 | 0.4 | 0.06—0.4 | 5 | 0.06—5 |
| Pantothenic acid, mg | 1 | 0.2—1 | 2 | 0.4—2 | 2 | 0.4—2 |
| Biotin, $\mu$g | 30 | 5—30 | 60 | 10—60 | | 10—60 |
| Ascorbic acid, mg | 3 | 0.5—3 | 6 | 2—6 | 20 | 20—25 |
| Retinol, $\mu$g (IU) | 100 (333) | 10—100 (33—333) | 100 (333) | 10—100 (33—333) | 150 (500) | 20—150 (67—500) |
| Vitamin D, $\mu$g (IU) | 2.5 (100) | 0.05—2.5 (2—100) | 2.5 (100) | 0.04—2.5 (2—100) | 2.5 (100) | 0.1—2.5 (4—100) |
| Vitamin K, $\mu$g | 50 | 2—50 | 50 | 2—50 | 150 | 2—150 |
| Tocopherol, IU | 1 | 0.5—1 | 1—1.5 | 0.75—1.5 | 1.5 | 1—1.5 |

[a]   Resting metabolism, specific dynamic effect, and some physical activity.
[b]   Postoperative state or depletion.
[c]   Burns, sepsis, or major trauma.

Table 15

OSMOTIC ACTIVITY OF PLASMA AND
SOME INFUSION SOLUTIONS

| Solution | Osmotic activity | |
|---|---|---|
| | mOsm/kg $H_2O$ | mOsm/$l$ |
| Plasma | 290 | 285 |
| NaCl 0.9% | 310 | 305 |
| Intralipid 10% | 300 | 260 |
| Intralipid 20% | 350 | 260 |
| Liposyn 10% | 340 | 300 |
| Liposyn 20% | 360 | 340 |
| Glucose 5% | 278 | 252 |
| Glucose 10% | 523 | 505 |
| Glucose 20% | 1250 | 1010 |
| Crystalline amino acids 5% | 520 | 500 |
| Crystalline amino acids 7% | 740 | 700 |
| Crystalline amino acids 10% | 1070 | 1000 |

Table 16

EXAMPLES OF REGIMENS FOR TOTAL PARENTERAL
NUTRITION

| Nutrients energy | Adults[a] | | | Pediatric Patient (per day) |
|---|---|---|---|---|
| | Standard[b] | Cardiac failure (patient)[c] | Renal failure (patient)[d] | Per kg of body weight |
| Water (m$l$) | 3000 | 1500 | 1500 | 120—150 |
| Energy (kcal | 2230 | 1625 | 1560 | 115—125 |
| or MJ) | 9.4 | 6.8 | 6.6 | 0.48—0.53 |
| Amino Acids (g) | 100 | 50 | 35 | 2.5—3.0 |
| Glucose (g) | 200 | 250 | 250 | 15—30 |
| Fat (g) | 100 | 50 | 50 | 0.5—3.0 |
| Sodium (Cl)[e] (meq) | 90 (90) | 35 (35) | 25 (25) | 3—4 (3—4) |
| Potassium (Cl, $PO_4$) (meq) | 82 (82) | 55 (55) | — | 2—4 (2—4) |
| Calcium (Glu) (meq) | 9 (4.5) | 9 (4.5) | 9 (4.5) | 1—4 (0.5—2) |
| Magnesium ($SO_4$) (meq) | 10 (5) | 10 (5) | — | 0.25 (0.125) |
| Manganese (Cl) (mg) | 0.4 (0.007) | 0.4 (.007) | 0.4 (0.007) | — |
| Zinc (Cl) (mg) | 4.0 (0.06) | 2.0 (.03) | 2 (0.03) | 0.150—0.300 (0.002—0.004) |
| Copper (Cl) (mg) | 1.5 (0.02) | 1.5 (0.02) | 1.5 (0.02) | 0.02—0.04 (0.0003—0.0006) |
| Chromium (Cl) ($\mu$g) | 12 (0.00022) | 6 (0.00011) | 6 (0.00011) | — |
| Chloride (Na,K) (meq) | 150 (150) | 70 (70) | 50 (50) | 5—6 (5—6) |
| Phosphate (K) | (15) | (15) | — | (1.36) |
| Thiamine (mg) | 3.0 | 3.0 | 3.0 | 15 |
| Riboflavin (mg) | 3.6 | 3.6 | 3.6 | 3 |
| Niacin (mg) | 40 | 40 | 40 | 30 |

Table 16 (continued)
## EXAMPLES OF REGIMENS FOR TOTAL PARENTERALNUTRITION

| Nutrients energy | Adults[a] | | | Pediatric Patient (per day) |
|---|---|---|---|---|
| | Standard[b] | Cardiac failure (patient)[c] | Renal failure (patient)[d] | Per kg of body weight |
| Pyridoxine (mg) | 4.0 | 4.0 | 4.0 | 4.5 |
| Folate ($\mu$g) | 400 | 400 | 400 | — |
| Vitamin B$_{12}$ ($\mu$g) | 5.0 | 5.0 | 5.0 | — |
| Pantothenic acid (mg) | 15 | 15 | 15 | 7.5 |
| Biotin ($\mu$g) | 60 | 60 | 60 | — |
| Ascorbic acid (mg) | 100 | 100 | 100 | 150 |
| Retinol (IU) | 3300 | 3300 | 3300 | 3000 |
| Vitamin D (IU) | 200 | 200 | 200 | 300 |
| Vitamin E (IU) | 10 | 10 | 10 | 15 |

[a]   Numbers in parenthesis are in millimoles.
[b]   Based on 2 *l* of TPN formula containing all water soluble nutrients and 1 *l* of 10% Intralipid®.
[c]   Based on 1 *l* of TPN formula containing all water soluble nutrients and ½ *l* of 10% Intralipid®.
[d]   Based on 1 *l* of TPN formula containing all water soluble nutrients and ½ *l* of 10% Intralipid®.
[e]   Signs in brackets represent ion used to form salt.

Table 17
## METABOLIC COMPLICATIONS ASSOCIATED WITH PARENTERAL NUTRITION

Carbohydrate metabolism
    Hyperglycemia
    Ketoacidosis
    Post infusion hypoglycemia
Protein metabolism
    Serum amino acid imbalance
    Hyperammonemia
    Prerenal azotemia
    Hyperchloremic metabolic acidosis
Fat metabolism
    Essential fatty acid deficiency
    Hypertriglyceridemia
Electrolytes
    Hyper- or Hypokalemia
    Hyper- or Hypocalcemia
    Hypophosphatemia
    Hypomagnesemia
Other
    Anemia (iron, folate or B$_{12}$ deficiency)
    Coagulopathy (vitamin K deficiency)
    Cholestasis
    Elevated SGOT, SGPT, and alkaline phosphatase

## Table 18
## MONITORING OF PATIENTS ON TPN

During the first period of parenteral nutrition or in unstable
patients
  Daily
    Vital signs (temperature)
    Body weight
    Fluid balance
    Glycosuria
  Two to three times per week
    Serum electrolytes
      (Na, K, Cl, Ca, P)
    Acid-base status
    Blood glucose
    Renal function (BUN, creatinine)
    Liver function (SGOT, SGPT, Alkaline Phosphatase)
    Total protein and albumin
    White blood count and hemoglobin
  Once a week
    Mg
    Zn
  Triglyceride level
    Prothrombin time
    Fe/total iron binding capacity
For stable patients or patients on home TPN, the parameters should
be checked monthly or as indicated

## REFERENCES

1. Elwyn, D. H., Nutritional requirements of adult surgical patients, *Crit. Care Med.,* 8, 9-19, 1980.
2. Grotte, G., Meurling, S., and Wretlind, A., Parenteral nutrition, in *Textbook of Paediatrics,* in press.
3. Shenkin, A. and Wretlind, A., Parenteral nutrition, *World Rev. Nutr. Diet.,* 28, 1-111, 1978.
4. Wretlind, A., Evaluation of carbohydrates in parenteral nutrition, *Nutr. Metab.,* 18 (Suppl. 1), 242-255, 1975.
5. Dudrick, S. J., MacFadyen, B. V., Van Buren, C. T., Ruserg, R. L., and Maynard, A. T., Parenteral Hyperalimentation. Metabolic problems and solutions, *Ann. Surg.,* 176, 259-264, 1972.
6. Kinney, J. M., Calorie and nitrogen requirements in catabolic states, in *Practical Nutritional Support,* Karran, S. J. and Alberti, K. G. M. M., Eds., Pitman Medical, Kent, England, 1980.
7. Levy, J. S., Winters, R. W., and Heird, W. C., Total parenteral nutrition in pediatric patients, *Pediatr. Rev.,* 2, 99-106, 1980.
8. Michel, L., Serrano, A., and Malt, R. A., Nutritional support of hospitalized patients, N. Engl. J. Med., 304, 1147-1152, 1981.
9. *Aktuelle Ernährungs Medizin,* Thieme, Stuttgart, West Germany.
10. *American Journal of Clinical Nutrition,* Williams & Wilkins, Baltimore, Md.
11. *American Journal of Intravenous Therapy and Clinical Nutrition,* Paramus, N.J.
12. *British Journal of Intravenous Therapy,* Medical News Tribune, Ltd., London, England.
13. *Infusiontherapie and klinische Ernährung — Forschung und Praxis,* S. Karger, Basel, Switzerland.
14. *Journal of Parenteral and Enteral Nutrition,* Williams & Wilkins, Baltimore, Md.
15. *Nutrition Research,* Pergamon Press, Oxford, England.
16. *Clinical Nutrition,* Churchill Livingstone, Edinburgh, Scotland.
17. **Nutritional Support Services,** North Hollywood, Calif.

# NUTRITIONALLY ADEQUATE VEGETARIAN DIETS

U. D. Register and Hulda Crooks

## INTRODUCTION

Edible plants form the basis of the diet of man in every country, whether they are consumed directly or after they have been eaten by animals and converted to meat, milk, or eggs. A rapidly rising world population presents an increasing threat to world food supplies, especially as more and more countries whose traditional diet has been mainly plant foods, adopt western-type diets rich in animal foods. Since an adequate diet can be compounded in many ways, we will consider in the following pages the adequacy of the simplest diet known to man — a diet composed largely or entirely of foods of plant origin.

## WHAT IS A VEGETARIAN DIET?

A consideration of the various types of nonflesh diets is requisite to any meaningful discussion of their nutritional adequacy, since many diets loosely designated "vegetarian" are not representative of meatless diets as commonly prepared in countries where an adequate food supply is available. Adherents to diets offering no flesh foods of any kind may be divided into three groups:

1. Lacto-ovovegetarians include dairy products and eggs in their diets
2. Lactovegetarians use only dairy products in addition to plant foods
3. Total or pure vegetarians avoid all animal products

Members of the total vegetarian group differ widely in their beliefs and practices. The dietary pattern of some differs little from the lactovegetarian pattern, the main difference being that they substitute soymilk and soy products for dairy products. Some total vegetarians (vegans) carry their nonanimal teaching beyond the matter of diet and refuse to use any animal products, refusing even to wear shoes made of leather. Few are lifetime vegetarians. Within this loosely knit group are found modern adherents of ancient religions similar to the teachings of Zoroaster, the founder of the Persian religion. Extreme and nutritionally unsound teachings are held by some. The bizarre and dangerous Zen Macrobiotic diet,[1] whose ultimate level of perfection consists in eating only cereals, mainly rice, and drinking as little water as possible, is a recent addition to the total vegetarian category. It is in no way representative of any common type of nonflesh dietary. Thus the term "vegetarian" covers a wide range and may connote much more than abstinence from flesh foods, being frequently associated with asceticism, philosophy, religion, or other specific beliefs.

When a variety of nonflesh foods is available in sufficient amounts, a vegetarian diet can be both tasty and nutritionally adequate. However, enforced vegetarianism due to inadequate food supplies or to economic limitations may be deficient both in quantity and quality as any other type of diet would be under similar conditions. Deficiency may also result when a diet is restricted (as the Zen Macrobiotic diet) due to gross misconception of the function of food in the body, taboos, superstition, or ignorance.

## PROTEIN REQUIREMENT

The most common concern regarding a diet without some kind of flesh food is the adequacy of its protein content. This concern stems largely from the 19th century misconception of the physiological function of protein in the animal body. Justus von Liebig (1803-1873), professor of chemistry at the University of Munich, theorized that physical activity or work used up muscle and that protein was required to replace the "worn out" tissues.[2] Thus every increase in physical activity required an increase in protein intake. Since animal tissues are high in protein, the term "meat" came to be equated with the term "protein", and a diet without meat seemed bound to be deficient in this nutrient.

Experimental research by another German physiologist, Carl von Voit (1831-1908), proved Liebig's teaching to be erroneous. He showed that dogs fed a diet of fat and carbohydrate without any protein did not break down an unusual amount of body protein to provide energy for vigorous exercise. Yet in spite of this clear evidence against the need of large amounts of protein for energy, the fear of a deficiency continued to dominate nutritional thinking. Voit himself set a human protein intake standard of 118 g/day based on his statistical finding that this was the average amount consumed by 1000 German laborers whom he studied.[2] However, this high recommendation was promptly challenged by physiologists in several countries. From different countries came evidence obtained through controlled feeding experiments that nitrogen balance can be maintained in normal subjects on a mixed diet with a protein intake of only 30 to 35 g/day.[3]

In 1902, Russel Henry Chittenden began nitrogen balance experiments with members of the University Faculty, college athletes, and a detail of 20 soldiers from the Hospital Corps of the U.S. Army. The results showed that good health and nitrogen balance could be maintained on 40 to 60 g of protein per day for periods of 6 months to several years. His subjects reported an increase in well being and demonstrated a gain in muscular power.[4] The results of Chittenden's work were largely responsible for paving the way for much lower protein intake recommendations.

In 1920, Henry C. Sherman did a critical analysis of 109 nitrogen balance experiments designed to determine the protein requirements of man.[5] He found that the apparent protein requirement for a 70-kg man averaged 44.4 g. Sherman concluded that his best data would yield a result not far from 0.5 g protein per kilogram body weight per day for normal maintenance. The Food and Nutrition Board of the National Research Council, in formulating its first Recommended Dietary Allowances (RDA), doubled this figure and recommended a gram of protein per kilogram of body weight, thus providing a most generous safety margin.[6] Later studies, however, revealed that this recommendation was unnecessarily high, and a step-wise lowering over the years has dropped it to 56 g for the reference man and 44 g for the reference woman.[7] This lower recommendation is regularly exceeded by any ordinary mixed diet and even by the total vegetarian diet, as we shall see below.

## LACTO-OVOVEGETARIAN DIET

In their study of 112 vegetarian and 88 nonvegetarian adults, adolescents, and pregnant women, Hardinge and Stare[8] found that a lacto-ovovegetarian diet does not differ markedly from the conventional American diet except in its omission of all kinds of flesh foods, including fish and fowl. The diet met all known nutritional needs with abundance for all classes. The protein intake of every lacto-ovovegetarian group considerably exceeded the RDA recommendations. Table 1 compares the intakes of calories and of animal and vegetable protein, and gives the heights and weights of the subjects on the vegetarian and nonvegetarian diets.

Table 1 shows that lacto-ovovegetarian protein intakes ranged from a low 82 g for the adult females (RDA recommends 44 g) to a high 141 g (RDA recommend 56 g) for the adolescent males. Not only was the total protein intake large for every group,

Table 1
COMPARISON OF CALORIE AND PROTEIN INTAKE AMONG
VEGETARIANS AND NONVEGETARIANS

| | | Protein intake | | | | |
| | Calorie | Animal | Plant | Total | Height | Weight |
| Groups | intake | (g) | (g) | (g) | (in.) | (lb) |
|---|---|---|---|---|---|---|
| | | Adult | | | | |
| Males | | | | | | |
| Lacto-ovovegetarian | 3020 | 41 | 57 | 98 | 68.0 | 162 |
| Nonvegetarian | 3720 | 86 | 39 | 125 | 69.5 | 170 |
| Pure vegetarian | 3260 | — | 83 | 83 | 68.0 | 146 |
| Females | | | | | | |
| Lacto-ovovegetarian | 2450 | 43 | 39 | 82 | 62.5 | 138 |
| Nonvegetarian | 2690 | 64 | 30 | 94 | 64.0 | 142 |
| Pure vegetarian | 2400 | — | 61 | 61 | 63.0 | 117 |
| | | Adolescent | | | | |
| Males | | | | | | |
| Lacto-ovovegetarian | 4450 | 69 | 72 | 141 | 68.0 | 141 |
| Nonvegetarian | 5350 | 116 | 63 | 179 | 68.5 | 142 |
| Females | | | | | | |
| Lacto-ovovegetarian | 3030 | 51 | 49 | 100 | 64.0 | 117 |
| Nonvegetarian | 4100 | 106 | 45 | 151 | 63.0 | 112 |
| | | Pregnant Women | | | | |
| Lacto-ovovegetarian | 2650 | 56 | 41 | 97 | 64.5 | 130 |
| Nonvegetarian | 3010 | 81 | 30 | 111 | 64.5 | 129 |

From Hardinge, M. G. and Stare, F. J., *Am. J. Clin. Nutr.*, 2, 76, 1954. With permission.

but the consumption of milk and egg protein alone was more than enough to meet the "safe level of intake" of the FAO/WHO Expert Committee on Nutrition, which is 29 and 31 g for adult and adolescent females and 37 and 38 g for adult and adolescent males, respectively.[9] The milk and egg protein exceeded the total protein intake recommended by the RDA for adult males and for adolescent males and females. Thus neither protein quantity or quality can be questioned when dairy products and eggs are used in the diet.

## LACTOVEGETARIAN DIET

This diet is quite similar to the preceding one, except that dairy products provide the only animal protein. It is less commonly used in western countries than is the lacto-ovovegetarian type.

Mirone[10,11] reported the nutrient intakes and blood findings of a community of men whose per capita total yearly animal protein intake was provided by 259 pt of milk, 286 oz of American cheddar cheese, and very few eggs (8 eggs) used in baking. The duration of the diet ranged from 12 to 47 years. The dietary mainstays were whole-wheat bread, skim milk and cheese, vegetables, and fruit. Blood findings were within normal range, and the men appeared in good health. They were classified as farmers, carpenters, lecturers, laborers, and teachers.

The diet of the Sherpas in the high mountains of eastern Nepal, whose men are famous for their unsurpassed endurance as carriers for Mount Everest expeditions, is essentially lactovegetarian. Tensing Norgay,[12] the Sherpa who accompanied Hillary on the first conquest of the world's highest mountain peak, writes that potatoes that grow in altitudes up to 14,000 ft are the mainstay of the Sherpa diet, as rice is in the Chinese diet. Wheat grows in altitudes up to 10,000 ft, and barley can grow in locations as high as those supporting potatoes.

These simple foods, supplemented with some milk from yak, goats, and sheep make up the sherpa diet. Meat is seldom eaten and not at all by the strict Buddhists among them. Yet young men raised on this diet are sought after for their endurance and strength in carrying heavy loads up steep trails at extreme altitudes in the world's highest mountains.

A study by Toomey and White[13] supports claims of the superior health of the Hunzas living in the high Himalayas north of Pakistan. The diet, described as "spartan", consists mainly of grains (barley, wheat, and millet), vegetables and fruits (mainly dried apricots), and some nuts together with a little goat or ewe milk. Meat, primarily mutton, is a treat once or twice a year for festive occasions only. The subjects of this study were 25 men believed to range in age from 90 to 110 years. They appeared to be in excellent health. Their blood pressures and serum cholesterol levels were low, and there was practically no evidence of heart or blood vessel disease.

Mehta et al. studied the serum vitamin $B_{12}$ and folic acid levels in 102 healthy vegetarian and nonvegetarian Indian medical students.[14] Of the subjects, 50 were lactovegetarian and lacto-ovovegetarian, and 45 were nonvegetarian. The results showed that the vegetarians had markedly lower serum vitamin $B_{12}$ and folic acid levels than matched nonvegetarians. The investigators pointed out, however, that the physiologically normal serum vitamin $B_{12}$ values are not well defined. The RDA recommends an intake of 3 $\mu$g/day for an adult. Many people in India live from childhood to old age on a lactovegetarian diet consisting mainly of rice, legumes, wheat flour for chappaties, green vegetables, fruits, and 5 to 10 oz of milk per person per day.

The weights and heights of Mehta's vegetarian and nonvegetarian subjects did not differ significantly, and the blood picture of the two groups was also similar. A recent analysis[15] found fresh milk and pasteurized milk to contain 1.6 and 1 $\mu$g of vitamin $B_{12}$ per cup, respectively. Thus 0.5 to 1 pt of milk per day could provide sufficient levels of the vitamin to prevent deficiency.

While on the topic of the central nutritional problems of our day, Dr. Arturri Virtanen, Director of the Biochemical Institute, Helsinki, Finland, said with reference to a diet of plant foods and dairy products: "Lactovegetarians can receive all the necessary nutrients from fruit, vegetables, potatoes, cereals, and milk low in fat."[16] He favored this type of diet for the prevention of overnutrition so prevalent in the developed countries.

## TOTAL VEGETARIAN DIET

Table 1 shows that the pure (total) vegetarians of the Hardinge and Stare study obtained an abundance of protein from whole-grain cereal, legumes, potatoes, vegetables, fruits, and nuts. The men averaged 81 g and the women 63 g daily. Not only did their protein intake exceed the recommended allowance in quantity, but it more than met Rose's finding of a "definitely safe intake"[17] for every essential amino acid except methionine.[18] However, the methionine intake met Rose's suggested minimum requirement and since, according to Rose, cystine is 80 to 89% capable of replacing methionine, the sum of the two sulfur amino acids surpassed his estimated safe intake, which is twice the highest minimum requirement observed in his subjects (Table 2).

The need for so high a methionine recommendation and the likelihood of a methionine deficiency problem in human nutrition has been questioned.[19]

Table 2
## ESSENTIAL AMINO ACIDS IN DIETS OF ADULT MALE VEGETARIANS AND NONVEGETARIANS[a]

Values Expressed in Grams

| Amino acid | Non-vegetarian | Lacto-ovo-vegetarian | Pure vegetarian | Recommendation[a] |
|---|---|---|---|---|
| Isoleucine | 6.6 | 5.4 | 4.0 | 1.4 |
| Leucine | 10.1 | 8.2 | 6.0 | 2.2 |
| Lysine | 8.3 | 5.4 | 3.7 | 1.6 |
| Phenylalanine + tyrosine | 10.4 | 8.8 | 7.0 | 2.2 |
| Methionine + cystine | 4.3 | 3.2 | 2.7 | 2.2 |
| Threonine | 5.0 | 3.8 | 2.9 | 1.0 |
| Tryptophan | 1.5 | 1.2 | 1.1 | 0.5 |
| Valine | 7.1 | 5.6 | 4.3 | 1.6 |
| Protein intake | 121.3 | 97.2 | 81.5 | 65.0 |

[a]   For average man.

From Hardinge, M. G., Crooks, H., and Stare, F. J., *J. Am. Diet. Assoc.*, 48, 25, 1966. With permission.

## ADEQUACY OF PLANT PROTEINS

The adequacy of plant protein was studied by Hegsted et al.[20] following World War II. Twenty-six subjects were placed on an all-plant diet in which 62% of the protein was supplied by cereals (mostly white bread), 30% by vegetables, and 8% by fruits. The authors concluded that 30 to 40 g of this protein per day met the requirement of an average-sized man.

Vegetable protein mixture (VPM) that simulate meat products have been prepared and used in human diets in this country for years. The protein of these mixtures is usually derived from wheat, soybean, peanut, yeast, or a combination of two or more. However, little information is available concerning the protein quality of such products. Studies in our laboratory have shown that selected VPMs compare favorably with meat in promoting growth in weanling rats,[21] as shown in Table 3.

Sanchez et al.[22] determined the biological value of selected meal patterns. The meals containing vegetable entrees compared favorably with similar meals containing meats (Table 4).

Register et al.[23] did nitrogen balance studies on three male and three female university students. The studies consisted of four 16-day periods in which total vegetarian, lactovegetarian, and nonvegetarian diets were tested. The VPM mixture prepared from soybean, yeast, and wheat proteins supplied a significant proportion of the protein in the all-plant diet; soymilk was also used. The lactovegetarian diet was adapted from the total vegetarian diet by replacing the soymilk and soy mayonnaise with dairy milk and commercial mayonnaise. The nonvegetarian diet was formulated by an exchange of ground beef for the commercial plant protein. At a level of 10 g nitrogen per day (approximately 60 g protein), there was no significant difference in the ability of the three diets to maintain nitrogen balance in the test subjects (see Table 5).

More recently, isolated soybean protein has been spun into fibers which can then be combined to make high-protein foods that closely resemble various types of meats in texture, appearance, composition, and taste.[24] Current technology, however, in-

Table 3

RAT GROWTH ON THE BASAL COLLEGE CAFETERIA DIET, WITH AND
WITHOUT ANIMAL FOODS AND WITH VARIED FAT COMPOSITION

| Diet | Average weight gain (g/week) | Net protein utilization[a] | Fatty acid composition (g/100 g crude fat) Total saturated | Total polyunsaturated | P:S ratio[b] | Percent of calories as fat |
|---|---|---|---|---|---|---|
| Basal college cafeteria[c] | | | | | | |
| + Vegetable entrées | 17.2[d] | 50 | 19 | 33 | 1.76 | 25 |
| + Vegetable entrées + skim milk | 37.2 | 61 | 19 | 33 | 1.76 | 25 |
| + Vegetable entrées + whole milk | 37.2 | 61 | 34 | 22 | 0.65 | 37 |
| + Vegetable entrées + soy milk[e] | 37.4 | 56 | 18 | 43 | 2.39 | 34 |
| + Meat entrées[f] | 32.4 | 64 | 28 | 22 | 0.79 | 33 |
| + Meat entrées + whole milk | 38.8 | — | 38 | 15 | 0.39 | 44 |
| Recommended diet for heart patients | — | — | — | — | 1.10—1.50 | 25 |
| Prudent diet | — | — | 20 | 30 | 1.50 | 30 |
| American diet | — | 49—67 | 39 | 17 | 0.44 | 44 |

[a]   Nitrogen retention/nitrogen intake × 100.
[b]   Polyunsaturated-to-saturated fatty acid ratio.
[c]   Composite of a week's diet composed of foods of plant origin without the entrees of the noon and evening meals and supplemented with vitamins and minerals.
[d]   Data based on 7 rats per group for 5 weeks.
[e]   Milk or soy milk (Soyagen®) was added at a level of 1 cup per meal.
[f]   Meat mixture as commonly consumed in the U.S.: beef, 56%; chicken, 17%; fish, 17%; and luncheon meats, 10%.

From Sanchez, A., Porter, G. G., and Register, U. D., *J. Am. Diet. Assoc.*, 49, 493, 1966. With permission.

cludes a large amount of egg albumin in the protein mixture to provide a suitable binder for the product.[25] Therefore, spun soybean products are not suitable for inclusion in total vegetarian test diets. Human subjects have been maintained in good health for 6 months on diets in which meat-like products made from soy protein fibers supplied 14% of the calories as protein.[26]

Fomon et al.[27] studied 13 female Caucasian infants on a soy-isolate formula. The babies were enrolled during the first 9 days after birth and observed unil they were 111 days of age. The formula was the sole source of nutrients during the first 28 days. Thereafter, certain strained plant foods were added. The subjects appeared in good health during the study period. Clinical observations, growth rates, and serum albumin concentrations were similar to those found in female, breast-fed infants and those fed a cow-milk formula providing greater protein intakes.

Kurtha and Ellis[28] and Ellis and Montegriffo[29] have reviewed the long-term effects of all-plant diets on the health of vegans. The investigators conclude that the general health of members of this vegetarian group is good and differs little from that of omnivores, providing the diet is supplemented with vitamin $B_{12}$ or with foods fortified with it. Total vegetarians tend to be lighter in weight than subjects who use animal foods. The reviewers considered this fact a possible advantage, since obesity is common in the general population and is associated with a higher incidence of coronary artery disease, hypertension, and diabetes mellitus.

Table 4
COMPARISON OF THE
POLYUNSATURATED-TO-
SATURATED FAT (P:S) RATIO
AND BIOLOGICAL VALUE OF
PROTEIN OF SINGLE MEALS

| Meal[a] | Biological value | P:S ratio |
|---|---|---|
| Basal II + VPM 2 + soybean milk[b] | 67 | 2.79 |
| Basal II + VPM 2 | 65 | 2.56 |
| Basal II + VPM 2 + skimmed milk | 70 | 2.50 |
| Basal I + beans and corn | 75 | 1.94 |
| Basal I + beans and rice | 79 | 1.72 |
| Basal II + VPM 2 + cow's milk | 70 | 0.90 |
| Basal II + veal | 73 | 0.32 |
| Average American diet | | 0.44 |

[a]  One pat of regular margarine was added to each meal.
[b]  Beverages, when indicated, were added in amounts equivalent to one glass per meal.

From Sanchez, A., Scharffenberg, J. A., and Register, U. D., *Am. J. Clin. Nutr.,* 13, 246, 1963. With permission.

In a review of the nature of the protein requirements and how these are to be met in the future, Scrimshaw[30] concludes: "Vegetable protein mixtures supplying the amino acids in appropriate proportions are as efficient in meeting protein needs at minimum levels of intake as proteins of animal origin, even though the concentration of essential amino acids in these mixtures is much lower." An understanding of these requirements, he says, "frees us from dependence on the concept of the need for animal protein or amino acids from conventional food alone . . . "

Wokes[31] has reported that, on a world basis in recent years, of some 69 million tons of protein produced yearly, cereals provided 33 million (nearly half), nuts and legumes provided 8 million, and fruits and vegetables provided 7 million tons. Of the 21 million tons of animal protein, milk and cheese yielded about 7.5 million tons. Thus the ratio of plant to animal protein for the whole world was 48:21 (about 2.3:1).

In a very recent article, Hegsted[32] suggests the modification of the American diet as one means of reducing major causes of death and disability in our population — coronary artery disease, diabetes, intestinal disease including cancer of the colon, and so on. He asks: "What risk is associated with a decrease in the consumption of meat and fat, particularly saturated fat and cholesterol, and greater consumption of vegetables, fruits, cereals? I submit that they are minimal. We could scarcely do worse than we are doing now."

The Food and Nutrition Board of the National Research Council issued a statement on vegetarian diets[33] in May 1974 which said: "Most nutritionists agree that vegetarian diets can be adequate, if sufficient care is taken in planning them." Obviously, careful planning is essential for good nutrition with every type of diet. As Harris[34] has so well observed:

Table 5
AVERAGE NITROGEN-BALANCE DATA FROM FOUR TESTS

| Test | Nitrogen intake (g/day) | Urinary nitrogen (g/day) | Fecal nitrogen (g/day) | Total nitrogen (g/day) | Nitrogen balance (g/day) | Creatinine excretion (g/day) | Percent true digestibility |
|---|---|---|---|---|---|---|---|
| Test I | | | | | | | |
| Pure vegetarian diet | 10.22 | 8.37 | 1.78 | 10.15 | +0.07 ± 0.20[a] | 1.32 | 87.3 ± 0.20[a] |
| Test II | | | | | | | |
| Lactovegetarian diet | 10.19 | 8.17 | 1.70 | 9.87 | +0.32 ± 0.21 | 1.35 | 88.1 ± 0.53 |
| Test III | | | | | | | |
| Nonvegetarian diet | 9.77 | 8.16 | 1.54 | 9.70 | +0.07 ± 0.22 | 1.63 | 89.1 ± 0.74 |
| Test IV | | | | | | | |
| Pure vegetarian diet | 10.05 | 7.73 | 1.89 | 9.62 | +0.43 ± 0.12 | 1.49 | 86.3 ± 0.66 |

[a]   Values are standard error of the mean.

From Register, U. D., Inano, M., Thurston, C. E., Vyhmeister, I. B., Dysinger, P. W., Blankenship, J. W., and Horning, M. C., *Am. J. Clin. Nutr.*, 20, 757, 1967. With permission.

"Man can formulate his diet from a wide variety of foods. Good nutrition is not assured necessarily by eating prescribed quantities of rice, wheat, milk, eggs, meat, maize and similar foodstuffs. Good nutrition results when an individual obtains adequate amounts of the various amino acids, vitamins, minerals, and calories required to meet his needs for growth and maintenance. It does not matter whether the calcium comes from milk or tortilla, whether the iron comes from meat or tampala, whether niacin comes from liver or peanuts, whether the tryptophane comes from eggs or soybeans, or whether the calories come from wheat or rice, so long as these nutrients are available . . . There is no indispensible food and it is now obvious that there are many ways to compound a good diet."*

## PLANNING THE VEGETARIAN DIET

Many an individual accustomed to the usual American diet looks upon a change to a vegetarian diet as difficult and perhaps hazardous. Actually, the one big difference is in omitting the meat and replacing it with a meatless entree. This is not difficult, but it does involve a change in dietetic habits. One accustomed to a steak as his main dinner dish may miss it for a while until he learns to enjoy the less familiar foods.

Planning a vegetarian diet requires the observation of the same basic principles as those used in planning the conventional diet. The four-food group meal pattern (meat, cereal and grains, milk and dairy products, and fruits and vegetables) may be adapted for use by omitting the protein-rich meat group and thus reducing the excess protein intake. More than sufficient protein can be obtained by the use of dairy products, some eggs, a variety of legumes, nuts, meat analogs made from soybean, and other plant proteins formulated to resemble meat products. Commercially prepared plant proteins are not essential for a well-balanced vegetarian diet, but they provide a pleasing variety and are easily and quickly prepared for serving.

Table 6 shows a range of food distribution that might be useful to others in planning a change to a nonflesh diet.[35] The data from Table 6 were considered in making the following recommendations:

1.  Reduce the use of "empty calories," i.e., foods which provide an excess of calories but are deficient in other needed nutrients. Such foods usually include sweets, soft drinks, jellies and jams, most desserts, etc. If a replacement is needed, substitute fruits (especially fresh fruits), vegetables, and nonsweet bakery products made from mostly unrefined flour.
2.  Sufficient vitamin $B_{12}$ should be available from a glass or two of either whole or skim milk. Eggs are good sources but should not be used freely because of their high cholesterol content.
3.  Substitute whole-grain breads and cereals for refined products. These high-energy foods can be increased or decreased as the needs indicate.
4.  Freely use fresh fruits and vegetables, either raw or cooked. Plan to use a variety from meal-to-meal and day-to-day rather than a great many at one meal. A mixture of fruits and coarse vegetables at the same meal may cause digestive disturbance and gas in some individuals. Serving them at separate meals often solves this problem.
5.  Planning a total vegetarian diet requires additional consideration. The change from a flesh diet is made easier if the first step is to a lacto-ovovegetarian or a lacto-vegetarian diet for a season before the final step is taken to adopt a diet devoid of any animal products including even milk. The following suggestions should be helpful:
a.  Maintain an adequate calorie intake. Many (but not all) plant foods are low in calories. This is especially true of the vegetables. However, breads and cereals,

* From Harris, R. S., Indigenous Edible Plants of Latin America, paper presented at El Congroso Internacional Sobre Vitamins, Havana, Cuba, January 1952. With permission.

Table 6
## DISTRIBUTION OF CALORIES OF ADULT NONVEGETARIAN, LACTO-OVOVEGETARIAN, AND PURE VEGETARIAN DIETS

| | Male | | | Female | | |
|---|---|---|---|---|---|---|
| Food | Non vegetarian | Lacto-ovo vegetarian | Pure vegetarian | Non vegetarian | Lacto-ovo vegetarian | Pure vegetarian |
| Milk | 10.6 | 16.6 | 2.1 (soy) | 8.2 | 17.7 | 4.9 (soy) |
| Cheese | 2.7 | 1.8 | 0.4 (soy) | 2.8 | 3.0 | 0.5 (soy) |
| Egg | 2.6 | 1.3 | — | 2.2 | 1.3 | — |
| Meat | 12.9 | — | — | 12.4 | — | — |
| Commercial vegetable protein | — | 1.6 | 1.0 | — | 2.0 | 1.1 |
| Cereal, dark | 5.5 | 16.0 | 13.8 | 4.8 | 8.2 | 11.8 |
| Cereal, white | 8.8 | 4.5 | 1.4 | 9.7 | 5.0 | 0.5 |
| Legumes | 1.2 | 4.0 | 5.7 | 1.0 | 3.2 | 5.2 |
| Nuts | 3.4 | 4.5 | 15.0 | 2.3 | 3.7 | 8.9 |
| Oil-rich seeds | — | 0.3 | 1.8 | — | 0.2 | 3.7 |
| Potatoes | 2.7 | 3.9 | 2.7 | 3.4 | 3.7 | 3.2 |
| Vegetables, other | 2.2 | 2.4 | 4.2 | 2.5 | 2.2 | 4.5 |
| Fruits | 9.3 | 19.0 | 30.8 | 10.0 | 17.3 | 28.9 |
| Soup | 1.5 | 3.6 | 0.9 | 2.4 | 2.4 | 0.9 |
| Fat, visible | 10.8 | 8.2 | 11.3 | 12.3 | 13.1 | 15.0 |
| Desserts (sweets) including honey, syrup, molasses, and soft drinks | 25.0 | 11.9 | 7.0 | 24.0 | 16.3 | 11.0 |
| Total protein (g) | 125 | 98 | 83 | 94 | 82 | 6 |
| Animal protein (g) | 86 | 41 | 0 | 64 | 43 | 0 |
| Total calories | 3720 | 3020 | 3260 | 2690 | 2450 | 2400 |

as well as legumes, carry a good supply of potential energy, and nuts and nut-like seeds (peanuts, sunflower seeds, soybeans, sesame seeds, and others) are high in calories because they are high in fat. There is no problem in getting sufficient calories if an individual changing from a diet of meat, dairy products, eggs, and rich desserts understands that such a change involves a sudden drop in highly concentrated foods and that the new diet needs proper balance. If caloric intake is too low, a prompt loss of weight will result. If this is not desirable, it can be stopped by the addition of the more concentrated foods already mentioned.

b.   Since there is no practical source of vitamins D or $B_{12}$ in plant foods commonly used in western countries, total vegetarians should obtain these from other sources. Vitamin D may be obtained by moderate exposure of some skin to sunlight. Vitamin $B_{12}$ can be provided by a supplement or by the use of such foods as fortified soymilk, meat analogs, cereals and other foods to which $B_{12}$ has been added. Planning lactovegetarian diets for children has been described by Vyhmeister et al.[41].

## MEAT ANALOGS

Food technology has produced vegetable-protein products textured and flavored to resemble beef, chicken, seafood, or ham and the many variations of their products.[36] These foods are made from edible plant proteins such as proteins of soybean, peanut, wheat, and other less common sources. These plant protein products contain less fat than what is found in meat. For example, ham analog has only 12% fat, compared to about 30 to 35% in real ham. About the same percentage holds true for plant protein wieners as compared to meat wieners. Beef analog contains about 13% fat, compared to 18% or more in beef.[37] When vitamins and other nutrients are added to the isolated protein, the final nutritional quality of these products is similar to the products they simulate.

Isolated soy protein foods made to resemble chicken, seafood, ham, or beef were well accepted by hospitalized, volunteer subjects. The experiment lasted for 24 weeks, during which time the patients maintained their normal weight and remained in good health. The results indicate that these soy proteins are both nutritious and acceptable as a major source of protein in the human diet.[38]

Various studies of the quality of the proteins of diets containing meat analogs, using different methods of comparison, have shown them to compare favorably with similar diets containing meat.[39]

Thus, as Harris[34] has observed: "Both the vegetarian type and carnivorous type of diet can adequately feed mankind. The realization of this fact by those who struggle with the food problem of the world is of terrible importance. There is not sufficient land in the world to feed all mankind the animal protein diet now consumed in the United States . . . People may prefer to eat diets rich in animal proteins, but those diets are not necessary, and most people cannot afford them."

Supplementary material, the book *How to Get the Most for Your Food Dollar,*[40] is now available.

# REFERENCES

1. Council on Foods and Nutrition, Zen Macrobiotic diets, *JAMA,* 218, 397, 1971.
2. Beach, E. F., Proteins in nutrition (historical), in *Proteins and Amino Acids in Nutrition,* Sahyun, M., Ed., Reinhold, New York, 1948, 1-26.
3. Mitchell, H. H., The biological utilization of proteins and protein requirements, in *Proteins and Amino Acids in Nutrition,* Sahyun, M., Ed., Reinhold, New York, 1948, 73-75.
4. Chittenden, R. H., *The Nutrition of Man,* Frederick A. Stokes Co., Norwood, Mass., 1907, 153-228.
5. Sherman, H. C., Gillet, L. H., and Osterberg, E., Protein requirement of maintenance in man and the nutritive efficiency of bread protein, *J. Biol. Chem.,* 41, 97-109, 1920.
6. NRC Recommended Dietary Allowances, Reprint and Circ. Ser. No. 115, National Research Council, Washington, D.C., 1943.
7. Food and Nutrition Board, *Recommended Dietary Allowances,* 9th ed., Publ. No. 2216, National Academy of Sciences-National Research Council, Washington, D.C., 1980.
8. Hardinge, M. G. and Stare, F. J., Nutritional studies of vegetarians. I. Nutritional physical, and laboratory findings, *Am. J. Clin. Nutr.,* 2, 73-82, 1954.
9. Joint FAO/WHO Ad Hoc Expert Committee, Energy and protein requirements, *WHO Tech. Rep. Ser.,* No. 522, 74, 1973.
10. Mirone, L., Blood findings in men on a diet devoid of meat and low in animal protein, *Science,* 3, 673-674, 1950.
11. Mirone, L., Nutrient intake and blood findings of men on a diet devoid of meat, *Am. J. Clin. Nutr.,* 2, 246-251, 1954.
12. Norgay, T. and Ullman, J. R., *Tiger of the Snows,* G. P. Putnam's, New York, 1955, 14.
13. Toomey, E. G. and White, P. D., A brief survey of the health of aged Hunzas, *Am. Heart J.,* 68, 841-842, 1964.
14. Mehta, B. M., Rege, D. V., and Satoskar, R. S., Serum vitamin $B_{12}$ and folic acid activity in lacto-vegetarian and nonvegetarian healthy adult Indians, *Am. J. Clin. Nutr.,* 15, 77-84, 1964.
15. Adams, J. F., McEwan, F., and Wilson, A., The vitamin $B_{12}$ content of meals and items of diet, *Br. J. Nutr.,* 29, 65-72, 1973.
16. Virtanen, D. M., Some central nutritional problems of the present time, *Fed. Proc. Fed. Am. Soc. Exp. Biol.,* 27, 1374-1378, 1968.
17. Rose, W. C., Wixom, R. L., and Lockhart, H. B., and Lambert, G. F., The amino acid requirements of man. XV. The valine requirement; summary and final observations, *J. Biol. Chem.,* 217, 987-995, 1955.

18. Hardinge, M. G., Crooks, H., and Stare, F., Nutritional studies of vegetarians. V. Proteins and essential amino acids, *J. Am. Diet. Assoc.*, 48, 25-28, 1966.
19. Hegsted, D. M., Variation in requirements of nutrients — amino acids, *Fed. Proc. Fed. Am. Soc. Exp. Biol.*, 22, 1424-1430, 1963.
20. Hegsted, D. M., Tsongas, A. G., Abbott, D. B., and Stare, F. J., Protein requirements of adults, *J. Lab. Clin. Med.*, 31, 261-284, 1946.
21. Sanchez, A., Porter, G. G., and Register, U. D., Effect of entree on fat and protein quality of diets, *J. Am. Diet. Assoc.*, 49, 492-496, 1966.
22. Sanchez, A., Scharffenberg, J. A., and Register, U. D., Nutritive value of selected proteins and protein combinations, *Am. J. Clin. Nutr.*, 13, 243-249, 1963.
23. Register, U. D., Inano, M., Thurston, C. E., Vyhmeister, I. B., Dysinger, P. W., Blankenship, J. W., and Horning, M. C., Nitrogen balance studies in human subjects on various diets, *Am. J. Clin. Nutr.*, 20, 753-759, 1967.
24. Irmiter, T. F., Foods from spun protein fibers, *Nutr. Rev.*, 22, 33-35, 1964.
25. Turk, R. E., Cornwell, P. E., Brooks, M. D., and Butterworth, C. E., Adequacy of spun soy protein containing egg albumin for human nutrition, *J. Am. Diet. Assoc.*, 63, 519-524, 1973.
26. Davis, S., Hodges, R. E., and Krehl, W. A., Use of isolated soybean protein (ISP) in experimental diets in man, *Fed. Proc. Fed. Am. Soc. Exp. Biol.*, 25 (Abstr.), 300, 1966.
27. Fomon, S. J., Thomas, L. N., Filer, L. J., Anderson, T. A., and Bergman, K. E., Requirements for protein and essential amino acids in early infancy, Studies with a soy-isolate formula, *Acta Paediatr. Scand.*, 62, 33-45, 1973.
28. Kurtha, A. N. and Ellis, F. R., The nutritional, clinical and economic aspects of vegan diets, *Plant Foods Hum. Nutr.*, 2, 13-22, 1970.
29. Ellis, F. R. and Montegriffo, V. M. E., The health of vegans, *Plant Foods Hum. Nutr.*, 2, 93-103, 1971.
30. Scrimshaw, N. S., Nature of protein requirements, *J. Am. Diet. Assoc.*, 54, 94-102, 1969.
31. Wokes, F., Proteins, *Plant Foods Hum. Nutr.*, 1, 23-48, 1968.
32. Hegsted, D. M., Protein needs and possible modifications of the American diet, *J. Am. Diet. Assoc.*, 68, 317-320, 1976.
33. Committee on Nutrition Misinformation, National Research Council, Vegetarian diets, *J. Am. Diet. Assoc.*, 65, 121-122, 1974.
34. Harris, R. S., Indigenous Edible Plants of Latin America, paper presented at the Congreso Internacional Sobre Vitaminas in Havana, Cuba, January 1952.
35. Hardinge, M. G. and Crooks, H., Non-flesh dietaries. III. Adequate and inadequate, *J. Am. Diet. Assoc.*, 45, 537-542, 1964.
36. Lockmiller, N., What are textured protein products?, *Food Technol. (Chicago)*, 25, 56-58, 1972.
37. Robinson, R. F., What is the future of textured protein products?, *Food Technol. (Chicago)*, 26, 59-63, 1972.
38. Koury, S. D. and Hodges, R. E., Soybean proteins for human diets? Wholesomeness and acceptability, *J. Am. Diet. Assoc.*, 52, 480-484, 1968.
39. Register, U. D. and Sonnenberg, L. M., The vegetarian diet, *J. Am. Diet. Assoc.*, 62, 253-261, 1973.
40. Wurlitzer, R. and Corry, W., *How to Get the Most for Your Food Dollar*, University Publishers and Distributors, Hauppague, N.Y., 1970.
41. Vhymeister, I. B., Register, U. D., and Sonnenberg, L. M., Safe vegetarian diets for children, *Pediatr. Clin. North Am.*, 24, 203-210, 1977.

# NUTRITIONAL STATUS AND ALTERNATIVE LIFE-STYLE DIETS, WITH SPECIAL REFERENCE TO VEGETARIANISM IN THE U.S.

Johanna Dwyer

## INTRODUCTION

This review summarizes the major work until 1977 on the nutritional status of vegetarians living in the U.S. The older literature on the subject has been dealt with in a series of excellent reviews.[1-19] The larger, somewhat more urgent problem of populations in developing countries that by dint of economic and ecological necessity, eat essentially vegetarian diets will be dealt with only peripherally. Environmental and social conditions are very different for vegetarians living in such settings. However, a number of authoritative reviews are available that admirably summarize the nutritional status of such populations.[20-27]

### Rationale for Concern About U.S. Vegetarian Diets

The rationale for concentrating upon a small but, perhaps, growing minority in one country rather than the vast vegetarian majority of the world's population needs explication.

First, in the last decade the popularity of vegetarianism has increased in this country. The rise is due to the adoption of new forms of vegetarianism coupled with other nontraditional dietary styles rather than to the growth of traditional vegetarian groups.[28-30]

These newer groups of vegetarians include the macrobiotics, fruitarians, raw food adherents, Zen Buddhists, Krishnas, Sufis, a number of different yogic groups, and American Hindus. They attract large numbers of young adults of child-bearing age. Characteristics and beliefs about diets among such adherents have recently been described.[30-33]

Second, the health effects of these diets are not well described. The alternative dietary styles adopted involve vegan or vegetarianism, as well as additional proscriptions on nonanimal foods in the diet.[34-39] "New" vegan or vegetarian diets are coupled with "natural", or organic, and "health" foods used by many such persons, with the end result being an eating pattern quite different from that which is usual in this country.

The food habits, beliefs, and nutritional status of traditional groups of vegetarians living in the U.S. and Western Europe have been extensively investigated.[1-15] The most extensive studies in this country are of lacto-ovovegetarian adults who were members of the Seventh-Day Adventist Faith[2,12] and lactovegetarian Trappist monks.[40-42] Several studies have also been reported on vegetarian children,[16,43,44] but these are confined for the most part to children over 5 years of age raised on lacto-ovovegetarian or other diets not completely devoid of animal protein. In such cases nutrient intakes and growth were satisfactory. With the appearance of new groups of American vegetarians, many of which adhere to totally vegan and alternative life-style diets rather than the lacto-ovovegetarian pattern which is common among Seventh-Day Adventists, the issue of what these persons eat has evolved from an interesting academic question to one with important practical implications.

Yet studies of "new" vegetarian groups (such as macrobiotics, various yoga sects, Krishnas, and raw food eaters) are less extensive. In the past few years several investigations of young adults who were adherents to these popular vegan-vegetarian groups have been published.[45-55] These include opinion surveys of adults on various types of alternative life-style diets that involve combinations of vegetarianism, "health", "natural", and "organic" food use[56-62] and a stratified, national sample of the opinions and attitudes toward health of onmivores, vegetarians, "natural", and "health" food users.[63] Studies on nutritional status are few, however, and are completely nonexistent in more than a few subject areas.[64-68] Recent reports of severe malnutrition and even death[64,65,69,70] have alerted health professionals to the dangers of some of these vegetarian regimes carried to excess while the low-serum lipids and favorable lipoprotein patterns characteristic of many vegetarians on less restrictive regimes suggest that such diets in moderation have much to recommend them.[71,72] Alterations in the type or amount of degradative products of the animal and plant sterols, bile acids, and related substances in the feces of persons on vegetarian diets are also being explored as of possible importance in altering the risks of colon cancer.[73-75] Variations in levels of dietary fiber, type of fat or carbohydrate, and protein sources between vegetarians and omnivores are also hypothesized as being of possible beneficial significance to health from the standpoint of such diverse conditions as obesity, diverticulosis, constipation, appendicitis, and osteoporosis.[76-83]

It is, therefore, important to delineate the health effects of these diets more fully, particularly among the so-called "vulnerable" groups such as children. Their parents might be carried away by overenthusiastic reports of the supposed health benefits of such diets without taking due caution to ensure against the risks involved in making uninformed and sweeping dietary changes. A number of reports in the literature suggest that the regimes advocated by certain groups, particularly macrobiotics, are associated with malnutrition in young children as well as in adults.[32,33,64,65,84] The types of diets suggested in the literature for young children of the macrobiotics[85] and some of the more restrictive yoga groups[86-89] would suggest that this might be the case. Among many of the parents who are members of those dietary group, smallness of children is considered desirable rather than undesirable, and is not a cause for concern or physician consultation.

These forms of vegetarianism are sometimes associated with other alterations in belief systems and lifestyle, which may have adverse as well as beneficial effects upon health. Smoking, use of illicit drugs, and alcohol abuse are seemingly less common among them, but there are also other less positive aspects of their behavior.

For example, in 1971 we studied the food intakes and living habits of 100 native born young American adults who were vegetarians of these types.[30] Our subjects differed from vegetarians of the Seventh-Day Adventist Faith in many respects, including dietary habits (veganism coupled with a strong tendency to eat foods considered to be "natural" or "organic"), less conventional current and past lifestyles, lack of formal religious affiliation, and negativistic attitudes toward health services. They lacked access to the special dietary advice involving vegetarian diets and were unaware of or refused to use the health network (e.g., hospitals serving vegetarian menus, etc.) that was available in the area. Moreover, many of them expressed an aversion to physicians and preferred to use lay healers, only seeking medical help when they or their children were very ill.

While a wide spectrum of dietary patterns were observed, 25 of the subjects were vegans who consumed no animal food. Most of these also had constraints on eating foods which they did not consider to be "natural";[46-47] these proscriptions often extended to all canned and frozen foods and other foods containing food additives. Several of these subjects were attempting to raise their young children on similar vegan diets. In our study we found that subjects reported an average duration of over 2 years on vegetarian and vegan diets. These findings tend to disprove the notion of some health professionals that such diets represent no more than transient eccentricities of a few months' duration.

A third reason for concern about vegetarianism in America is that it is considered by both its adherents and omnivore populations to be deviant from the sociocultural viewpoint. This being the case, it makes comparisons of similar dietary styles and their supposed health effects across cultures hazardous. Other aspects of lifestyle having a bearing on health may vary simultaneously. Therefore, it deserves careful study in itself.

The fact that vegetarians are deviant from the larger culure should not be taken to imply that they are therefore irrational. Human kind's food habits always exhibit a high degree of irrationality. In no culture have food patterns been based on a reasonable consideration and use of all the material available for human consumption. For example, the dominant carnivore pattern of Americans rejects dog, horse, and human flesh as food fit for human beings. Simoons[90] concluded his exhaustive study of food avoidances by stating that foods are chosen in accordance with culturally determined attitudes and patterns of behavior involving foodways rather than by solely ecological concerns. Therefore, the most surprising thing about American vegetarians is not that they do not eat certain animal foods, since no one eats all of the types of animal foods which are available in the environment, but that they fail to eat certain foods which have been sanctioned as appropriate foods for human beings by the larger society and culture.[90]

The means by which they are able to sustain these eating styles are of more than passing interest. Compliance to diets that are far less unusual for preventive and curative purposes as prescribed by health professionals is usually poor. Anything that can be learned from observing groups such as vegetarians may be helpful in developing more means of supporting patients who, for health reasons, must also consume diets that defy customary patterns and are often semivegetarian in fact if not in name.

This curious cultural anomaly and its potential ramifications on nutritional status and health are therefore the substance of this review. However, since vegetarianism is often associated with other unusual behavior, such as the use of "natural-organic" or health foods and high doses of of vitamin-mineral supplements, these other types of "alternative diets" will also be touched upon.

### Scope of the Review

We shall first briefly review the definitional and descriptive problems that arise in attempting to categorize unusual eating behavior of this type and suggest one possible classification. Second, the broad characteristics of alternative life-style diets of various types and how vegetarianism is related to them are sketched. Third, times of particular risk from the physiological standpoint and other factors influencing nutritional status are mentioned. Then specific aspects of nutritional status that may be problematic are attacked for vegetarians and, on a more general level, for other alternative dieters.

## DEFINITIONS

### Vegetarianism

A "vegetarian" is defined as "one who lives wholly or principally on vegetable foods; a person who on principle abstains from any forms of animal food, or at least such as it obtained by the destruction of life", or "a member of a fanatical Chinese sect, or other sects by attribution". "Vegetarianism" refers to "the doctrine or practice of vegetarians; abstention from eating meat, fish, or other animal products".[92]

### Definitional Problems

In this very definition lie formidable problems for the nutritionist. First, it is a negative definition, involving what is *not* rather than what is eaten. Traditionally, nutritionists have concerned themselves with what was eaten. It is difficult to describe what is avoided except in very broad terms in a society in which some 5,000 to 10,000 different food products are available in most supermarkets. The idiosyncrasy of food preferences is such that almost every individual in this country has certain foods he fails to eat. Therefore, avoidances can only be described in general terms and only when they reach such a level that the individual reporting them or the observer is aware that they exist. Some individuals living in sheltered or isolated environments, such as young children, inmates in institutions for the mentally retarded, or residents of remote, rural areas may not even have the opportunity to avoid foods which for all intents and purposes do not exist in their microenvironments.

A second problem is that the definition implies a philosophical, quasireligious, or other rationale for the avoidance. That is, the eating style is seen as reflecting conscious choice and committment at least at some point rather than simply habit. In a sense this simplifies the task, since it suggests that persons who are not consciously avoiding animal foods of one class or another are not truly vegetarians. Thus persons who avoid catfish, venison, rattlesnake meat, or some other specific animal food on the basis of food preferences are eliminated from consideration. But are we to say that a 5-year-old child who has never consumed any animal food other than milk is not a vegetarian because he himself has never abstained on principle? Certainly his dietary profile in terms of foods consumed and nutrient intakes are likely to be more equivalent to those of a 25-year-old lactovegetarian than they are to an omnivore. Nutrition scientists have not classically been concerned with the reasons for food patterns and avoidances unless they jeopardize nutritional status, yet the definition implies that unless one delves into the belief systems of persons adhering to these regimes, food practices will remain obscure and alteration via counseling difficult.

A third problem is hinted at by the fact that the principles governing abstinence apparently vary depending upon the sect or cult the individual adheres to. This suggests that an enormous amount of heterogeneity in food avoidance patterns is possible, and it at least alerts us to the possibility that other associated variations in belief systems or lifestyle may also be present. Again, we are faced by issues usually considered to be the province of the cultural or medical anthropologist rather than the nutrition scientist.

In the face of these unfamiliar problems it is not surprising that nutritional scientists, who are most accustomed to the task of analyzing diets for nutritional variations in foods, have developed a nomenclature for vegetarians that centers around alterations in the type of animal food eaten. Unfortunately, the terminology reflects a rather primitive conceptualization of reality. It is based upon animal food eaten when it has been known for over 100 years that other alterations in diet as well as lifestyle are the rule rather than the exception among many such persons. It is broadly descriptive rather than specific and quantitative with reference to nutrient consumption or the consumption of other substances in foods, going against the whole thrust of nutritional science over the same length of time. Words are not available in the traditional nomenclature to describe even the realities of animal food intake alterations existing in the population today. For these reasons we must define our terms very precisely and coin new terms when necessary if we are to even begin to understand and categorize what truly exists. This type of orderly description is the scientist's first obligation. Having developed a suitable nomenclature, it may then be possible to build models and hypothesize about the different effects of these various regimes upon nutritional status and health. But until it is quite clear exactly what type of vegetarian is being referred to when the term is used, little advance in the study of the physiological or psychological effects of these regimes is likely.

In view of the great interest in the asociation of vegetarian diets with the prevalence and incidence of various chronic diseases, this is a matter of great practical importance.

Use of present nomenclature may cause us to incorrectly attribute such associations to differences in animal food intakes when in fact some other variable that is different between vegetarians and omnivores is actually responsible for the correlations, such as type or amount of fat, dietary fiber, trace minerals, or other substances such as food additives.

### Animal Food Consumption

The terminology commonly used to describe persons whose usual diets diverge from dominant eating styles is currently in a state of flux because of the rise of dietary styles that were virtually unknown a decade ago.

Nutritionists traditionally described nonflesh dietarys as being "vegan", "lacto-" or "lacto-ovovegetarian". Until the early 1960s such terminology was apparently sufficient to describe animal food intake patterns of most vegetarians in this country. However, such latinizations do not reflect the reality of animal food intake behavior among American vegetrians today.

In the first place, there is a great deal of interest among health care professionals in diet modifications for preventive or curative purposes that involve decreased consumption of animal foods high in saturated fat, cholesterol, sodium, and perhaps other, as yet unidentified substances which may have an adverse effect upon health. For example, the American Heart Association[93] and more recently, the Senate Select Committee on Nutrition and Human Needs[94] have publicized recommendations involving decreased consumption of red meats, eggs, and whole milk coupled with increased consumption of chicken, fish, and plant protein sources. While these recommendations clearly do not involve the adoption of a "vegetarian" pattern as this is taken to mean a vegan or lactovegetarian diet, they do involve extensive alteration of both the type of animal protein consumed and, in some cases at least, alteration in: (1) the proportion of animal to vegetable protein, (2) possibly total protein as percent of calories, and (3) consumption of associated substances such as cholesterol if they are followed. Since the older classifications involve different alterations in the type of animal food and associated changes in the proportion of other nutrients and substances in the diet, they do not serve as well for describing the former patterns. Perhaps a better term for them would be *modified animal food diets*. Indeed, these suggestions are very close to patterns followed by Americans 4 decades ago.[95,96]

In the second place, there is no terminology to describe persons who make extensive use of the meat analogues which now have widespread distribution. Also, how are we to describe the milk analogues (such as soy-based formulas) which are increasingly popular in the feeding of infants? These products differ from their animal food counterparts in their protein composition but also with respect to type and, sometimes, amount of fat, trace elements, and sodium provided. At least in the case of infants fed such modified formulas in the first few months of life, these diets approximate a vegan pattern. Their nutritional realities are probably quite different than those of true vegans, however, since baby foods providing meat and other animal foods may be added. Moreover, the formulas provide vitamin $B_{12}$. Other persons using meat analogues as a major item in their diet hardly are likely to conform to any of the vegetarian patterns previously described with respect to their overall intakes, type, and amount of proximate constituents or nutrients, although as yet little or no information on this point is available. The term *animal analogue diets* will be used to refer to such patterns in this review.

One major reason the use of meat analogues or other specially formulated plant protein mixtures such as soy formula, special protein supplement mixes, etc. is important to document is that these products very often are designed especially to provide suitable complementary proteins in a single food. Theoretically, it might be suspected that if, in fact, protein quality was limited in the diet, these commercial products might provide protein of higher biological value than would reliance upon menu planning to provide complementary mixtures of separate plant foods. In practice, however, such a consideration may be moot since protein quality is rarely an issue. Rather, caloric adequacy has been a matter of much greater concern from the clinical standpoint than have the issues of either protein quantity or quality.

In the third place, many persons today eat all animal foods with the one exception of red meat. The term "nonflesh" does not describe their dietary realities since it implies that chicken (and perhaps fish) are also avoided, and it is not. These persons might better be referred to as "semivegetarians", although such a term is only appropriate if the proportion of animal food as percent of total calories is in fact altered from that usually consumed in this country as a result of these patterns, which may not always be the case.

In the fourth place, existing terminology lacks terms to describe persons who only eat fish or chicken to the exclusion of all other animal foods. Yet terms are needed to describe patterns involving fish as the sole animal food as followed by some macrobiotic vegetarians. Therefore, in line with the present forms, we must add "fish eating", "chicken eating" vegetarian and the various combinations of these to our repertoire.

None of these additions to our lexicon do anything more than to very grossly describe *qualitative* factors having to do with animal food intake, however; that is, which of the five groups of animal foods are eaten. *Quantitative* statements must be carefully worded since, unless dietary data are available, they are based only upon reasoning by analogy from the previous experience of persons having qualitatively similar animal food intake patterns. Yet we shall see that many and indeed probably most Seventh-Day Adventists who adhere to vegan or lactovegetarian diets exhibit a high degree of sophistication in nutritional knowledge. They are wont to use vitamin-mineral supplements in physiological doses and meat analogues. Therefore, the elimination of, say, red meat may have little impact on iron status. In contrast, vegan or lactovegetarian macrobiotics reject nutritional findings based on the Western scientific method, very rarely use vitamin mineral supplements, and avoid meat analogues with similar animal food restrictions that would be more likely to comprise their iron status. Since little data is available on this latter group, and none at all except very general observations have been published on the considerable number of vegans and lactovegetarians who belong to other cults, it is obvious that broad generalizations and extrapolations from a literature based almost exclusively upon Seventh-Day Adventists or Trappist monks is perilous and uncertain at best.

## A Better Nomenclature for Alterations in Animal Food Consumption

In order to understand the context of alterations in consumption of animal foods more fully, it may be helpful to briefly review the spectrum of alterations in the type or amount of animal foods consumed that have been reported in this country.

The most deviant of all practices in our culture, indeed in all cultures, is not animal food avoidances of various sorts but "cannibalism", or the eating of human flesh. Sporadic reports from Western countries, including the U.S., in times of famine and war are documented in the literature. The most recent example is the lurid, recent best seller entitled *Alive*, which describes cannibalism in a group of Uruguayan students who were stranded in the Andes Mountains for several months.[97] The exciting work elucidating the etiology of the slow virus disease Kuru, for which D. Carleton Gajdusek recently won the Nobel prize was based on his studies of ritual cannibalism amongst tribesman in New Guinea.[97a] Fortunately, in spite of the recent attention these reports have received in the new media, cannibalism is an exceedingly rare phenomenon.

Almost equally abhorrent to many people in this country is what we shall call, for a lack of a better term, "inappropriate carnivorous behavior". For example, roasting and eating of the family dog, cat, or parakeet would be considered by most Americans as reason enough to declare that the cook had taken leave of his senses. The eating of raw meat, with the possible exception of "steak tartare" (raw, lean ground beef) is also considered to be excessively vigorous omnivore behavior.

The normative individual in American society is the so-called "omnivore" who has no categorical restrictions on the broad types of animal foods he eats, although he may, and often does, have individual likes or dislikes that cause him to avoid certain animal foods such as lamb or shellfish.

Then we come to those whose diets are such that, for one reason or another the frequency of consumption varies from usual. Here would be categorized persons who adhere to *diets which modify the type of animal food* eaten but who totally avoid none of them.

From this point onward categorical restrictions on one or more classes or types of animal food come into play; the "Semivegetarians" avoiding only red meat, and dual and triple avoidance patterns which give rise to "lacto-ovo-fish", "lacto-ovo-chicken", "lacto-ovo", and "lacto-fish" eating styles. "Monovegetarians" commonly include lactovegetarians and fish eating vegetarians, who avoid all but one class of animal foods. Finally, we come to the vegans, who avoid all animal foods completely. Table 1 summarizes these definitions. Societal recognition of deviance in animal food consumption is sharpest the farther towards the polarities one goes from the omnivorous norm.

### Other Categorical Food Avoidances: "Processed" and "Nonorganic" Foods

Categorical avoidances also exist for other foods in the diet. One broad set of avoidances which has become popular in the past decade involves those who choose to eat only foods which are "organic" or "natural". Organically grown foods are defined by those who use them as foods which are grown without the use of chemical fertilizer, fumigants, fungicides, herbicides, or other toxic pesticides. "Natural" foods are usually defined by users as those foods which have not been highly refined, and/or those to which preservatives, emulsifiers, or other synthetic substances have not been added. Since most canned, frozen, and packaged foods fall in this later category, persons eating "natural" diets often avoid these products.[99-105] They may also avoid the use of artificial sweeteners, an issue of some interest today.

Just as was found to be the case with animal food avoidance patterns, people undoubtedly vary as to the universality of their avoidances of nonanimal foods. At one end of the spectrum are those who refuse to eat foods that are not organically grown but place no restrictions on whether foods are or are not "natural". At the other end of the spectrum are the raw food eaters, who abhor any food which is processed in any way. There are also those who avoid whole categories of food and only consume one or two classes of nonanimal foods, combining avoidance of animal, "nonorganic", and "processed" foods, e.g., fruitarians. Unfortunately, the literature is meager indeed on the avoidance patterns of such subjects. The reports that do exist concern themselves mostly with persons who are vegetarians and who also have proscriptions such as these. Therefore, until the time when better typologies can be developed on the basis of descriptive studies, we will refer to this heterogeneous group as "natural/organic food users".

### Use of Dietary Supplements and Health Foods

In addition to the vegetarians, who have categorical avoidances of some or all animal foods, and the natural/organic food users, who have similar categorical avoidances involving animal as well as plant foods in their diets, there are the health food users.

Table 1
## LEXICON FOR DESCRIBING PERSONS ENGAGING IN VARIOUS ALTERNATIVE LIFE-STYLE DIETS

### Terms Having to do with Animal Food Avoidance

**Omnivore** — an individual who has no formal restrictions or constraints on the eating of animal products

**Modified animal food dieter** — persons who have purposefully altered their consumption of certain types of animal food, such as red meat, whole milk, and eggs, for various reasons, but who have not totally eliminated such foods from their diets

**Animal analogue users** — persons who extensively use food products that are animal food analogues in their diets

**Semivegetarian** — an individual who has adopted a vegetarian pattern of eating involving the exclusion of only some foods of the animal type, such as red meat, fish, or poultry, etc.; sometimes also referred to as partial or mild vegetarians

**Vegetarian** — consumes few or no flesh products; may or may not consume other animal products such as eggs or dairy foods

**Monovegetarian** — vegetarians who consume only one group of animal foods

Examples of monovegetarians

    **Lacto-ovovegetarian** — consumes eggs and dairy products

    **Pescovegetarian** — consumes only fish and seafood

    **Pullovegetarian** — consumes only chicken

    **Lactovegetarian** — consumes only milk and dairy products

    **Vegan** — consumes essentially no animal foods

### Terms Having to do with Avoidances of Other Foods

**Organically grown foods** — foods grown without the use of chemical fertilizer, fumigants, fungicides, herbicides, or other toxic pesticides

**"Unprocessed" or "natural foods"** — foods that have not been highly refined or processed, such as foods to which preservatives, emulsifiers, or other synthetic substances have not been added

**Natural/organic food users** — persons who use organically grown foods or foods they regard as being unprocessed or natural.

### Terms Applying to Health Food or Nutrient Supplement Use

**"Health" foods** — foods claimed by those who sell them to have special health-giving properties

**Vitamin-mineral supplement use** — use of vitamin or mineral supplements in prophylactic amounts

**Megadose supplement use** — use of vitamin or mineral supplements that involves amounts five to ten times Recommended Dietary Allowances on a regular basis

### Terms Applying to Groups Adhering to Alternative Life-Style Diets

**Seventh-Day Adventists** — an adherent to the Seventh-Day Adventist sect; the majority of Seventh-Day Adventists are lacto-ovo- or lactovegetarians if they adhere to vegetarian diets at all; a small proportion of Seventh-Day Adventists are vegans; prophylactic use of vitamin-mineral supplements is quite common; "natural/organic" food use is rare

**Macrobiotics** — adherents of a sect founded by Georges Ohsawa that employs a dietary pattern of a vegan or vegetarian type coupled with natural/organic food use; ten different diets, varying in restrictiveness, are suggested; these diets grow progressively more restrictive with respect to both animal and other foods used; tamari, misco, and various seaweeds are used as health foods and endowed with special properties; fluid restriction is also common; vitamin-mineral supplement use is rare

**Hare Krishnas or Krishnas** — adherents to an American Hindu sect who adhere to a lactovegetarian diet coupled with natural/organic food use; health food use is minimal, as is use of vitamin-mineral supplements

**Yogic vegetarians** — adherents of various American yogic sects, such as Divine Light Mission (followers of Guru Maharaji), Ananda Marga yogic sect, One Horse Commune, Baba Ram Dass, Healthy Happy Holy yogic sect etc.; these sects vary with respect to animal food avoidances from semivegetarian to lactovegetarian; Natural/organic food use similarly varies, as do vitamin-mineral supplement use and health food use

**Idiosyncratic vegetarians** — persons who do not adhere to the philosophy of a particular dietary group but adopt their own individualistic pattern of eating

Health foods are defined as foods that are claimed by those who sell them to have special health giving properties.[106-112] Protein supplements and bone meal are two examples of products which are widely touted as having such properties. Dietary fiber supplements such as bran or wheat germ are others which are currently in vogue.

While by definition, pure vegetarianism or natural/organic food use implies avoidances of certain categories of food, health food use does not. Health food use sometimes simply involves additive behaviors, i.e., averting supposed risks stemming from the usual diet by adding these special "health" foods. The foods may be seen as protecting or ensuring the eater against health risks, neutralizing the presumably adverse effects of other substances which are consumed. For definitional purposes this type of behavior will be referred to as "health food use".

Another type of supplementation involves nutrients assumed to have beneficial effects on health rather than foods. This will be referred to as "vitamin-mineral supplement use". The vast majority of persons who use vitamin or mineral supplements use over-the-counter multivitamin preparations, which provide amounts approximating the Recommended Dietary Allowances for nutrients. However, another smaller group of consumers purchase much higher potency preparations or use low-potency preparations in very large dosages.[112-114] When use of micronutrients is such that it exceeds the recommended dietary allowances by five or more times for one or more nutrients, such a pattern may appropriately be referred to as "megadose use". It is necessary to distinguish between the physiological dose levels approached by moderate use of vitamin-mineral supplements and the pharmacological dose levels often achieved by megadose users.

## ALTERNATIVE LIFE-STYLE DIETS

### Describing Alternative Life-Style Diets

Having established our definitions, we can now attempt to catalogue the habits of persons indulging in alternative life-style diets.

The most striking finding, one which has escaped many nutrition scientists until recently, is that the four major alternative life-style dietary patterns (e.g., vegetarianism, natural/organic food use, health foods use, and vitamin-mineral supplement use) are by no means mutually exclusive. "Pure" vegetarianism with no other dietary alteration is seemingly exceedingly rare. Table 2, for example, presents data collected on 252 alternative dieters in the Boston area in the summer of 1974 by Dwyer et al.[115] The vast majority of all subjects engaged in several alternative dietary styles simultaneously.

Of all those surveyed on alternative life-style diets, 43% claimed to involve vegetarianism of one sort or another. Yet only 2% of all the alternative dieters engaged only in vegetarianism; more often it was coupled with natural/organic food use and the use of vitamin mineral supplements. Only very rarely did vegetarianism reach the extent of veganism.

Insofar as both vegetarianism and natural/organic food use involve avoidance patterns, which may or may not be coupled with substitution behaviors, (e.g., adding similar foods to make up for those avoided) it can be seen that it is important to investigate both these dimensions of food avoidances in describing vegetarians. Health food and vitamin-mineral supplement use both involve adding substances to the diet which also may or may not be coupled with substitution behaviors with respect to other foods selected. Some persons, for example, might simply add a protein supplement to their regular diet, others might cut down on animal food simultaneously. The use or nonuse of these foods and/or nutrients is also vital for accurate description of vegetarian diets. Needless to say, dietary adequacy will reflect the overall balance of additions, subtractions, and substitutions of foods.

Table 2

ASSOCIATION BETWEEN SELF REPORTS OF VARIOUS DIETARY STYLES
AND USE OF VITAMIN-MINERAL SUPPLEMENTS AMONG 252 PERSONS
WHO CLAIMED TO ADHERE TO ALTERNATIVE LIFE-STYLE DIETS
(BOSTON 1974)[115]

| | Health food user | | Nonhealth food user | |
|---|---|---|---|---|
| Self report of dietary style | Vitamin-mineral supplement user | Not a vitamin-mineral supplement user | Vitamin-mineral supplement user | Not a vitamin-mineral supplement user |
| Vegetarian | 0 | 2 | 1 | 6 |
| Natural/organic | 60 | 37 | 15 | 30 |
| Vegetarian and natural/ organic | 36 | 40 | 11 | 13 |
| Neither and | 5 | 6 | — | — |
| Total vitamin-mineral sup- plement | 101 | 85 | 27 | 49 |
| Total | 186 | | 76 | |

Table 3

SELF-REPORTED DIETARY STYLES BY
PERSONS SURVEYED LEAVING VARIOUS
FOOD STORES IN METROPOLITAN BOSTON IN
AUGUST 1974[115]

| | Percent | |
|---|---|---|
| Reported dietary style(s) | Natural or health Food Store[a] | Supermarket[b] |
| Health | 5 | 3 |
| Vegetarian | 6 | 3 |
| Natural/organic | 14 | 9 |
| Combinations | | |
| Health-vegetarian | 1 | 20.3 |
| Natural-vegetarian | 7 | 1 |
| Health-natural | 16 | 3 |
| Health-vegetarian natural | 16 | 3 |
| Omnivore | 36 | 78 |

[a]   778 subjects were approached; 520 or 67% agreed to return the questionnaire and 259 or 32% did so.

[b]   1127 persons were approached; 518 or 47% agreed to return the questionnaire and 224 or 19% did so.

Thus it is important to ascertain the interrelationships and overlays between the different alternative dietary patterns. While the overlays may vary from group to group, it is likely that this general picture of multiple alternative life-style behaviors is the rule rather than the exception today in this country.

A second finding which quickly emerges when all of these behaviors are inventoried was that the prevalence of alternative life-style diets was probably somewhat greater than might be supposed. For example, in the same study during a week in 1974, a group of persons leaving supermarkets and natural/health food stores in the Boston area were surveyed with a short questionnaire. Cooperation and resulting self-descriptions of dietary style are given in Table 3. While response rates in comparison to the total of all subjects approached were low, it is nonetheless interesting to note that the vast majority of persons shopping in health or natural food stores classified themselves as adherents to alternative life-style diets. More surprising, however, is the fact that a substantial minority of subjects (e.g., 22%) shopping in supermarkets who volunteered information also adhered to alternative life-style diets. No doubt those who did so overresponded to the questionnaire, since the items on it involved this very topic. However, the response bias notwithstanding, it is hardly conceivable that such results could have been obtained a generation ago.

What might explain the growth of the alternative diet movement? A recent review of 32 consumer surveys prepared by General Mills, Inc. may provide some answers.[116] This review reveals that while consumers have traditionally considered cost, convenience, and family taste preferences in their food choices, in recent years an increasing concern about the overall "healthfulness" of the food supply, nutritional quality, and food safety has developed. Many consumers now tend to classify foods as "bad" based on the presence of "negative" nutrients or ingredients. For example, the review cited shows that some consumers think of "man-made" foods as "bad" because of the presence of artificial additives in them and the perceived removal of "natural" nutrients in processing. Conversely, "God-made" or basic agricultural commodities that are unaltered by processing are perceived as good for the opposite reasons.

These negative attitudes are particularly pronounced with respect to additives, processing, and energy-providing nutrients. Consumers relate excessive ingestion of calories, fat, and cholesterol to increased risk of heart disease, for example, and many choose to limit it.

It follows from surveys such as these that consumers are likely to modify their diets in ways they believe will prove healthful. The fact that they may have misconceptions about how best to do this may lead to some of the more bizarre alternative dietary styles which are now in evidence. Table 4 illustrates the medical indications for certain types of dietary alterations and possible homeopathic efforts on the part of consumers to achieve the same healthy effects. Also listed are some possible measures which might serve to better inform consumers about the nutritional realities of the food they eat and thus clear up at least some of the misconceptions that currently exist in their minds.

### "Establishment" Types of Alternative Diets

At one end of the spectrum within the alternative diet movement are the people within the "orthodox" health and medical care system who believe that the American diet must be changed for preventive or public health reasons. The types of changes desired or advocated vary from one group to another. The American Heart Association's Prudent Diet for Better Heart Health, measures to reduce dental caries by dietary means advocated by public health dentists, and many other examples could be given. The latest example of fairly respectable suggestions is the list of "Dietary Goals for the United States", which resulted from the National Nutrition Policy Hearings in the U.S. Senate.[94] This diet is similar to the "prudent diet" and involves decreased total calories from fat, especially saturated fat, increased total calories from complex carbohydrate (and decreased calories from refined carbohydrates), decreased caloric density of the food supply, and so forth. The wisdom of its adoption is being sharply debated at the present time.

Many "establishment" people are asking questions about the "American diet". For example, analysis of recent literature on the possible health implications of changing dietary patterns in the U.S. reveals that many health scientists have called for more careful study of the etiology of a number of diet-related diseases that constitute major health problems in the U.S. These include obesity and diseases associated with it, (such as diabetes mellitus), gall bladder disease, gout, kidney and digestive diseases, and

## Table 4
## COMPARISON OF WAYS NUTRIENTS ARE PROVIDED TO CONSUMERS, ATTEMPTS BY CONSUMERS TO CONSUME THAT ACCOMPLISH THESE SAME PURPOSES, AND IMPLICATIONS FOR CONSUMER EDUCATION

| Different forms consumers encounter nutrients in the market place and the purpose of these forms | "Diet" used by consumers | Implications for education and regulations |
| --- | --- | --- |
| As medicine by prescription, including prescription drugs which are nutrients, such as $B_{12}$ shots, intramuscular iron injection, etc. <br><br> As curative or preventive medicine; vitamin pills, minerals, and hematinics sold over the counter | Megadoses to "cure" cancer, schizophrenia, etc. <br><br> Vitamin pill use as "preventive" medicine, use of remedies for tired blood, etc.; the "insurance" idea or protective medicine idea of building up a backlog against possible misfortune while otherwise continuing usual behavior patterns is stronger here than the preventive medicine concept as it is understood by health professionals; the preventive medicine concept involves decreasing risk by behavior change; it also involves averting risk by adding some action to the already-existing behavior repertoire | Conduct appropriate clinical trials and communicate results to both health professionals and the lay public <br><br> Review efficacy of various O.T.C. preparations and publish results both in scientific monographs and in forms easily understandable to public; develop mass media educational campaigns as well, which stress the concept that "protective medicine" and preventive medicine are not synonymous |
| Dietetic foods for special dietary uses, including iron-fortified infant formula, LoFenelac® or other special formula products, protein supplements, etc. | "Natural", "organic", "nonprocessed", or "health" foods, foods classified by regulations as being for special dietary use may or may not be thought of as such by consumers; in some cases, especially among those who object to processed foods or additives, those foods so classified by the regulations as special dietary foods may be considered "bad" or "unnatural" foods; thus we see people resorting to "natural" homemade baby foods instead of commercially available foods in order to safeguard their young infants Homeopathic remedies, such as herbal teas, hot whiskey, etc., may be used here also for colds, as well as in the first two categories <br><br> Self-prescribed elimination diets or other special diets as self-diagnosed (for hypoglycemia, "allergy to foods", "lactose intolerance") | Label P/S ratios, cholesterol; label sodium potassium; develop data base for professional access on food's content with respect to other nutrients and substances such as lactose, etc., which may cause adverse reactions; develop a method that expresses something that better reflects the relative cariogenicity of various foods than a simple statement of concentrated carbohydrates or sucrose; *more vigorous and specific consumer education by public sector in particular* |

| | | |
|---|---|---|
| **"Downwardly" modified foods**, including low- or reduced-calorie foods, low- or reduced-sugar of "diabetic" foods, low-fat and cholesterol foods, low-sodium foods; these foods are used for a variety of health reasons | Physician/nutritionist prescribed diets for actual, nutrition-related health problems | Better education of health professionals in clinical nutrition |
| | Diets that eliminate or cut down on one or more of the following: "Processed" or "nonorganic" foods, such as the "Feingold Diet" eliminating foods with artificial colors and flavors purported to be of help for hyperkinetic children | Nutrient labeling of all foods; percent ingredient labeling; listing of food colors by number and flavors by "artificial or natural" or by number as well. Better clinical trials to determine effectiveness of such diets; more vigorous consumer education efforts on risks, benefits of additives |
| | Vegetarian or vegan regimes cutting down on animal or flesh foods, but also a wide variety of other foods considered "nonnatural", "organic", or processed and addition (usually) of "health" foods | Nutrient labeling; percent ingredient labeling<br>More vigorous consumer information and nutrition education efforts, particularly by public sector |
| | Reducing diets eliminating high-calorie foods or foods thought to be fattening (note that this approach, rather than total calorie reduction is usual — that is, consumers "diet" by using special foods instead of simply cutting down on all foods across the board) | Universal nutrient and calorie labeling<br>More vigorous consumer information and nutrition education efforts |
| | "Killer" or "bad" foods, foods considered to be high in some other undesirable substance, be it sugar, cholesterol, fat, salt, pesticide residues, molds, or food additives | Labeling for cholesterol, saturated fat, P/S ratios, sodium, potassium<br>Develop index of relative cariogenicity of foods, which is more useful than simply percent ingredient labeling for concentrated carbohydrates or sugar |
| **Foods that have been restored, enriched, or fortified** | Use of foods believed to be especially healthy or "natural" and, therefore, better or more powerful than a usual mixed diet; again, since "natural" vitamins and mineral are not seen as the same as "synthetic" vitamins and minerals, and consumers have other worries about "junk"/"nonjunk" and processed and "nonorganic" foods, the "fortification" race, sugar, food additives, etc.; the foods chosen as "rich" sources may not in fact be the ones most highly restored, enriched, or fortified | Better nutrition education of the consumer, especially comparisons by price and nutrient content between these products and ordinary foods |
| **Ordinary, unmodified fresh or processed foods** | Basic 4 and other food guides | Develop better guides for good eating that are intelligible to laymen; develop bias-free consumer information and educational materials; adopt universal nutrient labeling, percent ingredient labeling, unit pricing, etc. |

possibly hypertension and coronary artery disease. Questions have been raised about the possible relationships of diet to cancer and diseases of the gastrointestinal tract, although data is not yet firm on such associations.

Questions particularly pressing in the view of experts might include the following:

1.    Does the higher-caloric density, high-fat, low-dietary fiber diet Americans eat, coupled as it is with low-energy expenditure and a mealing pattern (as opposed to a snacking pattern) lead to greater incidence of obesity?
2.    Does obesity contribute to the development of certain chronic illnesses?
3.    Does the relatively low proportion of dietary fiber we eat have anything to do with changes in the gastrointestinal tract and can this explain the higher incidence of certain diseases of this system such as colon cancer and diverticulosis?
4.    Is the high proportion of calories from refined sugar (about 16%), visible fats and oils (about 18%), alcohol, and highly processed baked goods consumed by Americans today associated with low intakes of trace elements (Zn, Cr, Fe, etc.) or certain vitamins such as folic acid?
5.    Do imbalanced nutrient intakes contribute to major health problems?

The difference between these "orthodox" views and the nonestablishment views is that the former consider these questions as hypotheses in need of testing. The latter often regard the questions as statements of fact and embark with vigor upon equally hypothetical courses of treatment.

### Nonestablishment Types of Alternative Diets

At the other end of the spectrum in terms of advocacy from the health professional establishment are various alternative movements which place heavy emphasis on diet such as Krishnas, macrobiotics, and fruitarians. Preventive medicine and medical cures are much more closely intertwined with these philosophical or quasireligious systems than is usual in the U.S., and it is difficult to separate out what is simply diet from what is a very deeply held philosophical or religious belief expressed through diet.

These groups are often very deeply committed to their ideologies, which are formally stated and include dietary prescriptions. Leaders of groups are often persons who, at least in their own eyes, have a mystical vision and hope by prosyletizing and evangelism to gain widespread support for a type of overall social revitalization. Personal, social, and formal organizational ties unite various persons in the group.

### The Genesis of the Nonestablishment Alternative Diet Movement

There are many different ways of looking at the alternative diet movement in the U.S. One way to look at it is as an alternative health maintenance system in which the patient or some other lay person becomes the healer — the quintessence of preventively oriented consumer behavior in health, if you will. A second way to look at it is as a mechanism for social revitalization or transformation, having little to do directly in terms of health. Rather, health issues are used as examples of such notions as self-help preventive efforts, restructuring of societal institutions, consumer activism, nonreliance on authority figures, reacting against society's structures, and so forth. A third way of looking at the movement is to say it incorporates a little of both of these models, and that it cannot be regarded as a "movement" at all, but rather as "movements" of different groups or branches having widely divergent aims and motivations. While there may be ideological unity on a few basic ideas, these notions are operationalized many different ways. Surveys of such groups clearly indicate that this is so. Let us assume that the third syncretistic model has the most to be said for it and explore the commonalities between the various kinds of "alternative" dieters.

### Views That are Fairly Common in Nonestablishment Alternative Diet Movement

First, there is great reliance on the natural food idea. Natural foods are believed to be of positive value and diets are chosen to include them. Persons who use large amounts of vitamin or mineral supplements consider these substances to be of positive value. Others put special trust in organically grown foods and make special efforts to obtain them. While unanimity exists toward the positive gains to be had from eating one or more of these types of food, there is disparity in judgments of which foods have negative values or are outright deleterious. While some people avoid all processed or nonorganic foods, others feel that as long as they include the "good" foods, these will cancel out the "bad". So while most health food users are characterized by "additive" behaviors, their tendency to "subtract" or avoid certain foods from their diets is less uniform.

A second idea that widely permeates the groups is cutting down and sometimes eliminating animal foods. This tends to be semivegetarianism rather than vegetarianism in many cases, since only one group of animal foods (such as red meats) may be avoided. In fewer cases it involves true lacto-ovovegetarianism or veganism (in which no animal foods whatsoever are eaten).

A third common idea is that diet is seen as one means to achieving or expressing a good life. Those who see diet as a means to the end of a balanced and righteous life may see other means as being important as well, but dietary alteration is an essential ingredient. The "ideal balance" in the food confers "ideal balance" to the eater. Some macrobiotics appear to conceptualize diet in this way, assuming that transference from food to feeder occurs. Some yogic persons believe that adherence to lactovegetarian or lacto-ovovegetarian diets increases receptivity to meditation. Then there are the people who see diet not so much as an essential means to an end but as an expression of their underlying philosophy. For example, the position of the person who avoids red meat because he is opposed to the slaughter of animals might be thus. Of course, this is the subject of Butler's *Erewhon,* in which great disputes about whether eating cabbage was cannibalism wracked the society. (If one believes cabbages are living beings with the further proviso that all living beings are brothers, then harvesting a cabbage is decapitation and eating it is cannibalism).

A fourth common characteristic is a tendency to use foods with special properties as the pharmacopoeia in an alternative type of medical system in which the patient is the physician for preventing illness and the physician's role is reserved for curative aspects. This idea is similar to that being bruited about today in other, more orthodox circles, in which the patient is charged with greater responsibility for preventing illness and promoting health by his own efforts. The major problem arising with alternative dieters is probably one of definition. Many health problems that orthodox physicians might see as needing curative care are seen by these persons not as being illness or disease, but as preventable by diet.

A fifth common element is the "groupiness" of people in the alternative dietary style movements. Food coops, communal living arrangements, courses or classes on these ways of looking at the world, etc. all exist and are patronized by those in the various movements. In some cases these efforts are devoted to health and mental well being in addition to traditional moral concerns such as proper conduct and moral intervention efforts. In others, the whole emphasis is on health and mental well being.

## FACTORS INFLUENCING NUTRITIONAL STATUS AMONG VEGETARIANS

### Diets Eaten

Vegetarian groups in this country clearly differ from one another both in the degree and types of dietary avoidances they practice. Among the groups suggesting more ex-

treme and inclusive proscription patterns, one would expect to find a higher prevalence
of poor nutritional status and dietary intake with respect to some nutrients. Infants,
young children, and women in the reproductive years might be particularly vulnerable.

Animal foods are not necessary in the diet to ensure optimal growth. It is the adequacy of the nutrient intake (rather than the presence of certain foods in the diet)
coupled with the ability of the organism to utilize them by which diet influences growth
and health. Theoretically, a well-planned vegan diet (supplemented by a source of vitamin $B_{12}$) might be expected to be adequate.[119] Indeed, vegetable protein mixtures
have been used as the only source of protein for older infants and adults with success
in the U.S. as well as many developing countries.[22-26,117-128] The vegan diets consumed
in this country are, however, occasionally associated with a number of other adverse
practices. Among these are the use of vegetable proteins that do not supplement each
other well, the disuse of vitamin and mineral supplements when medically indicated,
certain health practices (little or no medical supervision), and perhaps, in some cases,
other deficits, such as inadequate sanitation.[125] These, taken *in toto*, might act to adversely affect health.

Whether dietary adequacy will be assured or compromised by such alternative diets
depends on the degree to which animal foods and other groups of foods are systematically avoided and the extent to which vitamin-mineral supplements or foods high in
missing nutrients are added. If the pattern is essentially a semivegetarian one, excluding
only the eating of meat, little difficulty is experienced in achieving adequate intakes
of most nutrients.[126-129] If, on the other hand, it rules out all animal foods and imposes
additional constraints on intakes of other foods (such as "processed" foods, or groups
of foods like grains, legumes, or fruits,) as well as upon the use of vitamin-mineral
supplements, the situation becomes more difficult. Risks of dietary inadequacy in
calories, vitamins, protein, $B_{12}$, vitamin D, iron, and other minerals such as calcium
and iodine are heightened.[125-128] Unfortunately, the paucity of data in the literature
makes it exceedingly difficult to describe the risks and benefits of the various permu-
tations and combinations of alternative life-style diets in any but the most general
terms.

### Health Practices

A number of the adherents of the stricter regimes among new dietary styles (particularly the macrobiotics, raw food eaters, and members of certain yogic groups) have
negative attitudes to health professionals and usual types of medical care, preferring
to obtain advice about health and illness from leaders of the dietary group, homeo-
paths, and other lay healers.[32,33,46-48,130] While very serious illness might provoke a visit
to orthodox sources of medical treatment, medical advice for minor illnesses, other
life events (such as birth), and usual preventive measures (such as immunizations, periodic well child visits, etc.) are often dispensed with.

Thus a substantial proportion of the "new" vegetarians differ not only in dietary
practices but in health care behavior as well as in other aspects of lifestyle from their
omnivore peers. While such behavior might be prejudicial to the health of adults
following such regimes, it is likely that the ill effects, if present, would be more pronounced in their children.

### Past History with Respect to Nutrition and Health

Perhaps the most obvious effect of past history with respect to nutrition and health
is its effects on anthropometric measurements. Size at a given time will be affected by
a wide variety of genetic, congenital, and environmental influences that have acted in
the past as well as in the present. The most obvious effect is perhaps that observed on
linear growth. As Thompson[131] has described so well, growth during early childhood

is perhaps best thought of as a three-phase process, with different influences having striking effects from one time to another. While catch-up growth can occur, it can rarely compensate for prolonged states of chronic malnutrition and their inevitable sequellae upon size, particularly if the timing of the nutritional insult coincides with periods of exceedingly rapid growth.[132] Thus, it is possible that a child who is short, say, at 6 years of age is growing at normal velocity, but that his small size relative to others of a similar age reflects past nutritional insults rather than present ones.

Body stores are another result of past rather than present nutritional history that can influence present nutritional status. For example, fetal stores of iron are sufficient to assure satisfactory nutritional status with respect to this nutrient during early infancy even when the infant is fed foods which are exceedingly low in iron. Owing to body stores, the clinical signs of vitamin B-12 deficiency may not become apparent even on diets totally devoid of this nutrient until several years later.

Growth represents at the same time a great reservoir and a drain for nutrients. Diets which are borderline with respect to the protective nutrient may, in a child who is not growing, be associated with few biochemically or clinically apparent problems. In contrast, a growing child may quickly develop apparent signs and symptoms of deficiency owing to the increased needs of growth. Hegsted has demonstrated that growth needs for energy and protein actually represent only a relatively small proportion (e.g., 20%) of total intakes even in rapidly growing infants, with a lesser proportion applying to older patients.[133] While similar and seemingly small proportions of minerals and vitamins may be necessary for growth, at least in the case of some nutrients, the body's capacities to regulate intake, storage, or excretion may not be as efficient as they are for calories or protein. Thus, especially in situations involving disease, the body's ability to cope with a paucity or excess of nutrients may be severely compromised. In view of the fact that past as well as present nutrition and health status may contribute to size and other objective indices of nutritional status observed among vegetarians, careful history taking is extremely important in pinning down the causes of these various problems.

## Socioeconomic Status

Insofar as both diet and health care are associated with socioeconomic status, the latter variable must be accounted for before drawing conclusions about differences between vegetarians and omnivores. In developing countries it is often the poorest and least educated whose diets are vegetarian by reason of economic necessity. Vegetarians in this country are rarely so poverty stricken that a vegetarian diet must be adopted, nor are they necessarily persons with little formal education. Therefore, different causes and remedies for problems that may arise as a result of the vegetarianism can be considered. At the same time, however, it must be recognized that various vegetarian groups vary quite widely with respect to income, education, and social status. Therefore, it is important to carefully describe these variables when these groups are studied.[134]

## Membership in Diet-Related Groups

A sizeable majority of American vegetarians are affiliated with diet-related groups or organizations.[31-33,62] These groups are often quasireligious or philosophical groups such as the yogic, Krishna, macrobiotic, and Seventh-Day Adventist sects. Group members usually share similar beliefs about diet, the food supply, the health care system, and perhaps other aspects of lifestyle. Insofar as these factors can all have an influence on health status, it is useful to know the individual's affiliation in this respect.[46-48,135]

## Groups at Special Physiologic Risk from Vegetarian Diets
### Pregnant Women

Calorie intakes and the establishment of positive energy balance are of special importance among vegetarians. Both prepregnancy weight and weight gain during pregnancy have been shown to be associated with outcomes as measured by birth weights. Low-birth weight outcomes are likely to be associated with higher rates of morbidity and mortality in newborns.[136] Information on weight gain in pregnancy among vegetarians is scanty, but weight gains appear to be the same or less than is usual for pregnant women. In view of the fact that prepregnancy weights are lower and weight gains may thus be less than recommended, careful surveillance of weight status is particularly important.

On vegetarian diets, risks of iron deficiency anemia are somewhat heightened. Pregnancy represents a drain on iron stores of some 600 mg. Iron supplementation or increased dietary intakes of iron are therefore advisable among pregnant vegetarians. If milk is not consumed, calcium supplementation should also be considered.

Vitamin $B_{12}$ nutriture may also pose a problem since the need to provide for the development of the fetus arises. Vegan pregnant women in India have often been reported to have a high prevalence of megaloblastic anemia. Vegans may therefore need vitamin $B_{12}$ supplements during pregnancy.[138]

An excellent review on meeting dietary needs during pregnancy in a manner compatible with the dietary habits of vegans and vegetarians has recently been published.[137]

### Lactating Women

Common among vegetarians are a prolonged period of breast feeding (often 6 months or longer) and late introduction of supplemental foods as compared to the omnivore populations.[134] The infant, therefore, depends primarily on breast milk as a source of energy and nutrients for a much longer period than does the omnivore American infant, who is usually weaned by a few days or months after birth and is routinely introduced to supplemental foods by three months or earlier.[139,140] Possibly the volume or composition of the milk these "vegetarian" babies receive is significantly affected by the nature of the vegetarian mothers' diet. Since the infants of vegetarian parents are much more likely to be dependent upon breast milk as a source of energy and nutrients than omnivore infants, it is particularly important to ascertain if quality and quantity are adequate.

### Quantity

A fairly extensive literature attests to the adequacy of breast milk production, at least in the first 4 to 6 months of life, among women eating vegetarian diets.[141-145] Assuming caloric intakes are adequate, the volume of milk produced appears to be satisfactory to sustain good growth in the infant.

Somewhat more problematic is whether production is sufficient to sustain growth after this time without supplementary feeding. This is not unique to vegetarian mothers but applies to all mothers. As Hegsted[133] demonstrated, after several months of age, depending upon the size of the infant, breast milk may not be provided in sufficient amounts to fulfill energy needs. Given the same volume of milk produced (for example, 1000 m$l$ which provides 720 cal and 11 g of protein), an infant at the 10th percentile would have all of his needs met until 4.5 months, but the needs of an infant at the 90th percentile would exceed production after 2.5 months. One would expect, therefore, that these large, rapidly growing infants would be the first to show slowed growth. Since breast milk production generally averages 800 to 1000 m$l$/day, if supplementary feeding is not provided, calorie needs may not be met for some infants at the breast — even under 4 to 6 months. Additionally, if calorie needs are not met, protein nutriture will also be compromised.

The breast milk production of poorly nourished mothers may be compromised, as suggested by the study of Bailey.[146] Other workers have found that breast milk production is a good deal less than had previously been imagined, even in privileged populations.

For example, Swedish workers ascertained daily milk volume in Swedish women to be 500 to 600 m$l$ in early lactation and between 700 and 800 m$l$ late (170 days) in lactation.[142] None of the mothers was supplementing the infants' intake at the breast. As Hegsted's data show,[133] if outputs do not exceed 800 m$l$, regardless of the size of the infant, after roughly 6 months of life breast milk supplies will be inadequate to permit growth unless supplementation with other foods occurs. Therefore, any infant who is not supplemented with additional foods after 6 months of life runs the risk of compromise in growth. This so-called "late marasmus" or marasmus at the breast is well known in developing countries. In particular supplies may be insufficient to permit rapid growth of large infants, and it is they who may thus be the first to suffer growth decreases.

*Quality*

We have seen that, since breast milk supplies are not infinitely expandable, vegetarian infants who are breast fed for well into the second half of the first year of life run the risk of undernutrition if supplementary feedings are not provided. One might also ask if the composition of the milk they drink is different.

Lönnerdal et al.[14] also found that few significant differences in either volume or proximate constituents existed between Swedish and Ethiopian women consuming largely vegetarian diets, whether they were adequate or inadequate in protective nutrients. Therefore, composition appears to be well preserved although milk outputs are not infinitely expandable.

The altered type of fat and perhaps the lowered fat content of the diet consumed by vegetarian mothers might influence the lipid content or, more likely, the composition of the milk. Insull et al. have demonstrated a relationship between the total lipid and fatty acid pattern of human milk and the amount and composition of fat in the diet.[147] Other investigators have also found maternal diet to affect fatty acid composition and total lipid content of secreted milk.[148,149]

Although the qualitative alteration in the lipid content of milk obtained from women following different types of vegetarian dietary regimes in several developing countries is known,[150-154] reports on the lipid content of human milk in the U.S. have not included samples from lactating women following a vegetarian diet.[155-157]

The study of Potter and Nestel[158] on the effects of alterations of dietary fatty acids and cholesterol on milk lipids of lactating women and the plasma cholesterol of breast-fed infants is also of interest. These workers provided two diets to the women. One diet was high in animal foods, saturated fat, and cholesterol. The other diet was low in cholesterol and higher in polyunsaturated fatty acids. Later, a third diet high in other polyunsaturated fats but equivalent in cholesterol to the high-animal food diet was fed. The cholesterol content of the milk did not change with dietary alteration and appeared to be related to the process of milk secretion rather than being dependent upon plasma cholesterol levels in the mother. However, moderate increases in polyunsaturated fatty acids increased the linoleic content of the milk, and infants' plasma cholesterol levels fell. Therefore, certain maternal dietary factors do influence milk composition and infant metabolism, polyunsaturates being one of them.

A final aspect of possible variation in human milk which has received a good deal of attention is that of nonprotein nitrogen content of the breast milk of women consuming largely vegetarian diets. Wurtman[159] amassed preliminary data suggesting that nonprotein nitrogen fractions may in fact be different in Guatemalan low-income women consuming diets high in maize and beans and also in American vegetarian women consuming vegan-like, macrobiotic diets, as opposed to omnivores in either society.

*Infants and Children*

Little is known about the diets or growth of vegans or vegetarian children living in the U.S., although concerns about their nutritional adequacy are frequently expressed.[2,7,28,33,37] Until recently such dietary patterns were rare, except among families in which the parents were foreign born. While there is data available on the diets and growth of preschool children who eat vegan or nearly vegan diets in some developing countries,[23] it is difficult to separate the dietary effects from other adverse environmental influences on their growth.[160]

The largest single group of children raised on vegetarian diets in this country are the Seventh-Day Adventists. Only a few studies have been reported that describe the growth of these children.[161,162] Diets are usually lacto-ovo- or lactovegetarian. The Seventh-Day Adventist Church operates a network of hospitals and the children of church members are usually under close pediatric surveillance. Vitamin-mineral supplementation is frequently employed as a prophylactic measure, and diets are carefully planned to fulfill nutrient needs.[124] The studies available on the growth and diets of these children suggest that nutritional status is satisfactory. This interpretation is further buttressed by the fact that the adult heights of Seventh-Day Adventists raised on vegetarian diets since childhood do not appear to differ from those of omnivores.[127]

Only a few studies of the dietary patterns of children of "new" vegetarian parents or those adhering to other vegetarian patterns have been published.[64-68,163] Such parents feed their infants and children similar, but not identical diets, and, therefore, each group must be investigated. The elements of both ill-chosen vegan diets and lack of medical supervision might represent potential threats to health and growth in the children of such persons. While the studies to date have been useful in identifying their potential nutrition and health problems, they have been limited in scope, involving only small numbers of subjects, short term in nature, exclusively concerned with severely ill patients who presented for hospital care, or based on anecdotal observations.[32,33,64,66-68]

The reported health effects of the regimes range from severe malnutrition and rickets in a few children to less dramatic deficits in length, weight, and biochemical indicators of nutritional status in others. Positive aspects such as relative leaness are also apparent.

Three major criticisms may be leveled at the small series of children referred to in these reports. First, patients were only those whose parents sought pediatric guidance for their children (an unusual phenomenon in a group generally so opposed to medical treatment) and hence are probably unrepresentative. Second, only meager cross-sectional data was cited as evidence that growth was not affected. Third, it is not clear if these children were all actually being raised on similar diets. Vegan, as opposed to lacto-ovovegetarian diets, have quite different risks from the nutritional standpoint.

Three recent investigations have overcome many of these objections and permit us to make more definitive statements about the effects of alternative diets on infant and child growth and size.[66,68,164] It must be remembered, however, that some of these subjects follow vegan or lactovegetarian patterns while others eat lacto-ovo- or semi-vegetarian diets.

Perhaps of greatest concern, since diets are most limited, are the effects of vegan diets in early life. The effects of a vegan diet during pregnancy on birth weights of infants are difficult to predict. Although calorically inadequate diets of this type might lower birth weights slightly, so many factors influence birth weights that it is difficult to detect differences that might exist unless extremely large populations are used.

We found that birth weights, lengths, and gestational age were within the normal range for the infants of most vegans and vegetarians we studied.[164] An inadequate vegan diet during early infancy when growth needs are high would undoubtedly have profound effects. Vegans, however, do not usually proscribe human milk. It is regarded as natural and healthy to lactate until the child's teeth come in. Lactation actually is prolonged in most cases much beyond the 3rd or 4th month post partum. The children of the vegans we have studied almost universally receive animal food in the form of human milk for at least the first 6 months of life. Growth and size are within normal limits to at least 6 months of age.

Reasoning from a knowledge of the nutrient requirements of infants and their growth patterns, it might be predicted that the breast-fed infants of vegan parents would have essentially normal growth patterns for the first few months of life, and, at least in our studies, they do.[164,165] If they were weaned between the 3rd and 6th month post partum to a weaning diet inadequate in calories and/or protein, or very low in the vitamins and minerals mentioned elsewhere in this review, growth might be retarded. This is a common finding among young infants and children fed in this way in developing countries.[66] The infants of American vegetarian parents studied by both of us[164] and Trahms[68] were generally weaned much later, however, and such size deficits were not apparent. In contrast, Robson reported two cases of gross undernutrition in macrobiotic infants who had been weaned in early infancy, and their sizes were indeed affected profoundly.[64]

It is only after 6 months of age that differences in size become apparent between vegan and omnivore infants, although it is possible that differences in growth velocities appear before that time.[164-168] A particularly sharp decrease in growth velocity was found in the period from roughly 6 months to 2 years of age, which coincides roughly with weaning and the consequent adaptations that would have to be made to a totally vegan or a vegetarian diet during this time. After this period, growth was not affected as dramatically. Seasonal variations in height and growth velocities that differed from that of omnivore infants were also noted.[167] Vegetarian children showed greater deviations in size from omnivores than children on totally vegan diets. The vegan children whose parents reported adequate medical supervision, as opposed to those who did not, might also show lesser deficits, but this has not yet been ascertained.

To what might these decrements in size and growth be attributed? A number of possible explanations exist. Before discussing them, however, it is important to point out that the deviations are relatively mild and not suggestive of frank failure to thrive on protein-calorie malnutrition of the type seen in developing countries. Moreover, in contrast to children suffering from failure to thrive, the vegetarian childrens' appearances and parent-child interactions are not suggestive of neglect, abuse, or antipathy.

Although the "new" vegetarians frequently breast feed their children and wean late (thereby furnishing at least some animal protein even if no other source is provided), they fail to use iron or vitamin D-enriched/fortified foods; nor do they employ vitamin-mineral supplements as a rule.

Diets at weaning appear to be low in nutrient density, low in animal protein, high in complex carbohydrates (starch and dietary fiber), and low in iron, and weaning is late, all reminiscent of Victorian times.[132] Particularly at weaning, such diets may be low in calories and perhaps in protein (but only secondarily to inadequate calories), vitamin $B_{12}$, iron, vitamin D, and calcium, especially in children who are small and growing poorly.

Both reports in the literature and popular guides distributed by alternative diet groups suggest, that especially in the stricter groups like macrobiotic and certain yoga sects, parents have misconceptions about the special dietary needs of pregnant women and young children. They may reject as irrelevant concepts prevalent in the wider society.[28-33,46-56,89-91]

These results with respect to physical measurements are reminiscent of the falling off of growth observed among children in developing countries who are weaned to vegetarian-type diets. Decrements in size are much less profound among American vegetarian children, however, and decreases in growth velocities are only apparent until roughly 2 years of age. This is in contrast to what is commonly observed in developing countries.[168]

After two years of age, growth velocities are within the normal range, although on the low side. Size continues to lag slightly behind norms as well but is rarely outside normal limits. This is in sharp contrast to the characteristic stunting and continued depressed growth velocities that are observed among poor preschool children living in developing countries, which result in much greater effects upon size.

The American preschool vegetarians studied to date[66-68,164,165] show as a group only slight differences in anthropometric measurements from omnivores, but these differences are consistent and remain at least to age 6. There are probably differences between vegans and vegetarians, but as yet these analyses have not been performed.

What is not entirely clear is why it is that sufficient catch-up growth does not occur to recoup the losses suffered earlier on in life.[169] Two possible explanations are differences in diet and disease experience.

Likely causes of diet-related, slowed growth with failure to catch up in these children might be infrequent feeding, offering of diets low in caloric density, and other special feeding practices followed by some parents in the population studied. Other causes of smallness related to diet might include low dietary intakes of a number of nutrients (e.g., iron, vitamin $B_{12}$, vitamin D, and calcium) coupled in some cases with increased losses in the feces of iron, calcium, and zinc due either to the form in which the nutrients occur in foods or a "washing out" because of the high fiber content of the diet. Thus diets may be adequate without being sufficient to permit catch up. Assuming the type of diet remains constant in the 3rd year of life, physiological requirements on a per-kilogram basis are somewhat less than they were in the earlier months of life, and the child is less dependent on his mother feeding him to obtain his food. The diet may be sufficient to permit growth rates closer to normal so that further slowing does not occur, but previous deficits are not remediated.[170]

It also is likely that health care practices and the perception of illness by the "new" vegetarian parents are quite different from those of omnivore parents. Infections, disease, congenital defects, and emotional illness are all possible causes for small measurements or slowed growth.[171] The parents of macrobiotic children tend to be the most at odds with orthodox health care attitudes. These opinions, coupled with differing perceptions of the dietary needs of young children, may adversely affect their childrens' growth. In view of the lack of prenatal care, possible low weight gains during pregnancy, home deliveries, and failures to have infants immunized or enrolled in on-going pediatric care, which were more common in the "strict" alternative diet groups than among the "lenient" alternative diet groups or controls, the possibility of differences cannot be ignored. At present, however, diet furnishes a more satisfactory explanation.

The final explanation for continued smallness lies in the nature of growth itself. Losses in length from genetically determined potentials are less easily recouped than losses in weight. Thus they persist even longer after the insult.

The final effects of these diets on adult size cannot be foretold, since their effects on the timing of and growth at puberty have not been ascertained and that growth spurt also has profound effects on adult size. Table 5 summarizes what evidence is available from our own work[164] and that of Trahms[68] about the relationship between the vegan diet and growth among infants and children. Table 6 summarizes some of the risks thought to be inherent in the infant and child feeding practices of vegan parents.

Table 5

QUESTIONS ON DIET, HEALTH CARE, AND GROWTH IN THE CHILDREN
OF VEGAN PARENTS AND SOME TENTATIVE ANSWERS

| Questions | Answers |
|---|---|
| Are birth weight, length, and gestational age within the normal range if the mother was on a vegan diet during her pregnancy; was weight gain during pregnancy unusually low? | Gestational age does not seem to be affected; birth weights reflect prepregnancy weights, and weight gain during pregnancy tended to be lower among vegans than among other vegetarians; birth weights, while usually within the normal range, also were lowest among the infants of vegan as opposed to vegetarian mothers |
| Do vegan mothers breast feed their infants more frequently than nonvegan controls, and, if so, what is the duration of lactation? | Vegan and indeed vegetarian mothers in general virtually all breast feed their infants; duration of lactation ranges, but the norm is 6—15 months. |
| Do vegan mothers feed their infants vegan diets after weaning, and, if so, is the growth of such infants retarded? If they do not feed totally vegan diets, do they prefer a lacto-ovovegetarian regime, or is some other pattern different from that of meat-eating parents adopted? | Vegan mothers usually feed vegan diets after weaning; growth velocities are depressed for infants under 2 years of age in weight and length; if vegan diets are not adopted vegetarian patterns usually are; very few vegan or vegetarian parents feed their infants omnivore type diets; with the exception of the Seventh-Day Adventists, vitamin-mineral supplements are also avoided |
| Is the medical supervision of the children of vegan parents adequate? | The medical supervision for the children of some macrobiotics is inadequate, as evidenced by lack of immunizations and, frequently, no contact with the orthodox health care system unless acute illnesses of a serious nature arises; Seventh-Day Adventists generally have very close medical supervision |
| Do vegetarian parents modify their childrens' diets to approximate similar to their own patterns? | Yes, after weaning; but long breast feeding is the rule (e.g., 6—18 months) |
| Are mean birthweights, lengths, and gestational ages similar in the children of vegetarian parents as opposed to omnivore parents? | Yes, although birthweights are slightly, but not significantly, lower. |
| Are length, weight, triceps, and subscapular skinfolds lower in vegetarian or omnivore children of similar ages? | Vegetarians and omnivores are similar under 6 months of age; from 6 months onward, weight, length, and triceps are all lower than norms and lower than simultaneous controls; subscapular measurements are lower, but not significantly so |
| Do mean head circumferences differ between vegetarian and omnivore preschool children? | No |
| Is velocity of growth in weight or length different for vegetarians than for omnivores? | Yes; breast-fed infants, in general, have slower weight-gain velocities, and since all vegetarians are breast fed, this difference is more likely to be apparent than in omnivores, many of whom do not breast feed; under 2 years of age vegetarians exhibit depressed weight and length velocities; over 2 years of age, velocities are within the normal range |
| Do vegan and vegetarian children show different seasonal variations in growth than omnivore children? | They follow the expected seasonal patterns of maximal weight gain in the fall and winter; yet length velocities are most depressed in the spring, which is contrary to usual findings of maximal growth in length during the spring; the reasons for these differences are not apparent |

Table 5 (continued)

## QUESTIONS ON DIET, HEALTH CARE, AND GROWTH IN THE CHILDREN
## OF VEGAN PARENTS AND SOME TENTATIVE ANSWERS

| Questions | Answers |
|---|---|
| Are children eating essentially vegan diets smaller than those eating vegetarian diets? | Yes; vegan children are slightly shorter, lighter, and leaner than vegetarian children |
| Do children eating essentially vegan diets have lower intakes of calories, percent of calories as total protein, animal protein, saturated fat, refined carbohydrate cholesterol, vitamins D, $B_2$, $B_{12}$, calcium, and iron? | Energy intakes and total protein as percent of calories do not appear to differ; the percent of calories from animal protein and animal fat total iron, animal sources of iron, and vitamin D are lower among vegans; percent of calories from carbohydrates is higher, and presumably this is from increased complex (as opposed to refined) carbohydrate; Cholesterol, $B_{12}$, and $B_{12}$ intakes as well as calcium intakes are lower |
| Are intakes of vegetarian and vegan children of vegetable protein, total carbohydrate, and vitamins A and C higher than usual intakes of children of these ages adhering to omnivore diets? | Intakes of weaned vegetarian and vegan children are clearly higher for total carbohydrate; intakes of vitamins A and C are comparable but not necessarily higher |
| Is growth and size more or less variable in vegetarian, as opposed to omnivore, children? | Both growth and size are more variable among the children of vegetarians |

Table 6

## POSSIBLE THREATS TO DIETARY ADEQUACY IN THE DIETS OF
## CHILDREN OF VEGAN PARENTS

**Protein intake** — vegetable proteins of low-biological value may be fed, in combinations do not take advantage of the supplementary ability of certain vegetable protein combinations; they may be inadequate in the amounts fed to support normal growth, particularly under 1 year of age if the infant is not breast fed; however, protein intakes usually appear to be adequate

**Calorie intakes** — may be low, particularly in the weaning period when foods of very low-caloric density may be introduced in large amounts, necessitating consumption of large quantities of food at a time when teething problems may make the child anorexic

**Vitamins D, A, $B_{12}$ and iron** — possibly low-dietary intakes coupled with lack of iron or vitamin D supplements are usually recommended for this age group

**Low-fluid intakes** — particularly possible are among macrobiotics, since this movement advocates limitation of fluids

**Medical care only as a last resort** — if child is very ill, and little or no continuing medical supervision — this might give rise to more extensive periods of anorexia with untreated, low-grade infections; also increase duration of severity of gastrointestinal disturbances, fever, etc., which affect utilization of nutrients

In summary, it is clear that at least some types of vegetarian regimes do have effects upon size and growth in childhood, but the effects are exceedingly variable and depend not only on the type of diet but when it is adopted and for how long it continues. For example, vegan parents do not always feed their children vegan regimes at an early age. Some of the vegans may not place their children on a vegan regime until the child is 4 or 5 years of age. In others, the vegan diet may be only a transient phenomenon that the parents give up after a few months, so that the child is exposed to a vegan regime for only a short time. Whether these new types of vegetarian diets will ultimately affect adult size is not yet clear.

## Table 7
## QUESTIONS AND ANSWERS ABOUT ADULTS FOLLOWING VEGETARIAN DIETS

| Questions | Answer |
|---|---|
| Do vegan and vegetarian adults exhibit greater reported weight losses from highest adult weights and lower present weights for their height than omnivores? | Yes |
| Do vegan and vegetarian adults exhibit lower fatness as measured by triceps skinfolds than omnivores? | Yes |
| Do vegan and vegetarian adults who are parents exhibit different beliefs about suitable feeding practices for preschool children, which they reflect in the diets they feed their children? | Yes, they believe that long breast feeding and late introduction of solids are appropriate |
| Do vegan and vegetarian adults exhibit different attitudes toward and less utilization of health services for themselves and for their children than omnivores? | Yes |

In addition to effects on size and growth velocities, there are a number of other, more specific health effects both for good and ill that may arise when vegetarian diets are fed to children. They include alterations in energy balance and fatness status, and bowel function; and possible risks of certain types of chronic disease, iron deficiency anemia, rickets, and dental caries. Each will be discussed in detail in the following section.

### Adults with Special Problems

The effects of vegetarian diets on adults have been discussed elsewhere in this paper. Additional associations of interest are detailed in Table 7. In the reviewer's opinion, the greatest risks exist among the emotionally dependent, those with underlying and often-unrecognized health problems, and the poorly educated.

### The Elderly, Especially if They are Ill

While they are not commonly recognized as being vegans because of their previous omnivore habits and lack of affiliation with vegan-type groups, the dietary realities of many elderly people who subsist on "tea and toast" because of depression, lack of teeth, and economic constraints are in fact just that. Therefore, their special risks must also be mentioned when discussing vegan and vegetarian diets.

## NUTRITIONAL STATUS OF VEGETARIANS

### Energy

Data on energy intakes obviously mean little in comparisons between populations unless one can assume that energy outputs are similar in the two groups. Studies between vegetarian and omnivore populations have concentrated on energy intakes rather than outputs, so that it is difficult to know if this assumption is valid, but both factors need to be considered. Garrow has recently reviewed this topic at length.[173]

### Energy Outputs

The two major variables in energy output are resting metabolism and the level of physical activity. Amongst sedentary populations it is the component of energy expenditure that goes to resting metabolism that accounts for the greatest proportion of energy output. Individuals vary considerably in their resting metabolic rates, but vegetarians behave no differently than omnivores in these respects. In the last decade, however, a new factor which may explain variations in resting metabolism has been studied, and it may have particular significance for vegetarians.

In the past few years a great deal of work has been done on the metabolism of thyroid hormone. It is becoming increasingly clear that just as is the case with vitamin D, an exceedingly active form of thyroid hormone is produced in the process of metabolism with greater physiological effects than $T_4$ thyroxine, the major secretory product of the thyroid gland itself. This extremely active metabolite, known as $T_3$, or 3,5,3'-triiodothyronine, and another inactive metabolite, R (reverse) $T_3$ or 3,3',5'-triiodothyronine are of particular interest since the ratios of the two substances vary during fasting.[174]

The decreases in $T_3$ and increases in $RT_3$ appear to explain the fact that resting metabolism falls more adequately during fasting than does a hypothesis based on simple alterations in $T_4$ production. It is not known whether these ratios are the result of variation at the central level (e.g., by changes in the rate of secretion of the substances by the thyroid gland itself) or whether the alterations are due to peripheral changes either in the relative proportions of $T_4$ being deiodinated peripherally to $T_3$ and $RT_3$, or in altered clearance of the two substances. Even of greater interest with respect to vegetarianism, however, is the possibility that, at least on hypocaloric diets, dietary carbohydrate helps to maintain serum $T_3$ levels.[175,176] Reductions in dietary carbohydrate decrease $T_3$, and total fasts decrease it still further. These findings suggest that the metabolism of $T_4$ is influenced peripherally by the presence or absence of carbohydrate, or that the turnover of $T_3$ increases on low-carbohydrate isocaloric diets. It raises the question of whether alterations in proximate composition of diet, particularly with respect to levels of carbohydrate, affect the peripheral metabolism of $T_4$ even when diets are not hypocaloric. Since vegetarian diets are usually a good deal higher in carbohydrate than those of omnivores, resultant alterations in peripheral $T_4$ metabolism would offer another possible (and as yet untested) explanation for the relative leanness of many vegetarian subjects. Since data are not available on resting metabolic rates or $T_4$, $T_3$, or $RT_3$ metabolism in subjects on various types of vegetarian diets, but this is a hypothesis worthy of investigation.

The second major variable in energy expenditure is physical activity. This component is exceedingly variable. While healthy individuals only show small differences in basal metabolic rates, differences in energy expenditure related to physical activity may be twice or three times as much in one person than in another. These variations are considered even in sedentary populations such as our own, particularly among children.

No evidence is available in the literature on the energy outputs of vegetarian populations living in this country vis à vis omnivores. In view of the different attitudes and beliefs vegetarians have on other health-related questions, it cannot be assumed that they do not differ in their physical activity. This question needs to be explored.

*Energy Intakes*

Vegetarian adults, particularly vegans and those on alternative life-style diets, have been found by a number of investigators to have low-energy intakes.[1,2,4,7-9,11,15,17] These are reflected in their leanness as a group when compared to omnivores.

*Implications for Health*

Of all the nutritional problems likely to be present among very lean or small vegetarian children, low energy intakes are the most likely to be observed. This is not to say that all vegetarian children are in negative energy balance; indeed, while vegetarian children and adults appear to be somewhat leaner as a group than omnivores, some are fat.[134] However, low-energy intakes among children, if they do exist, are of particular concern since they may compromise growth. In view of the relationship between weight and pregnancy outcomes, pregnant women are also of particular concern.

The anthropometric measurements of a substantial proportion of the vegetarian children[66-68,164] are also suggestive of energy intakes that are on the low side as compared to need, at least during some periods of growth.[177]

The reasons for low energy intakes are not entirely clear, either in adults or in children, although a number of explanations have been suggested. First, vegetarian infants are breast fed for long periods of time. Breast-fed infants as a group have lower caloric intakes than bottle-fed infants.[178] A second possible explanation applying to infants is the relatively late introduction of solid foods, which is associated at least in some studies with lesser gains in weight or fatness, and presumably, decreased total caloric intake.[179,180] A third explanation is that parents may differ in their attitudes toward feeding, i.e., they may be less likely to overfeed their infants. At least in our own experience, vegetarian parents seem less apt to equate "bigness" and high rates of weight gain with positive health than the omnivore parents in our pediatric clinics. Most adult vegetarians are also very much aware of the positive benefits of relative leanness vis à vis obesity in their own lives.

A fourth reason for low-energy intakes is the poverty of certain vegetarians. Diets of poor vegetarians and nonvegetarians alike in developing countries sometimes do not provide sufficient energy,[181] but even in such settings this is likely only among the poorest of the poor. Therefore, such an explanation is unlikely in this country.

Fifth, it may be that low-energy intakes reflect decreased energy outputs in physical activity. It is well known that voluntary exertion is avoided by persons who are undernourished, and Graves recent study has shown that this also occurs in infants and children.[182] It has long been known that the growth of infants and children is extraordinarily sensitive to caloric restriction.[183]

But it is also exceedingly difficult to detect inadequate calorie intakes from dietary data alone, because of the enormous variability in individual needs resulting from differences in energy outputs.[184] Nevertheless, this possibility must be seriously considered, at least among vegetarian infants and children who fail to show satisfactory growth.

A sixth possibility is that in view of the extensive proscriptions such diets impose, eating outside the home is sharply cut back owing to the lack of suitable food. Since most Americans eat a great deal of food away from home, if one maintains a "Kosher" diet yet must be away from home a good deal of the time, food intake might be curtailed among such vegetarians.

A seventh but somewhat unlikely explanation is that some vegetarians engage in periodic fasts on a regular basis. While fasting has been reported among a few groups, it does not appear to be a generalized phenomenon. At least one recent study in omnivores has shown a negative correlation between fatness and the frequency of eating.

Perhaps appetite is frequently compromised by illness. There is no evidence to support this contention in the literature, however.

Eighth, if frequency of eating and time spent eating are constant, one might assume that with low-caloric density plant food diets, it would be hard to overeat.

A final possibility is that the frequency of feeding and time devoted to eating is less than that of omnivore populations, or that other sociocultural factors encourage undereating.

Our own bias is to favor the theory first expounded by Nichol,[185] namely that the bulk of the diet, especially in the early years of life, and infrequency of meals on such high-bulk diets might overtax the young child's capacity to consume food, resulting in low-caloric intakes. Calorie values per unit weight, and perhaps even more dramat ically per unit volume, would appear to be much higher on vegan preschool diets than on omnivore diets, and thus might be daunting to the appetite of the eater by their sheer bulk, as well as making it physiologically more difficult to overeat.

Not all vegetarian children or adults are lean, however. Some, in fact, are obese. Therefore, again we must distinguish between different types of regimes. And certainly the above-mentioned theory does not appear to be proven out by experience with Chinese-American infants, whose growth is satisfactory in spite of a diet quite high in bulk.[186] It is entirely possible, however, in view of the exceedingly high-energy intakes necessary to recover from periods of undernutrition, that with such high-bulk diets sufficient energy intakes to allow for catch-up growth in weight will not be possible.[187,188]

### Protein

The three major influences on protein utilization are the total energy value of the diet, protein quantity, and protein quality. Another factor sometimes mentioned is the time at which protein is fed.

#### Protein Calorie Ratios

It is impossible to have satisfactory protein nutriture if energy needs are not met. The question of safe ratios of protein to calories has received a great deal of attention in the past decade, owing to the growing realization that in many parts of the world the energy intakes of infants and children might be both inadequate and a much more common reason for protein-calorie malnutrition than had previously been suspected.[180-190] Therefore, the recent report of Ferro-Luzzi et al.[191] is of particular interest. These workers found that even amongst a population subsisting on a staple diet of starchy roots and tubers providing only 2 g of protein per 100 g, energy intakes were more commonly limited than was protein. They further suggested that either ad aptations had occurred among these children or energy standards were too high. There fore, even on vegetarian diets low in protein in which bulk is high it is primarily energy rather than protein that appears to be problematic.

#### Protein Quantity

Since vegetarians do not eat or restrict their consumption of three major sources of protein in the American diet (i.e., flesh food, dairy products, and eggs)[192-197] it is not surprising that they are usually found to eat less animal protein than omnivores.[15,199,200] This does not necessarily mean that they are protein deficient,[201], however, since ani mal protein intakes in this country are generous and have risen in the past 15 years as beef consumption has reached new highs.

#### Protein Quality

Vegetable protein diets that might be entirely satisfactory for adults may not be so for children, owing to the quantity and quality of protein available, even if energy intakes are adequate. In addition to the fact that infants and young children need greater amounts of protein on a per-kilogram basis, there are important qualitative differences in requirements for amino acids as well.

The need for total essential nitrogen as percent of total nitrogen is much higher in infants than adults. Arroyave[202] recently showed that the nutritional quality of a pro tein will vary according to the age of the individual consuming it. His group has shown, for example, that different corn-bean mixtures might be satisfactory for achieving ni trogen balance in 2-year-old infants and in adults. The type of mixture eaten of various plant proteins or of animal and plant protein affects biological value quite profoundly, although most diets contain mixes of several different plant proteins,[203] even among vegetarians. Most vegetable proteins have amino acid deficiencies if consumed as the sole source of protein: usually lysine, methionine, tryptophan, and threonine. These can be overcome by the addition to the diet of other proteins rich in these amino acids. If eaten raw, many legumes, including soybeans, lima beans, navy beans, and peanuts, contain trypsin inhibitors. These interfere with the digestion of the protein and availability of the limiting amino acid, methionine.

Protein quality is not likely to be problematic among American vegetarians since a wide variety of plant foods are eaten. Popular books on vegetarianism nevertheless stress the need for complementary sources of protein, so that most American vegetarians are very much aware of the need to use a variety of plant foods. The mixtures of plant protein fed by some macrobiotic vegan parents are not always of the type that would be expected to be optimal on the basis of studies in experimental animals and more limited trials in humans for purposes of complementation, however. But overall intakes of protein appear to be high enough to compensate for such effects as long as energy supplies are adequate.

### Timing of Feeding Protein Vis à Vis Calories

A fourth factor sometimes suggested as affecting nitrogen retention is the time at which protein is fed. A recent study showed satisfactory nitrogen retentions and weight gains among children receiving protein mixtures in one feed.[204] Thus on a practical basis, this does not seem to be a problem in either children or adults.

### Implications for Health

While evidence suggests that most vegans eat a broad variety of plant protein sources in seemingly adequate amounts, their calorie intakes may be insufficient, thereby compromising protein nutritional status. Also, in the case of prematurely born children or children who are frequently ill or recovering from serious illness on vegan diets, intakes may be insufficient to compensate for the relatively low biological values of some of the protein mixtures eaten.

### Fat
#### Quantity

Since approximately 90% of the fat in the American diet is from fats and oils, meat, poultry, and dairy products, it is not surprising that vegetarians have lower fat intakes than do omnivores.[15,205] Animal fat provides roughly a quarter of total calories in omnivore diets; since animal products account for a lesser proportion of the diet among vegetarians, animal fat as a percentage of total calories is usually lower[71,205-208] especially among vegans.

#### Quality

In the usual American diet approximately 40% of the fat is comprised of saturated fatty acids, 12% of polyunsaturated fatty acids, and the remainder from other fatty acids and glycerol. Cholesterol intakes are 500 or more milligrams per day. Substantial reductions in total and saturated fat intake are best achieved by reducing consumption of meat, fish and poultry, fats and oils, and dairy products, which furnish the greatest amounts of fat in the diet. Vegans, of course, eliminate all animal foods and therefore have usually lowered cholesterol and fat intakes. Semivegetarians may have a slightly lower intake of total fat, but if a lacto-ovovegetarian pattern is adopted, saturated fat consumption might still be high.[71]

*Implications for Health*

It is a common observation in studies of vegetarians, particularly vegans, that they have lower plasma lipid values and different plasma lipoprotein patterns from those of comparable omnivore populations in the same geographic areas.[15,72,205] A recent study of long-term vegetarian diets on blood lipids bears this out. Chen[209] studied 394 vegans living in Formosa who had adhered to such a diet for a median of 15 years. Serum cholesterol levels were exceedingly low; lower than among the local nonvegetarian population.

The vast bulk of evidence suggests that these effects on blood lipids are associated with the type of fat and amount of cholesterol consumed. But it may be that other, less obvious factors such as the presence of larger amounts of dietary fiber may also be at least partially responsible for the lowered levels of serum lipids observed. Several investigators have proposed the theory that atherosclerosis is a dietary fiber deficiency disease.[210-213] The evidence for this theory is by no means conclusive. In any event, it is clear that the many types of dietary fiber are not similar in their hypolipidemic effect,[212] wheat bran differing from lignins, lignins from bagasse (a sugar cane residue of a fibrous nature), and these from pectins both in their apparent influence on serum cholesterol and on fecal excretion of sterols and bile acids.[214,215]

The phytosterols in some types of fiber may also inhibit cholesterol absorption. It has been suggested that some fraction in whole-wheat bread has an effect in raising serum cholesterol levels.[212]

It has also been suggested that vegetarian diets alter the type of degradative products of animal and plant sterols, bile acids, and their degradation products found in the feces, and that these may be of significance from the standpoint of potential carcinogenicity.[216-218] The type of diet eaten influences the distribution of bacteria in the lower gut, but at least in man, attempts to change the bacteria flora by dietary manipulation have not been successful, at least as measured by cultures of fecal specimens.[218] While Drasar and Irving[216] reported large differences in cultures of fecal specimens between groups on essentially vegetarian, high-carbohydrate, low-fat diets in developing countries as opposed to Americans or Englishmen on "usual" omnivore diets. When they examined differences in fecal specimens between vegan and omnivore Englishmen living in London, however, cultures were quite similar. Other groups have now also shown that a changeover to a vegetarian diet produced no demonstrable changes in predominant fecal flora.[219,220]

Alterations in diet may change the composition of the mixture of intestinal secretions and residues that enter the colon. Alterations in dietary constituents that usually follow a change over to a vegetarian diet have already been seen as probably having little effect on the bacterial species and genera comprising the colonic microflora. However, the gut microflora are known to be important in the metabolism of lipids and sterols. Eysson,[221] for example, cites evidence that their functions include transformation of primary bile acids into secondary bile acids, reduction of the bile acid pool in the intestine, and alterations in metabolism and turnover of the bile acids, thereby resulting in a more rapid catabolism of cholesterol to bile acids. The metabolic activity of the flora may be altered due to changes in the dietary compounds reaching them. Several workers[73,75,77,210] have suggested the possibility that the presence of certain animal sterol or bile acid degradation products or, perhaps, other potentially carcinogenic substances in the Western diet but present in lesser amount or concentration in vegetarian-type, non-Western diets may account for the differences in rates of colon cancer which are observed from region to region. This hypothesis has not been confirmed as yet.

Nonetheless, it is clear that fecal animal sterols such as cholesterol are proportionately lower among vegetarians than they are among omnivores, and the fecal plant sterols are higher.[216,221] In vegetarians, a lesser percentage of the cholesterol is degraded to coprastanone and coprostanol,[217] and bile acid levels in the feces tend to be higher.[221] Whether these changes are important from the standpoint of human health remains to be ascertained.

Clearly, a number of different dietary constituents may affect the types of sterols and amounts of bile acids found in the feces. For example, Antonis and Bersohn[222] found that quadrupling the fiber content of the diet from 4 to 15 g increased fecal bile acids from 24 to 43%, but this was only true when the diet was low in fat; on a high-fat diet it did not occur. While these effects on health remain obscure, the potential effects of alterations in serum lipids by modifications of the type of fat consumed by at least some vegetarians are more convincing. However, Heaton[223] attributes these effects to fiber depletion, although he holds a distinct minority opinion.

## Carbohydrate
### Total Carbohydrate
On the basis of percent of calories, vegetarians eat more carbohydrate than do omnivores.[7,15,224]

### Type of Carbohydrate
"Available" carbohydrates: complex and refined — Of the metabolizable carbohydrate eaten, vegetarians' intakes of complex carbohydrates are higher than that of omnivores.[15,225] Intakes of simple sugars (e.g., mono- or disaccharides) may be lower in some groups. Macrobiotics, for example, avoid sugar and any formulated or fabricated foods containing it, so that intake of sticky sweets in the diet is probably reduced. Among other groups, honey or "raw" sugar is popular. While the metabolic effects of increased intakes of complex (as opposed to simple) carbohydrates and their significance on health status are not yet entirely clear, decreased intakes of sticky, sugary sweets in the contact diet to which the teeth are exposed is regarded as beneficial by virtually all dental authorities at present.[225-227] Risk of dental caries might be reduced by such a dietary pattern.

"Unavailable" carbohydrates: dietary fiber — Vegetarians also eat more "unavailable carbohydrate" than do omnivores.[15] Dietary fiber is analogous to the "unavailable fiber" in the diet as it is usually defined, although it does contain certain noncarbohydrate substances such as lignins as well. It represents a different group of substances than that obtained by crude fiber analysis, which includes hemicelluloses, cellulose, and lignins, in that pectins are also included.[215,228] While it is true that the digestibility of the supposedly unavailable carbohydrates may vary from one individual to the next, depending upon differences in the extent to which these substances are acted upon by the secretions of the digestive tract or by intestinal flora, variations in transit times, size of particle, frequency of feeding, and other factors, individual variations are quite small. On a practical basis, it is therefore possible to arrive at a fairly good estimate of the dietary fiber present in foods.

While it is widely recognized that the biologically available carbohydrates are heterogeneous with respect to structure and function, dietary fiber is often thought of as a single substance. The fact is that dietary fiber is not a homogeneous entity with respect to chemical composition, associated materials and their proportions from one source to the next. It is thus of great importance in assessing the biological effects of dietary fiber to specify the type of dietary fiber and its constituents as clearly as possible.[229] For example, the pectins and other water-absorbing substances like psyllium seeds have very different effects than bran.[230,231]

Crowther et al.[232] have recently shown that chemically defined, fiber-free diets reduced fecal bacterial flora, interaction of the intestinal steroids with the colonic flora, and excretion of both acidic and neutral steroids, as well as fecal bulk.

### Possible Health Effects of Alterations in Proximate Composition on Vegetarian Diets

**Alterations in serum lipids** — These have already been discussed. It is evident that the heterogeneity of vegetarian diets is such that, without carefully ascertaining the type of fat eaten and intakes of cholesterol, it is impossible to assume that reductions in serum lipids will be automatic. Others[231] have recently reviewed the effects of dietary fiber on plasma lipids and these too must be considered.

**Alterations in risk of colon and breast cancer** — In addition to the numerous references that have already been cited on the Burkitt hypothesis, a whole spate of papers have recently been published that explore the interrelationships between bacteria, diet, and large bowel cancer.[233-237] Current hypotheses concern themselves largely with dietary fat and fiber intakes, their interactions with gut flora, and how these various factors may vary between vegetarian and omnivore populations as well as with different disease states. Similarly, the influence of dietary factors on bacterial metabolism and their links to estrogen metabolism and their potential links to breast cancer are being very actively explored.[238] Findings are tantalizing but insofar as they are based primarily upon epidemiological evidence, they must still be regarded as hypotheses rather than facts. Again, the very heterogeneity of vegetarian regimes makes it likely that, even if vegetarians were demonstrated to be at lower risk, rates might differ substantially from one type of diet to another.

**Fecal bulk** — The varying effects of different kinds of fiber on fecal bulk illustrate the importance of specifying the type of dietary fiber clearly when attempting to relate dietary fiber to various biological effects. The various types of fiber are disparate in their abilities to absorb water, thereby differing in the degree to which they increase fecal bulk. In both experimental animals and man, agar, carrots, cabbage, and bagasse increase stool weights more than do bran, lucerne leaf meal, or cellulose.[239]

Diets high in dietary fiber have been shown by many investigators to increase fecal bulk.[232,233,239,240] The effects observed depend both on the type of diet as well as amounts present. Alterations in fecal mass are due not only to the residue of undigested fiber itself, but to water (both free and bound) and bacteria. For example, wheat bran's laxative effect is due in large part to its property of absorbing and retaining water, so that stool wet weight increases although intestinal transit time and stool frequency do not. Spiller et al.[241] have suggested that fecal weight be used to establish recommendations for intakes of dietary fiber, an optimium being approximately 150 g/day. Not all scientists agree with Burkitt's[242] belief that fecal bulk is the common mediating factor between a series of diseases. MacDonald argues that some of the effects of dietary fiber are adverse rather than positive.[243] Before either risks or benefits are ascertained, it is clear that more adequate chemical methods for characterizing dietary fiber will be needed, as was stressed in a recent symposium on the topic.[244,245]

Dietary fiber intakes among vegetarian children living in this country are not directly available in the literature. Indeed, they are scanty for omnivore children as well. After over 3 decades, the most complete study of dietary fiber intakes of young children remains that of Macy[246]. Children in that study were found to have average intakes of 6 to 7 g of dietary fiber per day, ranging from 0.33 g/kg/day for the younger children to 0.20 g/kg/day for the older children. At the time those analyses were done, as at present, the definition of dietary fiber was not standardized, but in essence the Macy analyses approximate present analyses for unavailable carbohydrate. These values for dietary fiber intake are lower on an absolute basis than those reported for American[247] adults, but understandably so in view of the lesser amounts of food consumed by infants and children.

On the basis of current evidence and preliminary analysis of the dietary data from our subjects, it is reasonable to assume that the fecal bulk of vegetarian children and adults is higher than that of omnivores, and that this accounts for the low prevalence of reports of constipation among them.

**Other alterations in bowel function** — Vegetarians sometimes mention a greater prevalence of diarrhea when they change from omnivore diets to these regimes. Fiber may be implicated in these effects.[248-251] Fordtran[252] has suggested that the diarrhea associated with large fiber intake caused by the poor absorption of the organic acids once they have been produced by the intestinal bacteria. These acids retard water absorption and thus contribute to producing a watery feces. Fiber of the type that is readily attacked by the enteric bacteria and produces large quantities of these acids provokes diarrhea more readily than does fiber resistant to bacterial degradation, as was observed by Williams and Olmsted[253] and Hoppert and Clark[254] decades ago.

**Flatulence** — Omnivores who have changed to a vegetarian diet often report "gas". Flatus production is sometimes considered a socially undesirable side effect of vegetarianism. Calloway's[255] review of this topic suggests that the greatest offenders are brussels sprouts and beans, owing to their high contents of stachyose and raffinose. If bean consumption increases as a vegetarian diet is adopted, this may account for the greater flatus experienced. Other types of intestinal gases such as hydrogen and carbon dioxide may also be produced in greater amounts if nonabsorbable-but-fermentable substances are eaten in greater quantity.

**Fatness status** — American vegetarians tend to be leaner than omnivores. This does not seem to be a matter simply of self-selection of leaner persons into these groups, since persons who were previously omnivores and became vegetarians in adulthood also report weight loss rather than weight gain.[46,47] The possible mechanisms by which caloric intakes might favor weight loss have already been discussed. Energy outputs owing to alterations in lifestyle with respect to physical activity may also play a part in this process, although studies on this point are not available. The beneficial effects of leanness as opposed to obesity have been extensively documented in many recent publications.[256]

Occasionally cases of neanness to the point of emaciation have been reported, particularly among vegans adhering to exceedingly restrictive regimes.[31] In general, however, this does not appear to pose problems. For some persons, such as those with adult onset diabetes mellitus, high-fiber, high-carbohydrate diets may have particularly beneficial effects over and above their effects on fatness per se.[257]

**Dental health** — No conclusive evidence is yet available on the dental health status of vegetarians as compared to omnivores. On regimes that encourage the use of coarse foods that might cleanse the teeth and discourage the consumption of sugar (particularly sticky sweets) and high-sugar snack foods, one might anticipate reductions in dental caries risk. Of course, oral hygiene, fluoridation of water supplies, and dental care may also influence caries rates, and these parameters might also vary between the two groups.

## Minerals
### General Issues

Several recent reviews have summarized the problems of mineral nutriture that may arise among persons consuming diets largely of plant origin. Vegetable fiber, being the heterogeneous complex of polysaccharides and lignins, is capable not only of sequestering water, but also of binding cations and anions, depending upon the chemistry of the particular vegetable fiber. It follows that not only stool weight, but also the content of bile acids, electrolytes, or other constituents normally reabsorbed as the remnants of digestion pass through the gut, may vary depending upon both the content of dietary fiber and the constituents of the dietary fiber in the diet. Fernandez et al.[258] tripled dietary fiber intakes of a group of adult volunteers and found that in addition to increasing fecal weight, potassium concentration in the stool nearly doubled, sodium excretion increased, and so did daily output of organic acids.

Gums or hydrophilic colloids such as kelp are used by some vegetarians in their daily diets. In addition to exerting a bulk-producing, laxative effect and increasing fecal weight and water content, absorption of calcium is slightly but clearly reduced with doses of 4 g of sodium alginate, the active laxative agent in kelp.[259] Decreased absorption of magnesium iron, copper and zinc, have also been noted, and workers suggested that prolonged administration of 10 g of kelp might deplete the organism of essential nutrients such as these. Red algae seaweed is another hydrophilic colloid eaten by vegetarians. This contains large amounts of carrageenan. Its effects on absorption of minerals are not documented at present. Calcium, iron, and zinc eaten in plant and particularly grain sources may form unabsorbable complexes with fiber and phytate (inositol hexaphosphate). Fiber is suspected of being quantitatively the more important of the two substances with respect to the losses it engenders, at least in this country, but until now phytates have received more attention in the literature. It is not clear today if the increased level of intake of these substances among vegetarians is great enough to have mineral-depleting effects.

*Iron*

A number of recent studies in this country[260-264] have reported marginal dietary intakes of iron and/or biochemical indices indicative of poor iron status among adults, infants, and preschool children on omnivore dietary patterns when such foods and supplements were not purposefully avoided by parents. Therefore, it should come as no surprise that vegetarians also are iron deficient; poor iron status is even more common among vegans.[15] Research in the past few years has clarified why this occurs.

*Iron Content*

The first and most obvious cause of poor iron nutriture is dietary shortage. Many foods high in iron such as red meat are not eaten by vegetarians; the substitutes employed (such as milk) may be lower in iron. Some vegetarians eschew the use of iron supplements that may be prescribed by physicians at times of especially high need, such as during pregnancy.[266] Others who adhere to natural/organic alternative dietary styles as well as vegetarianism may find such products as iron-fortified formulas or infant cereals unacceptable. Generalization is dangerous, however, since some vegetarians, such as Seventh-Day Adventists, are careful to provide iron supplements at times of high physiological need, and owing to the extensive use of enriched or whole-grain foods, total iron intakes are often equal to those of omnivores.

*Iron Availability*

The iron in vegetarian diets may be in a form more difficult to absorb. The old dictum that iron from animal sources is more available than that from plant sources, although generally correct, has proven to be much more complicated in actual practice than was formerly anticipated. The form of the iron and other dietary factors exert influences. These will be discussed in turn.

It is well known that the bioavailability of iron is highest for diets rich in animal foods, and that it decreases as the proportion of vegetable foods in the diet increases. Moore[266] and Layrisse and associates[267-270] have reviewed this problem at length. Different animal foods were not equivalent in their effects on the enhancement of iron absorption.[271] Milk, cheese, and eggs brought about relatively little increase in absorption, while animal tissues such as beef, lamb, pork, liver, fish, etc. brought about increases ranging from two- to fourfold. These researchers suggest a better distinction than animal and vegetable sources of protein would be animal tissues vs. other sources, since it is the animal tissues that bring about the greatest increases in absorption. Although the mechanisms are not clear, animal tissues somehow enhance the availability of dietary iron. In contrast to meats, from which absorption ranges from 7 to 22%, the bioavailability of iron in eggs is lower than that of other animal foods.[272] Milk iron also shows a lower bioavailability than meat as well as being low in iron to begin with.

Takkunen and Seppänen[273] studied dietary factors associated with iron deficiency in Finland. Not surprisingly, in line with the above findings, those persons who consumed less meat and more milk were most at risk. Equally important from the standpoint of vegetarian diets is the fact that the addition of even small amounts of meat to meals providing iron from plant sources greatly increases the absorption of iron from plant foods, perhaps because of the cystine it provides.[267]

Iron absorption has recently been studied among Burmese subjects on high-rice diets;[274] iron absorption from a basal meal of rice, vegetables, and spices providing roughly 8 mg of iron was only 1.4%. Addition of 40 g of fish increased absorption three to four times. Even with less fish, absorption was much higher than from the basal meal. The authors concluded that absorption on a rice and vegetable diet would be insufficient to maintain iron balance. They further maintained that consumption of meat and fish even in the small and variable quantities may be sufficient to maintain iron balance in many persons, although the rates of iron-deficiency anemia are exceedingly high.

Therefore, it seems likely that persons consuming predominantly vegetarian diets based on corn or rice are especially likely to develop iron deficiency because of the low bioavailability of iron on such diets.[275] Indeed, if the usual absorption of iron from individual vegetable foods is 1 to 6%, it is easy to see how diets high in one of these staples could be risky.

But there are myriad other factors which also influence iron absorption. Ascorbic acid increases the absorption of nonheme iron in foods.[276,277] Insofar as many vegetarians have high-ascorbic acid intakes, this may be beneficial to iron absorption.

Monsen and Cook[278] found that both calcium and phosphorus salts added to the diet in large amounts reduce iron availability from nonheme sources, but not when calcium salts or phosphate salts were added simultaneously. Since the world's supply of food iron is in predominantly nonheme forms, this is a matter of some importance. Dairy products are high in both calcium and phosphate salts, and thus they need examination in this respect, particularly for lactovegetarians.

It is readily apparent that all vegetarian diets are not alike. They may vary by iron content, iron availability, and the influence on the iron availability from the plant sources of other foods ingested simultaneously. Animal tissues may exert a greater positive effect in this latter manner than they do by the iron they themselves supply. One would, therefore, expect the risk of poor iron status to be especially high with diets including no animal tissues.

In view of the better absorption of most forms of animal iron sources, one can see how vegan, or even lacto-ovovegetarian diets devoid of meat, would place the eater at potential risk of iron-deficiency anemia. Those individuals with especially high iron needs (e.g., young children of 6 to 18 months, menstruating women, and pregnant women) would be at particularly high risk.

### Effects on Health Status

The health effects of iron deficiency anemia among these or other subjects is more difficult to ascertain. The question of marginal or suboptimal intakes of micronutrients is a thorny one. But even at more frankly deficient levels seen in some vegans, the health effects are entirely clear. Recent evidence suggests that, at least in certain situations, iron-deficiency anemia is associated with a seeming protective effect against certain bacterial infections,[279,280] and investigators are exploring its association with lessened immune function and response. The negative effects of iron-deficiency anemia have been reviewed at length elsewhere[263] and include possible effects on work performance. A major scientific problem remaining to be solved is the determination of long-term consequences of marginal intakes not only of iron, but also of chromium, zinc, and perhaps other micronutrients.

*Zinc*

The original reports of zinc deficiency in humans were on a population that had high-sweat losses and low concentrations of zinc in their water supply, and in which geophagia for clay was common.[281] The high-phytate content of the bread consumed was suggested as one of the reasons why children and adolescents eating such diets became zinc and iron deficient. Recently, the failure of zinc supplementation to reverse the hypogonadal dwarfism thought to be due to zinc in the Shiraz experiment has also been attributed to the sequestering action of phytate and fiber on the zinc in the unleavened, whole-meal bread consumed in large amounts by the children tested.[282,283] The study of Reinhold et al.[284] on alterations in zinc, calcium, phosphorus, and nitrogen balances in Iranian villagers after a change from a phytate-rich to a phytate-poor diet offers support for this interpretation. A subsequent study casts doubt on this, however.[285] Pica for clay is an alternative explanation.[286]

Working in the U.S., Hambidge et al.[287] reported that several small children in Denver had low levels of zinc in their hair samples and suggested that their smallness might be due to zinc deficiency. However, the methodology involved in using zinc levels in hair has proven to be questionable unless different sections of the shaft are all sampled and analyzed, since values may vary from one point to another.[288] While values may be low in some diets, the health significance is not yet clear.[289-292]

Most of the vegetarians in the U.S. appear to eat high-vegetable protein, high-fiber diets, but a more varied diet than has been observed among populations where zinc deficiency is suspected of being common. In most but not all parts of the U.S., water supplied appear to be adequate in zinc, and no geophagia has been reported in the vegetarian population. Thus the possibility of zinc deficiency is considered remote.

Walravens and Hambidge[289] have suggested that some infant formulas may have zinc levels below that of human milk and increase risks of poor nutritional status with respect to zinc among infants consuming them. Since most vegetarians infants are breast fed for long periods of time, at least until weaning, this does not appear to be relevant.

Mahloudji et al.[285] supplemented the high-phytate, high-fiber semivegetarian diets of Iranian children with zinc, iron, or both metals. The zinc supplementation did not lead to alterations in serum zinc or increased growth.

In view of the lack of evidence that vegetarian subjects in this country are subject to zinc deficiency and with clear knowledge that zinc intoxication is possible, it would be unwise to recommend supplementation until data is more convincing.

**Vitamin Intakes**

*Vitamin D, Calcium, and Phosphorus*

**Bone formation** — In order for normal bone to form, there must be proper synthesis and mineralization of osteoid with appropriate remodeling. The first identifiable mineral deposits are amorphous tricalcium phosphate. After continued exposure to extracellular fluid, hydroxyapatite and amorphous phosphate form the crystalline phase of bone mineral.

**Vitamin D deficiency rickets** — In the absence of vitamin D, among other physiological effects, the absorption of calcium from the upper small intestine is compromised. In children a deficiency of vitamin D results in rickets, which is characterized by an excess of uncalcified osteoid, most probably owing to decreased calcium absorption. Vitamin D deficiency rickets occurs most frequently during periods of rapid skeletal growth when calcium needs are high. Thus it is most often seen in infancy from approximately 3 to 6 months to 2.5 years and again, but more rarely, during adolescence.

**History of vitamin D deficiency rickets in the U.S.** — At the turn of the century rickets was a common problem in many parts of the U.S.[293] For example, in 1900, Morse[294] reported that in 400 poor Boston infants under 2 years of age, over 80% had one or more rachitic changes. Only a few years later, Lovett identified over 500 cases in that same city using X-rays.[295] Even earlier than this, Haven[296] had noted the greater frequency of cases in black children living in the Boston area. Other cities showed similar high incidence rates. The vast majority of these infants had been breast fed and after weaning received supplemental foods and milks devoid of vitamin D. Apparently, the sun's ultraviolet radiation alone could not be relied upon in this northern climate as a means of assuring vitamin D nutriture, owing no doubt to cultural factors that prevented infants from being "sunned".

Also apparent to sapient pediatricians at the turn of the century were the association of rickets with iron deficiency anemia, the relative paucity of cases in infants who were failing to thrive, the high prevalence of cases in the latter part of the first year of life, and the difficulty of making the diagnosis without careful clinical inspection because of the relative rarity of full-blown cases with genu varus or genu valgum. It was only after public health campaigns were mounted to encourage the use of cod liver oil that the incidence of this disease began to drop.[297-299] The introduction of vitamin D-fortified milk in the 1930s dealt rickets its final blow. As late as the 1930s deaths from rickets averaged 400 or more cases per year, By the 1950s rickets was a rare disease;[300] its conquest was pointed to as one of preventive medicine's triumphs. In the 1960s the incidence rate in the U.S. was less than 0.3/1000 pediatric admissions, according to data reviewed by the American Academy of Pediatrics.[301]

**Vitamin D deficiency rickets in the U.S. today** — The question of vitamin D deficiency rickets has received less complete study in the U.S. than it has in Great Britain in recent years,[301-312] although various inborn errors of metabolism affecting vitamin D metabolism have been more extensively explored here.

One reason for the relative lack of emphasis upon dietary deficiency is presumably the fact that the prevalence of problems is somewhat less in the U.S., particularly in areas of the country with benevolent climates. Indeed, 25 hydroxy-vitamin D levels do appear to be higher among infants and children in the U.S. as whole than they do in the U.K.

A second reason for the inattention to studies of vitamin D deficiency rickets in this country is the lack of a large, easily identifiable group of persons at particular risk. The influx of Pakistani and Asian immigrants in the U.K. coincided nicely with the rise in the prevalence of rickets there, and it was only a matter of time until this group was ascertained as being at high risk.

There is still reason to suspect that there is no cause for complacency. Because of a variety of factors, simple vitamin D deficiency rickets has not been diagnosed or treated with the alacrity its potentially serious sequellae deserve in at least one minority group within the American population — vegetarians.

**Conditioning factors** — Vitamin D deficiency rickets is a nutritional disease heavily conditioned by the microenvironment in which the individual lives. Therefore, each of the various causes that contribute to its expression needs close examination.

### Vitamin D from Dietary Sources

Most foods are exceedingly low in vitamin D unless they are fortified artificially. The most notable exceptions to this general rule are human milk, which provides 2 to 100 IU/$\ell$, unfortified cow's milk, which provides 3 to 50 IU/$\ell$, calf and beef liver, providing 100 to 400 IU/100 g, and egg yolk, providing 100 to 500 IU/100 g. The livers of certain fatty fish, e.g., the cod, also are extraordinarily rich sources of the vitamin as well as of vitamin A. Therefore, with the exception of fish liver oils, food sources are exceedingly poor unless the vitamin is added to them. Even fish liver oils vary greatly in their vitamin D content. Both the variety of the diet and breed of animal may lead to very large variations. On a usual adult mixed diet consisting of unfortified foods, contributions from sources other than fish liver oils rarely exceed 100 IU/day and infants or young childrens' intakes are even lower. It is for this reason that fortification of certain foods in the diet with vitamin D is necessary.

Public health measures to prevent rickets usually involve fortification of one or more staple foods, particularly foods that groups at high risk of rickets are likely to consume. The most commonly fortified foods are milk (400 IU/qt), infant cereals (approximately 100 IU/cup), cod liver oil (which naturally provides varying amounts, but approximately 100 IU/g), margarine (about 60 IU/Tsp), and bread (only in the U.K. and Germany). Since milk is a commonly consumed staple food in this country, consumption of such fortified foods generally assures adequacy of vitamin D nutriture from dietary sources so that the vagaries of climate can be ignored. Fortification of foods has made rickets a rare disease in many countries. For example, during World War II the British distributed a national dried milk containing 700 IU of calciferol per pint if it were reconstituted correctly, and they also provided cod liver oil to infants through clinics. This caused a sharp drop in rickets unti 1960, according to Arneil.[313] Vitamin supplementation at levels of 400 IU/day are recommended for breast-fed infants who may not consume these foods. When neither of these measures is feasible, as is the case in some developing countries, the cheaper but more dangerous method of providing "megadoses" is used. These involve doses of 200,000 IU/6 month. Such large doses are not physiological and may therefore increase the incidence of idiopathic hypercalcemia syndrome amongst some infants.[314]

One of the reasons that other factors have been searched for in attempting to explain the high prevalence of rickets in certain groups is that the correlation between rickets and vitamin D intake has not proven to be close in epidemiological studies. For example, in Great Britain, while children of Indian and Pakistani immigrants had very much lower mean vitamin D intakes than native Caucasian English children, vitamin D intakes among the "Asian" children were not associated with either alkaline phosphatase or other, more pronounced biochemical signs of rickets.[303] A survey of children living in Glasgow, Scotland showed few differences in dietary intakes between native Scots and children of Asian immigrants.[315] A survey of apparent dietary intakes of vitamin D and 25 hydroxy-vitamin D levels among healthy white adults living in London also failed to show significant correlations.[316]

O'Hara-May and Widdowson[317] observed that the diets of Asian children living in England with and without rickets did not differ in that all had high-calcium and low-vitamin D intakes. If exposure to sunlight was minimal, as it was suspected to be in all of the children, the children who developed rickets were postulated as being those with highest vitamin D requirements. Since requirements for vitamin D are not linked to size, these children could not necessarily be identified by anthropometric measurements. Again we see the principle that those whose needs are highest suffer the most.

However, when apparent intakes are so low as to be essentially nil, as was the case in the patient with a 30 IU/day intake studied by Dent,[318] correlations improve.

### Calcium and Phosphorus in the Diet

Total dietary lack of calcium or phosphorus may result in rickets. Human dieters are almost never totally devoid of calcium and phosphorus, however, although they may be devoid of vitamin D. Thus the deficiency disease is most often associated with vitamin D deficiency. Nevertheless, lacks of calcium and phosphorus have been thought by many investigators to contribute to the problem.

Deficient calcium absorption alone has never proved to lead to rickets or osteomalacia, although it is at least theoretically possible in premature infants. Even on virtually calcium-free diet, apparent healing of nutritional rickets resulting from administration of vitamin D alone has been observed.[319] Absorption rates appear to be sufficiently adaptable so that if vitamin D nutriture is assured even on diets very low in calcium, as in many developing countries, rickets does not develop. However, when nutritional status with respect to vitamin D is compromised along with dietary levels of calcium and phosphorus, the risk of rickets appears to be much greater.

Human milk provides approximately 32 mg/100 ml of calcium and 15 mg phosphorus per 100 ml. Cow's milk (undiluted) provides roughly 120 mg calcium and 100 mg phosphorus, and usual formula dilutions approximate half that amount. Thus breast-fed infants are provided with lesser amounts of these nutrients than are bottle-fed infants. Yet if vitamin D is provided in adequate amounts they rarely develop rickets.* Apparently, calcium absorption is exceedingly efficient in the breast-fed infant — more so than it is among bottle-fed infants.

The composition of the diet after weaning may also influence the efficiency of calcium and phosphorus absorption as well as the total amounts of these minerals in the diet. Most items, other than dairy foods (and with the exception of almonds and hazel nuts which are high in both nutrients) in usual American diets are much lower in calcium than is milk, although many items are rich in phosphorus. Red meat, eggs, and cereals are examples. The addition of dried milk and improvers to bread increases the calcium and phosphorus contents of this staple. Hard water also contributes a fair amount of calcium to the diet and soft water about half this amount. Waters of medium hardness usually provide about 5 mg/100 ml, and hard water has been reported to run as high as 11 mg/100 ml. Under conditions of very low-calcium intakes, hard water might make a significant contribution to the calcium content of diet.

The ratio of calcium to phosphate may influence calcium absorption, and ratios between 2:1 and 1:2 are usually suggested. As long as vitamin D intakes are adequate, this seems to have little practical importance. When this is not the case, however, widely variant ratios may also have adverse effects on calcium absorption.

Alterations in protein intakes also affect calcium metabolism. Urinary calcium losses increase when protein intakes are high.

In the U.S. the vast majority of usual calcium intakes come from dairy products. People such as some vegetarians who do not like dairy products therefore usually exhibit lower calcium intakes than the rest of the population. Similar calcium intakes are observed in parts of the world where people subsist on vegetarian diets. However, the protein intakes of American semivegetarians are usually much higher than are those of people in the developing countries of Asia and Africa. It has recently been shown that as protein intakes increase, calcium excretion increases, and it is difficult to overcome losses by use of calcium supplements.[326] On such high-protein, low-calcium diets, risks of osteoporosis may be increased.

### Substances that Chelate or Complex Calcium

Oxalic acid in certain foods and phytic acid in cereals unite with calcium to form insoluble salts. While this is unlikely to be problematic if calcium intakes are suffi-

---

* The recent findings of Lakdawala and Widdowson[411] that a water-soluble form of vitamin D also exists in human milk, suggests that vitamin D intakes of breast-fed infants are higher than was previously supposed, and this also may help to protect against rickets. However, a number of other even more recent reports show that in fact there is no rickets protective effect which is attributable to the substance.

ciently liberal in vegetarian cereal-based diets, the presence of these substances may hinder absorption.

Phytates tend to reduce absorption by binding a certain proportion of dietary calcium in the gut, but it is still unproven that the phytate content of the diet has a richitogenic effect in man. Mellanby's[321] classical study on the effect of phytates involved puppies, not human beings. Species differences with respect to calcium: phosphorus ratios and other factors associated with rickets are known to be considerable, so that it is difficult to assume that this is the case in human beings.

A number of recent studies have investigated the potential of diets high in phytates as contributory to rickets in persons eating vegetarian diets.

Reinhold[322] suggests that in rural areas of Iran the consumption of unleavened bread with high levels of phytates may be important in interfering with calcium absorption from the lumen and that this further compromises an already acute situation with respect to vitamin D. Willis et al.[323] believe that it is possible to cure some cases of rickets observed among immigrants of Pakistani or Indian origin by cutting out the unleavened bread they eat. These immigrants eat chappatis, flat cakes of whole-meal flour made without yeast. Leavening reduces the phytic acid content of the food, but unleavened breads such as chappatis retain their high levels.

Dent et al.[324] studied a 14-year-old English adolescent of Kenyan-Asian origin who had florid rickets and ate a vegan diet providing 30 IU/day of vitamin D with a great deal of chappatis. The omission of chappatis for two 4-day periods during early healing and the use of a white bread substitute allowed calcium and phosphorus intakes to be held virtually constant while testing the theory that the high phytate content of the chappatis altered absorption and led to rickets. In fact no changes in plasma, calcium, or phosphorus or calcium balance were observed. However, if his skin was irradiated daily with UV light even on the high-chappatis diet, healing of the rickets proceeded rapidly. Therefore, the vitamin D provided rather than the presence or absence of phytates appeared to be critical in bringing about cure or causing deficiency. Upon further screening, several adults and sibs in this boy's family were also found to be suffering from minimally active rickets.

Others,[325] however, have tested the chappatis theory and found that upon withdrawal of these breads high in phytate from the diet, serum calcium, phosphate and serum alkaline phosphatase all increased, whereas they decreased upon reintroduction of chappatis. In view of the possible seasonal changes over the course of the study, which raise the possibility of exposure to sufficient UV light to cure the rickets, it is questionable if the effects observed can be attributed to the withdrawal of chappatis. There is also the possibility that dietary vitamin D intakes changed over the course of the study.

*The Physical Environment*

Vitamin D deficiency rickets has long been associated with atmospheric and climatic factors. These include pollution of the atmosphere, which may prevent the penetration of UV rays, high latitudes at which little UV light reaches the earth, and cold climates, which further reduce exposure.

There are two major sources of vitamin D available to human beings. One is diet; it includes fortified foods. The second major source is UV wavelengths of 290 to 320 m$M$ from sunlight. These permit the hydroxylation of 7-dehydrocholesterol in the stratum granulosum of the skin. One in vitro experiment suggested that a square centimeter of Caucasian skin could synthesize 18 IU of vitamin D in 3 hr in sunlight.[326] Therefore, it was assumed that an adult with 1.5 m² of surface area exposed to the sun would synthetize 800,000 IU in 6 hr if exposed to UV wavelengths of 290 to 320 m$M$.

Since sunlight stimulates the endogenous production of the vitamin, it can be seen that only very rarely, in the absence of metabolic disease, is it likely that environmental factors will coincide so as to produce rickets. Although the potential for such synthesis is enormous, several factors may interfere with it.

The first is insufficient exposure to UV light. Rickets have frequently been reported even in tropical environments among infants who were heavily swaddled or otherwise prevented from being exposed to sunlight.

Second, smoke, dust, or other atmospheric factors may exert a powerful filtering action. For example, at 40° north latitude or higher, when the winter sun is less than 20° above the horizon, most of the needed UV radiation is filtered out by the atmosphere through which the slanting rays of the sun have to pass.[328] London and Glasgow are even more northerly than this. Most of the continental U.S. is at 40° north or less, so that one would expect conditions for the development of rickets to be more suitable in Northern Europe and the U.K. At the same latitude one might expect a greater prevalence of rickets in heavily polluted atmospheres, particularly those polluted with $SO_2$, since this chemical is associated with decreased UV light penetration.

A third interfering factor is the barrier provided by a heavily pigmented or keratinized stratum corneum, as is the case with negro skin.[328] Thus even in Nigeria rickets have been reported, as Oke has demonstrated.[329,336]

It is therefore puzzling that only one report of nutritional rickets in Great Britain involves the very dark-skinned West Indians,[302] while many reports indicate greatly elevated prevalence of the disorder in lighter Hindu persons of Gujarati origin from Pakistan or India. The differences in apparent prevalence are probably due to the fact that West Indians are rarely vegetarians while the Hindu subjects are virtually all vegetarians. Differences in exposure to sunlight are also possible, of course, but in view of the fact that the transmission of UV light to the deeper layers of the epidermis is theoretically most compromised in Negroes, one would expect the West Indians to be at a disadvantage unless dietary intakes of vitamin D differed. However, traditional clothing covering the limbs completely and the habit of avoiding direct sunlight may deprive the Asians of exposure to UV light more than does the dark skin of the West Indians.

A fourth factor that interferes with the endogenous synthesis of vitamin D is a cold climate, which reduces exposure of the skin to UV rays. Seasonal variations in the incidence of rickets in Great Britain has long been reported.[331-333] At the turn of the century, Schmorl[334] also reported the same thing in Germany. Gupta et al.[333] recently assessed signs of "biochemical rickets" (serum calcium, phosphorus, and 25-hydroxy-vitamin D) in 21 Indian vegetarians living in Great Britain. Assays were carried out in the spring (the month of April) and in the fall (early October). A striking tendency toward hypocalcemia was observed in the early spring. By the fall, a spontaneous rise in plasma 25-hydroxy-vitamin D had occurred. A control group of healthy, Caucasian, nonvegetarians living in the same environment showed no such changes.

It appears that subclinical vitamin D deficiency among these subjects, as indicated by hypocalcemia and in some cases by raised alkaline phosphatase levels, resolved itself spontaneously during the summer months. Thus one can expect sharp seasonal variations in vitamin D nutritional status in vegetarians and nonvegetarians alike. However, it was[333] also found that the vegetarians maintained much lower levels of 25-hydroxy-vitamin D throughout the study and that serum values seemed to rise less sharply, suggesting that inadequate bodily exposure to summer sunlight or some other factor may also be involved. They explain the presence of hypocalcemia in the spring in these subjects as being due to a relative vitamin D deficiency severe enough to become the limiting factor in maintaining normal plasma calcium levels. In contrast, when vitamin D nutriture is not compromised there is little correlation between 25-hydroxy-vitamin D and serum calcium levels.

In assessing vitamin D nutriture in vegetarian subjects, it is therefore important to take the time of year into account. Patients who appear perfectly normal in the fall after a summer of exposure to sunshine may show relative vitamin D deficiency at the end of the winter.

### The Sociocultural Environment

We must consider the sociocultural microenvironment, which may act in concert with factors already mentioned to produce rickets.[335] It has usually been assumed that rickets is exceedingly rare in the tropics and other warm climates. In Greek rural areas, however, the prevalence of rickets reaches as high as 15% under 1 year of age.[336] It is also high in some Moslem countries in the Mediterranean area where women and infants rarely go out of doors without heavy clothing.[314]

### Clinical Picture in Rickets

The clinical signs and symptoms of rickets are several. In the early states of the disease the child may be weak and apathetic. Some of the diagnostic clinical signs are craniotabes with softening of the occiput, the rachitic rosary due to enlargement of the costochondral junction and beading of the ribs, and Harrison's groove (an indentation of the lower ribs at the site of attachment of the diaphragm). With continued disease, abnormal curvatures of the spine (scoliosis and/or thoracolumnar kyphosis) may develop. Angular deformities due to enlargement at the ends of the long bones of the extremities with standing or walking may result in genu varum (bowed legs) or, more rarely, genu valgum (knock knees). If the deficiency is long-standing, general growth is retarded and the child develops short structure. Such children may also be particularly susceptible to fractures. Dental development may be slow and abnormal. In extreme cases, hypocalcemia tetany may occur.

Our group in Boston has just completed a review of the nutritional status of some 30 infants and children adhering to macrobiotic type vegan diets.[337] Residual bowing of the legs was present in one subject, four subjects' parents revealed a history of bowed legs that reversed after administration of cod liver oil, and one child showed radiographic evidence of rickets. Three other children were reported to show florid rickets confirmed by radiographs at earlier times in their lives by a colleague who was the personal physician to many of these subjects.

### Theories on the Physiology and Biochemistry of Rickets

A three-stage progression of human rickets is generally accepted. The vitamin D deficiency is first seen to produce hypocalcemia. This leads to the development of a reactive hypoparathyroidism, which in turn leads to hyperphosphaturia and hypophosphatemia. Finally, bone rickets become evident along with the accompanying chemical signs of hypocalcemia, hyperphosphaturia, and hypophosphatemia.[338-340]

Bronner[341] has recently proposed that human nutritional rickets is the result of a nutritional vitamin D deficiency that aggravates the expression of a preexisting metabolic defect in phosphate transport. That is, he regards vitamin D deficiency and rickets not to be similar, although on histological, clinical, and dietary grounds many might object to his interpretation. He claims that simple, nutritional vitamin D deficiency unaccompanied by rickets may occur but that it has probably always been rare.

According to Bronner, three possible situations may occur in children:

1.  Simple deficiency in vitamin D resulting from either a nutritional deficiency or a metabolic defect leading to deficient production of the active vitamin D metabolite.
2.  A phosphate deficiency, either nutritional in origin or resulting from a defect in phosphate metabolism.

3.   A combination of both deficiencies, a double efficiency, resulting from human nutritional rickets.

Since low intakes of phosphorus are rare, Bronner suggests that children exhibiting clinical rickets have both low intakes of vitamin D and some defect in phosphate transport either in the kidney or intestine. Owing to the environmentally induced vitamin D deficiency, this defect would be symptomatic. Industrial smoke pollution filtering out UV rays, child rearing practices involving infrequent exposure to the sunlight, use of clothing preventing exposure to UV light of any portion of the body, poor dietary practices, and prolonged breast feeding by relatively poorly nourished mothers are all environmental factors that might contribute to the problem, according to Bronner. His theories have not yet been confirmed.

It remains to be seen whether the pathophysiology of human rickets arises simply from a vitamin D deficiency as Frazer et al.[338] propose or whether preexisting defects in phosphate transport predispose the infant to react in this way to a vitamin D deficiency as Bronner suggests.[341]

One might synthesize the two theories and propose that nutritional rickets be classified as those exhibiting both vitamin D deficiency and calcium deprivation in the diet (i.e., a calciopenia) as opposed to those exhibiting vitamin D deficiency and phosphate transportation defects (phosphopenia). Until such notions are demonstrated clinically, the most parsimonious explanation for rickets remains a simple, single deficiency of vitamin D.

### Risks of Vitamin D Deficiency Rickets in Various Groups

**Infants born of vegetarian mothers** — The infants of vegan-vegetarian Asian mothers living in Asia apparently are subject to a high incidence of neonatal hypocalcemia. Temporary immaturity of the parathyroid glands in the newborn, especially if the infant is premature, may be responsible for the condition. It may also be due to high dietary phosphate intakes if the infant is given cow's milk formula.[343] Similar findings of neonatal hypocalcemia have been reported by Rosen et al.[344] among nonvegetarian Negro- and Puerto Rican-American infants. In vegetarians the condition is precipitated by the mothers' exceedingly low vitamin D dietary intakes.[345] Transfer of 25-hydroxyvitamin D is good across the placenta, with infant hormones approximating 87% of maternal levels. Thus only if maternal levels are very low is neonatal vitamin D deficiency likely to be a problem.[346,347]

**Children of vegetarian parents** — Roughly 100 IU (2.5 μg) of vitamin D prevents rickets and assures adequate absorption of calcium in the gut, satisfactory growth, and normal mineralization of bone in infants. At a level of 300 to 400 IU (7.5 to 10 μg), however, calcium absorption and slightly increased growth velocities are apparent. These levels are recommended, taken either through diet or vitamin supplement.

Greece is an unlikely location for vitamin D deficiency rickets, yet several cases have recently been reported,[336] seemingly due to low dietary intakes and insufficient exposure of the infants to sunlight.

Vegan parents usually (but not always) feed their children a diet similar to their own. Therefore, vegan and vegetarian children may run special risks from the dietary standpoint with respect to vitamin D. In contrast, in omnivore American children vitamin D deficiency rickets is an exceedingly rare disease for which the cure is known, easily available, and inexpensive. The Preschool Nutrition Survey of 1968 to 1970[260] exhibited exceedingly low prevalence rates of signs suggestive of rickets upon physical examination. Out of 2118 children examined, 5% exhibited bossing of the skull, less than 1% had pot bellies, less than 0.2% (5 children) exhibited epiphyseal swelling at the wrists, and less than 0.1% (2 children) exhibited beading of the ribs. In view of the nonspecificity of these signs and the lack of radiographic or biochemical confirmation of rickets, it seems that the prevalence was exceedingly low if present at all. Similarly, the Ten-State Nutrition Survey of 1969 and 1970 found little evidence of either florid or subclinical vitamin D deficiency rickets,[261] although some cases were evident among omnivores.

Over a decade ago, Scottish and British workers noted that the incidence of child-hood rickets was on the increase, chiefly among the children of immigrants to Scotland from Pakistan, India, and Asian countries.[309-318,348,349] These children subsisted on largely vegetarian or vegan diets and failed to use vitamin D-fortified foods. Owing perhaps to the unfamiliarity of the signs and symptoms of florid rickets, the rareness of classical deformity, and the failure to use the radiological and biochemical tests necessary to diagnose subclinical or minimally active rickets (which is far more com-mon), many cases went unrecognized.

Subsequent careful investigations that included plasma assays of 25-hydroxy-vitamin D[350] revealed that dietary vitamin D intakes were exceedingly low (e.g., <50 IU) in about one third of Asian children in English and Scottish cities, although not all of these children developed rickets. Low dietary intakes and low 25-hydroxycorticosterol levels were particularly common in the winter and spring.[333] These were not confined to infants and toddler-aged children but persisted into adolescence.[351] Low prevalence rates were found in Chinese and African children living in these same locales. In com-parison, relatively higher prevalences of both florid and subclinical rickets were evident in Pakistani and Indian children.[302] This finding argued against the hypothesis that the skin pigment of these noncaucasian groups impaired conversion of 7-dehydrocho-lesterol to vitamin $D_3$ and suggested that some environmental factor associated with diet that increased risks might be involved. Indeed, the group with the highest intakes of phytates, substances that might bind calcium, were the very ones having the highest prevalence of rickets.[325] Others[352,353] suggested that making ghee might destroy what vitamin D was present in butterfat and that this is what led to the particular predispo-sition to rickets among the Pakistanis.

Milk was not fortified in Canada in the mid-1960s. Very much higher rates of rickets were reported in the 1960s than in the U.S.[354] For example, 100 cases were admitted to the Montreal Sick Childrens' Hospital[355] in a year's time in 1965 and 1966. Later surveys in Canada also indicated that 30% of infants and children were receiving less than the usual recommended levels of 400 IU/day.[356] These low intakes were appar-ently due to failure to use supplements rather than to vegan or vegetarian dietary hab-its. Fortunately, since the more widespread use of vitamin D supplements and fortifi-cation, this situation has been remedied in Canada.

Recent evidence amassed by our group suggests that the prevalence of rickets in at least one group of vegan-vegetarians living in the Boston area is exceedingly high.[337] Other workers in the U.S.[32,33] have recently reported vitamin D deficiency rickets in infants subsisting on diets devoid of fortified foods, and rickets of this type were re-ported in Boston prior to the advent of fortified foods and the widespread use of supplements.

How is it that such cases are missed by our sophisticated medical care system? There are probably several reasons. These include the low prevalence of such unusual dietary habits, the fact that the parents of these children are perhaps somewhat less likely to seek medical care than omnivore parents, the enormous number of care providers, the unfamiliarity of many providers with the disorder except in its most acute forms, and the confidential relationship that exists between physician and patient that may inhibit publication of findings, and the ease with which parents can treat the illness them-selves. All of these factors have led to failure to ascertain or report such cases when present.

In the light of these relationships, we will consider the possible factors possibly predisposing vegan children to rickets in our own population. Unfortunately, dietary data are incomplete for subjects who were breast fed in our study, since the volume of breast milk secreted was not recorded. Complete dietary analysis of supplementary foods given is available, however. For the macrobiotics with essentially vegan patterns of food intake, vitamin D intakes over and above that supplied by the breast milk they drank were essentially nil.

Among vegan macrobiotic subjects over a year of age, dietary calcium intakes were approximately 430 mg/day; in the other vegetarian they were 471 mg/day, as opposed to the recommended daily allowance of 800 mg. The contribution of plant foods, especially cereals, to total calories was high. The calcium:phosphorus ratio was 0.9:1.0 for the vegan macrobiotic subjects and 0.6:1.0 for the other subjects. Protein intakes were low in comparison to usual children of this age but approximated the recommended dietary allowances. However, vitamin D from dietary sources was exceedingly low, e.g., <40 IU in the vegan macrobiotics, and 270 IU for the other vegetarians.

Clearly, if calcium absorption rates rose, even on these diets fairly low in calcium, one would not anticipate the development of rickets. The exceedingly low intakes of vitamin D rather than dietary lacks of calcium or phosphorus, protein, or distorted calcium:phosphorus ratios apparently predispose the macrobiotics to rickets, particularly after weaning when the contribution of the Vitamin D in breast milk is lost.[412]

In view of the fact that clear clinical and radiologic evidence of florid rickets is corroborated by dietary history in a number of these children, histories of cure with cod liver oil in others, and confirmatory radiologic evidence in still others, there is little doubt that the three cases of rickets seen were due to vitamin D deficiency. It is puzzling that these subjects did not obtain sufficient vitamin D from the sunlight during the summer. This is partially explained by the practice of at least some subjects of bundling infants up with clothing even in the summer months.

Adolescents — The precise requirement for vitamin D in older children and adolescents is unknown. Therefore it is usually recommended that they consume at least 400 IU from dietary sources. The recent reports from London of both florid rickets and minimally active rickets in vegan-vegetarian Indian and Pakistani immigrant children suggest that at least some dietary sources of vitamin D are necessary at this time of life and that supplements should be provided if dietary sources are lacking.

The study of Birmingham, England adolescents showed that of 569 adolescents in various ethnic groups surveyed, 51 (8%) showed signs of rickets; 47 had radiological evidence; 4 had marked genu valgum, with bone biopsy showing excess osteoid tissue.[357] Of the 51 adolescents, 15 were vegetarians. These children were also exceedingly short, their heights falling between the 10th and 25th percentiles. Birmingham has fewer hours of sunlight than many other English cities, including London, and at least in summer, Glasgow.

This investigation was contrasted to that done in the London area by Round[358] on the heights and weights of adolescents. The Birmingham children's heights were no different at 14 years of age but were shorter at both 15 and 16 years.

Another report by Cooke et al.[351] showed that calciferol therapy administered for a year to Caucasian, Asian, and West Indian school children resulted in a highly significant increase in both height and weight when compared with school children who were not treated. Mean dietary intakes were less than 100 IU, which is the usual amount provided by mixed dietary sources in Great Britain. Levels of 25-hydroxy-vitamin D were low (e.g., less than 3.8 $\mu$g/m$\ell$) in 40% of those studied, most of these low values being Asian children subsisting on vegan-vegetarian diets. Mean calcium levels for the groups as a whole were 780 mg. Phytate levels showed a mean of 160 mg but averaged 230 mg for Asians, as opposed to 85 mg for West Indians and whites. Except for biochemical signs of rickets, the children appeared to be well nourished.

Also interesting was the fact that the rickets or relative vitamin D deficiencies seemed to be cured when the physiological growth spurt came to an end.[351] In untreated children, however, height and weight were lessened by 3 cm and 3 kg, respectively.

These studies suggest that, at least in England, the prevalence of biochemical rickets in school children and adolescents is high, particularly in vegetarian Asians.[359,360] Supplements need to be provided, especially around the period of the adolescent growth spurt. For American vegan children approaching adolescence, especially those who live in cold climates, similar precautions may be advisable.

**The risk of osteomalacia during pregnancy on vegan-vegetarian diets** — The nonpregnant, nonlactating adult female is assumed to require roughly 70 to 100 IU of vitamin D per day. During pregnancy and lactation 400 IU are recommended, although they are not for other adults. This is based upon the assumption that vitamin D requirements may rise during pregnancy.

Dent and Gupta[346] studied 25-hydroxy-vitamin D levels in pregnant Caucasian omnivores, Hindu vegetarian immigrants, and Hindu nonvegetarian immigrants living in England. The vegetarian group exhibited the lowest levels throughout pregnancy.

The failure to observe decreases in plasma 25-hydroxy-vitamin D levels over the course of the pregnancy even among the vegetarian women disproved the hypothesis that pregnancy increases the vitamin D requirement and therefore predisposed to osteomalacia. Rather, it appears that florid osteomalacia is precipitated in pregnancy only when both dietary levels of vitamin D and serum levels of 25-hydroxy-vitamin D are exceedingly low, and when this is coupled with extremely low intakes of calcium or a series of recent pregnancies that place a drain on the women's nutrient stores in many respects. Such conditions apparently applied in classical studies of severe osteomalacia and resulting pelvic deformities in the 1920s in China. Asians living in Asia do indeed have much lower dietary intakes of vitamin D.[362] Reports such as that from a study of Indian vegetarians living in Delhi do suggest that the incidence of osteomalacia is high, and that in many it first became evident during pregnancy.[362]

Various workers have studied the Bedouins of the Negev desert in Israel. Some years ago it was suggested that the low-calcium and high-phytate content of their diets might be causative of the osteomalacia observed.[363,364] More recent work[365] suggests that while 25-HCC levels are low today among pregnant women, they are not indicative of a deficiency of vitamin D, and little osteomalacia is now seen. Apparently, changes in social customs have resulted in women being exposed to more sunlight than before, and thus risks of osteomalacia are lessened, although other aspects of diet do not appear to have changed.

Another recent study described the effects of maternal malnutrition on bone density of neonates in Indian mothers.[366] The poverty-group mothers were vegetarians, consuming 40 g of protein (mostly from vegetable sources), 1600 to 1800 cal, 200 mg of calcium, 60 to 70 g of protein, and 700 to 800 mg of calcium per day. Radiodensities of mother's and neonates' bones were lower in the poor groups, and birth weights were also lower, although prematurity was not reported.

### Other Forms of Rickets

The prevalence of environmentally caused rickets and osteomalacia was so high early in this century that it was not until the late 1930s that various hereditary and metabolic bone diseases that resulted in rickets became apparent. In the 1930s Albright et al.[367] published the now classic paper on rickets that were refractory to treatment with the relatively small doses of vitamin D considered necessary to prevent nutritional rickets (e.g., 40 to 100 IU or 1.0 to 2.5 $\mu$g) of vitamin $D_2$, ergo-calciferol, or vitamin $D_3$, cholecalciferol. Since that time it has become apparent that clinical rickets can result from many causes that lead to a defect in calcium and phosphorus metabolism.

For example, rickets may be secondary to:

1. One of the fat malabsorption syndromes.
2. Congenital lack of enzymes required to transform vitamin D into an active form.
3. Interference with such conversion by administration of antagonistic agents, such as some anticonvulsants.
4. Defective renal function leading to losses of phosphorus.
5. Osteodystrophy associated with chronic renal insufficiency.
6. A variety of other possible disease states.

In view of this wide range of possible explanations for these characteristic changes in the bony skeleton and the relative rareness of the simple vitamin deficiency causing the disorder, elaborate and costly differential diagnosis may be necessary before the cause of the problem can become apparent.

More recently Scriver[368] proposed that one might classify all of the various causes of rickets refractory to vitamin D into those which are calciopenic and phosphopenic in nature by examining their fundamental aberrant processes, and by so doing the rationale for preferring one mode of treatment over another might be made more clear. Fraser and Scriver have further developed this concept in a subsequent communication.[369]

## Vitamin A

The Ten-State Nutrition Survey revealed a high prevalence of persons under 16 years of age with low-plasma vitamin A levels, and dietary data also suggested low intakes. Vegetarians usually have higher intakes of carotenes and lower intakes of preformed vitamin A due to their dietary patterns. Studies have seldom revealed blood chemistries indicative of deficiency. However, a recent report of a macrobiotic adult who presented in hospital with severe xerophthalmia and soon died[370] suggests that lack of variety of foods as well as protein-caloric malnutrition may, in extreme cases, cause additional dietary problems such as this one. Fortunately, xerophthalmia has never been reported among vegetarian-vegan children in the U.S.

Recent work in developing countries with malnourished children[371] indicates that ability to mobilize and transport vitamin A from the liver may be compromised in under- or malnutrition. Cases appear in some developing countries in the 3rd and 4th years of life. For example, among children in Indonesia and India on rice staple diets low in vitamin A, xerophthalmia is often precipitated by a series of infectious diseases and protein-calorie malnutrition. Marasmic infants in India, the Middle East, and Asia often develop xeropthalmia even earlier on in life.[372, 373]

## Vitamin $B_{12}$

Nutriture with respect to vitamin $B_{12}$ is of interest, particularly among the vegans, because of their animal food devoid diets.

Vitamin $B_{12}$ is ultimately of bacterial origin, although man obtains most of his vitamin $B_{12}$ indirectly from animal sources such as meat, milk, eggs, and fish. Ruminants have $B_{12}$ synthesizing bacteria in their rumens, and it is synthesized if the diet contains cobalt. Fish eat plankton rich in the vitamin. Chicken must obtain preformed $B_{12}$ in their diets, which is transferred to flesh or eggs. Plant foods and even drinking water sometimes contain assayable $B_{12}$. This usually represents contamination from soil bacteria.

Seaweeds of certain types are believed by certain vegetarians, particularly macrobiotics, to be rich in vitamin $B_{12}$ and to obviate the necessity of animal food intake. This belief is based on the fact that some seaweeds have assayable vitamin $B_{12}$, due to their contamination with plankton.[396,397] Unfortunately, the samples vary greatly, and in any event the amount present is relatively slight. Therefore, seaweed cannot be considered a substitute for a reliable source of vitamin $B_{12}$.

Omnivores, especially those eating diets high in animal protein, consume up to 100 $\mu$g of the vitamin per day and have sufficient stores to meet the body's requirement for 3 to 5 years.[374] Vegetarians consume much less (0.3 to 0.4 $\mu$g), the amount depending upon the dietary proscriptions imposed, and have much smaller stores. If dietary supplies of the vitamin are unavailable, overt deficiency may develop within a few weeks or months. The 0.3 to 0.4 $\mu$g usually present are enough to maintain health, although not enough to keep stores at optimal levels. However, such intakes are virtually impossible to obtain on vegan diets unless they are supplemented.

It is well known that the Indian Hindus who adhere to a lactovegetarian diet frequently exhibit lowered serum $B_{12}$ levels[375,376] and that megaloblastic anemia and early neurological complications of dietary $B_{12}$ deficiency have been observed among Hindu immigrants to Great Britain.[377,378] It is not surprising that similar findings might occur among other persons adhering to such diets.[379]

Vegans sometimes develop complications of vitamin $B_{12}$ deficiency after continued adherence to these diets. Because most of them eat very high amounts of fruits and vegetables, folic acid nutriture is likely to be good, and the megaloblastic anemia characteristic of $B_{12}$ deficiency is therefore masked. While serum $B_{12}$ levels are usually diagnostic, the test is not available in most hospitals and must be specially ordered. Therefore, the first indication may come from a carefully taken dietary history rather than clinical examination. A number of workers have recently reported complications of vitamin $B_{12}$ deficiency in British vegans.[378-382] What is particularly unsettling about the cases Gleeson and Graves[382] reported is that the complications were not ascertained as being linked with the nutritional disorder until after almost 2 years of highly specialized medical care when someone thought to take a dietary history, and veganism of some 10 years or more standing was revealed. Subsequent $B_{12}$ therapy reversed these findings.

Dastur et al.[383] recently reported several cases of a neuromyelopathy among lactovegetarians living in Bombay, India. The vitamin $B_{12}$ deficiency was associated with similar lacks of riboflavin and pyridoxine, but with elevated serum folate levels. Folate levels fell upon treatment, consistent with the hypothesis that "methyl/tetra hydro folate trap" existed, which was remedied by supplying vitamin $B_{12}$.

Folic acid deficiency is rare among vegetarians because of the fact that most of them eat large amounts of fresh, green vegetables and other foods high in the vitamin. The only group that might conceivably be at risk in this respect would be edentulous elderly persons who adopt a vegetarian diet but use cooked foods that are softer and easier to eat. Folic acid toxicity is also rare, in spite of the fact that some vegetarians indulge in megadose supplementation.

The reason for concern about folic acid nutriture among vegetarians chiefly involves its interrelationship with vitamin $B_{12}$ metabolism. Therapeutic doses of folic acid or, conceivably, the very high intakes of the vitamin among vegetarians cause remission of the hematopoetic signs of vitamin $B_{12}$ deficiency. Since dietary vitamin $B_{12}$ deficiency may occur amongst vegans, the megaloblastic anemia may thus be masked. However, only administration of vitamin $B_{12}$ prevents or relieves the neurological manifestations of the deficiency, and these may continue to progress even in the absence of the characteristic anemia if dietary folate levels are high. Since the most commonly used clinical diagnostic sign of vitamin $B_{12}$ deficiency is the anemia, cases may be overlooked among vegans. Therefore, routine assay of serum $B_{12}$ is suggested for vegans to ascertain vitamin $B_{12}$ nutriture.

Fortunately, at least in adults, serum vitamin $B_{12}$ values among vegans have not proven to be as low as many investigators expected.[384,385] Among adults, dietary $B_{12}$ deficiency usually develops among those on very strict vegan diets. Yet the largely vegetarian diet consumed by persons in many parts of India still contains enough of the vitamin to meet the body's needs. One possible reason is the high level of contamination of food and water supplies in that country with soil microorganisms. In the U.S., which provides a more protected environment, such contamination is much less likely, and perhaps greater caution on similar diets is warranted in this regard. Pregnant women are of particular risk,[386] but stores of folic acid and vitamin $B_{12}$ are present in human fetal livers at term. These stores serve to cushion the infant against the dietary changes of early life.[387]

Infants born of vitamin $B_{12}$-deficient mothers start life with low-body stores. If they are breast fed by the same mother, they will not be able to make up for the antenatal deficiency and develop signs and symptoms of $B_{12}$ deficiency between 8 and 18 months.[388] These signs include developmental regression and tremors of limbs, head, and trunk, with ultimate coma and death in extreme cases.

Lampkin and Saunders[389] provide an alarming case report of dietary vitamin $B_{12}$ deficiency of a 10-month-old Caucasian infant whose mother was a Seventh-Day Adventist and had adhered to a vegan type diet for 12 years. The mother had seven pregnancies, three carried to term, of which this infant was the last. While she had taken multivitamins providing 1 $\mu$g of vitamin $B_{12}$ per capsule during her pregnancies, neither she nor the infant received any nutrient supplements after birth. Pernicious anemia and intestinal malabsorption of vitamin $B_{12}$ were ruled out, and the infant responded well to a therapeutic dose of vitamin $B_{12}$. Apparently the mother's breast milk was low in vitamin $B_{12}$ due to decreased oral intakes of the nutrient. This emphasizes the importance of administration of exogenous vitamin $B_{12}$ to infants breast fed by mothers who are vegan-vegetarians.

Obviously, vitamin $B_{12}$ supplementation is a simple prophylactic to the problem if only such vegans can be induced to comply. An alternative to vitamin $B_{12}$ tablets is food fortified with the vitamin as long as these are acceptable and available. Supplementation of vegan diets with vitamin $B_{12}$ reverses low serum $B_{12}$ levels, while untreated vegans continue to have subnormal serum $B_{12}$ levels.[390]

Among American vegan groups, macrobiotics are the group most likely to be heavy smokers. The combination of smoking and veganism may affect vitamin $B_{12}$ metabolism.[391] Dastur et al.[392] found that both smoking and vegetarianism affected the type and distribution of the forms of vitamin $B_{12}$ appearing in the body.

Gleeson and Graves[382] suggest that optic atrophy associated with dietary vitamin $B_{12}$ deficiency due to veganism might be associated with the fact that low vitamin $B_{12}$ levels may predispose to cyanide neurotoxicity. Hydroxocobalamin is required for the detoxification of cyanide,[393] and the metabolism and excretion of vitamin $B_{12}$ is affected by tobacco smoking.[391,395] This matter is of some practical importance since many macrobiotics who exist on essentially vegan diets are heavy smokers, and thus they may be at special risk of cyanide neurotoxicity.

## HEALTH PROBLEMS OBSERVED WITH INCREASED FREQUENCY AMONG PERSONS ADHERING TO OTHER TYPES OF ALTERNATIVE LIFE-STYLE DIETS

### Use of Homeopathic Remedies

Virtually all of the studies of persons using alternative life-style diets reveal a heavy reliance on the special preventive and curative properties of certain foods or nutrients. The particular substances used vary from herbal teas and seaweed to large doses of vitamins and mineral supplements. The major difference between the more deviant beliefs in this respect and those of omnivores is the extraordinary efficacy that some alternative dieters regard these substances as having, and the enormous range of diseases (including, in some cases, cancer, diabetes, brain damage, and heart disease) that they believe can be cured by such use. They may persist in the use of homeopathic remedies until illness is severe and seek treatment in late rather than early stages of illness.[45,59,63,112,113,398,399] Such generalizations are appropriate for alternative dieters in general, but again, various types and subgroups among them probably vary greatly. Thus it is important to ascertain attitudes toward the use of homeopathic remedies on an individual basis if one is attempting to deal with such patients.

## Inappropriate Use of Vitamin Supplements and "Health" Foods
### Inappropriate Vitamin Mineral Supplements

For some alternative life-style dieters whose philosophical or religious beliefs proscribe the consumption of animal foods or other groups of foods, judiciously prescribed vitamin-mineral supplements may be helpful. Self prescribed use of vitamin-mineral supplements is unlikely to serve as an effective prophylactic against real risks of nutrient lacks, however, and may further engender a sense of false security that gets in the way of seeking health care advice. Multivitamin capsules sold over-the-counter that such persons would be likely to obtain on their own provide superfluous amounts of some nutrients and insufficient amounts of others. The risks ensuing from these dietary patterns involve specific nutrients, and medical advice on choice of supplement is mandatory since patients may not purchase the correct types of supplements without direction.

### Failure to Use Prophylactic Supplements

Persons adhering to other alternative life-style dietary patterns may fall into difficulty because they fail to use supplements that are usually prescribed at certain periods of life or for physiological conditions such as pregnancy or prematurity. Premature infants have increased needs for a number of nutrients, as well as metabolic difficulties that make it necessary to design diets particularly suitable for their needs. The younger and lighter the exterogestate fetus is, the more nutritional adjustments are likely. If the parents' alternative life-style dietary philosophy rules out the use of such special measures, infant health status may be severely compromised.

It has long been pediatric practice to prescribe vitamin D on a prophylactic basis for breast-fed infants or those being fed nonfortified milk formulas. Failure of vegans to use such supplements increases risks of vitamin D deficiency rickets. It is usual to prescribe iron supplements or an iron-fortified formula after 4 months of life, since dietary intakes are generally not sufficient to meet the iron needs of young infants. Persons whose philosophies are such that they will not administer such supplements run higher risks of their infants developing iron deficiency anemia. These risks are sizeably increased — probably doubled — if infants and young children adhere to vegan or vegetarian diets, as well-absorbed sources of iron from animal foods such as red meat are not eaten. Also, the high phytate content of the diet may lead to binding of iron, rendering what little iron present less absorbable. Therefore, iron supplementation should be strongly encouraged if full-blown iron deficiency anemia is to be avoided.

A similar situation exists among pregnant women. They are routinely prescribed iron supplements to compensate for the increased drain on iron stores due to the growing fetus.

It is only good preventive medicine to prescribe vitamin $B_{12}$ supplements to persons whose diets include no animal protein. If for some reason the patient refuses to take the supplement, risks of megaloblastic anemia and irreversible neurologic sequelae are increased.

## Megadose Use and Its Associated Risks

Health food users and other alternative dieters who use very large doses of vitamin-mineral supplements are subject to risks associated with toxicities of these substances. The use of vitamin-mineral supplements has been widespread in the U.S. for many years. In 1973, American spent over $600 million on over-the-counter products of this sort.[397,398] A national survey of a representative sample of the population in 1972 revealed that 22% were currently taking them and 50% of the respondents had, at some time in their lives, taken vitamin mineral supplements.[63]

Information on the regularity with which these supplements are used and the doses employed is more difficult to come by. The widespread popularity of books advocating megadoses of vitamins, the rapid growth of the health food industry, the fact that many proponents of these products and health food consumers advocate megavitamin use;[51,60] and the increased popularity of other alternative life-style diets involving vegetarian, natural/organic, or health food use all suggest that a growing proportion of persons are indulging in these practices and that at least some of them may be using large doses on a regular basis.

Since alternative diet patterns encompass a whole variety of different eating styles; it is difficult to generalize. The majority of health food users have been reported to use large doses of vitamin-mineral supplements.[4,5,8] Yet vegetarians and natural food users are apparently much less homogeneous in their self-prescribed usage patterns of these substances.

For purposes of this review, nutrient supplement users have been defined as persons who use vitamin, mineral, or nutrient supplements under their own volition. "Megadose" users are operationally defined as those who take a vitamin-mineral preparation that supplies approximately five times the recommended dietary allowance *in toto* on a daily basis.

Alternative dieters who do indulge in megadose use are subject to all of the risks that such use might engender in omnivore subjects. We will consider only the most potentially dangerous megadose use, that of high doses of vitamins D and A, and the currently popular use of ascorbic acid.

## Hypervitaminosis D

There is a maximum over which increasing the amount of vitamin D provided will have no effect in increasing calcium absorption from the gut. Very large doses of vitamin D result in increased bone resorption and increased intestinal absorption, which in turn leads to hypercalcemia, increased renal excretion, and the possibility of kidney stones.

Clinical signs of toxicity may include anorexia, constipation and vomiting, polydypsia and polyuria; muscular hypotonia, and bradycardia with cardiac arrythmia. With continued hypercalcemia, metastatic calcifications appear in the soft tissues, especially the kidney, leading to nephrocalcinosis and irreversible renal tubular damage if the insult is long continued. This potentially irreversible kidney damage is the most serious effect of megadoses.

Toxicities have been reported in adults upon chronic administration of doses of 100,000 IU/day, or 1,000 to 3,000 IU/kg. This would be equivalent to a dose of 10,000 to 30,000 IU/day for a 12-month-old infant by extrapolation on a per-kilogram basis. Effects on growth or other suggestive signs have been reported at even lower levels, however. For example, Arneil[302a] reported an increased incidence of hypercalcemia amongst children receiving more than 4000 IU/day from dietary sources in England, where fortification levels of a number of foods are exceedingly high.

The syndrome of idiopathic hypercalcemia in infants involving some of the symptoms of vitamin D toxicity described above and sometimes coupled with mental retardation and osteosclerosis received much attention a decade ago, particularly in Great Britain, where levels of vitamin D available from fortified foods are high.[400] Owing to an inborn error of metabolism some infants within the population are extraordinarily sensitive to the vitamin, as Frazer suggests.[340] Other normal infants ingested toxic levels of the vitamin, owing to overly ambitious food fortification schemes and maternal vitamin dosing.

Vitamin D toxicity is difficult to treat. The first step is to withdraw the vitamin to reduce calcium intakes and to dehydrate the patient if necessary. Prednisone has been used by some workers to block the intestinal action of vitamin D. Other treatments, such as the intravenous or intramuscular administration of diphosphate to correct the hypercalcemia are still in trial stages.

Prevention of vitamin D toxicity is the first aim with alternative dieters who are potentially susceptible to such misuse. Toxicity from usual diet alone is exceedingly rare in this country. Perhaps somewhat more common in infants and children than adults, yet presenting a potential health problem of some magnitude for both groups, is the oversupplementation of diet with cod liver oil or more purified sources of vitamin D. Since the manifestations of hypercalcemia may develop in utero, excessive vitamin D intakes should also be avoided by pregnant women. This unfortunate problem usually results from good intentions upon the part of the mother or caretaker, it being assumed that if some is good, more is better. Owing to the widespread use of vitamin D-fortified foods in the U.S., pediatricians rarely prescribe vitamin D supplements. They are not a common homeopathic remedy except among a small proportion of the population. It is only the most dedicated vitamin-mineral megadose users and the uninformed who overuse this particular vitamin today.

If a patient is known to be using megadoses (e.g., doses ranging from 5 to 10 times the recommended dietary allowances) on his own, the very real dangers of vitamin D intoxication should be stressed. If this alone is not enough to convince the patient that such behavior is unwise, his health status should be carefully monitored in a manner similar to that for patients on large doses of the vitamin for medical reasons.

Another cause of hypervitaminosis D is therapogenic, due to physician misuse of the vitamin. The most common causes of the disorder are secondary to the treatment of hypoparathyroidism, resistant rickets, or osteodystrophy associated with chronic renal failure. These problems can be avoided by taking the following precautions when pharmacologic doses are prescribed:[401,402]

1.    Warn the patient of potential dangers and the need to report unusual symptoms promptly.
2.    Keep such patients under close medical supervision for the entire time they are receiving the vitamin. All such patients should have blood calcium levels monitored quarterly, and more often when dosages are being adjusted. Vitamin D intoxication may develop suddenly even in patients who have been well controlled for years.
3.    If vitamin D intoxication does ensue, an acute sensitivity to the vitamin may remain for many months after serum calcium levels have returned to normal. Maintenance of normocalcemia may be achieved by the use of calcium supplements in the interim. Even slight degrees of hypercalcemia due to vitamin D overdoses may be associated with toxicity and irreversible renal damage, so the presence of other signs and symptoms also needs to be investigated.

### Hypervitaminosis A

The potentially harmful effects of vitamin A toxicities are somewhat less profound than those of vitamin D. Clinical experience with single massive doses (e.g., 200,000 IU at two 6-month intervals) administered to large numbers of children in developing countries has shown that these doses are well tolerated.[372] Megadoses of 100,000 IU of water-miscible vitamin A are administered orally on a quarterly basis for the first 2 years of life. Lactating women receive a single oral dose of the same magnitude after delivery[373] to protect against xeropthalmia. Indeed, such prophylactic treatment appears to be quite successful.

However, while true signs of toxicity rarely result from such schedules of use, adverse reactions suggestive of intolerance have been reported. These include gastrointestinal distress and headaches of a few days' duration. Persons at particular risk of developing toxicities from self dosing are those whose liver function is abnormal, as it is in hepatitis. Patients recovering from hepatitis should therefore be particularly cautioned against such megadosing practices.

### Megadoses of Vitamin C

Dietary intakes of ascorbic acid are usually more than adequate among vegetarians. Moderate excess is excreted in the urine after tissue saturation levels are reached, and side effects are few.[403-405]

Some vegetarians or other alternative dieters use megadose amounts (e.g., 1 to 15 g/day) of ascorbic acid, however, usually in the hope that it exerts a prophylactic effect upon the common cold. Common side effects of large doses include diarrhea, nausea, and general gastric upset.[406-408] A number of legitimate uses in medicine exist for the nutrient.[409] There is no conclusive evidence about the efficacy of large doses of ascorbic acid in either preventing or ameliorating symptoms of the common cold. Indeed, the clinical trials and studies to date suggest little or no effect.[410-417] Yet, there is solid evidence that megadoses of ascorbic acid are not as innocuous as was previously thought. Therefore, there is little rationale for such supplementation from the standpoint of preventive medicine.

### Fiber Supplements

Many alternative dieters indulge in various types of dietary fiber supplements, bran perhaps being the most common. The literature on the effects of bran was reviewed extensively in a previous section, but special aspects pertaining to effects observed when it is used as a supplement will be considered here.

In a recent experiment confirming the extensive previous literature on the subject, raw and cooked bran supplements were found to differ in their effects.[251] Raw bran increased transit times and stool volume but only when 20 g/day were fed. Cooked bran in equal doses had no such effects, suggesting that the cereal manufacturing process altered the bran. Cummings et al.[250] fed subjects various types of wheat cereals that increased their dietary fiber intakes from 17 to 45 g/day and found a fourfold increase in fecal weight, largely due to water, and shortened mean transit times. Fecal bile acid output also increased, as did that of the volatile fatty acids.

Kahaner et al.[249] supplemented subjects on their usual diets with 3 oz of a high-fiber breakfast food for 3 weeks. During the supplementation period, subjects ate less eggs, butter, and breakfast meats because they chose to eat the cereal instead at breakfast. On these same subjects also showed increases in stool weight and total anaerobe counts in the feces.

When dietary fiber supplements are used, fecal bulk usually rises, but not always. Additional effects stemming from the substitution of one food for another may be seen if high-fiber foods are used rather than high-fiber supplements. The physiological effects of these supplements or dietary changes would probably be similar to those already discussed for vegetarians, although somewhat less in effect owing to the lesser doses probably involved in most cases.

## Lack of Trust in Physicians

We have seen that nontraditional or alternative life-style dieters often hold skeptical or negativistic attitudes toward physicians and other orthodox health care professionals. For example, in our studies of "new" vegetarians subjects believed that orthodox physicians are unsympathetic to vegetarian diets, that they failed to practice preventive medicine, and that their fees were excessive.[46,47] Glyer's studies of natural/organic food users revealed that these persons generally felt physicians know little about nutrition, treat symptoms rather than disease, and fail to practice preventive medicine.[51] Health food users in the Glycer study as well as in that of New and Priest[53] believed that physicians underemphasize healthy diets because they are afraid that their widespread use would "run them out of business". All groups are characterized by negativistic attitudes, with the sole exception of Seventh-Day Adventists.

## Failure to Utilize Orthodox Health Services

The alternative dieters also often differ in their attitudes toward alternative practitioners such as chiropractors, acupuncture experts, etc., as well as in habits of self-medication and their utilization of health care services.[33,45-48,51,53,396,397] Unfortunately, no systematic studies of the differences between vegans, vegetarians, natural/organic, and health food users have as yet been reported to allow comparisons between these groups to be made with certainty.

The fragmentary evidence which does exist suggests that: (1) vegans are exceedingly resistant to seeking treatment even for rather serious health problems,[33,130] (2) natural/organic food users and less restrictive vegetarians use orthodox health services for what they regard as serious illnesses,[130] and (3) health food users visit physicians somewhat more often than these other groups.[59] Utilization of health care services may be widely different even within these various dietary styles, however. This has been demonstrated in studies of both health food users and vegans by Calvert and Calvert[59] and our group,[130] respectively. It depends in part upon membership in structured groups that either favor or discourage such use. For example, lactovegetarian Seventh-Day Adventists make extensive use of pediatric services for their children, while lactovegetarian macrobiotics and Krishnas do not. These various groups of alternative dieters may also vary in the extent to which they follow medical advice that has been proffered.

## Use of Lay Healers Whose Advice is at Variance with Scientific Fact

Alternative dieters as a group rely on self-diagnosis and lay healers to a greater extent than the general population.[130] From the public health standpoint it is therefore important to reach these lay healers and the adherents themselves with health-related information which will help them to avert health catastrophes. For example, lay practitioners and teachers in one vegan group are convinced that vitamin $B_{12}$ is present in sufficient amounts in seaweed to make any other source of the vitamin unnecessary. They also believe that sea salt prevents and cures rickets if taken on a regular basis. These teachings are obnoxious since they are at variance with the tenets of preventive medicine and thus may result in needless morbidity. Other teachings may be less dangerous or even health promotive in some cases. Therefore, it is necessary to carefully study these belief systems and to attempt to change only those attitudes and teachings that militate against the maintenance of positive nutritional and health status while fostering those which already work for it.

## CONCLUSION

Alternative dieters' eating habits and lifestyles are positive in many respects. At the same time they are subject to certain risks not commonly recognized. For this reason it is suggested that all patients be asked if they indulge in these practices during intake interviews or screening in health care visits.

The curious paradox of simultaneous deficiency and excess that may exist among persons adhering to vegan-type diets and using nutrient supplements in megadose amounts (for the very nutrients they are not likely to be short in) means that these patients may present very odd clinical and biochemical profiles to the clinician. Their diets and lifestyles must not be condemned or praised indiscriminately. Rather, they should be carefully and objectively evaluated. Individually designed diets conforming to both scientific reality and quasireligious or philosophical beliefs must then be developed in conjunction with the patient. Since many of these patients are likely to raise their children on such diets, it is doubly important to neutralize the effects of potentially harmful practices as quickly as possible and to keep these persons under ongoing health surveillance. This is no mean task.

## ACKNOWLEDGMENT

The author is grateful for grants in aid NICHD08958 and Research Career Development Award K04AM00272, which supported much of the research reported in this review done in our clinical facilities. She also thanks her former students, particularly Barbara Zavitz, Lorraine Kwok, Marilyn Watanabe, Sherrie Sondel, Margaret Sexton, and Linda Swenson, as well as her colleagues Ruth Palombo, Alice Lichtenstein, Halorie Thorne, Jane Smithers, Linda Miller, Nancy Lally Arduino, and William Dietz, M.D., whose help and insights have made these investigations a pleasure.

## REFERENCES

1. Kurtha, A. N. and Ellis, F. R., The nutritional, clinical, and economic aspects of vegan diets, *Plant Foods Hum. Nutr.,* 2, 13, 1970.
2. Hardinge, M. G. and Stare, F. J., Nutritional studies of vegetarians. I. Nutritional, physical and laboratory studies, *Am. J. Clin. Nutr.,* 2, 73-83, 1954.
3. Mirone, L., Blood findings in men on a diet devoid of meat and low in animal protein, *Science,* 111, 673, 1950.
4. Ellis, F. R. and Montegriffo, V. M. E., Veganism: clinical findings and investigations, *Am. J. Clin. Nutr.,* 23, 249, 1970.
5. McCullagh, E. P. and Lewis, L. A., A study of diet, blood lipids and vascular disease in Trappist monks, *New Engl. J. Med.,* 263, 569, 1960.
6. Groen, J. J., Tijong, K. B., Koster, M., Willebrands, A. F., Verdonck, G., and Pierloat, M., The influence of nutrition and ways of life on blood cholesterol and the prevalence of hypertension and coronary heart disease among Trappist and Benedictine monks, *Am. J. Clin. Nutr.,* 10, 456, 1962.
7. Guggenheim, K., Weis, Y., and Fostick, M., Composition and nutritive value of diets consumed by strict vegetarians, *Br. J. Nutr.,* 16, 467, 1962.
8. Wokes, F. J., Badenoch, F., and Sinclair, H. M., Human dietary deficiency of vitamin B-12, *Am. J. Clin. Nutr.,* 3, 375, 1955.
9. Smith, A. D. M., Veganism: a clinical survey with observations on vitamin B-12 metabolism, *Br. Med. J.,* 1, 1655, 1962.
10. Ellis, F. R. and Wokes, F., The treatment of dietary deficiency of vitamin B-12 with vegetable protein foods, *Nutr. Dieta,* 9, 81, 1967.
11. McKenzie, J., Profile on vegans, *Plant Foods Hum. Nutr.,* 2, 79, 1971.
12. Hardinge, M. G. and Crooks, H., Non-flesh dietaries. I. Historical background 2. Scientific literature, *J. Am. Diet. Assoc.,* 43, 545-551, 1963.
13. McKenzie, J. C., Social and economic implications of minority food habits, *Br. J. Nutr.,* 26, 197, 1967.
14. West, E. D., The psychological health of vegans compared to two other groups, *Plant Foods Hum. Nutr.,* 3, 147, 1972.

15. Miller, D. S. and Mumford, P., The nutritive value of western vegan and vegetarian diets, *Plant Foods Hum. Nutr.*, 2, 201, 1972.

16. Foote, R. and Eppright, E. S., A dietary study of boys and girls on a lacto-ovo vegetarian diet, *J. Am. Diet. Assoc.*, 16, 222, 1940.

17. Ellis, F. R. and Montegriffo, M. E., The health of vegans, *Plant Foods Hum. Nutr.*, 2, 93, 1971.

18. Dwyer, J. T., Vegetarian, "health" and "junk" foods, in *Handbook of Clinical Nutrition*, Paige, D. and Young, V. R., in press.

19. Hardinge, M. G. and Crooks, H., Non-flesh dietaries: adequate and inadequate, *J. Am. Diet. Assoc.*, 45, 537, 1964.

20. LeRiche, H., Kenaear, A. A., and Smit, R. J., The Dilpkoof nutrition and health study on Bantu boys, South Africa, *Can. Med. Assoc. J.*, 74, 130, 1956.

21. Jelliffe, D. B., Child Nutrition in the Developing Countries; A Handbook for Fieldworkers, Publ. No. 1822, U.S. Department of Health, Education and Welfare, Public Health Service, Washington, D. C., 1968.

22. Shaw, R. L., Incaparina: a low cost vegetable mixture and its commercial application, *Plant Foods Hum. Nutr.*, 2, 99, 1969.

23. Scrimshaw, N. S. and Bressani, R., Vegetable protein mixtures for human consumption, *Fed. Proc. Fed. Am. Soc. Exp. Biol.*, 20 (Part 3, Suppl. 7), 80, 1961.

24. Dean, R. F. A., The nutritional adequacy of a vegetable substitute for milk, *Br. J. Nutr.*, 5, 269, 1951.

25. Graham, G. G., Cordano, A., Morales, E., Acevedo, G., and Placko, R. P., Dietary protein quality in infants and children. V. A wheat flour wheat concentrate mixture, *Plant Foods Hum. Nutr.*, 2, 23, 1970.

26. Jensen, J. H., Protein calorie malnutrition and centrally processed vegetable based protein-rich weaning foods in *Priorities in Child Nutrition*, Vol. 2, Mayer, J. and Dwyer, J., Eds., Harvard University School of Public Health, Boston, 1975, 276-291.

27. Beaton, G. H. and Bengoa, J. M., *Nutrition in Preventive Medicine*, World Health Organization, Geneva, 1974, 349-460.

28. Erhard, D., Nutrition education for the "now" generation, *J. Nutr. Educ.*, 2, 135, 1971.

29. Gardiner, B., Celestial food and scientific nutrition, *Order of the Universe*, 4(2), 24, 1972.

30. Dwyer, J. T., Mayer, L. D. V. H., Kandel, R. F., and Mayer, J., The new vegetarians: who are they? Food and other avoidances and attitudes toward health services of 100 young vegetarians, *J. Am. Diet. Assoc.*, 62, 503, 1973.

31. White, P. L., Ed., Nutrition misinformation and food faddism, *Nutr. Rev.*, 32 (Suppl. 1), 1-73, 1974.

32. Erhard, D., The new vegetarians part 1, *Nutr. Today*, 8(64), 12, 1973.

33. Erhard, D., The new vegetarians part 2, *Nutr. Today*, 9(1), 20-27, 1974.

34. Henderson, L. M., Nutritional problems growing out of new patterns of food consumption, *Am. J. Public Health*, 62, 1194, 1972.

35. Frankle, R. T., McGregor, B., Wylie, J., and McCann, M., The door: a center of alternatives, *J. Am. Diet. Assoc.*, 63, 269, 1973.

36. Majumder, S. R., Vegetarianism: fad, faith or fact, *Am. Sci.*, 60(2), 175, 1972.

37. Wolff, R. J., Who eats for health?, *Am. J. Clin. Nutr.*, 26, 438, 1973.

38. Shimoda, N., Observations of a nutritionist in a free clinic, *J. Am. Diet. Assoc.*, 63, 273, 1973.

39. Todhunter, E. N., Food habits, food faddism, and nutrition, *World Rev. Nutr. Diet.*, 16, 287, 1973.

40. Sanchez, A., Porter, G. G., and Register, U. D., Effect of entree on fat and protein quality of diets, *J. Am. Diet. Assoc.*, 49, 492, 1960.

41. Strom, A. and Hensen, R. A., Mortality from circulatory disease in Norway 1940-45, *Lancet*, 260, 126, 1951.

42. Barrow, J. G., Quinlan, C. B., Cooper, G. R., Whitner, V. S., and Goodloe, M. H. R., Studies in atherosclerosis. III. An epidemiological study of atherosclerosis in Trappist and Benedictine monks: a preliminary report, *Ann. Int. Med.*, 52, 368, 1960.

43. Nagy, M., Teenage vegan, *J. Am. Med. Assoc.*, 211, 306, 1970.

44. Widdowson, E. M. and McCance, R. A., Studies on the nutritive value of bread and on the effect of variations in the extraction rate of flour on the growth of undernourished children, *Med. Res. Council (G.B.) Spec. Rep. Ser.*, 287, 1954.

45. Anderson, M. A. and Standal, B. R., Nutrition knowledge of health food users in Oahu, Hawaii, *J. Am. Diet. Assoc.*, 67, 116, 1975.

46. Dwyer, J. T., Kandel, R. F., Mayer, L., and Mayer, J., The new vegetarians: relationship of group affiliations and dietary structures to diet and life style, *J. Am. Diet. Assoc.*, 64, 376, 1974.

47. Dwyer, J. T., Kandel, R. F., Mayer, L., Dowd, K., and Mayer, J., The new vegetarians: the natural high?, *J. Am. Diet. Assoc.*, 65, 529, 1974.

48. Dwyer, J. T., How to counsel today's vegetarians: a nutritionists' practical guide, *Med. Opinion,* 33, March 1975.
49. Dwyer, J. T. and Mayer, J., Vegetarianism in drug users, *Lancet,* 2, 14291, 1971.
50. Sherlock, P. and Rothschild, E. O., Scurvey produced by a zen macrobiotic diet, *J. Am. Med. Assoc.,* 199, 794, 1967.
51. Glyer, J., Diet healing: a case study in the sociology of health, *J. Nutr. Educ.,* 4, 163, 1972.
52. Frankle, R. T. and Heussenstamm, F. K., Food zealotry and youth-new dilemmas for professionals, *Am. J. Public Health,* 64, 11, 1974.
53. New, P. K. and Priest, R. P., Food and thought: a sociologic study of food cultists, *J. Am. Diet. Assoc.,* 51, 13, 1967.
54. Prout, C., Dietary restriction: the New Nirvana, *Trans. Am. Clin. Climatol. Assoc.,* 83, 218, 1971.
55. Blix, G., Ed., *Food Cultism and Nutrition Quackery: VII Symposium Swedish Nutrition Foundation,* Almqvist Wikseels, Stockholm, 1972.
56. Fleshman, R. P., Symposium on the young adult in today's world; eating rituals and realities, *Nurs. Clin. North Am.,* 8, 9, 1973.
57. Schaefer, R. and Yetley, E., Social psychology of food faddism, *J. Am. Diet. Assoc.,* 66, 129, 1955.
58. Bernard, V. W., Why people become the victims of medical quackery, *Am. J. Public Health,* 55, 1142, 1975.
59. Calvert, G. P. and Calvert, S. W., Intellectual convictions of "health" food consumers, *J. Nutr. Educ.,* 7, 95, 1975.
60. Bremer, M. and Weatherholz, W., Nutrition attitudes in a university community, *J. Nutr. Educ.,* 7, 60, 1975.
61. Demby, E. H., Over the counter lifestyle, *Psychol. Today,* 5, 75, April 1972.
62. McBean, L. D. and Speckmann, E. W., Food faddism: a challenge to nutritionists and dietitians, *Am. J. Clin. Nutr.,* 27, 1071, 1974.
63. National Technical Information Service, A Study of Health Practices and Opinions, U.S. Department of Commerce, U.S. Government Printing Office, Washington, D.C., 1972.
64. Robson, J. R. K., Konlande, J. E., Larkin, F. A., O'Connors, P. A. and Liu, H., Zen macrobiotic problems in infancy, *Pediatrics,* 53, 320, 1974.
65. Berkelhamer, J. E., Thorp, F. K., and Cobbs, S., Kwashiokor in Chicago, *Am. J. Dis. Child.,* 129, 1240, 1975.
66. Brown, P. T. and Bergan, J. G., The dietary status of "new" vegetarians, *J. Am. Diet. Assoc.,* 67, 4555, 1975.
67. Brown, P. T. and Bergan, J. G., The dietary status of practicing macrobiotics: a preliminary communication, *Ecol. Food Nutr.,* 4, 103, 1975.
68. Trahms, C. M., Dietary Patterns of Vegan Vegetarian and Nonvegetarian Preschool Children, Master's thesis, University of Washington, Seattle, 1975.
69. Bernhardt, I. B. and Dorsey, J., Hypervitammosis A and congenital renal anomalies in a human infant, *Obstet. Gynecol.,* 15, 750, 1974.
70. Anon., Presentment of Passiac grand jury, *Public Health News,* 132, June 1966.
71. West, R. O. and Hayes, O. B., Diet and serum cholesterol levels: a comparison between vegetarians and nonvegetarians in a Seventh Day Adventist group, *Am. J. Clin. Nutr.,* 21, 853, 1968.
72. Sacks, F. M., Castelli, W. P., Donner, A., and Kass, E. H., Plasma lipids and lipoproteins in vegetarians and controls, *New Engl. J. Med.,* 292, 1148, 1975.
73. Burkitt, D. P., Epidemiology of cancer of the colon and rectum, *Cancer,* 28:3, 1971.
74. Hill, M. J., Draser, B. S., Hawksworth, G., and Arees, V., *Lancet,* 1, 95, 1970.
75. Reddy, B. S. and Wynder, E. L., Large bowel carcinogenesis: fecal constituents of populations with diverse incidence rates of colon cancer, *J. Natl. Cancer Inst.,* 50, 1437, 1973.
76. Malhotra, S. L., Serum lipids dietary factors and ischaemic heart disease, *Am. J. Clin. Nutr.,* 20, 462, 1967.
77. Burkitt, D. P., Walker, A. R. P., and Painter, N. S., Divertiscular disease of the colon: a deficiency of western civilization, *J. Am. Med. Assoc.,* 229, 1068, 1974.
78. Mendeloff, A. I., Dietary fiber nutrition reviews, *Br. Med. J.,* 33, 32, 1975.
79. Almy, T. P., Diverticular disease of the colon — the new look, *Gastroenterology,* 49, 109, 1965.
80. Ellis, F. R., Holesh, S., and Ellis, J. W., Incidence of osteoporosis in vegetarians and omnivores, *Am. J. Clin. Nutr.,* 25, 555, 1972.
81. Ellis, F. R., Holesh, S., and Sanders, T. A. B., Osteoporosis in British vegetarians and vegans, *Am. J. Clin. Nutr.,* 27, 769, 1974.
82. Reilly, R. W. and Kirsner, J. B., Eds., *Fiber Deficiency and Colonic Disorders,* Plenum Press, New York, 1975.
83. Haenszel, W., Berg, J. W., Segi, M., Kurihara, M., and Lock, P. E., Large bowel cancer in Hawaiian Japanese, *J. Natl. Cancer Inst.,* 51, 1965, 1973.

84. Council on Foods and Nutrition, Zen macrobiotic diet, *J. Am. Med. Assoc.*, 218, 397, 1971.

85. Ohsawa, G., *Zen Macrobiotics,* Ignoramus Press, Los Angeles, undated.

86. Needleman, J., *The New Religions: The Teachings of the East and Their Special Meaning for Young Americans,* Pocket Books, New York, 1972.

87. Roberts, R. E., *The New Communes: Coming Together in America,* Prentice Hall, Englewood Cliffs, N.J., 1971.

88. Vassi, M., *The Stoned Apocalypse,* Pocket Books, New York, 1973.

89. Shelton, H. M., *The Hygienic Care of Children,* Natural Hygiene Press, Chicago, 1970.

90. Simoons, F. J., *Eat Not This Flesh: Food Avoidances in the Old World,* University of Wisconsin Press, Madison, 1961.

91. McKenzie, J. C., Mattinson, J., and Yudkund, J., Milk in schools: an experiment in nutrition education, *Br. J. Nutr.*, 21, 811, 1967.

92. *Oxford English Dictionary,* Oxford University Press, Oxford, 1964.

93. American Heart Association, Diet and Coronary Heart Disease, American Heart Association, New York, 1973.

94. Senate Select Committee on Nutrition and Human Needs, Dietary Goals for the United States, U.S. Senate Committee Prints, Washington, D.C., January 1977.

95. Anon., Family Food Consumption in the United States Spring 1942, Misc. Publ. #550, U.S. Department of Agriculture, U.S. Government Printing Office, Washington, D.C., 1944.

96. Stiebling, H. K., Monroe, D., Phipard, E. F., Adelson, S. F., and Clark, F., Family Food Consumption and Dietary Levels Five Regions, Misc. Publ. #452, Bureau of Home Economics in Cooperation with the Work Projects Administration, U.S. Department of Agriculture, Washington, D.C., 1941.

97. Reid, P. P., *Alive: The Story of Andean Survivors,* Pocket Books, New York, 1975.

97a. Gajdusek, D. C. and Wiesenfeld, S. L., Genetic structure and heterozygosity in the Kuru region, eastern highlands of New Guinea, *Am. J. Phys. Anthropol.*, 45, 177, 1976.

98. Lopez, H., *They Lived on Human Flesh,* Pocket Books, New York, 1975.

99. Kamil, A., How natural are those natural vitamins?, *J. Nutr. Ed.*, 4, 92, 1972.

100. Jukes, T. H., The organic food myth, *J. Am. Med. Assoc.*, 230, 276, 1974.

101. Anon., *Food Faddism. Dairy Counc. Dig.*, 44, January - February 1973.

102. Bruch, H., The allure of food cults and nutrition quackery, *J. Am. Diet. Assoc.*, 57, 316, 1972.

103. Roebuck, J. B. and Hunter, B., The awareness of health care quackery as deviant behavior, *J. Health Soc. Behav.*, 13, 162, 1972.

104. Schneider, H. A. and Hesla, J. T. The way it is, *Nutr. Rev.*, 31, 233, 1973.

105. Schroeder, H. A., Loss of vitamins and trace minerals resulting from processing and preservation of foods, *Am. J. Clin. Nutr.*, 24, 562, 1971.

106. Young, J. H., The persistence of medical quackery in America, *Am. Sci.*, 60, 318, 1972.

107. Stare, F. J., "Health foods": definitions and nutrient values, *J. Nutr. Educ.*, 4, 94, 1972.

108. Butler, R., Why are older consumers so susceptible?, *Geriatrics*, 23, 85, 1968.

109. Sinclair, H. M., Health and health foods, in *Nutritional Problems in A Changing World,* Hollingsworth, D. and Russell, M., Eds., Halsted Press, New York, 1973, 255-263.

110. Sinclair, H. M., The rationale of health foods, in *Health and Food,* Birch, G. C., Green, L. F., and Plaskett, G. L., Eds., Halsted Press, New York, 1972, 11-25.

111. Appledorf, H., Wheeler, W. B., and Koburger, J. A., Health foods vs. traditional foods, *Food Technol. (Chicago)*, 36, 242, 1973.

112. Margolius, S., *Health Foods: Facts and Fakes,* Walker Publishing, New York, 1973.

113. Barret, S. and Knight, G., Eds., *The Health Robbers,* George F. Stickley Co., Philadelphia, 1975.

114. Deutsch, R., *The Nuts Among the Berries,* Ballantine Books, New York, 1965.

115. Dwyer, J. T., Ross, D., Rosenberg, R., Zabitz, B., and Watanabe, M. K., unpublished manuscript, Boston, 1977.

116. General Mills, Inc. *A Survey of Consumer Knowledge Attitudes and Practice,* General Mills, Inc., Minneapolis, Minn., 1977.

117. Anon., Symposium on the role of plant foods in solving the world food problem, *Plant Foods Hum. Nutr.*, 1, 11, 1968.

118. Cameron, M. and Hofvander, Y., *Manual on Child Feeding,* Protein Advisory Group of the United Nations, New York, 1972.

119. Bressani, R., Viteri, F., Elias, G. G., deZaghi, S., Alvarado, J., and Odell, A. D., Protein quality of a soybean textured food in animals and children, *J. Nutr.*, 93, 349, 1967.

120. Dutra de Oliveira, J. E., Scatena, L., de Oliveira Netto, N., Duarte, G. G., The Nutritive value of soya milk and cow's milk in malnourished children: a comparative study, *J. Pediatr.*, 69, 670, 1966.

121. Fomon, S. J., Comparative study of human milk and a soya bean formula on promoting growth and nitrogen retention, *Pediatrics*, 24, 577, 1959.

122. Jelliffee, E. F. P., A new look at weaning mixtures in the contemporary Caribbean, *J. Trop. Pediatr.,* 17, 135, 1971.
123. Technical Staff, *Vegetarian Diets,* Am. J. Clin. Nutr., 27, 1095, 1974.
124. Veymeister, I. B., Register, U. D., and Sonnenberg, L. M., Safe vegetarian diets for children, *Pediatr. Clin. North Am.,* 24, 203, 1977.
125. Robson, J. R. K., Food faddism, *Pediatr. Clin. North Am.,* 24, 189, 1977.
126. Marsh, A. G., Food, D. L., and Christensen, D. K., Metabolic responses of adolescent girls to a lacto-ovo-vegetarian diet, *J. Am. Diet. Assoc.,* 51, 441, 1967.
127. Register, U. D. and Sonnenberg, L. M., The vegetarian diet, *J. Am. Diet. Assoc.,* 62, 253, 1973.
128. Smith, E. B., A guide to good eating the vegetarian way, *J. Nutr. Educ.,* 7, 109, 1975.
129. Armstrong, B. K., Davis, R. E., Nicol, D. J., Van Merwyk, A. J., and Larwood, C. J., Hematological, vitamin B-12 and folate studies on Seventh Day Adventist Vegetarians, *Am. J. Clin. Nutr.,* 27, 712, 1974.
130. Zavitz, B., *Attitudes Toward Health Among Alternative Dieters,* Senior thesis, Frances Stern Nutrition Center, New England Medical Center Hospital, Boston, unpublished, 1977.
131. Thompson, A. M., The evolution of human growth patterns, *Am. J. Dis. Child.,* 120, 398, 1970.
132. Aykroyd, W. A., Nutrition and mortality in infancy and early childhood: past and present relationships, *Am. J. Clin. Nutr.,* 24, 480, 1971.
133. Hegsted, D. M., Theoretical estimates of protein requirements of children, *J. Am. Diet. Assoc.,* 33, 226, 1957.
134. Pellett, P. E., Nutritional problems of the Arab world, *Ecol. Food Nutr.,* 5, 150, 1976.
135. Committee on Nutrition, American Academy of Pediatrics, Nutritional aspects of vegetarianism, health foods and fad diets, *Pediatrics,* 59, 460, 1977.
136. Jacobson, H. N., Nutrition, in *Scientific Foundations of Obstetrics and Gynecology,* Philipp, E. E., Barnes, J., and Newton, M., Eds., William Heinemann Medical Book, London, 1977.
137. Register, U. D. and Sonnenberg, L. M., The vegetarian diet, *J. Am. Diet. Assoc.,* 62, 253, 1973.
138. Baker, S. J., Jacob, E., Rajan, K. T., and Swaminathan, S. P., Vitamin B-12 deficiency in pregnancy and the puerperium, *Br. Med. J.,* 1, 1658, 1962.
139. Filer, L. J. and Martinez, G. A., Intakes of selected nutrients by infants in the U.S., *Clin. Pediatr.,* 3, 633, 1964.
140. Fomon, S. J., Infant Nutrition, 2nd ed., W. B. Saunders, Philadelphia 1974, 1-20.
141. Lönnerdal, B., Forsum, E., Gebre-Medhin, M., and Hambraeus, L., Breast milk composition in Ethiopian and Swedish mothers II Lactose, nitrogen, and protein, *Am. J. Clin. Nutr.,* 29, 1134, 1976.
142. Lönnerdal, B., Forsum, E., and Hambraeus, L., A longitudinal study of the protein, nitrogen, and lactose contents of human milk from Swedish well nourished mothers, *Am. J. Clin. Nutr.,* 29, 1127, 1976.
143. Wray, J. D., Maternal nutrition, Breast Feeding and Survival in *Nutrition and Fertility,* Moseley, H., Ed., Plenum Press, 1977.
144. Hytten, F. E. and Thomson, A., Nutrition of the lactating woman, in *Milk: The Mammary Gland and Its Secretion, Vol. 2,* Kon, S. K. and Cowie, A. T., Eds., Academic Press, New York, 1961, 3.
145. Hanafy, M. M., Morsey, M. R. A., Seldick, Y., Habib, Y. A., and el Lozy M., Maternal nutrition and lactation performance, *Environ. Child Health,* 187, September 1972.
146. Bailey, K. V., Quantity and composition of breast milk in some New Guinean populations, *J. Trop. Pediatr.,* 11, 35, 1965.
147. Insull, W., Hirsch, J. and James, T., The fatty acids of human milk. II. Alterations produced by manipulation of caloric balance and exchange of dietary fat, *J. Clin. Invest.,* 38, 443, 1959.
148. Read, W. W., Lutz, P. G., and Tashjian, A., Human milk lipids II influence of dietary carbohydrates and fat on the fatty acids of mature milk. A study in 4 ethnic groups, *Am. J. Clin. Nutr.,* 17, 180, 1965.
149. Kon, S. K. and Cowie, A. T., *Milk: The Mammary Gland and Its Secretions,* Academic Press, New York, 1967.
150. Larson, B. and Smith, V., *Lactation: A Comprehensive Treatise,* Academic Press, New York, 1974.
151. Bracco, U., Human milk lipids and problems related to their replacement, in *Dietary Lipids and Postnatal Development,* Galli, C., Jacini, G., and Pecile, A., Eds., Raven Press, New York, 1973, 23-40.
152. Kamal, L., Hafhawi, F., Ghoneim, M., Talleta, M., Youni, S. H., Tqui, A., and Abdalla, M., Clinical biochemical & experimental studies on lactation, *Am. J. Obstet.,* 105, 314, 1969.
153. Underwood, B. A., Hepner, R., and Abdullah, H., Protein lipid and fatty acids of human milk from Pakistani women during prolonged periods of lactation, *Am. J. Clin. Nutr.,* 23, 400, 1970.
154. Jelliffe, D. and Jelliffe, E. F. P., *Human Milk in the Modern World,* Oxford University Press, London, 1977.

155. Macy, I. G., Kelley, H. J., and Sloan, R. E., Nutrition and Chemical Growth of Children, Publ. No. 254, National Research Council—National Academy of Sciences, Washington, D.C., 1953.

156. Committee on Nutrition, American Academy of Pediatrics, Statement, *Pediatrics,* 26, 1039, 1960.

157. Hytten, F. E., Diurnal variation in major constituents of milk, *Br. Med. J.,* 1, 176, 1954.

158. Potter, J. M. and Nestel, P. J., The effects of dietary fatty acids and cholesterol on the milk lipids of lactating women and the plasma cholesterol of breast-fed infants, *Am. J. Clin. Nutr.,* 29, 54, 1976.

159. Wurtman, J., personal communication, 1977.

160. Graham, G. G. and Andrazian, T. B., Growth, inheritance and diet, *Pediatr. Res.,* 5, 691, 1971.

161. Foote, R. and Eppright, E. S., A dietary study of boys and girls on a lactovegetarian diet, *J. Am. Diet. Assoc.,* 16, 222, 1940.

162. Lane, D. E., The nutrition of twins on a vegetable diet, during pregnancy, the nursing period, and infancy, *Am. J. Dis. Child.,* 43, 1384, 1931.

163. Jaffa, M. E., Nutrition investigation among fruitarians and Chinese, *U.S. Dep. Agric. Bull.,* 107, 1901.

164. Dwyer, J. T., Palombo, R., Thorne, H., Valadian, I., and Reed, R., Diet and growth among vegetarian children, *J. Am. Diet. Assoc.,* 72, 264, 1978.

165. Shull, M., Reed, R. B., Valadian, I., and Dwyer, J. T., Velocities of growth in Vegetarian preschool children, *Pediatrics,* 60, 410, 1977.

166. Wills, L., The clinical picture in children fed after weaning on a predominantly vegetable diet, *Br. J. Nutr.,* 5, 265, 1951.

167. Shull, M., Valadian, I., Reed, R. B., Palombo, R., Thorne, H., and Dwyer, J., Seasonal variations in growth velocity in vegetarian children, *Am. J. Clin. Nutr.,* 31, 1, 1978.

168. Baertl, J. M., Adrianzen, B. T., and Graham, G. G., Growth of previously well nourished infants in poor homes, *Am. J. Dis. Child.,* 130, 33, 1976.

169. Graham, G. G. and Adrianza, T. B., Late catchup growth after severe infantile malnutrition, *John Hopkins Med. J.,* 131, 204, 1972.

170. Williams, C. D. and Jelliffe, D. B., *Mother and Child Health: Delivering the Services,* Oxford University Press, London, 1972.

171. Apley, J. and MacKeith, R., *The Child and His Symptoms: A Comprehensive Approach,* 2nd ed., Blackwell Scientific Publications, Oxford, 1972, 168.

172. Sacks, F. B., Rosner, B., and Kass, E. H., Blood pressure in vegetarians, *Am. J. Epidemiol.,* 100, 390, 1974.

173. Garrow, J., *Obesity and Energy Balance in Man,* Elsevier, Amsterdam, 1973.

174. Palmblad, J., Levi, L., Burger, A., Melander, A., Westgren, U., Von Schenck, H., and Skude, G., Effects of total energy withdrawal (fasting) on the levels of growth hormone, thyrotropin, cortisol, adrenaline, noradrenaline, T4, T3 and RT3 in healthy males, *Rep. Lab. Clin. Stress Res. Dep. Med. Psychiatr. (Karolinska Institute),* No. 47, Stockholm, May 1976.

175. Spaulding, S. W., Chopra, I. J., and Sherwin, R. S., Effect of caloric restriction and dietary composition on serum T3 and reverse T3 in Man, *J. Clin. Endocrinol. Metab.,* 42, 197, 1976.

176. Vagenakis, A. G., Burger, A., Portnay, G. I., Rudolph, M., O'Brian, J. T., Asizi, F., Arky, R. A., Nicad, P., Ingbar, S. H., and Braverman, L. E., Diversion of peripheral thyroxine metabolism from activating to inactivating pathways during complete fasting, *J. Clin. Endocrinol. Metab.,* 41, 191, 1975.

177. McCance, R. A., The effect of calorie deficiencies and protein deficiencies on final weight and stature in *Calorie Deficiencies and Protein Deficiencies,* McCance, R. A. and Widdowson, E. M., Eds., Churchill, London, 1968, 319.

178. Neumann, C. G. and Alpaugh, M., Birthweight doubling time: a fresh look, *Pediatrics,* 57, 469, 1976.

179. Taitz, L. S., Obesity in pediatric practice: infantile obesity, *Pediatr. Clin. North Am.,* 24, 107, 1977.

180. Dwyer, J. T. and Mayer, J., Obesity and over feeding in infancy and childhood, *Bibl. Nutr. Dieta,* 18, 123, 1973.

181. Matter, S. K. and Wakefield, L. M., Religious influences on dietary intakes and physical condition of indigent pregnant Indian women, *Am. J. Clin. Nutr.,* 24, 1097, 1971.

182. Graves, P. L., Nutrition, infant behavior and maternal characteristics: a pilot study in West Bengal, India, *Am. J. Clin. Nutr.,* 29, 305, 1976.

183. Macy, I. G. and Hunscher, H. A., Calories: a limiting factor in the growth of children, *J. Nutr.,* 45, 189, 1951.

184. Widdowson, E. M., *A Study of Individual Childrens Diets,* MRC Special Rep. Ser. #257, Her Majesty's Stationary Office, London, 1947.

185. Nichol, B., Protein and calorie concentration, *Nutr. Rev.,* 29, 83, 1971.

186. Lin, S., King, J., and Leune, V., Diet, growth and cultural food habits of Chinese American infants, *Am. J. Clin. Nutr.,* 3, 125, 1975.

187. Spady, D. W., Payne, P. R., Picon, D., and Waterlow, J. C., Energy balance during recovery from malnutrition, *Am. J. Clin. Nutr.,* 29, 1073, 1976.

188. Ashworth, A., Bell, R., James, W. P. T., and Waterlow, J. C., Calorie requirements of children recovering from protein-calorie malnutrition, *Lancet,* 2, 600, 1968.

189. Payne, R. R., Safe protein-calorie ratios in diets: the relative importance of protein and energy intakes as causal factors in malnutrition, *Am. J. Clin. Nutr.,* 28, 281, 1975.

190. Anon., Energy and protein requirements: report of a Joint FAO/WHO Ad Hoc Expert Committee, *WHO Tech. Rep. Ser.,* No. 522, 1973.

191. Ferro-Luzzi, A., Norgan, N. G., and Durnin, J. G. V. A., Food intake, its relationship to body weight and age, and its apparent nutritional adequacy in New Guinean children, *Am. J. Clin. Nutr.,* 28, 1443, 1975.

192. Lee, K. T., Kin, D. N., Han, Y. S., and Goodale, F., Geographic studies of arteriosclerosis: the effect of a strict vegetarian diet on serum lipid and electrocardiographic patterns, *Arch. Environ. Health,* 4, 4, 1962.

193. Ellis, F. R. and Mumford, P., The nutritional status of vegans and vegetarians *Proc. Nutr. Soc.,* 26, 205, 1967.

194. de Wijn, J. F., Donath, W. F., and Meulen van Eysbergen, H. D., A study of the effects of completely vegetarian diets on human subjects, *Proc. Nutr. Soc.,* 13, 14, 1954.

195. Tso, E., A vegetable milk substitute for North China, *Am. J. Physiol.,* 90, 542, 1929.

196. Lane, D. E., The nutrition of twins on a vegetable diet during pregnancy, the nursing period, and infancy, *Am. J. Dis. Child.,* 42, 1345, 1931.

197. Ritinger, F., Dembo, L. H., and Torrey, G. G., *J. Pediatr.,* 6, 417, 1935.

198. Brown, R. G., Possible problems of large intakes of ascorbic acid, *J. Am. Med. Assoc.,* 224, 1259, 1973.

199. Hardinge, M. G., Crooks, H., and Stare, F. J., Nutritional studies of vegetarians. V. Proteins and essential amino acids, *J. Am. Diet. Assoc.,* 48, 25, 1966.

200. Doyle, M. D., Morese, L. M., Gowan, J. S., and Parsons, M. R., Observation on nitrogen and energy balance in young men consuming vegetarian diets, *Am. J. Clin. Nutr.,* 17, 368, 1965.

201. Herman, R. O., Introduction: the economics of protein, in *Nutrients in Processed Foods: Proteins,* White, P. L. and Fletcher, D. C., Eds., Publishing Sciences Group, Acton, Mass., 1974, 21.

202. Arroyave, G., Amino acid requirements by age and sex, in *Nutrients in Processed Foods: Proteins,* White, P. L. and Fletcher, D. C., Eds., Publishing Sciences Group, Acton, Mass., 1974, 15-29.

203. Bressani, R., Complementary amino acid patterns, in *Nutrients in Processed Foods: Proteins,* White, P. L. and Fletcher, D. C., Eds., Publishing Sciences Group, Acton, Mass., 1974, 149.

204. MacLean, W. C., Jr., Morales, E., and Graham, G. G., The effect of uneven dietary protein to calorie distribution on nitrogen retention and weight gain, *Pediatrics,* 54, 312, 1974.

205. Hardinge, M. G., Crooks, H., and Stare, F. J., Nutritional studies of vegetarians. IV. Dietary fatty acids and serum cholesterol levels, *Am. J. Clin. Nutr.,* 10, 516, 1962.

206. Oelze, F., Fielder, H., Fuhr, J., and Verhoeven, J., A clinical contribution to the problem of atherosclerosis and fat metabolism, *Med. Ernaehr.,* 6, 51, 1965.

207. Feeley, R. M., Stanton, A. L., and Moyer, E. Z., Fat metabolism in preadolescent children on all vegetable diets, *J. Am. Diet. Assoc.,* 47, 396, 1965.

208. Mironne, L., Nutrient intake and blood findings in males on a diet devoid of meat, *Am. J. Clin. Nutr.,* 2, 246, 1954.

209. Chen, I., Effects of a long term vegetarian diet on blood components in adults, *J. Formosan Med. Assoc.,* 72, 158, 1975.

210. Burkitt, D. P., Epidemiology of large bowel disease: the role of fiber, *Proc. Nutr. Soc.,* 32, 51, 1973.

211. Trowell, H., Dietary fiber, ischaemic heart disease and diabetes mellitus, *Proc. Nutr. Soc.,* 32, 51, 1973.

212. Anon., Dietary fiber and plasma lipids, *Lancet,* 2, 353, 1975.

213. Eastwood, M. A., Dietary fiber and serum lipids, *Lancet,* 2, 1222, 1969.

214. Van Soest, P. J., and McQueen, R. W., The chemistry and estimation of fiber, *Proc. Nutr. Soc.,* 32, 123, 1973.

215. Eastwood, M. A., Vegetable fiber: its physical properties, *Proc. Nutr. Soc.,* 32, 137, 1973.

216. Drasar, B. S. and Irving, D., Environmental factors and cancer of the colon and breast, *Br. J. Cancer,* 27, 167, 1973.

217. Eastwood, M. A., Kirkpatrick, J. R., Mitchell, W. D., Bone, A., and Hamilton, T., Effects of dietary supplements of wheat bran and cellulose on feces and bowel function, *Br. Med. J.,* 4, 392, 1975.

218. Wynder, E. L., Kalitani, T., Ishikawa, S., Dodo, H., and Takano, A., Environmental factors of cancer of the colon and rectum, *Cancer,* 23, 1210, 1969.

219. Moore, W. E. C., Human fecal flora: the normal flora of 20 Japanese Hawaiians, *Appl. Microbiol.*, 27, 961, 1974.
220. Goldin, B., Dwyer, J., Gorbach, S. L., Gordon, W., and Swenson, L., The influence of diet and age on fecal bacterial enzymes, *Am. J. Clin. Nutr.*, in press.
221. Eysson, H., Role of gut microflora in metabolism of lipids and sterols, *Am. J. Clin. Nutr.*, 11, 142, 1962.
222. Antonis, A. and Bersohn, I., The influence of diet on fecal lipids in South African white and Bantu prisoners, *Am. J. Clin. Nutr.*, 11, 142, 1962.
223. Heaton, K. W., Fiber, blood lipids and heart disease, *Am. J. Clin. Nutr.*, 29, 125, 1976.
224. Hardinge, M. G., Chambers, A. D., Crooks, H., and Stare, F. J., Nutritional studies of vegetarians III Dietary levels of fiber, *Am. J. Clin. Nutr.*, 6, 523, 1958.
225. Bender, A. E. and Damji, K. B., Some effects on dietary sucrose, *World Rev. Nutr. Diet.*, 15, 106, 1972.
226. Stahl, S. S., Nutritional influences on periodontal disease, *World Rev. Nutr. Diet.*, 32, 131, 1973.
227. Bibby, B. G., *J. Am. Dental Assoc.*, 70, 121, 1975.
228. Southgate, D. A. T., Fiber and other unavailable carbohydrates and their effects on the energy value of the diet, *Proc. Nutr. Soc.*, 32, 131, 1973.
229. Eastwood, M. A. and Smith, A. W., Nomenclature and definition of dietary fiber, *Am. J. Clin. Nutr.*, 20, 658, 1977.
230. Stanley, M., Paul, D., Gocke, D., and Murphy, J., Effects of cholestranine, metamucil and cellulose on bile salt excretion in man, *J. Gastroenterol.*, 65, 889, 1973.
231. Kay, R. M. and Truswell, A. A., Effect of citrus pectin on blood lipids and fecal steroid excretion in man, *Am. J. Clin. Nutr.*, 30, 171, 1977.
232. Crowther, J. S., Drasar, B. S., Goddard, P., Hill, M. J., and Johnson, K., The effect of a chemically defined diet on the fecal flora and fecal steroid conversion, *Gut*, 14, 790, 1973.
233. Drasar, B. S. and Jenkins, D. J. A., Bacteria, diet and large bowel cancer, *Am. J. Clin. Nutr.*, 29, 1410, 1976.
234. Walker, A. R. P., Effect of high crude fiber intake on transit time and absorption of nutrients in South Africans, *Am. J. Clin. Nutr.*, 29, 1417, 1976.
235. Wynder, E. and Reddy, B., Metabolic epidemiology of colon rectal cancer, *Cancer*, 34, 801, 1974.
236. Burkitt, D. and Trowell, H. C., *Refined Carbohydrate Foods and Disease: Some implications of Dietary Fiber*, Academic Press, London, 1975.
237. Drasar, B. J., Jenkins, D. J. A., and Cummings, J., The influence of a diet rich in wheat fiber on the human fecal flora, *J. Med. Microbiol.*, in press.
238. Armstrong, B. and Doll, R., Environmental factors and cancer incidence and mortality in different countries, with special reference to dietary practices, *Cancer*, 15, 617, 1975.
239. Littman, A., Nutritional consequences of nondigestable carbohydrates, in *Nutrients in Processed Foods: Proteins*, White, P. L. and Fletcher, D. C., Eds., Publishing Sciences Group, Acton, Mass., 1974, 120.
240. Hodgkinson, A., Nordin, B. E. C., Hambleton, J., and Oxby, C. B., Radiostrantum absorption in man: suppression by calcium and sodium alginate, *Can. Med. Assoc. J.*, 97, 1139, 1967.
241. Spiller, G. A., Chernoff, M. C., Shipley, E. A., Beigler, M. A., and Briggs, G. M., Can fecal weight be used to establish a recommended intake of dietary fiber (Plantix)?, *Am. J. Clin. Nutr.*, 30, 659, 1977.
242. Burkitt, D. P., Relationships between diseases and their etiological significance, *Am. J. Clin. Nutr.*, 30, 262, 1977.
243. MacDonald, I., The effects of dietary fiber: are they all good?, in *Fiber in Human Nutrition*, Spiller, G. A. and Amen, R. J., Plenum Press, New York, 1976, 263-267.
244. Throne-Holst, J., Trowell, H., Van Soest, P. J., et al., Food and Fiber 5th Annual Maribou Symposium, *Nutr. Rev.*, 35(3), 1-71, 1977.
245. Trowell, H., Definition of dietary fiber and hypothesis that it is protective in certain diseases, *Am. J. Clin. Nutr.*, 29, 417, 1976.
246. Macy, I. G., *Nutrition and Chemical Growth in Childhood*, Charles C Thomas, Springfield, Ill., 1942.
247. Darfman, S. H., Ali, M., and Floch, M. H., Fiber content of Connecticut diet, *Am. J. Clin. Nutr.*, 29, 87, 1976.
248. Fuchs, H. M., Dorfman, S., and Floch, M. H., The effect of dietary fiber supplementation in man. II. Alteration in fecal physiology and bacterial flora, *Am. J. Clin. Nutr.*, 27, 1443, 1976.
249. Kahaner, N., Fuchs, H. M., and Floch, M. H., The effect of dietary fiber supplementation in man. I. Modification of eating habits, *Am. J. Clin. Nutr.*, 29, 1437, 1976.
250. Cummings, J. H., Hill, M. J., Jenkins, D. J. A., Pearson, J. R., and Wiggins, H. S., Changes in fecal composition and colonic function due to cereal fiber, *Am. J. Clin. Nutr.*, 29, 1468, 1976.

251. Wyman, J. B., Heaton, K. W., and Manning, A. P., The effect on intestinal transit and the feces of raw and cooked bran in different doses, *Am. J. Clin. Nutr.*, 29, 1474, 1976.
252. Fordtran, J. S., Organic anions in fecal contents, *New Engl. J. Med.*, 284, 329, 1971.
253. Williams, R. D. and Olmstead, N. H., The effect of cellulose, hemicellulose and lignin and the weight of the stool: a contribution to the study of laxation in man, *J. Nutr.*, 11, 433, 1936.
254. Hoppert, C. A. and Clark, A. J., Digestibility and effect on lactation of crude fiber and cellulose in certain common foods, *J. Am. Diet. Assoc.*, 21, 157, 1945.
255. Calloway, D. H., Gas in the alimentary canal, in *Handbook of Physiology: Alimentary Canal,* Vol. 5, Code, C. F., Ed., Williams & Wilkins, Baltimore, 1968, 2839-2859.
256. Bray, G., Ed., Obesity in Perspective: Proceedings of the Conference, DHEW Publ. No. (NIH) 75-708, U.S. Government Printing Office, Washington, D.C., 1975.
257. Kiehm, T. G., Anderson, J. W., and Ward, K., Beneficial effects of a high carbohydrate, high fiber diet on hyperglycemic diabetic men, *Am. J. Clin. Nutr.*, 29, 895, 1976.
258. Fernandez, L. B., Gonzalez, E., Marzi, A., and Paolo, M. I., Fecal acidorhea, *New Engl. J. Med.*, 284, 295, 1971.
259. Hodgkinson, A., Nordin, B. E. C., Hambleton, J., and Oxby, C. B., Radiostrontium absorption in man: suppression by calcium and sodium alginate, *Can. Med. Assoc. J.*, 97, 1139, 1967.
260. Owen, G. M., Kram, K. M., Garry, P. J., Lowe, J. E., and Lubin, A. H., A study of the nutritional status of preschool children in the United States 1968-1970. II, *Pediatrics*, 53(4), (Suppl.), 1974.
261. U.S. Department of Health, Education and Welfare, Highlights: Ten State Nutrition Survey 1968-1970, DHEW Publ. No. (HSM) 72-8134 HSMHA/CDC, U.S. Government Printing Office, Washington, D.C., 1972.
262. Eppright, E. S. et al., Nutrition of infants and preschool children in the North Central region of the United States of America, *World Rev. Nutr. Diet.*, 14, 269, 1972.
263. Wadsworth, G. R., Nutrition factors in anemia, *World Rev. Nutr. Dietet.*, 21, 75, 1975.
264. Fox, H. M., Fryer, B. A., Lamkin, G., et al., Diets of preschool children in the North Central Region, *J. Am. Diet. Assoc.*, 59, 233, 1971.
265. Martinez-Torres, C. and Layrisse, M., Interest for the study of dietary absorption and iron fortification, *World Rev. Nutr. Diet.*, 19, 52, 1974.
266. Moore, C. V., Iron nutrition, in *Iron Metabolism,* Springer-Verlag, Berlin, 1964, 244.
267. Layrisse, M., Martines-Torres, C., and Roche, M., The effect of interaction of various foods on iron absorption, *Am. J. Clin. Nutr.*, 21, 1175, 1968.
268. Layrisse, M. and Martinez-Torres, C., Iron absorption from food. Iron supplementation of foods, *Progr. Hematol.*, 137, 1971.
269. Layrisse, M., Cook, J. D., Martinez-Torres, C., Roche, M., Kuhn, I. N., and Finch, C. A., Food iron absorption: a comparison of vegetable and animal foods, *Blood*, 33, 430, 1969.
270. Martinez-Torres, C. and Layrisse, M., Effect of amino acids on iron absorption from a staple vegetable food, *Blood*, 35, 669, 1970.
271. Cook, J. D. and Monsen, E. R., Food iron absorption in human subjects. III. Comparison of the effect of animal proteins on nonheme iron absorption, *Am. J. Clin. Nutr.*, 29, 859, 1976.
272. Callender, S. T., Marney, S. R., and Warner, G. T., Eggs and iron absorption, *Br. J. Haematol.*, 19, 657, 1970.
273. Takkunen, H. and Seppanen, R., Iron deficiency and dietary factors in Finland, *Am. J. Clin. Nutr.*, 28, 1141, 1975.
274. Batu, A.-T., Thein-Than, and Thane-Toe, Iron absorption from Southeast Asian rice based meals, *Am. J. Clin. Nutr.*, 29, 219, 1976.
275. Layrisse, M., Roche, M., and Baker, S. J., Nutritional anemias, in *Nutrition in Preventive Medicine,* Beaton, G. H. and Bengoa, J., Ed., World Health Organization, Geneva, 1973, 68-101.
276. Sayers, M. H., Lynch, S. R., Jacobs, R., Charlton, R. W., Bothwell, T. H., Walker, R. B., and Mayer, F., The effects of ascorbic acid supplementation on the absorption of iron in maize, wheat, and soya, *Br. J. Haematol.*, 24, 209, 1973.
277. Cook, J. D. and Monsen, E. R., Vitamin C, the common cold, and iron absorption, *Am. J. Clin. Nutr.*, 30, 235, 1977.
278. Monsen, E. R. and Cook, J. D., Food iron absorption in human subjects. IV. The effects of calcium and phosphate salts on the absorption of nonheme iron, *Am. J. Clin. Nutr.*, 29, 1142, 1976.
279. Taylor, C. E. and de Sweemer, C., Nutrition and infection, *World Rev. Nutr. Diet.*, 16, 204, 1973.
280. Gopalon, C. and Srikantia, S. G., Nutrition and disease, *World Rev. Nutr. Diet.*, 16, 98, 1973.
281. Halsted, J. A., et al., Zinc deficiency in man, *Am. J. Med.*, 53, 277, 1972.
282. Rheinhold, J. G. et al., Binding of zinc to fiber and other solids of wholemeal bread, in *Trace Elements in Human Health and Disease,* Vol. 1, Prasad, A. S. and Oberleas, D., Ed., Academic Press, New York, 1976, 163-180.

283. Reinhold, J. G., Ismail-Beigi, F., and Faradji, B., Fiber versus phytate as determinants of the availability of calcium, zinc, and iron in breadstuffs, *Nutr. Rep. Int.,* 12, 75, 1975.
284. Reinhold, J. G., et al., Zinc, calcium, phosphorus and nitrogen balances of Iranian Villagers following a change from phytate-rich to phytate-poor diets, *Ecol. Food Nutr.,* 2, 157, 1973.
285. Mahloudji, M., Reinhold, J. G., Haghshenass, M., Ronaghy, H. A., Spivey-Fox, M. R., and Halsted, J. A., Combined zinc and iron compared to iron supplementation of diets of 6-12 year old village school children in Southern Iran, *Am. J. Clin. Nutr.,* 28, 721, 1975.
286. Ronaghy, H. A. and Halsted, J. A., Zinc deficiency occurring in females, *Am. J. Clin. Nutr.,* 28, 831, 1975.
287. Hambidge, K. M., Walravens, P. A., Brown, R. M., Webster, J., White, S., Anthony, M., and Roth, M. L., Low levels of zinc in hair, anorexia, poor growth and hypoguesia in children, *Pediatr. Res.,* 6, 868, 1972.
288. Anon., Zinc in human medicine, *Lancet,* 2, 351, 1975.
289. Walravens, P. A. and Hambidge, K. M., Growth of infants fed a zinc supplemented formula, *Am. J. Clin. Nutr.,* 29, 1114, 1976.
290. Sandstead, H. H., Zinc nutrition in the U.S., *Am. J. Clin. Nutr.,* 26, 1251, 1973.
291. Davies, N. T. and Williams, R. B., Zinc balance in pregnancy and lactation, *Am. J. Clin. Nutr.,* 30, 300, 1977.
292. Klevay, L. M., Coronary Heart disease-the zinc copper hypothesis, *Am. J. Clin. Nutr.,* 28, 764, 1975.
293. Weick, M. T., A history of rickets in the United States, *Am. J. Clin. Nutr.,* 20, 1234, 1967.
294. Morse, J. L., The frequency of rickets in infancy in Boston and vacinity, *J. Am. Med. Assoc.,* 34, 724, 1900.
295. Lovett, R. W., The roentgenographic appearance in rickets, *J. Am. Med. Assoc.,* 65, 2062, 1915.
296. Haven, H. C., The etiology of rachitis, *Boston Med. Surg. J.,* 115, 27, 1886.
297. Eliot, M. M., The control of rickets, *J. Am. Med. Assoc.,* 85, 19, 1925.
298. Eliot, M. M., The control of rickets, *J. Am. Med. Assoc.,* 85, 656, 1925.
299. Eliot, M. M. and Park, E. A., Rickets, in *The Cyclopedia of Medicine,* Vol. 11, Piersol, G. M., Ed., F. A. Davis, Philadelphia, 1935, 1-59.
300. Harrison, H. E., Symposium on homogenized vitamin D milk: disappearance of rickets, vitamin D milk as related to mineral nutrition, *Q. Rev. Pediatr.,* 8, 323, 1953.
301. American Academy of Pediatrics, The relation between infantile hypercalcemia and vitamin D: public health implications in North America, *Pediatrics,* 40, 1050, 1967.
301a. Richards, I. D. G., Sweet, E. M., and Arneil, G. C., Infantile rickets persists in Glasgow, *Lancet,* 1, 803, 1968.
302. Goel, K. M., Logan, R. W., Arneil, G. C., Sweet, E. M., Warren, J. M., and Shanks, R. A., Florid and subclinical rickets among immigrant children in Glasgow, *Lancet,* 1, 1141, 1976.
302a. Arneil, G. C., Rickets in Glasgow today, *Practitioner,* 210, 331, 1973.
303. Stamp, T. C. B., Vitamin D metabolism, *Arch. Dis. Child.,* 48, 2, 1973.
304. Arneil, G. C. and Crosbie, J. C., Infantile rickets returns to Glasgow, *Lancet,* 2, 423, 1963.
305. Swan, C. H. J. and Cooke, W. T., Nutritional osteomalacia in immigrants in an urban community, *Lancet,* 2, 456, 1971.
306. Ford, J. A., Calhoun, E. M., McIntosh, W. B., and Dunnigan, M. G., Rickets and osteomalacia in the Glasgow Pakistani community, *Br. Med. J.,* 2, 677, 1972.
307. Hoffer, A., Ascorbic acid and toxicity, *New Engl. J. Med.,* 285, 635, 1971.
308. Richards, I. D. G., Hamilton, F. M. W., Taylor, E. C., Sweet, S. M., Bremner, E., and Price, H., A Search for subclinical rickets in Glasgow children, *Scott. Med. J.,* 13, 297, 1968.
309. Moncrief, M. W., Lant, H. R., and Arthur, L. J. H., Nutritional rickets at puberty, *Arch. Dis. Child.,* 48, 221, 1973.
310. Ford, J. A., MacIntosh, W. B., and Dunnigan, M. G., Aetiology of Asian rickets and osteomalacia in the United Kingdom, *Arch. Dis. Child.,* 48, 827, 1973.
311. Preece, M. A., Tomlinson, S., Ribot, C. A., Pietrick, J., Korn, H. T., Davies, D. M., Ford, J. A., Dunnigan, M. G., and O'Riordan, J. L. H., Studies of vitamin D deficiency in man, *Q. J. Med.,* 44, 575, 1975.
312. Preece, M. A., Ford, J. A., MacIntosh, W. B., Dunnigan, M. G., Tomlinson, S., and O'Riordan, J. L. H., Assessment of vitamin D status in man using measurement of serum 25 hydroxycholecalciferol concentration, *Lancet,* 1, 907, 1973.
313. Arneil, G. C., The return of infantile rickets to Britain, *World Rev. Nutr. Diet.,* 10, 239, 1969.
314. Paunier, L., Rickets and osteomalacia, in *Nutrition in Preventive Medicine,* Beaton, G. and Bengoa, J., Eds., World Health Organization, Geneva, 1975, 140-149.
315. Dunnigan, M. G. and Smith, C. M., The aetrology of late rickets in Pakistani children in Glasgow. Report of a diet survey, *Scott. Med. J.,* 10, 1, 1965.
316. Holmes, A. M., Eroch, B. A., Taylor, J. L., and Jones, M. E., Occult rickets and osteomalacia amongst the Asian immigrant population, *Q. J. Med.,* 42, 125, 1973.

317. O'Hara-May, J. and Widdowson, E. M., Diets and living conditions of Asians boys in Coventry with and without signs of rickets, *Br. J. Nutr.,* 36, 23, 1975.

318. Dent, C. E., Rickets (and osteomalacia) nutritional and metabolis, *Proc. R. Soc. Med.,* 63, 401, 1970.

319. Stadler, G., Schmid, R., Held, U., and Rossier, R., Sero chemical and radiological improvement of vitamin D deficiency rickets on treatment with vitamin D in spite of a calcium free diet, *Ann. Pediatr.,* 199, 215, 1962.

320. Chu, J. Y., Margen, S., and Costa, F. M., Studies of calcium metabolism. II. Effects of low calcium and variable protein intake on human calcium metabolism, *Am. J. Clin. Nutr.,* 28, 1028, 1975.

321. Mellanby, E., Rickets — producing and anticalcifying action of phytate, *J. Physiol.,* 109, 488, 1949.

322. Reinhold, J. G., Nutritional osteomalacia in immigrants in an urban community, *Lancet,* 1, 386, 1972.

323. Willis, M. R., Day, R. C., Phillippo, J. B., and Bateman, E. C., Phytic acid and nutritional rickets in immigrants, *Lancet,* 1, 771, 1972.

324. Dent, C. E., Round, J. M., Rowe, D. J. F., and Stamp, T. C. B., Effect of chappatis and ultraviolet radiation on nutritional rickets in an Indian immigrant, *Lancet,* 1, 1282, 1973.

325. Ford, J. A., Calhoun, E. M., MacIntosh, W. B., and Dunnigan, M. G., Biochemical response of late rickets and osteomalacia to a chupatty free diet, *Br. Med. J.,* 3, 446, 1972.

326. Beckmeier, H. and Heminsdorf, G., Metabolites of vitamin D3 and their biological activity, *Physiol. Chem.,* 214, 720, 1958.

327. Loomis, W. F., Rickets, *Sci. Am.,* 223(6), 77, 1970.

328. Loomis, W. F., Skin pigment regulation of vitamin D biosynthesis in man, *Science,* 157, 501, 1971.

329. Oke, O. L., Rickets in developing countries, *World Rev. Nutr. Diet.,* 15, 86, 1972.

330. Thomson, M. L., Relative efficiency of pigment and horney layer thickness in protecting the skin of Europeans and Africans versus solar ultraviolet radiation, *J. Physiol.,* 127, 236, 1955.

331. Underwood, M. A., With general directions for the management of infants from the birth, *A Treatise on the Disease of Children,* Vol. 1, J. Mathews, London, 1789, 313.

332. Schwartz, A. R., Togo, Y., Hornick, R. B., Tominaga, S., and Gleckman, R. A., Evaluation of the efficacy of ascorbic acid in prophylaxis of induced rhinovirus 44 infection in man, *J. Infect. Dis.,* 128, 500, 1973.

333. Gupta, M. M., Round, J. M., and Stamp, T. C. B., Spontaneous cure of vitamin D deficiency in Asians during summer in Britain, *Lancet,* 1, 586, 1974.

334. Schmorl, G., Über die Beziehungen der Knorpelmarkkanale zu der bei Rachitis sich findenden Störung der endochondralen Ossifikation, *Verh. Dtsch. Pathol. Ges.,* 40-48, 1909.

335. Aykroyd, B., *Conquest of the Deficiency Diseases,* Freedom from Hunger Campaign Basic Study #24, United Nations, New York, 1970.

336. Lapantsanis, P., Deliyanni, V., and Daxiadis, S., Vitamin D deficiency rickets in Greece, *J. Pediatr.,* 73, 195, 1968.

337. Dwyer, J. T., Dietz, W., Hass, G., and Susskind, R., The return of rickets to Boston, *New Engl. J. Med.,* in press.

338. Frazer, D., Koch, S. W., and Scriver, C. R., Hyperparathyroidism as the cause of hyperaminoaciduria and phosphaturia in human vitamin D deficiency, *Pediatr. Res.,* 1, 425, 1967.

339. Fraser, D. and Salter, R. B., The diagnosis and management of the various types of rickets, *Pediatr. Clin. North Am.,* 5, 417, 1958.

340. Committee on Nutrition, American Academy of Pediatrics, The relationship between infantile hypercalcemia and vitamin D — public health implications in North America, *Pediatrics,* 40, 1050, 1967.

341. Bronner, F., Vitamin D deficiency and rickets, *Am. J. Clin. Nutr.,* 29, 1307, 1976.

342. Fairney, A., Jackson, D., and Clayton, B. E., Measurement of serum parathyroid hormone, with particular reference to some infants with hypocalcamia, *Arch. Dis. Child.,* 48, 419, 1973.

343. Pincus, J. B., Gittleman, I. F., Marius, N., and Bachra, B., The effects of graded doses of vitamin D on the serum calcium and phosphorus levels, *Am. J. Dis. Child.,* 96, 16, 1958.

344. Rosen, J. F., Roginsky, G., Nathenson, G., and Finberg, L., 25 hydroxy vitamin D:plasma levels in mothers and their premature infants with neonatal hypoglycemia, *Am. J. Dis. Child.,* 127, 220, 1974.

345. Watney, P. J. M., Chance, G. W., Scott, P., and Thompson, J. M., Maternal factors in neonatal hypocalcemia: a study in 3 ethnic groups, *Br. Med. J.,* 2, 432, 1971.

346. Dent, C. E. and Gupta, M. M., Plasma 25-hydroxy-vitamin-D levels during pregnancy in Caucasians and in vegetarian and non-vegetarian Asians, *Lancet,* 2, 1057, 1975.

347. Hillman L. S. and Haddard, J. G., Human prenatal vitamin D metabolism. I. 25 hydroxyvitamin D in maternal and cord blood, *J. Pediatr.,* 84, 742, 1974.

348. Benson, P. F., Stround, C. E., Mitchell, N. J., and Nicoliades, A., Rickets in immigrant children in London, *Br. Med. J.,* 1, 1054, 1963.

349. Stewart, W. K. R., Mitchell, R. G., Morgan, H. G., Lowe, K. G., and Thompson, J., The changing incidence of rickets and infantile hypercalcemia as seen in Dundee, *Lancet,* 1, 679, 1964.

350. Haddad, J. G. and Stamp, T. C. B., Circulating 25-hydroxy vitamin D in man, *Am. J. Med.*, 57, 57, 1974.
351. Cooke, W. T., Asquith, P., Rusk, N., Melikan, V., and Swan, C. H. J., Rickets, growth and alkaline phoshatase in urban adolescents, *Br. Med. J.*, 2, 293, 1974.
352. Wills, M. R., Day, R. C., Phillips, J. B., and Bateman, E. C., Phytic acid and nutritional rickets in immigrants, *Lancet*, 1, 771, 1972.
353. Ford, J. A., Davidson, D. C., MacIntosh, W. B., Fyfe, W. B., and Dunnigan, M. G., Neonatal rickets in an Asian immigrant population, *Br. Med. J.*, 3, 211, 1973.
354. Barsky, P., Rickets: Canada 1968, *Can. J. Public Health*, 60, 29, 1969.
355. Anon., 250 cases annually: Montreal reports high rickets rate, *J. Am. Med. Assoc.*, 207, 1269 and 1272, 1969.
356. Broadfoot, B. V. R., Trenholme, M. L., McClinton, E. D., Thompson, S. H., and Cowin, E. J., Vitamin D intakes of Ontario children, *Can. Med. Assoc. J.*, 94, 332, 1966.
357. Cooke, W. T., Swan, C. H. J., Asquith, P., Melikian, V., and McFeeley, W. E., Serum alkaline phosphatase and rickets in urban school children, *Br. Med. J.*, 1, 324, 1973.
358. Round, J. M., Plasma calcium magnesium, phosphorus and alkaline phosphatase levels in normal British school children, *Br. Med. J.*, 3, 137, 1973.
359. Reddy, V. and Srikantia, S. G., Serum alkaline phosphatase in malnourished children with rickets, *J. Pediatr.*, 71, 59, 1967.
360. Cooke, W. T., Asquith, P., Ruck, N., Melikian, V., and Swan, C. H. J., Rickets, growth and alkaline phosphatase in urban adolescents, *Br. Med. J.*, 2, 293, 1974.
361. Maxwell, J. P., Further studies in osteomalacia, *Proc. R. Soc. Med.*, 23, 639, 1930.
362. Patwardhan, V. N., *Nutrition in India*, 2nd ed., Indian Journal of Medical Sciences, Bombay, 1961, 1-150.
363. Groen, J. J., Echchar, D., Ben Ishay, W. J., Alkan, T., and Ben Assa, B. I., Osteomalacia in Negev Bedouins, *Arch. Int. Med.*, 116, 195, 1965.
364. Berlyne, G. M., Ben Ari J., Nord, E., and Skaikin, R., Bedouin osteomalacia due to calcium deprivation caused by high phytic acid content of unleavened bread, *Am. J. Clin. Nutr.*, 26, 910, 1973.
365. Shany, S., Hirsch, J., and Berlyne, G., 25 hydroxycholecalciferol levels in Bedouins in the Negev, *Am. J. Clin. Nutr.*, 29, 1104, 1976.
366. Krishnarnachari, K. A. V. R. and Iyengar, L., Effect of maternal malnutrition on the bone density of the neonate, *Am. J. Clin. Nutr.*, 28, 482, 1975.
367. Albright, F., Butler, A. H., and Bloomberg, E., Rickets resistant to vitamin D therapy, *Am. J. Dis. Child.*, 59, 529, 1937.
368. Scriver, C. R., Rickets and the pathogenesis of impaired tubular transport of phosphate and other solutes, *Am. J. Med.*, 57, 43, 1974.
369. Frazer, D. and Scriver, C. R., Familial forms of vitamin D resistant rickets revisted. X linked hyperphosphatemia and autosomal recessive vitamin D dependency, *Am. J. Clin. Nutr.* 29, 1315, 1976.
370. Anon., personal communication, Imogine Bassett Hospital, Cooperstown, N.Y., 1975.
371. Underwood, B. A., The determination of vitamin A and some aspects of its distribution, mobilization and transport in health and disease, *World Rev. Nutr. Diet.*, 19, 124, 1974.
372. Gopalan, C., Venkatachalom, P. S., and Bhavani, B., Studies of vitamin A deficiency in children, *Am. J. Clin. Nutr.*, 8, 833, 1960.
373. Anon., Hypovitaminosis A in the Americans, Rep. PAHO Tech. Group Meet. Sci. Publ. #198, Pan American Health Association, Washington, D.C., 1970.
374. Grasbeck, R., Physiology and pathology of vitamin B-12 absorption, distribution, and excretion, *Adv. Clin. Chem.*, 3, 299, 1960.
375. Banarjee, D. K. and Chatterjee, J. B., Serum vitamin B-12 in vegetarians, *Br. Med. J.*, 2, 992, 1970.
376. Baker, S. J., Human vitamin B-12 deficiency, *World Rev. Nutr. Diet.*, 8, 62, 1967.
377. Stewart, J. S., Roberts, P. D., and Hoffbrand, A. V., Response of dietary vitamin B-12 deficiency to physiological oral doses of cyanocobalamin, *Lancet*, 2, 542, 1970.
378. Britt, R. P., Harper, C., and Spray, G. H., Megaloblastic anemia among Indians in Britain, *Q. J. Med.*, 40, 499, 1970.
379. Smith, A. D. M., Veganism: a clinical survey with observations on vitamin B-12 metabolism, *Br. Med. J.*, 1, 1655, 1972.
380. Bourne, M. and Olesky, S., Dietary deficiency of vitamin B-12, *Br. Med. J.*, 2, 511, 1960.
381. Misra, H. N. and Followfield, J. M., Subacute combined degeneration of the spinal cord in a vegan, *Postgrad. Med. J.*, 47, 624, 1971.
382. Gleeson, M. H. and Graves, P. S., Complications of dietary deficiency of vitamin B-12 in young Caucasians, *Postgrad. Med. J.*, 50, 462, 1974.

383. **Dastur, D. K., Santadeve, N., Quadros, E. V., Gagrad, B. M., Nadia, N. H., Desai, M. M., Singhal, B. S., and Bharalha, E. P.,** Interrelationships between the B vitamins in B-12 deficiency neuromyopathy. A possible malabsorption malnutrition syndrome, *Am. J. Clin. Nutr.,* 28, 1255, 1975.

384. **Kurtha, A. N. and Ellis, F. R.,** Investigation into the causation of electroencephalographic abnormality in vegetarians, *Plant Foods Hum. Nutr.,* 2, 55, 1971.

385. **Wokes, F., Badenoch, J. L., and Sinclair, H.,** Human dietary deficiency of vitamin B-12, *Am. J. Clin. Nutr.,* 3, 375, 1955.

386. **Baker, S. J., Jacob, E., Rajan, K. T., and Swaminathan, S. P.,** Vitamin B-12 deficiency in pregnancy and the puerperiam, *Br. Med. J.* 1, 1658, 1962.

387. **Pinto-Vaz, A., Torras, V., Sandoval, J. F. F., Dillman, E., Mateos, C. R., and Cordova, M. S.,** Folic acid and B-12 determination in fetal liver, *Am. J. Clin. Nutr.,* 28, 1085, 1975.

388. **Jadhav, M., Webb, J. K. G., Vaishnava, S., and Baker, S. J.,** Vitamin B-12 deficiency in Indian infants: a clinical syndrome, *Lancet,* 2, 903, 1963.

389. **Lamkin, B. C. and Saunders, E. F.,** Nutritional vitamin B-12 deficiency in an infant, *J. Pediatr.,* 75, 1053, 1969.

390. **Linnell, J. C., Hoffbrand, A. V., Peters, T. J., and Matthews, D. M.,** Chromatographic and bioautographic estimation of plasma cobulamine in various disturbances of vitamin B-12 metabolism, *Clin. Sci.,* 40, 1, 1971.

391. **Matthews, D. M.,** Effects of smoking on the metabolism and excretion of vitamin B-12, *Br. Med. J.,* 2, 237, 1968.

392. **Distur, D. K., Quadros, E. V., Wadia, N. H., Desai, M. M., and Bharucha, E. P.,** Effect of vegetarianism and smoking on B-12, thiocyanate, and folate levels in the blood of normal subjects, *Br. Med. J.,* 3, 260, 1972.

393. **Boxer, G. E. and Richards, J. C.,** Studies on the metabolism of the carbon of cyanide and thiocyoinate, *Arch. Biochem. Biophys.,* 39, 7 1952.

394. **Darty, P. W. and Wilson, J.,** Cyanide, smoking and tobacco amblyopia: observations on the cyanide content of tobacco smoke, *Br. J. Ophthalmol.,* 36, 336, 1967.

395. **Wilson, J. and Matthews, D. M.,** Metabolic interrelationships between cyanide, thiocyanate, and vitamin B-12 in smokers and non-smokers, *Clin. Sci.,* 31, 1, 1966.

396. **Ericson, L. E. and Banhidi, Z. G.,** Bacterial growth factors relation to B-12 and folinic acid in some brown and red seaweeds acta, *Chem. Scand.,* 7, 167, 1953.

397. **Ericson, L. E. and Lewis, L.,** On the occurrence of B-12 factors in marine algae, *Arkiv. Kemi,* 6, 427, 1955.

398. **Takton, D.,** *The Great Vitamin Hoax,* Macmillan, New York, 1973.

399. **McKenzie, J.,** Profile on vegetarians, *Plant Foods Hum. Nutr.,* 2, 49, 1971.

400. **Committee on Nutrition, American Academy of Pediatrics,** The prophylactic requirement and the toxicity of vitamin D, *Pediatrics,* 31, 512, 1963.

401. **DeLuca, H.,** Current concepts: vitamin D, *New Engl. J. Med.,* 281, 1103, 1969.

402. **Yendt, E. R., DeLuca, H. F., Garcia, D. A. and Cochanin, M.,** Clinical aspects of vitamin D, in *The Fat Soluble Vitamins,* De Luca, H. and Fond Suttie, J. W., Eds., University of Wisconsin Press, Madison, 1969, 125.

403. **Baker, E. N., Hodges, R. E., Hood, J., Sauberlech, N. E., March, S., and Canham, J. E.,** Metabolism of 14 C and 3H labeled L-ascorbic acid in human scurvy, *Am. J. Clin. Nutr.,* 24, 444-454, 1971.

404. **Harris, L. J., Ray, S. W., and Ward, A.,** The excretion of vitamin C in human urine and its dependence of the dietary intake, *Biochem. J.,* 27, 2011-2015, 1933.

405. **Goldsmith, G. A. and Ellinger, G. F.,** Ascorbic acid in blood and urine after oral administration of a test dose of vitamin D, *Arch. Int. Med.,* 63, 531-536, 1939.

406. **Goodhart, R. S. and Shils, M. E.,** Ascorbic type acid, in *Modern Nutrition in Health Disease,* 5th ed., Wohl, M. G., Goodhart, M., and Shils, M., Eds., Lea & Febiger, Philadelphia, 1973, 250.

407. **Wilson, C. W., Loh, H. S., and Foster, F. G.,** The beneficial effect of vitamin C on the common cold, *Eur. J. Clin. Pharmacol.,* 6, 26, 1973.

408. **Herfindal, E. T. and Hirschmon, J. L.,** *Clinical Pharmacy and Therapeutics,* Williams & Wilkins, Baltimore, 1975, 432.

409. **Riccitelli, M. L.,** Vitamin C — a review and reassessment of pharmacological and therapeutic uses, *Conn. Med.,* 39, 609-614, 1975.

410. **Clegg, K. M. and McDonald, J. M.,** L-ascorbic acid and D-isoascorbic acid in a common cold survey, *Am. J. Clin. Nutr.,* 28, 973, 1975.

411. **Lakdawala, D. R. and Widdowson, E. M.,** Vitamin D in human milk, *Lancet,* 1, 167-168, 1977.

412. **Charleston, S. S. and Clegg, K. M.,** Ascorbic acid and the common cold, *Lancet,* 1, 1401, 1972.

413. **Anderson, T. W., Reid, D. B. W., and Beaton, G. H.,** Vitamin C and the common cold: a double blind trial, *Can. Med. Assoc., J.,* 107, 503, 1972.

414. Krishnamachari, K. A. V. R. and Laxmaiah, N., Lack of effect of massive dose of vitamin C on fluoride excretion in fluorosis during a short clinical trial, *Am. J. Clin. Nutr.,* 28, 1234, 1975.
415. Chalmers, T. C., Effects of ascorbic acid on the common cold: an evaluation of the evidence, *Am. J. Med.,* 58, 532-536, 1975.
416. Anon., Vitamin C and the common cold, *Med. Lett. Drugs Ther.,* 16, 85, 1974.
417. Wilson, C. W. M., Greene, M., and Loh, H. S., The metabolism of supplementary vitamin C during the common cold, *J. Clin. Pharmacol.,* 16, 19, 1976.

# FOOD MIXTURES FOR COMBATING CHILDHOOD MALNUTRITION

## Peter L. Pellett and Amira S. Pellett

## INTRODUCTION

It remains a truism that a major cause of ill health and high mortality in infants and young children is inadequate and/or improper feeding. General views of causation, nevertheless, have changed considerably in recent years, nutritional problems in the past have been seen as being specifically nutrient related, a deficiency of a nutrient resulting in a deficiency syndrome. Present views, however now, increasingly recognize that infantile malnutrition may be caused less by food and nutrient deficiency as such and more by many interrelated socioeconomic and hygienic factors.[1] Nevertheless, correct selection of acceptable forms of feeding which are also nutritionally sound, economically feasible, and relevant to the situation in developing countries can lead to considerable reductions in infant morbidity and mortality. Problems and their resolution, however, differ from age group to age group and from country to country and holistic solutions are probably not possible.[2]

Some definition of the scope of this review is necessary since the title could be considered, in its widest interpretation, to include all feeding from birth to adolescence. Food mixtures in this context mean mixtures of foods of high-nutritional value often supplemented with minerals and vitamins that are mixed in such a way that the protein sources used, complement each other to give higher protein quality than any of the major individual components.

Food mixtures also must be cheap since they are designed for use in poor countries. The protein sources will thus be of predominantly vegetable origin, small amounts of animal protein foods (e.g., milk powder) may be present, cost factors will, however, generally preclude this proportion being very high. While manufactured mixtures will be a major concern, consideration will also be given to mixtures of recommended proportions for home preparation.

Milk products, milk substitutes, humanized milk, and similar products designated for the feeding of neonates and young babies whose mothers are unable or do not desire to breast feed are not considered within the scope of this review. As will be elaborated below, the main focus will be upon relatively low cost, nutritionally adequate protein foods that can be used to supplement breast feeding.

The early discontinuance of breast feeding by mothers in low-income groups in urban areas of most developing countries has been a serious concern for some years.[3-5b] Protein Advisory Group (PAG) Statement No. 23 — promotion of special foods for vulnerable groups[5] was a reaction to this concern. This statement emphasized the critical importance of breast feeding under the sociocultural and -economic conditions that prevail in many developing countries. Infants of more affluent socioeconomic groups in industrialized and developing countries, in the absence of breast feeding, suffer no nutritional disadvantage when fed properly constituted and hygienically prepared processed commercial formulas. However, the early abandonment of breast feeding by mothers among lower socioeconomic groups has often proved to be disastrous to infants. This is particularly true when financial resources are inadequate to purchase sufficient formula and when knowledge of and facilities to follow hygienic practices necessary to feed infants adequately and safely with breast milk replacements are not available. Under such circumstances, and where animal milk and other supplementary protein resources are expensive or in short supply, an important function of the food industry, in close cooperation with governments and physicians, should be the development and marketing of relatively low-cost, nutritionally equivalent proteins foods that can be used to supplement breast feeding. Much has already been done in this area, but there have been problems and disagreements.

In order to resolve some of these problems, a seminar was promoted by the Protein-Calorie Advisory Group of the United Nations[6] to recommend policies and practices for feeding infants and young children and also to identify the roles of medical and health professions, the infant food industry, and the government agencies in promoting desirable policies and practices. A further aim was to devise a permanent machinery for collaboration among these groups so that they could carry out effectively their identified roles in the region and in the individual countries.

Recommendations[6] for feeding policies and practices were

A.  Young Infants (0 to 6 months)
    1.  The food of choice for this age group is mother's milk; thus, breast feeding should be promoted among all mothers and should be stressed in teaching in medical, nursing, and paramedical schools; such education should also be extended to community leaders
    2.  Since there is a small proportion of women who for recognized reasons are unable to breast feed at all or can do so only inadequately, professional aid to correct this situation or to arrange for an alternative feeding method should be made available; even if a mother works, she should be encouraged to breast feed whenever possible
    3.  Alternative feeding of young infants should be viewed as a critical risk situation regardless of the type or nature of the food substituted for mother's milk; the four basic essentials for alternative feeding are sufficient money, proper use of substitute food, adequate food hygiene, and proper maternal education; problems can occur when any one is lacking[7]

B.  Older Infants (6 or 12 months) and Young Children (12 to 24 months)
    1.  Breast feeding should be continued for as long as possible, but the declining supply of breast milk must be reckoned with; therefore, breast milk, although beneficial, should not be considered the primary source of nourishment for infants beyond 6 months of age
    2.  The primary role should be taken over by nourishing foods other than breast milk; they must be introduced into the diet gradually, and their selection should be in stages, based on the physical consistency of the food used
    3.  Suitable recipes and menus should be worked out locally in each country or region by the appropriate nutrition and health personnel according to the special conditions prevailing in the area; efforts should be undertaken to prepare for each country a manual of homemade nutritious foods for weaning; as often as possible these foods should be part of the entire family's diet.
    4.  Inexpensive nutritious foods should be developed and marketed for young children because of the tremendous importance of the weaning phase; such foods should, as far as possible, be prepared and blended locally in the countries, using commodities available in the area; these foods should play a major nutritional role, similar to the role of milk in more affluent populations

Within this review, the rationale behind, and history of food mixtures will be discussed together with some reasons for their success or failure and their possible future role in a world of limited energy, limited food, and even increasing population.

Food mixtures are sometimes considered as if they are exclusively manufactured products, an alternative approach, advocated by many over a long period and discussed in detail by Cameron and Hofvander,[8] lies in the home mixing of components so as to produce more balanced mixtures for the feeding of infants and young children. While this is much more in the domain of infant feeding practice than in food mixture technology, the approach is highly relevant and eliminates many of the limitation and dangers inherent in the food mixture approach.[9]

Soon after World War II, awareness of the prevalence of protein-energy malnutrition (PEM) resulted in massive research activity in all areas related to protein. With the availability of amino-acid analytical data and biological methods for the assay of protein quality[10-12] the concepts of supplementation, complementation, and amino-acid fortification[13-15] became increasing widely known and the development of protein-rich food mixtures grew to be one of the major areas in programs designed to alleviate the scourge of PEM. The projects carried considerable prestige and high-level support and funding became widely available. Later it became almost mandatory for any nutrition research unit working on the problems of the developing world to have its own mixture. With hindsight, it is easy to see that the enthusiasm may have been misplaced; complex problems do not usually have simple solutions and the problems of malnutrition are overwhelmingly complex. For too long, an implicit assumption has been that malnutrition was caused by ignorance and that scientific methodology would, when effectively marshalled, overcome it. A corollary of this viewpoint was that malnutrition was primarily food and nutrient related. We now realize that malnutrition, especially infantile malnutrition, may be caused more by absence of clean water than by low-protein quality and more dependent upon flies and infection than protein intake.[1] The solutions thus lie in the areas of preventive rather than curative medicine, in economics rather than in nutrition, and in land reform rather than in food technology.

All this is not to say that "food mixtures" do not have a place: with the recent realization that world energy (fossil fuel) supplies and food production are highly interrelated and not independent, their place may become more important. While the concept of complementation of proteins has only received scientific explanation since amino-acid data have become available, the principle has been traditional in the dietary habits of most peoples of the world since antiquity.[16] Just as soybean and rice have been part of the Far Eastern dietary pattern, wheat bread with legumes has been a hallmark of the Middle Eastern diets.[17]

The development of food mixtures has, throughout its history, had close association with several United Nations agencies, notably WHO, FAO, and UNICEF, and led to the development of the PAG. Brief histories exist on the development of protein foods and the involvement of the United Nations agencies.[18,19] In addition, a series of statements and guidelines relevant to food mixtures have been produced by the PAG (Table 1 ), and extensive reviews and critiques of the whole field have appeared recently.[20-24]

## COMPLEMENTARY PROTEIN MIXTURES

### Available Sources of Vegetable Protein

Animal foods are expensive partially because of the inefficiencies of conversion of feed protein into protein for human consumption.[25] Rich regions of the world have traditionally supplemented their cereal staples with animal products especially milk and eggs, adequate supplementation is also possible with vegetable mixtures.

Some 70% of the worlds supply of edible protein comes from plant sources, of this, nearly 70% is from cereals and 18% from grain legumes.[26] In the developing regions of the world, a rather larger proportion of total protein comes from plant sources most being directly consumed by humans. In the rich regions of the world, i.e., North America, Europe, U.S.S.R., and Oceania, the major proportion of the cereals (except wheat and rice) and almost all of the grain legumes are used for animal feed.

Table 1

SOME RELEVANT DOCUMENTS FROM THE PROTEIN-CALORIE
ADVISORY GROUP OF THE UNITED NATIONS

| Statement No. | Title | Year | PAG Bull. Publ.[a] | PAG Compendium reference[b] |
|---|---|---|---|---|
| 3 | Nature and magnitude of the protein problem | 1971 | Vol. 1, No. 12, 1971 | 13/3: F 749—754 |
| 5 | Marketing and distribution of protein-rich foods | 1971 | Vol. 1, No. 12, 1971 | 13/5: G 397—401 |
| 9 | Amino acid fortification of foods | 1970 | — | 13/9: B 367—387 |
| 19 | Maintenance and improvement of nutritional quality of protein foods | 1972 | — | 13/19: B 111—112 |
| 20 | The protein problem | 1973 | Vol. 3, No. 1, 1973 | 13/20: F 785—794 |
| 22 | Upgrading human nutrition by the improvement of food legumes | 1973 | Vol. 3, No. 2, 1973 | 13/22: D 127—169 |
| 23 | Promotion of special foods (infant formula and processed protein foods) for vulnerable groups | 1972 | Vol. 2, No. 3, 1972 | 13/23: E1 623—630 |
| 24 | The green revolution and protein supplies | 1973 | — | 13/24: D 171—180 |
| 25 | The global maldistribution of protein | 1973 | Vol. 2, No. 3, 1973 | 13/25: F 795—798 |
| 2 | Preparation of food-quality groundnut flour | 1970 | — | 14/2: C2 1519—1522 |
| 4 | Preparation of edible cottonseed protein concentrate | 1970 | — | 14/4: C1 1137—1140 |
| 5 | Edible, heat-processed soy grits and flour | 1969 | — | 14/5: C2 1945—1953 |
| 6 | Preclinical testing of novel sources of protein | 1972 | Vol. 4, No. 3, 1974 | 14/6: D 785—809 |
| 7 | Human testing of supplementary food mixtures | 1972 | Vol. 3, No. 3, 1973 | 14/7: D 933—946 |
| 8 | Protein-rich mixtures for use as weaning foods | 1972 | Vol. 1, No. 12, 1971 | 14/8: E1 631—636 |
| 9 | Fish protein concentrate | 1971 | Vol. 1, No. 12, 1971 | 14/9: C1 469—474 |
| 10 | Marketing of protein-rich foods in developing countries | 1971 | — | 14/10: G 405—500 |
| 11 | Sanitary production and use of dry protein foods | 1972 | Vol. 2, No. 3, 1972 | 14/11: D 1041—1056 |
| 12 | Production of single-cell protein for human consumption | 1972 | Vol. 2, No. 2, 1972 | 14/12: CD 2249—2253 |
| 13 | Preparation of milk substitutes of vegetable origin and toned milk containing vegetable protein | 1972 | Vol. 3, No. 1, 1973 | 14/13: E1 637—645 |
| 14 | Preparation of defatted edible sesame flour | 1973 | Vol. 3, No. 1, 1973 | 14/14: C2 1625—1632 |
| 15 | Nutritional and safety aspects of novel protein sources for animal feeding | 1974 | Vol. 4, No. 3, 1974 | — |
| 16 | Protein methods for cereal breeder as related to human nutritional requirements | 1975 | Vol. 5, No. 2, 1975 | — |
| Documents | | | | |
| 1.14/5 | Feeding the Preschool Child — Report of a PAG ad hoc Working Group | 1971 | — | 6.4.3/45 E2 1161—1225 |
| 1.14/26 | Manual on Feeding Infants and Young Children by Margaret Cameron and Yngve Hofvander, 1st Edition | 1971 | — | 6.4.3/46 — |
| No number | 2nd Edition | 1976 | — | 6.4.3/46 — |

[a] Not all statements and guidelines are available in the *PAG Bulletins*.

[b] *PAG Compendium* — the collected papers issued by the Protein-Calorie Advisory Group of the United Nations System 1956—1973. Nine volumes marked A, B, C1, C2, D, E1, E2, F, and G. Worldmark Press, Ltd., Halsted Press Division, John Wiley & Sons, New York, 1975. The first number describes the new classification while the letter and numbers describe the volume and pages within the Compendium where the document may be found.

Table 2

PROTEIN, FOOD ENERGY, AND ESSENTIAL AMINO ACIDS FOR
SELECTED STAPLE FOODS AND SUPPLEMENTS[a]

| Staples | Protein (g) | Food energy | | Essential amino acids (mg/g N) | | | | | Score[b] and limiting amino acid |
| | | kcal | kJ | Lys | Thr | Try | SAA | PER | |
| | | Per 100 g | | | | | | | |
| Corn Meal | 9.5 | 350 | 1465 | 167 | 225 | 40 | 217 | 1.2 | 0.49 L |
| Millet | 9.7 | 360 | 1510 | 214 | 241 | 110 | 302 | 1.6 | 0.63 L |
| Oats | 12.0 | 390 | 1630 | 232 | 207 | 80 | 272 | 1.9 | 0.68 L |
| Rice | 6.7 | 350 | 1465 | 226 | 207 | 84 | 229 | 1.5 | 0.66 L |
| Sorghum | 10.1 | 355 | 1485 | 126 | 189 | 70 | 181 | 0.9 | 0.55 L |
| Wheat | 12.2 | 355 | 1485 | 179 | 183 | 70 | 253 | 1.3 | 0.53 L |
| Supplements | | | | | | | | | |
| Egg | 12.4 | 150 | 630 | 436 | 320 | 93 | 362 | 4.7 | 1.00 + |
| Meat (lean) | 17.7 | 260 | 1090 | 556 | 287 | 70 | 249 | 3.2 | 1.00 + |
| Fish | 18.8 | 150 | 545 | 569 | 286 | 70 | 253 | 3.0 | 1.00 + |
| Dried skim milk | 36.0 | 360 | 1510 | 503 | 218 | 90 | 190 | 3.0 | 0.86 S |
| Soya flour (defatted) | 46.0 | 330 | 1380 | 380 | 267 | 96 | 193 | 2.0 | 0.88 S |
| Chickpea | 19.2 | 376 | 1575 | 428 | 235 | 54 | 140 | 2.0 | 0.64 S |
| Common bean (autoclaved) | 22.6 | 350 | 1465 | 450 | 249 | 63 | 119 | 1.9 | 0.54 S |
| Groundnut | 25.6 | 570 | 2385 | 221 | 163 | 65 | 150 | 1.7 | 0.65 L Thr |
| Cottonseed cake | 27.4 | 425 | 1780 | 259 | 205 | 90 | 182 | 1.7 | 0.82 L S |

*Note:* L = lysine, S = Total sulfur amino acids, Thr = threonine, and PER = protein efficiency ratio.

[a]  Data from FAO[27] and Pellett and Shadarevian.[28]
[b]  Score using FAO/WHO 1973 scoring system.[30]

The different areas of the world vary from each other not only in the amounts but also in the types of cereals consumed. The three most important cereals of the world are rice, wheat, and maize, rice and wheat being the staple foods to about four fifths of the world. The Far East is typically a rice consuming region. The Near East, the Mediterranean countries of Africa and Europe, as well as North America and Oceania are wheat regions, while South America and the coastal regions of Africa are maize consumers. The Savanna areas of Africa and the Near East use millet and sorghum. These natural distributions, originally dependent upon climate, now control to some degree through taste preference patterns, the preferred composition of feeding mixtures, whether manufactured or homemade, for different regions of the world.

In Table 2 are shown analytical and biological data for some selected cereals and supplementary protein foods. While the protein efficiency ratio (PER) is one of the least satisfactory procedures for assaying protein quality,[11,29] it does allow some degree of comparison between samples. Animal proteins (egg, meat, fish, and milk) are generally superior in quality to the vegetable proteins. There are also distinctions within the vegetable proteins not so much in their PER values but more in the proportions of amino acids present in their proteins. The cereals have relatively low levels of protein which also is of poor quality, being generally low in lysine and tryptophan. Rice, however, while having a lower content of total protein has a better balanced amino-acid pattern than wheat and corn. Chickpea, soybean, and cottonseed all have high levels of lysine and rather low levels of sulfur amino acids. Groundnut is an exception, while having a moderate level of protein (25%), it has a poor pattern of essential amino acids. The other legumes, however, seem almost designed by nature to supplement cereals since they have higher protein content, either high or adequate levels of lysine, and are themselves limited by sulfur amino acids which are present in moderate levels in cereals.

Despite the relatively low-protein quality and quantity in cereals such as wheat, calculations appear to show that a child's protein requirement[30] should be met by cereal diets provided that sufficient protein of the diet could be consumed to meet energy needs. Whitehead[31] has shown indeed that children can grow, albeit slowly, on diets with a protein-energy ratio of only 0.078 (Pcal% = 7.8). However, in practice, diets would frequently be so bulky that insufficient protein could be consumed.[32] Hegsted and Neff[33] have argued that the methods in current use for the determination of protein quality such as net protein utilization (NPU) have an inherent error when used to determine the quality of poor proteins such as cereals and will thus overestimate the true quality. It has been shown further that protein requirement of the cebus monkey is underestimated by the factorial method, and it has been claimed that if quality is determined by a slope-ratio technique then estimation of utilizable protein will better predict the growth obtained.[34] Problems relating to protein assay have recently been reviewed.[10-12,29]

Whatever the reasons for these discrepancies, i.e., bulk, protein quality, or even palatability, it would appear that cereal alone cannot meet protein needs and that either amino-acid fortification, the improvement of quality by addition of the limiting amino acids or complementation, and the mixing of other proteins with cereal protein to improve both quality and quantity, are necessary, especially for the infant whose needs are high. In the rich countries of the world, animal proteins fulfill this role but are not available to the poor nations on economic grounds. This is not to agree with the hypothesis that a world protein shortage in fact exists. Many authors have in recent years questioned the "impending world protein crisis" school of thought, claiming that a food crisis does indeed exist, but that with the exception of those communities existing on very low-protein staples such as cassava, protein needs would be met if energy needs were met.[35,36] The problem is compounded by the fact that at low-energy intake, protein is diverted into energy pathways and is burnt as fuel. A recent human study in Guatemala[37] has demonstrated that a food energy supplement could improve rate of growth as well as a protein supplement. FAO food availability data[38] tends to confirm this viewpoint. The shortfall of energy is far more obvious than that of protein, this appears true even for the developing countries as a whole where protein availability is 47% above requirements while energy needs are barely met. This trend appears to continue with the projections for 1980. For the high-income countries, protein availability is 129% above needs, while energy is only 21% in excess. These values, however, have only an indirect relation to the incidence of PEM where the cause lies much more in maldistribution of protein within the family and it is here that the protein-rich foods may play a role.

While legumes and cottonseed protein products are ideal as complementary protein sources, there are antinutritional factors which may be present, such as trypsin inhibitors, hemagglutinins and anticoagulant factors in legumes, and gossypol in cottonseed.[39,40] Vegetable protein concentrates are excellent natural media for the growth of microorganisms. Toxic aflatoxins were shown to be produced by *Aspergillus flavus* in peanut flour and this directly led to the demise of one protein mixture in Africa. A full discussion of these effects with many references to original work is given by Bressani and Elias[41] who also discuss the various technological advances which have solved many of the problems, allowing these protein sources to make a contribution to human diets.

### Protein Mixtures

The mixing of two or more proteins does not always lead to complementation. Four types of effects have been described by Bressani[14,15] and are illustrated in Figure 1.

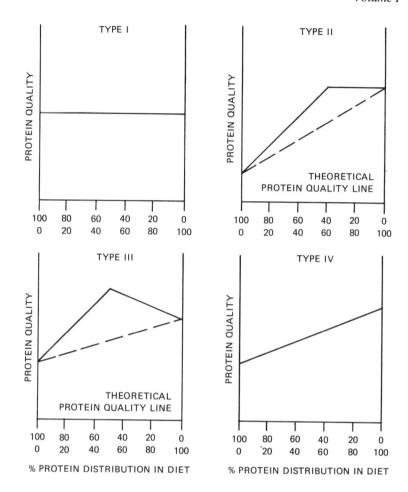

FIGURE 1.   Types of response lines obtained when mixing two protein sources. (From Bressani, R., in *Nutrients in Processed Foods - Proteins,* White, P. L. and Fletcher, D. C., Eds., Publishing Sciences Group, Acton, Mass., 1974, 149-166. With permission.)

The dotted line in the graphs represents the response to be expected if there was no complementary effect. Values above the line are due to complementation.

Of the four types of response shown, the only one which represents true complementation is Type III, where there is a synergistic effect between the two proteins. Type I results when the protein sources mixed have common essential amino-acid deficiencies at a similar level. The quality of such mixtures remains essentially unchanged.

Type II is usually the result of the combination of two protein foods with a common amino-acid deficiency, one of the two proteins having a higher level of the deficient amino acid than the other. This relatively higher amount of the deficient amino acid in one of the proteins is able to supply part of the deficiency of the same amino acid in the other protein — an effect observed only to a certain degree, thereafter, the protein quality value does not change. In Type IV the linear response is probably due to either an overall better essential amino-acid balance, or higher amino-acid availability, or both.

Figure 2 also from Bressani[14] further clarifies the differences between protein complementation and protein supplementation. The graph on the upper left (A) was obtained by mixing maize and soy protein in different proportions, but keeping protein content of the diet constant. On the other hand, the graph on the lower left (C) was

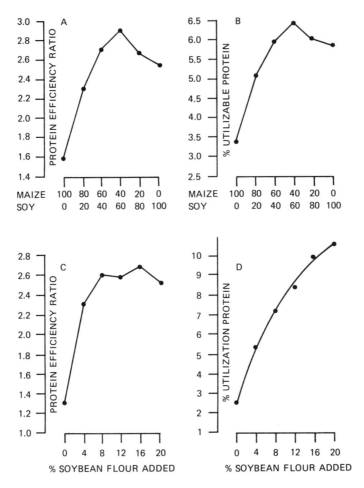

FIGURE 2. Protein complementation and protein supplementation. (From Bressani, R., in *Nutrients in Processed Foods — Proteins,* White, P. L. and Fletcher, D. C., Eds., Publishing Sciences Group, Acton, Mass., 1974, 149-166. With permission.)

obtained by adding to a fixed level of maize, increasing amounts of soy protein, therefore increasing the protein content of the diets. Graph A shows a complementary effect between maize and soy protein, while graph C shows a supplementary effect of soy to maize protein. The same results are shown on the right side. In this case, however, protein quality is not represented by PER, but is expressed as utilizable protein, a value which includes protein concentration. The shape of graph B is the same as graph A since only protein quality changed, protein quantity remaining constant. Graph D, however, is now almost linear since the protein-quality factor was corrected for protein content.

These considerations, then, indicate that Types II and III responses can be classified as complementary. Cereal-legume combinations are usually of Type III and as can be seen from Table 2, the low lysine of the cereal is effectively supplied by the legume. It will be noted that of the nine essential amino acids for the human, only lysine, threonine, tryptophan, and total sulfur amino acids are shown in Table 2. In practice, only these four amino acids are likely to be limiting in real dietaries. Of these four, methionine (total SAA) and lysine are by far the most frequent limiting amino acids. Some optimum mixtures are shown in Table 3. Mixtures giving maximum protein quality

## Table 3
### PROTEIN QUALITY VALUES FOR SOME SELECTED MIXTURES

| Mixtures | Proportions[a] | Protein quality | Ref. |
|---|---|---|---|
| **PER Data** | | | |
| Maize: peanut | 66:34 | 1.28 | 42 |
| Sorghum: beans | 70:30 | 1.77 | 43 |
| Corn: cowpea | 50:50 | 1.85 | 15 |
| Wheat flour: soybean flour | 50:50 | 1.98 | 15 |
| Pea: wheat germ | 50:50 | 2.00 | 15 |
| Pea: corn germ | 50:50 | 2.00 | 15 |
| Corn: black beans | 50:50 | 2.00 | 15 |
| Maize: beans | 50:50 | 2.10 | 44 |
| Millett: black gram | 70:30 | 2.10 | 45 |
| Black beans: cottonseed flour | 30:70 | 2.30 | 15 |
| Rice: beans | 70:30 | 2.37 | 46 |
| Pigeon pea: cottonseed flour | 40:60 | 2.38 | 15 |
| Torula yeast: corn | 40:60 | 2.40 | 15 |
| Corn: whole beans | 35:65 | 2.54 | 15 |
| Wheat: soya | 60:40 | 2.57 | 47 |
| Torula yeast: cottonseed flour | 20:80 | 2.58 | 15 |
| Opaque-2 corn: blackbeans | 50:50 | 2.60 | 15 |
| Rice: black beans | 80:20 | 2.63 | 15 |
| Rice: beans | 50:50 | 2.66 | 46 |
| Torula yeast: sesame flour | 60:40 | 2.70 | 15 |
| Wheat flour: casein | 55:45 | 2.74 | 15 |
| Opaque-2 corn: milk | 66:34 | 2.74 | 15 |
| Corn: soybean flour | 40:60 | 2.76 | 15 |
| Corn: milk | 50:50 | 2.81 | 15 |
| Opaque-2 corn: soybean flour | 40:60 | 2.82 | 15 |
| **NPU Data** | | | |
| Rice: beans | 40:60 | 0.61[b] | 48 |
| Wheat: beans | 50:50 | 0.62 | 48 |
| Wheat: bread, beans | 60:40 | 0.62 | 48 |
| Oats: beans | 60:40 | 0.67 | 48 |
| Egg: beans | 50:50 | 0.81 | 48 |

[a]    Proportions of protein.
[b]    Expressed as a fraction.

range between 60:40 to 50:50 for proportion of cereal protein to legume protein. This would correspond to about 70:30 proportion by weight of, for example, wheat and chickpea or corn and beans. Corn and cottonseed mixtures are of Type II complementation while for corn and groundnuts, both low in lysine, protein quality remains essentially constant (i.e., Type I response). Comparison with Table 2 shows that there is significant improvement in almost all cases as the result of complementation. In the case of maize-peanut, little improvement has occurred as would be expected by inspection of the amino-acid pattern. Further elaboration on the various types of response, including tables showing which mixtures produce which type of response, is given by Bressani.[15]

The considerations so far are for protein quality alone and the mixture with highest protein quality is not necessarily the best supplement to a poor diet. For the maximum response within mixtures of this type, higher proportions of the noncereal component are required than are present in the normal diet pattern of the region. Thus, if a mixture is consumed as a dietary supplement along with the staple diet of the region, whether it be corn or wheat, it can be seen that the effect of the legume will be much less in terms of the diet as a whole because of the further dilution of the legume with the cereal product. Only additions of high-protein products such as fish protein concentrate, skim milk powder, the limiting amino acid, or even the legume alone could be expected greatly to improve the overall dietary protein value in these circumstances. This means that the use of vegetable protein mixtures can have limitations when confronted with the unbalanced dietary patterns consumed in the real world. However, where a well-designed weaning mixture can replace the normal poor quality weaning food, benefits could follow provided that the hygienic environment is satisfactory and that because of cost considerations, a net decrease in protein and/or calorie intake does not follow.[9]

### Evaluation of Food Mixtures

While the early food mixtures were tested during their development by a variety of methods, a set of guidelines has been developed by the PAG for the use of investigators so that all products could undergo similar evaluation (Table 1). For those concerned with the development of food mixtures, Guideline Nos. 6, 7, and 8 are the most relevant. PAG Guideline No. 6[49] "Preclinical Testing of Novel Sources of Protein", is intended as a series of general recommendations rather than mandatory procedures, and the objective is to ensure the safety of any new product for human consumption. The document which is summarized in Table 4 discusses evaluation of nutritional values together with other criteria such as animal toxicity tests and microbiological evaluation. Further details of sanitary production and use of dry protein foods are given in Guideline No. 11.[58]

Human testing of supplementary food mixtures is discussed in Guideline No. 7[59] which is summarized in Table 5. The methods recommended are described as extensive, but flexible so that the fewest number of subjects possible can be used to obtain significant data. The document outlines methods for the determination of product acceptability and tolerance, detailing such considerations as age and number of subjects, duration of the experiment, method of food preparation, and the level of protein and energy in the test diets. Criteria are also suggested for the observations that should be made and how tolerance to the product should be judged. In addition, growth and nitrogen balance studies are described with the precautions necessary for accurate determinations. New methods, however, are now being recommended for human determinations of protein quality using variations of the slope-ratio assay technique.[11,62,63]

While testing of new products is of high importance, excessive testing of minor variations of normal foods can hamper progress. Two major categories of product are suggested. Those requiring full testing procedures and those requiring only limited clinical testing. Those requiring the full test procedures are divided into (1) processed or nonprocessed protein-containing foods which have not previously been considered in WHO/FAO/UNICEF programs and (2) products, previously considered as suitable, which have been subjected to different processing conditions which may raise questions regarding their nutritional or toxicological properties. Products requiring only limited clinical testing, for example, acceptability and tolerance only, are staples and protein sources which are well known or have been considered suitable to WHO/FAO/UNICEF programs and have not been subjected to processing which could cast doubts on their safety.

Guideline No. 8[65] is a recommendation on the composition of supplementary foods considering both the physical characteristics, i.e., flavor, taste, and packaging requirements, and also specifications for the levels of protein, energy, fats, minerals, and vitamins. With regard to the quantity of protein, the recommendations are that with protein of quality equivalent to cow's milk (NPU = 0.80), the level of protein should be at least 150 g/kg on a dry weight basis. With NPU less than 0.80, the quantity of protein should be increased *pro rata* to 200 g/kg at NPU = 0.60. It is further recommended that no products should have an NPU below 0.60 which is approximately

Table 4

GUIDELINES FOR THE PRECLINICAL TESTING OF NOVEL SOURCES OF
PROTEIN (ADAPTED FROM PAG GUIDELINE NO. 6)[49]

Introduction

| | |
|---|---|
| Categories of information | Safety; nutritional value; sanitation acceptability; and technological properties |
| Tests and procedures | Chemical analyses; microbiological examinations; safety evaluation; protein quality studies; acceptability; extensiveness of testing; choice of procedures; and limitation of tests and procedures |

Evaluation Procedures

**Chemical**
 Proximate composition

Moisture, total N, crude fiber, total ether extract

 Protein
  Amino acid composition

Protein should be hydrolyzed and determined for amino acid composition; alternative hydrolytic procedures may be needed for sulfur amino acids; and tryptophan must be separately determined

  Available amino acids

Lysine damage is the most likely, hence, available lysine value[50] (ALV) should be determined; other amino acids (e.g., methionine) can also be rendered nonavailable

  Nonprotein nitrogen

Glucosamines, amides, and amines

  Nucleic acids [for single-cell protein (SCP)]

With high levels of SCP alternative calculations for total protein content will be necessary[51]

 Fat

Triglycerides steroids and phospholipids; fatty acid profile by Gas Liquid Chromatography; and polyunsaturated to unsaturated fatty acid ratio

 Ash

Ca, P, Fe, I, alkali, and alkaline earth elements plus heavy metals should be determined; marine origin materials should also be examined for mercury

 Vitamins

All relevant major vitamins plus those anticipated as being low due to the nature of the material and its method of processing

 Food additives

Analyze for those permitted and for which tolerance limits have been set

 Processing damage

Available lysine as above, but also spectrophotometric examination for Maillard products, or in the case of legumes urease activity, lysinoalanine[52] determinations may be useful if alkaline processing is used

 Physical properties

Solubility, wettability, viscosity, etc. all necessary to establish technological utility as foods or food supplements

 Miscellaneous

Solvent residues, e.g., polycyclic or chlorinated hydrocarbons; pesticide residues; and natural toxicants, e.g., gossypol or hemagglutinins[39,40]

**Biological and biochemical**
 Microbiological

Number and types of organisms present are indicative of unsanitary conditions in production or processing

 Protein quality
  Predicative from amino acid data

Does not take into account digestibility of protein, but score in relation to FAO/WHO 1973 reference pattern[30] is a useful predictor of quality; major discrepancies between score and protein value determined biologically are a good indication of either poor amino acid availability or presence of toxins

 Bioassays
  PER

Most commonly used procedure for biological assay of protein quality, but subject to severe limitations and criticisms;[10-12,53] measures both digestibility and amino acid composition in a combined index; only functional for proteins that support growth; defined as weight gain per gram protein consumed; and often adjusted in relation to casein = 2.5

Table 4 (continued)
GUIDELINES FOR THE PRECLINICAL TESTING OF NOVEL SOURCES OF
PROTEIN (ADAPTED FROM PAG GUIDELINE NO. 6)[49]

Evaluation Procedures

| | |
|---|---|
| NPR and NPU | NPR measured using weight gain, NPU using carcass nitrogen loss on a nonprotein diet; also a combined index measuring both digestibility and amino acid composition (biological value) |
| Slope ratio procedures | Probably most accurate procedures for biologically evaluating proteins by growth or nitrogen retention; not widely used at present but have been demonstrated as superior in a collaborative assay[54] and have been recommended for use in a UNU book on assay of protein quality;[11] also a combined index including digestibility |
| Nitrogen balance | Can be used to determine NPU but by assay of fecal and urinary losses; hence, can determine both components of NPU, i.e., digestibility and biological value; the procedures are similar to those used for human studies; and current modifications include tests at multiple levels |
| Limitations | Results obtained do not necessarily apply to man; other limitations are in respect to (1) differentiation between maintenance and growth, (2) estimations of metabolic and endogenous losses, (3) ad-libitum vs. controlled food intake, and (4) dietary level of proteins, food energy, and other dietary components; a further point of major importance is that quality as determined alone may not bear any relation to the value when consumed as part of a dietary; and major reviews and texts[10-12,53-55] should be consulted in relation to all protein assay procedures |

Safety
Related factors

| | |
|---|---|
| Nutritional adequacy of test diet | Growth depression or any other adverse effect can be caused both by nutritional inadequacy or toxicity; as indicated above, gross discrepancies between protein quality score and growth response can be indicative of poor availability and/or presence of toxins |
| Identity of test materials | Materials tested must be identical to those used for production; many natural toxicants may be present in protein foods;[39,40] their presence can be avoided by care in the selection of raw materials, appropriate methods of storage, heat processing, or extraction |
| Microbiological toxins | Raw materials subject to microbial contamination and spoilage must be examined for the presence of pathogenic organisms (e.g., *Salmonella, Shigella, Staphylococci, and Clostridia*) and for the endotoxic and exotoxic substances they produce; raw materials exposed to warm, humid conditions which induce fungal growth must be examined for the presence of mycotoxins such as the aflatoxins |
| Extraction residues | Solvent residues should be examined for, if protein concentrates are used which have been solvent extracted; if any such residues and/or products formed from the use of reactive chlorinated hydrocarbons are present, toxicological data should be available to establish safe limits |
| Miscellaneous | If test protein source contributes high levels of lipid, ash or undigestible cellulose, adjustment may be required to balance these factors in test and control diets; for safety testing as high levels of protein as possible should be used; and it must be noted, however, that high levels of even high-quality proteins can depress growth and food efficiency |
| Testing protocol | Need for testing is dependent on the novelty of the protein as a food for man both with regard to its source and its method of production; this section assumes product to be sufficiently different from conventional dietary protein to require thorough toxicological appraisal; and most products for combatting childhood malnutrition based on conventional foods will not require this degree of testing |

**Table 4 (continued)**
**GUIDELINES FOR THE PRECLINICAL TESTING OF NOVEL SOURCES OF PROTEIN (ADAPTED FROM PAG GUIDELINE NO. 6)[49]**

## Evaluation Procedures

| | |
|---|---|
| Choice of animal species | Rats most widely used; mice less used because less known of nutritional requirements and size precludes obtaining sufficient blood or urine for examination; dogs, monkeys, and minature pigs have all been used for short-term, but not for chronic (life cycle) studies |
| Basal diet | For short-term (e.g., 3 months) tests either "synthetic" casein-starch or a commercial natural type ration is suitable; for long-term (e.g., 2 years) studies, latter is preferable; and basal ration must satisfy all nutritional requirements for the species in question |
| Dietary level of test protein | Two or three graded levels should be used, highest level being determined by its nutritional adequacy as a sole source |
| Equilibriation of test and control diets | If test protein is of high-ash content (e.g., certain fish protein concentrates), it may be advisable to balance this component in both test and control diets |
| Age, weight, sex, and assigning of animals to groups | Rodents are usually assigned to groups of equal size balanced with respect to litter distribution, sex, and average weight at or shortly after weaning; for short-term tests 10—15 animals of each sex, but at least twice this number should be used for long-term tests; for larger mammal groups should contain 3 and 6 of each sex for short- and long-term studies, respectively; the use of neonatal animals as toxicological test subjects for the evaluation of products which might be included in diets of infants is suggested; and it has been demonstrated that newborn animals have not yet achieved the capability of the adult for enzyme induction and, hence, lack the ability to metabolize or detoxify foreign substances |
| Individual or group housing | Animals should be housed individually during initial period of rapid growth so as to permit reliable measurement of food consumption; caging in pairs or larger groups can be used at later stages |
| Maintenance and sanitary controls | Animal quarters should be maintained in a sanitary condition and controlled with respect to temperature and humidity; the environment should be kept insect free without the use of pesticidal aerosols; and cages should be washed weekly |
| Nature and frequency | A whole series of observations upon the typical criteria used in toxicological evaluations are specified for both short- and long-term studies; these range from daily observations upon physical appearance, behavior, body weight, and food consumption to monthly determinations within the detailed areas of hematology, blood chemistry, and urine chemistry; at termination, gross pathological examination is required for both dead or sacrificed animals together with determinations of organ weights and histopathology of all major organs and tissues |
| Functional or metabolic studies | Tests for hepatic, gastrointestinal or renal function, metabolic balance studies, or neurological or behavioral tests may be suggested in special cases; SCP is present with high levels of nucleoprotein special studies on uricogenesis are additionally necessary |
| Reproduction and lactation, multigeneration studies | Tests of this type are probably unnecessary for foods derived for convention sources, but are probably necessary for novel sources such as SCP |
| Test duration | Short-term tests are generally 3—6 months, while long-term tests are from 1—2 years; if potential carcinogenicity is suspected, larger groups of animals should be used and studies must extend between 1.5 and 2 years |
| Teratogenic or mutagenic studies | Probably unnecessary unless protein source extremely unusual |

Table 4 (continued)
GUIDELINES FOR THE PRECLINICAL TESTING OF NOVEL SOURCES OF
PROTEIN (ADAPTED FROM PAG GUIDELINE NO. 6)[49]

Evaluation Procedures

| | |
|---|---|
| Statistical analyses and inter-<br>pretation of findings | For basic procedures involved in safety evaluation of food compo-<br>nents and their interpretation references is made to reviews of the<br>U.S. Food and Drug Administration;[56] the Food Protection Com-<br>mittee of the National Academy of Sciences—National Research<br>Council[57] and the reports of the Joint Expert Committee on Food<br>Additives of FAO/WHO |

equivalent to a PER of 2.1. The major features of this document are shown in Table 6 and the compositional recommendations are given in Table 7.

After satisfactory passing of the tests outlined in Guideline Nos. 6 and 7 and meeting the composition standards of Guideline No. 8, marketing tests would follow. Guideline No. 10[66] is an extensive monograph on the marketing of protein-rich foods in developing countries. Consideration is given to the protein food program as part of the country's total nutrition system, project planning, technical and economic feasibility studies, project implementation, and program evaluation. The emphasis of the last few years has been placed more and more on the need for marketing studies as a prerequisite for support of a project under the FAO/WHO/UNICEF protein food program.

## Introduction of Food Mixtures

The introduction of processed foods without proper safeguards may cause more harm than good for large segments of the childhood population. Just as promotion of processed-complete infant foods intended for formula preparation may cause mothers to abandon breast feeding, careless introduction of processed supplementary foods may also have an adverse effect on child feeding and health. Also, the indiscriminate promotion of "western-style" baby foods in jars may cause mothers to spend their limited cash on these foods which might easily and inexpensively be prepared at home at a much lower cost. Distribution of imported supplementary foods may also act to hold back local efforts to manufacture and distribute such foods.

Recommendations have been made by the PAG[67] in respect to the situation in developing countries. The recommendations are intended primarily for the processed, low-cost, protein-rich foods intended for older infants and young children as described earlier.[65] The views are, however, pertinent also to "western-style" processed products intended for this age group and already widely in use in developing countries.

1.  Products of this type should not be recommended for infants below six months of age.
2.  The introduction on the market and the promotion of these products should be carried out in close cooperation and contact with the health authorities, after obtaining the support of pediatric associations.
3.  Whenever possible, products of this kind should be produced within the country. If they are imported, and especially if they are donated and intended for free distribution, great care must be taken not to weaken the interest and possibility of initiating production on a national level.
4.  Simple but effective information with respect to the correct use of the product should always be found on the package or accompanying the package.
5.  Products distributed through health centers, well-baby clinics and other similar facilities, should be available in the market.

Table 5
# HUMAN TESTING OF SUPPLEMENTARY FOOD MIXTURES (ADAPTED FROM PAG GUIDELINE NO. 7)[59]

| | |
|---|---|
| Applicability of Guideline | Preliminary steps are necessary; for new components the Guidelines for preclinical testing of novel sources of protein should be followed[49] which are summarized in Table 4 |
| **Preliminary steps** | |
| Identification of sources of edible protein | Quantity available, economic studies on its development |
| Chemical evaluation of components | Quantity, quality, amino acid composition |
| Other consideration of components | Raw material costs, processing, anticipated packaging, storage, shelf-life, distribution, and profits |
| Value of mixture | Chemical and biological evaluation of mixture including possibilities of damage during processing |
| Bacteriological standards | Freedom from harmful microorganisms |
| Toxicity | Testing for freedom from toxicity, i.e., presence intentional or unintentional additives and infestation; FDA Guidelines[56] for acute and chronic toxicity trials are recommended |
| Extensiveness of testing procedures required | While there is no question as to the need for the clinical testing of really new sources of protein or of the results of new ways of processing protein concentrates, there is a real danger that excessive and unnecessary testing of minor variations in formulas using previously tested ingredients or processes could needlessly hamper progress |
| Products requiring full testing procedures | Processed or nonprocessed protein-containing foods which have not been subjected to different processing conditions which may raise questions regarding their nutritional or toxicological properties
Products, previously considered as suitable, which have been subjected to different processing conditions which may raise questions regarding their nutritional or toxicological properties |
| Products requiring only limited clinical testing | Acceptability/tolerance only, are staples and protein sources which are well known or have been considered suitable in FAO/WHO/UNICEF programs and not subjected to processing which could cast doubts on their safety; and it would be advisable, however, to ascertain the nutritional value (PER or NPU) of the final product by animal experimentation |
| **Categories of tests required with humans** | |
| **Acceptability and tolerance tests** | |
| Subjects | Numbers of subjects should be between 20—30 and ages should be similar to those for which the product is intended; the total volume fed, meal timing, and total intake should be consistent; test and control groups should be similar age and have similar weights for heights; and subjects in both experimental and control groups should be interrogated daily to determine any occurrence of diarrhea, vomiting, or other signs of intolerance |
| Duration of observation and feeding | Should be long enough to overcome any initial intolerance |
| Method of preparation | Suitably flavored gruel or incorporated into a local recipe; preparation procedure, however, should be practicable in conditions for which the mixture is recommended |
| Level of protein in feeding | Should attain 50% or more of FAO/WHO[30] recommended safe levels for the age of the subjects; an additional group fed ad libitum will provide information on maximal quantities acceptable per meal in the form supplied |
| Level of food energy | Should be sufficient to maintain constant weight in adults or adequate weight gain in children;[30] for previously malnourished children, 120—150 kcal (500—600 kJ)/kg/day may be needed |
| Observations to be made | Forcing of food must be avoided; tolerance judged by loss of appetite, flatulence, vomiting, undigested stool contents, and diarrhea; when legumes are involved extent of flatus and bloating should be observed |

Table 5 (continued)
## HUMAN TESTING OF SUPPLEMENTARY FOOD MIXTURES (ADAPTED FROM PAG GUIDELINE NO. 7)[59]

| | |
|---|---|
| Growth tests | Growth tests and N-balance trials are alternate approaches; if possible should be done in country of intended use and only performed in centers specialized in nutrition or allied disciplines |
| Observations to be made | Most common index is rate of gain of body weight; urinary creatinine output of over a timed period may provide additional information relevant to increases in muscle mass; height or body length may be more significant than weight gain but needs a longer period; and arm circumference may also be useful indicator |
| Age and type of subjects | Growth is faster with infants and young children who should be as normal as possible, i.e., above third percentile in height and should if possible have weight for height above 95% ideal;[60] weaning foods should be tested in children between 6 months—2 years; and substitutes for mothers milk should be tested in infants below 6 months, but no new product should be tested on young infants before being shown safe for older children |
| Duration of studies | With infants about 1 year of age under close supervision in a hospital ward, daily weighing for 2—4 weeks can give reasonably accurate indications of growth rate; for older children under well-controlled conditions 3—6 months may be necessary; and high-ambient temperatures and infectious epidemics will invalidate trials |
| Numbers of subjects | Depends on age and cooperativeness; institutional well-controlled studies can give valuable information with as few as 5 infants per group; for children between 1—2 years, 10—15 per group, are needed; and for preschool children, 20 per group may be necessary |
| Frequency of observations | Infants: weekly weighings are necessary or biweekly for height, biweekly measurements are suggested for older infants but between 1—3 months is adequate for height in older children |
| Level of feeding | Tests for protein value will be valueless if other dietary components are limiting; diet must thus supply an adequate intake of food energy from fats and carbohydrate and of vitamins and minerals; test protein should generally be the only source of protein in the diet and should meet the recommended allowance of FAO/WHO;[30] and control group should receive milk or egg as protein source with protein and food energy levels adjusted to be comparable |
| Nitrogen balance tests | Nitrogen balance studies require sophisticated staff and facilities for the data to be in any degree meaningful; even when all precautions are taken the conclusions from nitrogen balance studies can be inconclusive;[61,63] because of the controversial nature of this area of protein evaluation and also because of considerable changes in recommended procedures since the PAG Guidelines were prepared, no summary will be given and consultation of current literature[10-12,62-64] is recommended for those needing more detailed information |
| Other criteria | |
| Serum albumin | Changes in serum albumin concentration may give a rough indication of protein quality; blood sample should be taken at the same time in relation to meals |
| Creatinine-height index | A 24-hr creatinine excretion for a malnourished child compared with that for a well-nourished child of the same height is claimed to be a good measure of the reduction of lean body mass due to malnutrition and its recovery with refeeding |
| New Indices | Serum glutamic-oxaloacetate transaminase activity, 3-methyl-histidine excretion and the status of the immune system have been suggested as being indicative of long-term adequacy of dietary protein[62] |

The PAG have also published a statement on the marketing and distribution of protein-rich foods[68] in which they recommend training programs concerned with the development of a new and societally oriented discipline **nutrition-operations** in which

## Table 6
## GUIDELINES FOR PROTEIN-RICH MIXTURES FOR USE AS
## SUPPLEMENTARY FOODS (ADAPTED FROM PAG GUIDELINE NO. 8)[65]

| | |
|---|---|
| Protein level | At least 150 g/kg if protein quality equivalent to cows milk (NPU = 0.80); for poorer quality mixtures (NPU = 0.60) quantity should be increased to 200 g/kg |
| Food energy level | As high as possible, may be achieved by adding fat; poorly-digestible carbohydrate should be held to a practical minimum; starch modification (heat, mechanical processing, or enzymes) can be performed so that when water is added the food has minimal bulk, maximum energy density, and maximum protein availability |
| Fat | As high a level as possible without compromising keeping quality, up to ca. 250 g/kg of the food energy value to come from fat; linoleic acid content to be 10 g/kg; if packaging costs to give an adequate shelf-life are excessive at these fat levels, fat may be omitted but added when mixture is prepared |
| Vitamins and minerals | Sufficient amounts should be added to meet recommended allowances (see Table 7) |
| Physical characteristics | Formulation should be such that by addition of freshly boiled water or by boiling after adding water, can be prepared as a gruel or porridge at correct consistency for feeding; this can be accomplished by procedures such as amylase treatment, extrusion cooking, or pre-cooking followed by roller drying; such processing should reduce home-cooking time and allow reduction of viscosity and water retention capacity to allow feeding of a more concentrated preparation; and processing must not affect protein quality of the mixture |
| Flavor and taste | Sugar may be added provided cost is not greatly increased and that acceptability is enhanced; however, in general, such additions should be made in the home; and addition of salt is generally unnecessary |
| Food additives | The use of excessive amounts of flavoring agents should be avoided; if any additives are used they should be those cleared by the Joint FAO/WHO Expert Committee on Food Additives;[57] the amounts added should not exceed the minimum necessary to produce the desired effect; and the materials added should be specified on the label |
| Standards and purity | Ingredients should meet national and/or international standards with regard to purity (see PAG Guidelines Nos. 2, 4, 5, 9, and 14 and PAG Statements Nos. 2, 11, 21, and 22; Table 1) |
| Microbiological and sanitary standards | See PAG Guideline No. 11[58] |
| Packaging | Packages and the containers in which they are shipped should provide protection from inroads of insects, microorganisms, moisture, and contaminants; if foods are dispensed for bulk containers, proper sanitary procedures should be observed; and simple but effective information with respect to the correct use of the product should be on the package |
| Shelf-life | The packaged product should remain acceptable for food use in terms of palatability, nutritional availability, and freedom from toxic or other deleterious changes for a period of 6 months under tropical conditions |

the needs and interests of the consumer at all economic levels were considered uppermost.

The sequence of steps involved in the commercial introduction of protein-rich food mixtures (PRFM) have been described by Mauron[69] as follows:

1. Search for suitable raw materials
2. Formulation of product and manufacturing trials
3. Laboratory trials using rats
4. Clinical trials

Table 7

### COMPOSITIONAL RECOMMENDATIONS FOR PROTEIN-RICH FOOD MIXTURES (PER 100 G)

| | per 100 g | | | per 100 g | |
| --- | --- | --- | --- | --- | --- |
| Protein | g | 15—20 | Niacin | mg | 5.0 |
| Calories | kcal (kJ) | 370 (1550) | Folate | mg | 0.2 |
| Fat | g | 10 | Vitamin $B_{12}$ | $\mu$g | 2.0 |
| Moisture | g | 5—10 | Ascorbic acid | mg | 20 |
| Ash | g | 5 (max) | Vitamin D | IU | 400 |
| Vitamin A Retinol equivalent | $\mu$g | 400 | Calcium | mg | 300 (As phosphate or carbonate) |
| Thiamine | mg | 0.3 | Iron | mg | 10 (Food grade with adequate iron availability) |
| Riboflavin | mg | 0.4 | Iodine | $\mu$g | 100 (As iodate or iodide) |

*Note:* Under certain local conditions, the addition of Vitamin $B_6$ to levels approximately that of thiamine and of Vitamin E to that of $\alpha$-tocopherol may be considered. The values for vitamins and minerals should be considered minimal except for Vitamin D where no further increase is desirable. The excess of each vitamin added during processing should be no greater than that needed to maintain label requirements over the expected shelf-life of the product.

From FAO/WHO/UNICEF Protein Advisory Group, PAG Guideline on protein rich mixtures for use as supplementary foods, *PAG Guideline,* No. 8, 1972. With permission.

5. Approval of formula by UNICEF, FAO, and WHO (PAG)
6. Search for governmental support or sympathy
7. Market tests and cost study
8. Reappraisal of the situation and readaptation of formula
9. Final decision
10. Launching of product

Each of the stages has proved to be fraught with difficulties and despite the basic soundness of the scientific concepts behind development of products of this type, few have been unequivocally successful. The histories of some of the products will be described in a later section illustrating some of the problems involved. Because concepts as to the types of products needed were colored by the conventional wisdom of the time especially relating to the "protein problem", current views now accept that PRFM can contain considerably less protein than the 25 to 35% advocated a decade ago. For these earlier products containing high levels of protein, it was almost essential to use protein concentrates as the major component. These were often oil seeds which were concentrated by the process of extraction of a oil. Current products of lower total protein content can be based on cereals supplemented with milk, legumes, or oil-seed proteins.

### Nutritional Value of Mixtures

Discussion of nutritive value of these mixtures is less productive than consideration of nutritional value of normal foods since these products have been designed with maximum nutrition in mind. An extensive literature exists containing details of chemical analyses, animal feeding trials, and human feeding experiments. Some examples are from Latin America with the early testing of *Incaparina*\* vegetable protein mixtures,[70-73] for India,[75-77] and for the Middle East.[78-80] The book *Protein-Enriched Ce-*

---

\* All products indicated in bold italics are registered trademarks.

*real Foods for World Needs*[20] also contains many references to testing and developmental experiments throughout the world. A recent report[82] discusses the nutritional effectiveness of soy-cereal foods in undernourished infants and concludes that a variety of soy-cereal foods can be the major or only source of protein in the diet of growing infants and children. A PAG Symposium[83] reports on the use of legumes and green, leafy vegetables in the feeding of young children and several papers consider the nutritional aspects.

Thus, the vast majority of the products have high-nutritive value, the protein quality being usually close to that of casein, and feeding trials with human subjects have generally shown high-nitrogen retentions with both normal and malnourished children. It has, however, sometimes been reported that while short-term experiments showed little difference when the protein source was milk or a variety of vegetable proteins or protein mixtures, in long-term experiments, the weight gain was less regular on vegetable protein mixtures than on milk even though the total gain was similar.[84] No explanation of the irregularities in growth was given, however, and it was also observed, again without discussion, that the percentage of nitrogen excreted as urea was lower in all babies fed vegetable proteins as compared to those fed milk. Potential inaccuracies in short-term studies and the consequent need for long-term experiments have been emphasized by Young and Scrimshaw.[62]

Thus, in most cases, it is not a question of praising or condemning products on the basis of their nutritive value, but rather reporting on success or failure of the products on the basis of marketing acceptability and of their potential using economic criteria. Some details of nutritional evaluation of selected products are shown in Table 8. It must be emphasized that this collective approval is for products that have been developed following the general PAG Guidelines[49,59,65] outlined in Tables 4 to 6. The guidelines are reasonable and sensible, and products which survive the test procedures are likely to be beneficial unless, and unfortunately this is a large reservation, they may encourage even more the early abandonment of breast feeding.[3,4,5a,85,86]

## PRODUCT HISTORIES

### Manufactured Mixtures

A wide range of products has been developed over the years in many countries. Cereal-legume mixtures predominate as the major components and are mainly proposed for use as weaning foods or gruels. Some other mixtures of higher protein content, composed of legume and milk or mixtures of legume were designed as protein supplements. The current status and country of origin of many of these products are shown in Table 9. A comprehensive list of most of the internationally available mixtures is shown in Table 10. Details are given of the components used for the formulation together with the proportions when known and the protein-energy concentration of the final product. Most, if not all, of the products listed include additional vitamins and minerals.

Recently, 69 programs, originating from 36 countries, were evaluated.[21] Nearly half of the products were from Central and South America (324 million population cf. nearly 2000 million). This bears no relation to the incidence of PEM and probably reflects the fact that the initial development of these products came from INCAP in Central America. However, a very recent publication from India[87] describes a series of products developed there for infant feeding. The total quantities being produced there probably now exceed all products combined for the rest of the world.

It is obvious that products which have been developed, irrespective of their nutritional value and impeccable testing history, can have no effect on the incidence of malnutrition unless they are produced and consumed on a wide scale. It is thus salutary

Table 8

## PROTEIN NUTRITIONAL VALUE OF SOME SELECTED PRODUCTS

| Product | PER[a] | NPU | Remarks | Ref. |
|---|---|---|---|---|
| *Balahar* | 1.8—2.0 | — | Well accepted in field trials and found quite suitable for emergency feeding programs | 87 |
| *CSM* | — | — | In children, biological value was 60—65% that of casein | 114 |
| Dongo | — | — | Preliminary tests on 200 children, aged 6 months—4 years indicated that satisfactory growth was produced; further evaluation trials are in progress | 87 |
| *Faffa* | 3.0 | — | Acceptability and digestibility tests were conducted on children aged 1—4 years as well as weight gain, over a period of 2 weeks—4 months; analysis of data obtained indicated a decrease in the frequency of rickets and skin infection, and a definite increase in muscle mass during the initial 12 months of the trial | 89 |
| *Hyderabad mix* | — | — | Human test results, without details of numbers of subjects, levels fed, and composition of the remainder of the diet, demonstrate an average increase in weight of 0.66 kg over 4 weeks; reductions in edema and diarrhea and mental improvements were reported after 1 week on the diet | 87 |
| *Incaparina* Cottonseed flour | 2.12 | — | Protein value improved as higher levels of cottonseed were incorporated in the test mixtures replacing sesame flour; the limiting amino acid using the FAO 1957[94] scoring system was total SAA; if values are calculated using the FAO/WHO 1973[30] scoring system, lysine appears to be limiting with a score of 0.60; N-balance studies with children demonstrated that at intakes of between 2—3 g protein per kg per day the nitrogen retention obtained was similar to milk; at lower levels, however, (0.5—1.0 g/kg/day) milk was superior | 72 |
| Soya blend | 2.56 | — | Biological value of this mixture was 0.73 with a digestibility of 0.79; the limiting amino acid was methionine, this was confirmed by studies involving amino acid supplementation | 73 |
| Kuzhandi Amudhu | — | — | Feeding trials have shown a statistically significant increase ($P < 0.01$) in the height and weight of children receiving the product when compared to those receiving a control diet; no further details of the study are, however, given; acceptability trials revealed that the product made from local foods was better accepted than *CSM* | 87 |
| Leaf Protein Mixture | — | — | The product was very well accepted by children; height, weight, and hemoglobin levels improved as well as the general health of the children; no further details given | 87 |
| *Laubina* | | | | |
| 101 | 2.4 | 0.43 | N-balance studies were determined on *Laubina* 102, 103, 104, 105, and results were compared to those obtained by using simulated mothers milk (whey protein milk S-26 by Wyeth); highest N-balance was obtained with *Laubina* 103; blood protein values showed a quick response in the malnourished children after receiving *Laubina* 103 or 104 mixtures; chemical scores for *Laubina* 104 and 105 were 0.56 and 0.47 (FAO 1957)[94] or 0.69 and 0.58 (FAO/WHO 1973),[30] respectively | 17,78,79 |
| 102 | 2.0 | 0.49 | | |
| 103 | 2.3 | 0.49 | | |
| 104 | 2.7 | 0.51 | | |
| 105 | 2.2 | 0.43 | | |
| 106 | — | — | *Laubina* 106 is limiting in sulfur amino acids but is high in lysine; preliminary studies with infants showed good tolerance and acceptability; chemical score 0.60 (FAO 1957)[94] or 0.74 (FAO/WHO 1973)[30] | 17 |

## Table 8 (continued)
## PROTEIN NUTRITIONAL VALUE OF SOME SELECTED PRODUCTS

| Product | PER[a] | NPU | Remarks | Ref. |
|---|---|---|---|---|
| Nutriene V | 2.3 | — | Product was well accepted by children; tests were performed on children recuperating from malnutrition for a period of 4 months, mean age of children at the beginning of the feeding trial was 2 years, 4 months; each child was its own control; the diet fed had 60% of its protein from Nutriene V and it met 100% of the recommended daily allowance; daily intake was 18.7 g of protein per child; at the end of the 4-month period the mean body weight of the children increased, serum protein levels were significantly increased ($P < 0.05$) as well as serum albumin ($P < 0.01$); arm circumference had a mean increase of 1.6 cm; an improvement in psychomotor behavior, motor coordination, and language ability was also observed | 109 |
| *ProNutro* | 2.2 | 0.65 | B.V. = 0.71·digestibility = 0.92; in a field test on children age 6 months—3 years the diet was supplemented with 2 oz of *ProNutro* per day; after a 6-month period the mortality rate was greatly reduced and there were no kwashiorkor cases | 90 |
| *Superamine* | 2.4 | 0.71 | Product was fed to children ages 6 months—2 years for a 3-week period; it was well accepted and there were no digestive troubles | 18 |
| Swedish Emergency Food | | | | |
| A₁ | 3.9 | — | Chemical scores using the FAO (1965)[b] procedure based on | 88 |
| A₂ | 3.6 | — | the essential amino acids of egg ranged from 0.63—0.79; | |
| A₃ | 3.7 | — | limiting amino acids appear to be total sulfur amino acids | |
| A₄ | 3.1 | — | and isoleucine | |
| A₅ | 3.6 | — | | |
| B₁ | 2.9 | — | | |
| B₂ | 2.9 | — | | |
| B₃ | 3.0 | — | | |
| VPM | — | — | N-retention studies were conducted on 8 infants that were fed VPM and were compared with 11 infants fed a cow's milk diet and they compared favorably | 80 |

[a]  The PER values may not be directly comparable since not all have been standardized to a PER for casein = 2.5.

[b]  FAO/WHO protein requirements, FAO Nutrition Meetings Rep. Ser. No. 37, Food and Agricultural Organization, Rome, 1965.

to examine in some detail the history of some of the products to ascertain reasons for success or failure and the degree of impact, if any, that these schemes have had on the world incidence of PEM. The excellent monograph by Elizabeth Orr entitled "The Use of Protein Rich Foods for the Relief of Malnutrition in Developing Countries: An Analysis of Experience",[21] is recommended reading and has been used extensively in the preparation of this section.

The development of the various Incaparina formulations has been described,[21,24,70-74] but before the product could be offered to responsible food industry companies, it was important to demonstrate that a vegetable mixture containing cottonseed protein had no potential hazards in human nutrition[74a] and further that such products would be acceptable. Field acceptability trials and market testing were carried out in several Central American countries during 1959 and 1960. Production commenced in early 1961 in Guatemala by Cerveceria Centro American SA, the principal Guatemalan brewer and soft drink producer, a company which was known to wish to diversify into

Table 9
ORIGIN AND STATUS OF FOOD PRODUCTS FOR COMBATING CHILDHOOD
MALNUTRITION

| Country | Responsible organization | Production terminated | Production irregular/position unknown | In production | Main use | Remarks | Ref. |
|---|---|---|---|---|---|---|---|
| | | | | **North/Central America** | | | |
| El-Salvador | — | *Incaparina* (1962) | — | — | Cereal-based beverage | Acceptability of product was poor, its promotional approach wasn't appealing, and the packaging was unattractive | 21,24 |
| Guatemala | General Mills | — | — | *Incaparina* (1961) Protina | Gruel | In 1974 *Incaparina* sales increased to 2000 tons; Protina sells at twice the price of *Incaparina* | 21,24 |
| Mexico | General Foods (1969) Corn products (1969) | — | Soya products (Conasupo) Early 1960s | Protea (1950s) Conlac | Conlac:baby food | — | 21,24 |
| Nicaragua | Quaker Oats (1968) Nutrition Development Corp. (1969) | *Incaparina* (1962) | — | — | Gruel | Production ceased due to lack of demand as well as lack of funds and expertise | 21 |

| | | | | | | |
|---|---|---|---|---|---|---|
| Panama | — | *Incaparina* (1966) | — | Nutrebien (1970s) | *Incaparina* used as gruel and Nutrebien as a food supplement | Sales of Nutrebien have been limited to social welfare institutions | 21,24 |
| U.S. | — | — | — | CSM WSB | Food aid export used as basis of some locally mixed products | By 1971, 2 billion pounds of the two products had been produced for international distribution | 20,21 |
| **South America** | | | | | | | |
| Brazil | Coca Cola (1968) General Foods (1968) Nestle Company | Multipurpose food (1956) *Incaparina* (1965) Saci (1968) *Fortifex* (1970) | Solein (1963) — — — | Cerealina (1965) — — — | *Incaparina* a cereal-based beverage and a food supplement Cerealina: gruel Solein: gruel *Fortifex*: weaning food and a protein supplement | Cerealina is sold on a retail basis only; to reduce the cost of the product the company is proposing a somewhat different product where locally defatted soya flour will be used without DSM; a cheaper packaging will also be used Solein retail sales are mainly directed to higher income groups | 21,69 |

Table 9 (continued)
ORIGIN AND STATUS OF FOOD PRODUCTS FOR COMBATING CHILDHOOD
MALNUTRITION

| Country | Responsible organization | Production terminated | Production irregular/position unknown | In production | Main use | Remarks | Ref. |
|---|---|---|---|---|---|---|---|
| | | | | | | *Fortifex* was packaged in 100 g polyethylene bags for the public and in 1 kg bags for institutions; a 100 g bag costs 160 Cr = 10 U.S. cents | |
| Chile | University of Chile/USAID (1968) | — | — | Superchil Fortesan (1970s) | Superchil and Fortesan for children age 2—6 years | The ingredients in Superchil and Fortesan are skimmed milk powder, imported Wheat Soya Blend (WSB), and milk powder; both products are manufactured by private companies; production was 16,000 tons in 1975 | 21,24 |

| Country | | | | | | | Description | Comments | Ref. |
|---|---|---|---|---|---|---|---|---|---|
| Colombia | — | — | Pochito (1967) *Incaparina* (1975) | — | — | Colombiharina (1967) Duryea (1969) Bienesterian (1975) Nestum Pensal | Pochito: a cereal based beverage Duryea: gruel Bienesterina: infant feeding mixture Nestum: weaning food Pensal: a nutritional supplement | Annual sales of Colombiharina decreased from 150 tons in 1968 to 40 tons in 1976 Sales of Duryea have decreased to less than half its peak level Instituto Colombiano de Bienestar Familiar (ICBF) has been producing Bienestarina to be distributed through Social Welfare outlets; about 5000 tons were produced in 1975 Nestum HP is sold on a commercial basis without subsidy Pensal sold in 1977 only to governmental institutions | 21,24,69a |
| Guyana | — | — | — | Puma (1969) | Protein beverage | Retail sales in excess of 29,000 bottles/year | | | 21 |
| Peru | Agrarian University (1968) | *Peruvita* (sweet) (1968) | — | — | *Peruvita* (sweet): weaning food | Both products have government participation and also | | | 21,69a |

Table 9 (continued)
ORIGIN AND STATUS OF FOOD PRODUCTS FOR COMBATING CHILDHOOD MALNUTRITION

| Country | Responsible organization | Production terminated | Production irregular/position unknown | In production | Main use | Remarks | Ref. |
|---|---|---|---|---|---|---|---|
|  |  | *Peruvita* (salt) (1968) |  |  | *Peruvita* (salt): supplement for adults | UNICEF and FAO involvement; both products were sold to the public in 100 and 300 g paper bags and in polyethylene bags of 20 kg for institutions; 100 g bag cost = 2.25 soles, about 13 U.S. cents |  |
| Venezuela | Nutrition Development Corp. (1969) | *Incaparina* (1965) | — | — | Cereal-based beverage | Product did not fit in with the local dietary pattern; this plus the high cost of labor and packaging caused its failure | 21,22 |
| Africa |  |  |  |  |  |  |  |
| Algeria | — | *Superamine* (1967) | — | — | Weaning food | *Superamine* sales were up to 400 | 21,24 |

| Country | Sponsoring agency (year) | Trademark (year) | Product (year) | Type of food | Production | Remarks | Ref. |
|---|---|---|---|---|---|---|---|
| Arab Republic of Egypt | United Nations Agencies/Government (1969) | — | *Superamine* (1973) | Weaning food | During the first 3 years, *Superamine* production was about 900 tons | tons in 1969 and 523 tons in 1970; the Government distributes the product to malnourished children in institutions and to poor families as part of a Government free distribution program; production increased from 1500 tons in 1970 to 800 tons in 1974/75 | 21,24 |
| Ethiopia | Ethiopian Nutrition Institute | — | *Faffa* (1967) | Weaning food | | Sales of *Faffa* have increased from 400 tons in 1970/71 to 1500 tons in 1975; product is well accepted | 21,24,89,92 |
| Kenya | — | Supro (1976) | Simba (1959) | Simba and Supro used as a gruel | | Supro production ceased due to increase in cost and its | 21,24 |

Table 9 (continued)
ORIGIN AND STATUS OF FOOD PRODUCTS FOR COMBATING CHILDHOOD
MALNUTRITION

| Country | Responsible organization | Production terminated | Production irregular/position unknown | In production | Main use | Remarks | Ref. |
|---|---|---|---|---|---|---|---|
| | | | | | | being too expensive for school feeding programs | |
| | Medical Research Council of India Project | — | — | Weaning food "Dongo" | "Dongo" used for infant and child feeding | "Dongo" is available in blocks which are packed in high-density polyethylene bags; 500 mℓ of water usually added to the block; one block cost 25 c | 87 |
| Madagascar | United Nations Agencies/Government (1969) | — | — | Weaning food | — | — | 21 |
| Mozambique | — | — | — | Super Maeu (1965) | Drink, and is used in school feeding schemes | Super Maeu sales are about 200 tons/month, about half plant capacity | 21,24 |
| Nigeria | — | Amama (1961) | | | Protein supple- | The fact that Amama was | 21,22 |

| Country | | Product | Type | Comments | Ref. |
|---|---|---|---|---|---|
| Rhodesia | — | *Arlac*(1968) | ment | being marketed as a dietary supplement did not make it appealing to the consumer and this contributed to the failure of the product | — |
| Senegal | — | Nutresco (1963) | Drink | — | 21 |
| | | *Ladylac* (1966) | Weaning food | Product was too expensive for the low per capita income and purchasing processed food was not a common habit to the rural Senegalese | 21 |
| Sierra Leone | FAO/WHO | Bennimix (1976) | Food for young children | A pilot plant was set up for Bennimix production with a capacity of 250 tons/year with the assistance of FAO/UNDP and Freedom from Hunger/Action for Development; the product incorporates the locally available benniseed (Sesamum indi- | 24 |

## Table 9 (continued)
## ORIGIN AND STATUS OF FOOD PRODUCTS FOR COMBATING CHILDHOOD MALNUTRITION

| Country | Responsible organization | Production terminated | Production irregular/position unknown | In production | Main use | Remarks | Ref. |
|---|---|---|---|---|---|---|---|
|  |  |  |  |  |  | cum); it is well accepted by young children |  |
| South Africa | — | — | — | *ProNutro* (1962) | *ProNutro* breakfast food, soup, or eaten as powder Protone, soup powder | Retail sales of *ProNutro* account for 95% of output; annual production 3000—4000 tons Protone production is about 270 tons/year Kupangi Biscuit sales are mainly to institutions | 21 |
| Uganda | — | — | — | Soya products (1968) | Porridge or gruel | Full scale marketing began in 1968; price likely to be beyond those in need | 21,24 |
| Zambia | — | — | — | Milk Biscuits (1971) | Snack | Milk Biscuits were manufactured by the Dairy Produce Board of Zambia on plant do- | 21,24 |

**Middle East**

| Country | Sponsoring organization (date) | | Product (date) | Type | Remarks | Ref. |
|---|---|---|---|---|---|---|
| | | | | | nated by the Australian Government; too expensive for government feeding programs and cannot compete in taste with commercial biscuits | |
| Iran | United Nations Agencies/Government (1969) | — | *Yoo-Hoo* (1969) | Drink | *Yoo-Hoo* product was first produced in the U.S. and was being produced under license in Iran, and has proved successful | 21 |
| | — | | Weaning food | Weaning food | Weaning food should be produced during 1977 | 24 |
| Israel | — | | VPM | Infant feeding | — | 80 |
| Lebanon | Department of Food Technology and Nutrition at American University of Beirut | — | *Laubina* (1965) | Weaning food | Successfully tested in pilot studies but never reached commercial production | 22 |
| Turkey | United Nations Agen- | — | Sekmama (1971) | Weaning food | Sales extending beyond original | 21,24 |

## Table 9 (continued)
## ORIGIN AND STATUS OF FOOD PRODUCTS FOR COMBATING CHILDHOOD MALNUTRITION

| Country | Responsible organization | Production terminated | Production irregular/position unknown | In production | Main use | Remarks | Ref. |
|---|---|---|---|---|---|---|---|
| | cies/Government (1968) | | | | | test marketing areas by 1976 | |
| **Europe** | | | | | | | |
| Sweden | Swedish Nutrition Foundation and Swedish International Development Authority (SIDA) | — | — | Swedish emergency food (1973) (SEF) | Emergency food for relief programs | SEF mixture is in powdered form 10% moisture content; it is packaged in 2-kg polypropylene paper bags; the cost per kg is approximately 2.00 Swedish Crown or U.S. :0.44 (October 1973) | 88 |
| Portugal | — | — | — | Pensal | Weaning food | Packaged in paper bags in carton packs; produced on a commercial basis without subsidy | 69a |
| Hong Kong | — | — | — | Vitasoy (1940) | Protein beverage | Commercially successful; sold hot and cold | 21 |

| Country | Product | | Producer | Use | Description | Ref. |
|---|---|---|---|---|---|---|
| India | *Balahar* (1964) | — | Food Corporation of India | School feeding programs | It is distributed by CARE, UNICEF produced 25,000 t during 1975 for special relief programs; production during 1969/70 was 7,500 tons, 1976/77 was 43,362 tons; about 75 g of *Balahar* per child per day is recommended, which gives about 300 cal and about 15 g of good quality protein | 81,87 |
| | *Balamul* (1971) | — | Weaning Food Plant, Gujarat, Central Food Technological Research (CFTRI) | Weaning food | It started development as a farmers cooperative, but was supported by the government of India and assisted by UNICEF | 87 |
| | CINI Nutrimix (1976) | — | Child in Need Institute (CINI), Calcutta | Supplementary feed for children under 5 years of age | No special plant is required except cast iron pans and coal fired "Chulas" (ovens); the mixture is packaged in polyethylene bags of | 87 |

Table 9 (continued)
## ORIGIN AND STATUS OF FOOD PRODUCTS FOR COMBATING CHILDHOOD MALNUTRITION

| Country | Responsible organization | Production terminated | Production irregular/ position unknown | In production | Main use | Remarks | Ref. |
|---|---|---|---|---|---|---|---|
| | | | | | | 450 g; this packet provides 1735 cal and 84.5 g of protein; about 4000 children benefited from the program during January-December 1976; approximately 36,361 packets were distributed during this period | |
| | CFTRI, Mysore and National Institute of Nutrition, Hyderabad | — | — | Energy food (1974/75) | Child feedings program; age 6 months —2 years | The powder as such can be eaten by older children; for infants, the powder needs to cook for 5 min; the product can be stored for 3—4 months at 37°C; a sample with 5% fat was found very pop- | 87 |

| | | | | | |
|---|---|---|---|---|---|
| Indo-Dutch Project for Child Feeding, Hyderabad | — | *Hyderabad mix* | Mothers and children | ular but expensive / The mix can be fed as plain powder, porridge with jaggery; jaggery balls (laddus), bread, cakes (chappattis); it is distributed in 70 g packets; no special plant is needed; it is done locally by the women's organizations; monthly consumption is about 3000 packets (70 g) | 87 |
| Kerala Indigenous Food Project, Kerala (KIF) | — | KIF | Pregnant/nursing mothers | Widely used for school feeding and also the Special Nutrition Program; KIP made with tapioca and fish powder has proved that, if provided at cost to the consumer, it will be readily acceptable | 87 |
| Shri Avinashilingam | — | Kuzhandai Amudhu | Supplementary | The food is produced in the | 87 |

Table 9 (continued)
ORIGIN AND STATUS OF FOOD PRODUCTS FOR COMBATING CHILDHOOD
MALNUTRITION

| Country | Responsible organization | Production terminated | Production irregular/ position unknown | In production | Main use | Remarks | Ref. |
|---------|-------------------------|----------------------|----------------------------------------|---------------|----------|---------|------|
| | Home Science College for Women | | | | feeding programs | school premises where it is distributed to the children; it can be used as a porridge with 30 ml of water and 100 g of the formulation, or made into balls or biscuits | |
| | Kaira District Cooperative Milk Producers' Union. Ltd., Gujarat | — | K-Mix-2 (1966) | | Supplementary feeding programs | The product was initially manufactured abroad; oil is added to the mix before feeding; KM-4 and KM-5 are roller dried products but have properties comparable to K-Mix 2 | 87 |
| | Shri Avinashilingam Home Science College | — | Leaf protein mixture (1969) | | Supplementary food | No special plant is needed; the product is air dried at | 87 |

| | | | | | |
|---|---|---|---|---|---|
| for Women, Coimbatore, Tamil Nadu | | | | 40—50°C using a tray drier and then ground to fine powder; no large scale distribution has started | |
| CFTRI | — | *Miltone* (1970s) | Milk extender | Three plants in current production; two more planned with UNICEF assistance; extends milk with groundnut proteinate and can sell below the price of milk | 87 |
| Soya Production and Research Association | — | *Nutrinuggets* | Snack | — | 87 |
| Soya Production and Research Association | — | Paushtikahar | Feeding program for children and adults | Suggested for use when milk is in short supply; 160 tons of the product has been used by the State Government of Uttar Pradesh for their feeding programs | 87 |
| Soya Production and Research Association | — | Paushtikahar (Agra mix) (1976) | Supplementary feeding of chil- | About 80 g of the product is sufficient for supplementary feeding | 87 |

Table 9 (continued)
ORIGIN AND STATUS OF FOOD PRODUCTS FOR COMBATING CHILDHOOD
MALNUTRITION

| Country | Responsible organization | Production terminated | Production irregular/ position unknown | In production | Main use | Remarks | Ref. |
|---|---|---|---|---|---|---|---|
| | | | | | dren and pregnant/ nursing mothers | of a child and 125 g for the pregnant/nursing mother per day; the product is distributed to feed about 9000 children, 1000 pregnant/nursing mothers in 80 local primary schools, and 20 social organizations; Most children eat the powder as such or eat it mixed with hot water or milk; the school feeding is available 24 days/month. | |
| | Soya Production and Research Association | — | — | *Protein Plus* (1972) | Infant feeding | Instant product; it is used by the government for feeding programs in some | 87 |

| Product | | Organization | | Use | Description | Ref. |
|---|---|---|---|---|---|---|
| | | | | | states; the product is exempted from excise duty of the Government in India | |
| Shaktiahar (1973) | — | Soya Production and Research Association | — | Feeding programs | 75 g of the product would provide 300 cal and 15 g of protein; it has only to be mixed in water | 87 |
| Shakti Malt | — | Lakshimi Seva Sangh, Gandhigram, Tamil Nadu | — | — | It is sold in 350 g packets; "Ragotine" is a commercial product of this nature | 87 |
| Shishu Ahar | — | International Child Development Scheme (ICDS) Project Area | — | Food supplement for toddlers and preschool infants | The distribution of the product would be at the rate of 1.5 kg/month/child; the project covers 100 villages with a total population of 1 lakh; the total requirement for rural ICDS blocks comes out to 1230 t/year | 87 |
| *Sukhadi* (1970) | — | Sadguru Seva Sangh Trust, Bombay | — | Fed to children as porridge | CARE supplies the DSM and oil; the product is in granular, ready-to-eat | 87 |

## Table 9 (continued)
## ORIGIN AND STATUS OF FOOD PRODUCTS FOR COMBATING CHILDHOOD MALNUTRITION

| Country | Responsible organization | Production terminated | Production irregular/position unknown | In production | Main use | Remarks | Ref. |
|---|---|---|---|---|---|---|---|
| | Weaning Food Plant, Anand, Gujarat | | Special weaning food (*SWF*) (1974) | | Infant feeding, no cooking needed | form; it is readily accepted for its sweetness; in 1974, 175,000 preschool and pregnant/nursing mothers at over 1450 centers in 12 districts of Maharashtra received *Sukhadi* under the Special Nutrition Program; shelf-life of product is 3 months | |
| | | | | | | Production capacity of the food plant at Mopar is 6 tons/day; UNICEF used the product in 1974-76 for the Special Child Relief Program in India | 87 |

| Country | Institution | Product (year) | Form/Use | Comments | Ref. |
|---|---|---|---|---|---|
| | Gandhigram Institute of Rural Health and Family Planning, Tamil Nadu | Win Food (1970) | Preschool children | No special plant required; sales of product went up from 340 packets a month in May 1970 to 3250 packets by June 1971 | 87 |
| Indonesia | — | Saridele (1967) | Drink/gruel | Product was too expensive and was used by the wealthy only; United Nations support was withdrawn | 21 |
| Malaysia | — | Vitabean (1952) | Drink | — | 21 |
| Nepal | — | Super flour (Sarbottam Pitho) | Supplementary food, mixed as porridge for children | Product is well accepted and has been used at home by villagers to combat malnutrition | 87 |
| Singapore | — | Vitabean (1952) | Drink | — | 21 |
| Taiwan | Wei Chuan (1964) | — | — | — | 21 |
| Sri Lanka | Department of Health Services and Care | Thriposha | Supplementary food | Thriposha has two formulations based currently on WSB from the U.S. | 24 |
| Thailand | Kasetsart University, Bangkok | *Poluk milk* (1964) Vitamilk (1960s) | *Poluk:* drink Vitamilk: drink | Kaset infant food is a product similar to weaning foods in | 21,24 |

## Table 9 (continued)
## ORIGIN AND STATUS OF FOOD PRODUCTS FOR COMBATING CHILDHOOD MALNUTRITION

| Country | Responsible organization | Production terminated | Production irregular/ position unknown | In production | Main use | Remarks | Ref. |
|---|---|---|---|---|---|---|---|
| | | | | Soya Product (1963) | Kaset: infant food | Western countries; it is a complete infant food and is recommended as a snack for children over 9 months | |
| Peoples Republic of China | — | — | — | Formula No. 5410 (1973) | Milk institute | It compares favorably with milk in nutritive value and vitamin contents and it is less expensive; product is available in small cubes which can be mixed with the desired amount of water; 100 cal of the product provide 3.8 g of total protein | 91 |

Table 10

PROTEIN-RICH FOOD MIXTURES, COUNTRIES OF ORIGIN AND THEIR
COMPOSITION

| | | | Composition (%) | | | | |
|---|---|---|---|---|---|---|---|
| Product | Country | Formulation[a] | Protein (g) | Calories (kcal) | Fat (g) | CHO (g) | Ref. |
| *Amana* | Nigeria | Groundnut (mainly), casein, yeast | — | — | — | — | 21,22 |
| *Arlac* | Nigeris | Groundnut (75), DSM (25) | — | — | — | — | 21,22 |
| Baby food | Turkey | Soya (20), DSM (10), chickpea (20), wheat (40) | 25 | 53 | 2.9 | | 21 |
| *Balahar* (children's food) BH | India | Wheat, bulgur wheat, soya fortified bulgur (15% soya), defatted soya flour, groundnut flour, Bengal gram flour, maize | 21 | — | — | — | 87 |
| BH-1 | India | Soya fortified bulgur (SFB) (85), groundnut flour (15) | 21 | 345 | 1.0— 2.5 | 62 | 87 |
| BH-2 | India | SFB (85), Bengal gram flour (15) | 17 | 346 | 1.0— 2.5 | 66 | 87 |
| BH-3 | India | Maize semolina (70), defatted soya flour (15), groundnut flour (15) | 21 | 345 | 1.0— 2.5 | 62 | 87 |
| BH-4 | India | Maize flour (65), soya flour (25), Bengal gram flour (10) | 21 | 345 | 1.0— 2.5 | 62 | 87 |
| BH-5 | India | SFB (90), Bengal gram flour (10) | 17 | 344 | 1.0— 2.5 | 66 | 87 |
| BH-6 | India | Whole wheat flour (70), groundnut flour (15), soya flour (15) | 17 | 350 | 1.0— 2.5 | 62 | 87 |
| BH-7 | India | Whole wheat flour (65), soya/groundnut flour (25), Bengal gram flour (10) | 17 | 350 | 1.0— 2.5 | 66 | 87 |
| BH-8 | India | Rolled oats (89), skim milk powder (11) | 16—18 | 350—380 | 5 | 62 | 87 |
| BH-9 | India | Rolled oats (83), skim milk powder (17) | 16 | 350 | 5 | 62 | 87 |
| *Balamul* | India | Defatted soya flour (20—25), cereal (25), legume (20), DSM (15), sugar, vitamins, and minerals | 22—36 | 384 | 7 | 60 | 22,87 |
| CINI-Nutri-mix | India | Wheat/rice (70 parts), Moongdhal (20 parts), skim milk powder (5 parts) | 18—19 | 385 | — | — | 87 |
| Cerealina | Brazil | Soya, DSM, maize | 20 | 485 | 9.9 | 59 | 21 |
| Colombihar-ina | Colombia | Soya (30), rice (60) | 18 | 355 | 1.4 | 68 | 21 |
| Conasupo products | Mexico | Soya (30), kidney bean (70) | 31 | — | — | — | 21 |
| *CSM* | U.S. | Soya (25), DSM (5), corn (68) | 20 | — | — | — | 21,23 |

Table 10 (continued)
PROTEIN-RICH FOOD MIXTURES, COUNTRIES OF ORIGIN AND THEIR
COMPOSITION

| Product | Country | Formulation[a] | Composition (%) | | | | Ref. |
|---|---|---|---|---|---|---|---|
| | | | Protein (g) | Calories (kcal) | Fat (g) | CHO (g) | |
| Dongo (growth) | Kenya | Maize (62.5), sesame (17.5), groundnut (10), green gram (10), vegetable oil (9) | 16 | 502 | — | — | 87 |
| Duryea | Colombia | Soya, DSM, maize | 20 | 345 | 1.6 | 57 | 21 |
| Energy food | India | Wheat flour (60 parts), Bengal gram flour (10 parts), groundnut flour, (10 parts), jaggery (30 parts) | 12—15 | 400 | 2.3 | — | 87 |
| *Faffa* | Ethiopia | Soya (18), DSM (5), legume (10) wheat or teff (57) | 20—25 | 340 | 2.2 | 64 | 21,89 |
| *Fortifex* | Brazil | Soyflour (48), corn flour (46), mineral salts, DL-methionine, vitamins | 30 | — | 2.0 | 59 | 21,69a |
| *Hyderabad mix* | India | Wheat or jowar (35), Bengal gram (12), groundnut (6.0), jaggery (12), defatted soy flour (6) Vitamin A 72 IU | 14—15 | 370 | — | — | 87 |
| *Incaparina* | Brazil | Soya (38), maize (58) | — | — | — | — | 21 |
| | Colombia | Soya (30), rice (60) | 28 | 370 | 4.2 | 54 | 21 |
| | Colombia | Soya (21), cottonseed (20), maize (58) | — | — | — | — | 21 |
| | El-Salvador | Cottonseed (38), maize (58) | 28 | 370 | 4.2 | 54 | 21 |
| | Guatemala | Cottonseed (38), maize (58) | 28 | 370 | 4.2 | 54 | 21 |
| | Nicaragua | Cottonseed (38), maize (58) | 28 | 370 | 4.2 | 54 | 21 |
| | Panama | Cottonseed (38), maize (58) | 28 | 370 | 4.2 | 54 | 21 |
| | Venezuela | Soya (19), cottonseed (19), maize (58) | — | — | — | — | 21 |
| Kerala Indigenous Food (KIF)[c] | India | Tapioca (70), groundnut (30) | 15 | 400 | — | — | 87 |
| | India | Tapioca (60), groundnut (30), soya (10) | 23 | 410 | — | — | 87 |
| | India | Wheat (50), tapioca (25), groundnut (25) | 20 | 395 | — | — | 87 |
| | India | Tapioca (200 g), fish powder (15 g), oil (5 m*l*) | 12 | 395 | — | — | 87 |
| K-Mix 2[d] | India | Calcium caseinate (12), skim milk powder (28), sugar (56) | 26 | 400 | — | — | 87 |
| K-Mix-4[d] | India | Skim milk powder (20), sugar (30), wheat flour (10), full-fat flour (40) | 24 | 382 | — | — | 87 |

Table 10 (continued)
## PROTEIN-RICH FOOD MIXTURES, COUNTRIES OF ORIGIN AND THEIR COMPOSITION

| Product | Country | Formulation[a] | Composition (%) | | | | Ref. |
|---|---|---|---|---|---|---|---|
| | | | Protein (g) | Calories (kcal) | Fat (g) | CHO (g) | |
| K-Mix-5[d] | India | Skim milk powder (20), sugar (40), full-fat soya flour (40) | 24 | 382 | — | — | 87 |
| K-Mix-6[d] | India | Skim milk powder (62), sugar (37), potassium chloride (0.07), magnesium hydroxide (0.03) | 22 | 370 | — | — | 87 |
| Kupangi Biscuit | South Africa | Soya, DSM, wheat | 8 | 70 | — | — | 21 |
| Kuzhandi Amudhu (child's nutrition food) | India | Roasted jowar flour (38), roasted Bengal gram flour (25), roasted groundnuts (12), jaggery (25) | 12—14 | 375—400 | — | — | 87 |
| | India | Roasted jowar flour (38), roasted green gram flour (25), roasted groundnuts (12), jaggery (25) | 13 | 385 | — | — | 87 |
| | India | Roasted maize flour (38), roasted Bengal gram flour (25), roasted groundnuts (12), jaggery (25) | 13 | 387 | — | — | 87 |
| | India | Roasted maize flour (38), roasted green gram flour (25), roasted groundnuts (12), jaggery (25) | 14 | 382 | — | — | 87 |
| | India | Roasted ragi flour (38), roasted Bengal gram flour (25), roasted groundnuts (12), jaggery (25) | 12 | 382 | — | — | 87 |
| | India | Roasted ragi flour (38), roasted green gram flour (25), roasted groundnuts (12), jaggery (25) | 12 | 377 | — | — | 87 |
| *Laubina* | | | | | | | |
| 101 | Lebanon | Parboiled wheat (40), chickpea flour (35), decorticated sesame (10), dried skim milk (5), sugar (10) | 17 | 420 | 21 | | 17,78,79 |
| 102 | Lebanon | Parboiled wheat (60), chickpea flour (20), decorticated sesame (10), dried skim milk (10) | 18 | 410 | 22 | | 17,78,79 |
| 103 | Lebanon | Parboiled wheat (60), chickpea flour (20), dried skim milk (10), | 16 | 410 | 13 | — | 17,78,79 |

Table 10 (continued)
## PROTEIN-RICH FOOD MIXTURES, COUNTRIES OF ORIGIN AND THEIR COMPOSITION

| Product | Country | Formulation[a] | Protein (g) | Calories (kcal) | Fat (g) | CHO (g) | Ref. |
|---|---|---|---|---|---|---|---|
| | | vegetale oil (5), sugar (2), bone ash (1), citric acid (1), vitamin A and D in sugar (1) | | | | | |
| 104 | Lebanon | Parboiled wheat (62), chickpea flour (25), dried skim milk (10), bone ash (1), citric acid (1), vitamin A and D (1) | 16 | 400 | 7 | — | 17,78,79 |
| 105 | Lebanon | Parboiled wheat (68), chickpea flour (27), vegetable oil (2), bone ash (1), citric acid (1), vitamin A and D (1) | 15 | 400 | 14 | — | 17,78,79 |
| 106 | Lebanon | Burghol (60), lentil (28), DSM (10), bone ash (1), vitamin A and D in sucrose (1) | 16 | 400 | 7 | — | 17 |
| Leche Alim | Chile | Sunflower seed flour, DSM, fish protein concentrate | — | — | — | — | 21 |
| Leaf protein mixture | India | Leaf protein (18), tapioca (40), ragi (10), sesame (2), jaggery (30) | — | — | — | — | 87 |
| *Ladylac* | Senegal | Groundnut (15), DSM (20), millet (45) | 18—20 | — | — | — | 21 |
| Milk Biscuit | Zambia | Soya (7), casein (13), wheat (27), fat and sugar | 20 | 460 | 20 | 50 | 21 |
| Milk substitute Formula No. 5410 | People's Republic of China | Soybean flour (28), rice flour (45), eggyolk powder (5), cane sugar (16.5), soybean oil (3.0), fermented millet (0.5), bone meal (1.5), salt (0.5), vanilla powder is added for flavor | 17 | 448 | 12.8 | 66 | 91 |
| *Miltone* | India | Groundnut protein isolate, wholesome cows milk, water, sugar syrup, vitamin and mineral mix | 4 | — | 2.0 | 5 | 87 |
| Mirpur mix | Bangladesh | Rice, wheat, pulses, groundnut, dried fish | 17 | 360 | 5.6 | — | 87 |
| Nestum | Colombia and Chili | Wheat flour, soya flour, oat flour, barley flour, sucrose, yeast, mineral salts, vitamins | 30 | — | 1.5 | 60 | 21,69a |
| Noodles | Thailand | Soya, wheat | — | — | — | — | 21 |
| Nutribien | Panama | Rice and soya | — | — | — | — | 24 |
| Nutriene | Brazil | Macagar bean flour (i.e., blackeyed peas) (50), corn meal (24), whole | 22 | 397 | 7.7 | 60 | 109 |

Table 10 (continued)
## PROTEIN-RICH FOOD MIXTURES, COUNTRIES OF ORIGIN AND THEIR COMPOSITION

| Product | Country | Formulation[a] | Protein (g) | Calories (kcal) | Fat (g) | CHO (g) | Ref. |
|---|---|---|---|---|---|---|---|
| | | powdered milk (25), calcium carbonate (1) | | | | | |
| *Nutrinuggets* | India | Textured vegetable protein made from defatted soya flour | 50 | — | — | — | 87 |
| Paushtika-har (Agra mix) | India | Soya fortified bulgur or soya fortified wheat grits (17.0), butter oil (2.1), sugar (2.0) | — | — | — | — | 87 |
| Pensal | Chili | Skimmed milk, sucrose, malt extract, milk fat, vitamins, iron | 20 | — | 10.0 | 62 | 69a |
| | Portugal | Wheat flour, sucrose, carob germs, flour, maize starch, soya flour, cocoa, barley flour, mineral salts, vitamins | 18 | — | 2.7 | 71 | 69a |
| *Peruvita* Savoury | Peru | Cottonseed (52), DSM (4), quinoa (28), sugar, natural flavors, vitamins A, $B_1$, and $B_2$ | 30 | 363 | 4.1 | 50 | 21,69a |
| Sweet | Peru | Cottonseed (47), DSM (4), quinoa (23), sugar, natural flavors, vitamins A, $B_1$, and $B_2$ | 35 | 338 | 4.9 | 37 | 21,69a |
| *Poluk* | Thailand | Soya, DSM | — | — | — | — | 21 |
| *ProNutro* | South Africa | Soya, groundnut, DSM, maize, yeast, wheat germ | 22 | 413 | 11.5 | 56 | 21 |
| *Protein plus* | India | Corn, soya flour | 20 | 330 | — | — | 87 |
| Sarbottam Pitho (super flour) | Nepal | Roasted soya flour (50), roasted corn flour (25), roasted wheat flour (25) | 20 | 366 | 8.3 | 53 | 87 |
| Shaktiahar | India | Puffed maize (44), full-fat soya (40), sugar (14), salt (1), vitamins and minerals (1) | 20 | 448 | 20 | 40 | 87 |
| Shakti Malt | India | Ragi, wheat, palm sugar flavors | — | — | — | — | 87 |
| Shishu Ahar | India | Ragi (45), wheat (48), pulse (10) | — | — | — | — | 81 |
| Simba | Kenya | Maize (85), DSM (15) | — | — | — | — | 21 |
| Solein | Brazil | Soya, DSM | 33 | 469 | 18 | 41 | 21 |
| Soya porridge | Uganda | Soya (38), DSM (5), maize (42) | — | — | — | — | 21 |
| *Sukhadi* (Child's Nutritious Food) | India | CSM, salad oil, jaggery (60:10:30) | 20 | 317 | 13.5 | — | 87 |
| *Superamine* | Algeria | DSM (10), chickpea (38), lentils (19), wheat (28) | 20 | 317 | 3.5 | 51 | 21 |

Table 10 (continued)
## PROTEIN-RICH FOOD MIXTURES, COUNTRIES OF ORIGIN AND THEIR COMPOSITION

| | | | Composition (%) | | | | |
|---|---|---|---|---|---|---|---|
| Product | Country | Formulation[a] | Protein (g) | Calories (kcal) | Fat (g) | CHO (g) | Ref. |
| Super Maeu | Mozam- bique | Soya (10), DSM (8), maize (61) | 23 | 350 | 4.9 | — | 21 |
| Swedish Emergency Food (SEF) A₁ | Sweden | Wheat flour (71), fish protein concentrate (FPC) (5), whey protein concentrate (10), sugar (9), oil (4), salt and minerals (1) | 23 | 375—390 | — | — | 88 |
| A₂ | | Wheat flour (71), FPC (7.5), whey protein concentrate (7.5), sugar (9), oil (4), salt and minerals (1) | 23 | 375—390 | — | — | 88 |
| A₃ | | Wheat flour (70), FPC (6.25), whey protein concentrate (6.25), dried peas (7.5), sugar (5), oil (4), salt and minerals (1) | 23 | 375—390 | — | — | 88 |
| A₄ | | Wheat flour (64), FPC (7), defatted soy flour (15), sugar (9), oil (4), salt and mineral (1) | 24 | 375—390 | — | — | 88 |
| A₅ | | Wheat flour (67), FPC (7), rapeseed protein concentrate (12), sugar (9), oil (4), salt and minerals (1) | 24 | 375—390 | — | — | 88 |
| B₁ | | Wheat flour (69), FPC (7), DSM (10), sugar (9), oil (4), salt and minerals (1) | 19 | 375—390 | — | — | 88 |
| B₂ | | Wheat flour (60), oatmeal (10), FPC (6), DSM (10), sugar (9), oil (4), salt and minerals (1) | 19 | 375—390 | — | — | 88 |
| B₃ | | Wheat flour (70), FPC (7), whey protein concentrate (1), defatted soy flour (8), sugar (9), oil (4), salt and minerals (1) | 21 | 375—390 | — | — | 88 |
| Special Weaning Food (*SWF*)[b] | | | | | | | |
| SWF—1 | India | Wheat flour (69), soya flour (20), sugar (10), salt (1) | 15 | 360 | — | — | 87 |
| SWF—2 | India | Wheat flour (79), soya flour (20), salt (1) | 15 | 360 | — | — | 87 |
| SWF—3 | India | Wheat flour (71), soya flour (20), sugar (8), salt (1) | 15 | 360 | — | — | 87 |
| SWF—4 | India | Wheat flour (69), soya | 15 | 360 | — | — | 87 |

Table 10 (continued)
## PROTEIN-RICH FOOD MIXTURES, COUNTRIES OF ORIGIN AND THEIR COMPOSITION

| Product | Country | Formulation[a] | Composition (%) | | | | Ref. |
|---------|---------|----------------|---------|----------|-----|-----|------|
| | | | Protein (g) | Calories (kcal) | Fat (g) | CHO (g) | |
| | | flour (6), calcium caseinate (10), sugar (14), salt (1) | | | | | |
| SWF—5 | India | Wheat flour (61), skim milk powder (15), full-fat soya flour (10), butter oil (6), sugar (8) | 15 | 360 | — | — | 87 |
| SWF—6 | India | Wheat flour (61), skim milk powder (25), butter oil (6), sugar (8) | 15 | 360 | — | — | 87 |
| SWF—7 | India | Rolled oats (67), skim milk powder (25), sugar (8) | 15 | 360 | — | — | 87 |
| SWF—8 | India | Wheat flour (67), skim milk powder (25), sugar (8) | 15 | 360 | — | — | 87 |
| Weaning Food | Egypt | DSM (10), chickpea (25), broad beans (25), wheat (25) | 20 | 400 | — | — | 21 |
| | Madagascar | Soya (38), DSM (5), rice (40) | — | — | — | — | 21 |
| | Taiwan | Soya (30), maize (20), rice (20) | — | — | — | — | 21 |
| | Turkey | Soya (20), DSM (10), chickpea (20), wheat (40) | — | — | — | — | 21 |
| Win Food | India | Millet (Combu), green-gram dhal flour, groundnut, jaggery | 20 | 406 | 4.6 | — | 21 |
| WSB | U.S. | Soya (20), wheat (73) | 38 | 400 | — | — | 23 |
| VPM | Israel | Chickpea (47), defatted sesame flour (35), soya bean flour (18) | 38 | 400 | — | — | 80 |

[a]   All formulation are in g/100 mixture unless otherwise specified.

[b]   All formulations are enriched by adding per 1 ton of *Balahar* or *SWF*, vitamin-mineral mix containing the following: vitamin A, 26 g; vitamin $B_1$, 3 g; vitamin $B_2$, 4 g; niacin, 50 g; vitamin $B_{12}$, 34 mg; folic acid, 340 mg; and dicalcium phosphate, 4 kg.

[c]   Vitamin-mineral mix generally added in similar levels to that in *Balahar*.

[d]   Vitamin mix (no minerals) added: per 1 ton of food mixture: vitamin A, 26 g; vitamin $B_1$, 3 g; vitamin $B_2$, 4 g; vitamin $B_{12}$, 34 mg; and folic acid, 340 mg. All K-M formulations have oil added at feeding centers. Primarily used for treatment of malnutrition and used 2—3 times per day.

food production. It is of interest that a Guatemalan affiliate of a large U.S. concern which had handled the market testing for INCAP was initially offered the long-term exclusive authorization. The parent company, however, was not prepared to make an adequate investment in the project and INCAP then sought another producer. Sales were slow to develop, partly as a result of the initial distribution which was undertaken by the drivers of the company's beer trucks. In 1964, special vans and wholesalers were used and in 1969 a separate sales organization and increased promotion began. Initially, production was in a corner of the parent company's brewery with manual filling of the packages, in 1968 a factory solely for the production of Incaparina products was built with a capacity of nearly 8 ton/8-hour working day. These improvements allowed sales to increase from 228 tons in 1965 to 1284 tons in 1970. Increases in sales allowed a 20% reduction in price in 1966, and in 1967, an addition of synthetic L-lysine to the product to improve nutritional value was possible without a price increase. Sales in 1974 had reached about 2000 ton/annum and a new plant has been built using extrusion processing thus allowing product diversification. A precooked version called Protina® is also in production and costs about twice the price of the original product.[24]

From Table 9, it can be seen that *Incaparina* was introduced into several Latin American countries but that production has ceased in many of them. The experience of *Incaparina* in Venezuela is of interest, showing how failure can occur despite the involvement of a highly financed international company with a considerable degree of expertise in production and marketing. *Incaparina* was launched in Venezuela in the provincial city of Valencia by Productos Quaker de Venezuela C.A., but under INCAP supervision. Initial publicity was well planned and stimulated high demand for the product. INCAP, however, had given permission to only one private enterprise company to manufacture and market the product and no direct support could be given by the government. At the same time, USAID donated milk powder and was available free for governmental feeding programs. Sales soon slumped, fell further when the price was raised, and ceased the following year. The product did not appeal to Venezuelan culinary habits which call for a thicker "atole" than could be made from Incaparina. A further deterrent to sales may have been the name, since in the same city there was a large manufacturer of animal foods whose product names mostly ended in the suffic "ina".

The Nestlé Company has been involved in the launching of protein-food products in many different countries. Some history of the early Nestlé involvement has been documented by Mauron.[69] The first product that reached the level of extensive field trials during the late 1950s was a high-protein food (HPF) biscuit designed for distribution in schools and Welfare Centers in Senegal. The formula contained mainly sorghum with added peanut meal and fish flour. The product had good nutritional value and was well accepted, but was, however, abandoned primarily due to the lack of government support and political problems relating to decolonization. A product was planned for Brazil since the Nestlé Company had been firmly established in that country for many years. Following extensive nutritional food and economic surveys in North East Brazil, a formula was proposed in 1960 primarily containing corn meal supplemented with peanut meal, soybean meal, and methionine. This mixture underwent extensive human studies during 1961, but in the meantime it had been observed that Brazilian peanut flour was often spoilt by a strain of *Aspergillus flavus* which produced the toxic aflatoxin. The formula was thus revised and the peanut replaced by soya. This new formulation named *Fortifex* was no longer as acceptable due to the higher soya content, nevertheless, it underwent extensive manufacturing trials during 1962 together with laboratory and clinical tests. By 1964, the Brazilian government withdrew financial backing but extensive market trials were still undertaken. By 1966 since sales were poor, the product was discontinued with the exception of sales to Institutions. Mauron[69] observes "The consumer in the North East area of Brazil is not willing to pay much more for a product similar to corn and with a less familiar taste. He is not in a position to appreciate the value of the high-protein content of the food and sales were not promoted with sufficient vigor due to the limited amount of funds available for this purpose." Some reevaluation appears to have occurred, since it is now reported[24] that a new product of the same name with a very similar formula will be launched by the Nestle Company.

The Nestlé Peruvian operation began in 1962 with a survey of the dietary situation and of the available protein sources in the country. The basic ingredient selected was rice which was to be supplemented with cottonseed flour and skim milk powder. The formula was tested both with rats and with children and was judged excellent. During this period contacts had been established with the Peruvian government and it was learned of the development of a HPF based on quinoa, a cereal-like product of the High Sierra. This development had been jointly between the Peruvian government and FAO. It was subsequently agreed that a product based on quinoa, now called *Peruvita* should be manufactured by Nestlé in Peru. According to the 10 year contract, *Peruvita* for governmental and institutional use would be sold at cost plus 5% profit, while the price to the public would also include the expenses of distribution, promotion, and marketing. Two varieties were developed and launched in 1966, a sweet variety designed for a weaning food and a salt variety as a supplementary food for adults.[69a] Neither were successful and except for sales to Institutions, both were discontinued in 1968. The major reason for failure was organoleptic. Government and United Nations Agency involvement had been extensive. Planning and publicity led to good initial sales, but these were followed by no second purchases. Initial consumer testing had been extremely poor since the product appeared to be completely unacceptable in taste, color, and smell.[21] A major factor was the use of quinoa, a cereal-like product which was often used for feeding chickens and pets and regarded at best as a poor man's food. Repeat sales are usually only generated when a product is liked, not because it has high-nutritional value. In view of these unfortunate histories, it is not surprising that a 2-year informal involvement between the Nestlé organization and the American University of Beirut for the proposed commercial production and marketing of *Laubina* never got beyond some minor changes in the formulation and very small-scale pilot production.

From Africa can be cited moderate success stories for *Faffa* in Ethiopia and **Pro-Nutro** in South Africa, and failures for *Amama* in Nigeria and *Ladylac* in Senegal. *Amama* was produced by the British pharmaceutical company, Glaxo, and was one of the earliest protein-food schemes in operation; it consisted of mainly groundnut with some added milk protein. It was designated as a dietary additive and the approach appeared to have been more toward its role as a medicine rather than as a food. As with the Nestlé HPF biscuit in Senegal, the discovery of aflatoxin affected the possibilities of production. However, sales were already declining before aflatoxin caused termination of production in 1961. A rather similar product, *Arlac* was produced in Northern Nigeria in 1963 with both government and UNICEF support, production continued for some 5 years and final closure was precipitated by political problems in the area and withdrawal of UNICEF support.

*Ladylac* was also produced with government involvement and United Nations assistance in the planning stages; however, production ceased within 6 months. The main reasons given for failure were the high costs of the product in relation to local wages. It was estimated that the minimum economic scale for production was over 200 tons/year while the prospective market was less than 20 ton/year. The introduction of a convenience-type food within the cultural pattern of Senegal may well have been before its time.

*ProNutro* had estimated sales in 1967 of about 7000 tons and a quote from the company that "Sales of product beyond expectations and have led to capacity problems" is cited by Orr.[21] Thus, further increases in production would have been expected. In fact total sales have fallen somewhat and are presently less than 4000 ton/year. However, retail sales as distinct from institutional purchases now account for 95% of output.[24]

*Faffa* is manufactured by the Ethiopian Nutrition Institute which is jointly sponsored by the Ethiopian and Swedish governments. Sales commenced in 1968 and had risen to some 400 tons by mid-1971. Throughout development, market research has been an integral component. A change in formulation to improve the "image" was made with wheat replacing teff as the cereal when the product was marketed in the lowlands. The consultant involved throughout the project was Dr. B. Wickstrom, author of the recent PAG Guideline on the marketing of protein-rich food in developing countries.[66] The problems to be overcome are those of low income, lack of the concept of the needs for special foods for children, lack of the habit of buying packaged foods, and a distribution network of a multitude of small stores with a passive retailer attitude. About 1000 ton/year will be needed for the project to be self-supporting on a nonprofit basis.

The product is still manufactured by the Ethiopian Nutrition Institute, not a commercial company, as had been planned.[24] The major outlet in recent years has been in emergency relief programs and production rose to 1500 ton/year in 1974.[92] Unfortunately, the retail trade in this product has dropped to about 25% of the 1971 sales.[24]

The introduction of *Superamine* in Algeria was widely assisted by the U.N. Agencies, followed closely most of the PAG Guidelines and took into account many of the lessons of the past. The World Food Program donated skim milk powder and sugar to the project until 1975, thus giving some degree of subsidy. In 1970 some 75% of total production (523 tons) was purchased by the government for direct-free distribution to malnourished children in institutions and in the lower socioeconomic groups. It is believed, however, that a new retail market will need to be developed so that the product can establish itself as part of a normal feeding pattern for the weaning of infants. Plant capacity has recently been increased for the free distribution program, and reached about 800 ton/year in 1974 and 1975,[24] the development of a retail market, however, remains disappointing.

In India, some of the worlds largest quantities of food mixtures have been produced, for example, in 1969, 26,000 tons of *Balahar* (children's food) were produced and in 1970, it constituted two thirds of all the special foods produced in low-income countries.[21] Current production (1976 and 1977) is some 43,000 tons.[87] *Balahar* exists in several different formulations, as are listed in Table 10. They are manufactured in many wheat flour mills in various parts of India under the Guidance of the Food Corporation of India. Amongst the raw materials used are wheat, bulgur wheat, defatted soya flour, maize, groundnut flour, and Bengal gram flour. The raw materials are crushed, ground, and blended with a vitamin/mineral mixture. The protein content has a minimum value of 21% (N × 6.25) while the PER ranges between 1.8 to 2.0 depending on the formulation. Many special feeding programs have been launched in India and are in operation under the auspices of the Central and State governments. A detailed booklet on *Supplementary Foods for Combatting Child Malnutrition in India* has been produced by Rao[87] on behalf of Food and Village Technology. UNICEF, Southeast Asia region, which lists 21 named products, many of which have various formulations, together with compositional, nutritional, and manufacturing details. *Hyderabad mix* contains wheat/flour supplemented with Bengal gram, groundnut, soya flour, and skim milk powder. It is produced as a womans activity in an India/Dutch project planned both to supply an inexpensive food for children and also to improve the earnings of poor women. The *Sukhadi* Feeding program commenced in 1970 and uses CARE supplied *CSM* mixed with salad oil and jaggery (a coarse brown Indian sugar). Production in 1970 was 40,000 tons and has been distributed both for nutritional improvement and partly for wages in kind. In 1974, 175,000 preschool and pregnant/nursing mothers received *Sukhadi* under the Special Nutrition Program. *Balamul* produced in Gujarat by a farmers cooperative supported by both the Government of India and UNICEF has been in production since 1971. The product contains cereals, legumes, soya, skim milk powder, and sugar together with vitamins and minerals. The plant has a capacity of 6000 tons/year. The formulation conforms to PAG Guidelines and has been successfully tested by the Central Food Technological Research Institute (CFTRI) in Mysore at the Vellore Hospital. There is an excellent marketing organization and the product sells throughout India on a commercial basis.

An additional cereal-milk food product *SWF* (special weaning food) commenced production in 1974. Eight different formulations have been used (see Table 10), but the most widely used variety contains wheat, soy, and sugar together with salt, minerals, and vitamins and provides 15 g protein and 360 kcal/100 g. The raw materials in the mix were mainly provided by UNICEF thus keeping the cost low to the consumer. In addition to these more traditional infant food products, extrusion technology has been used to produce nutritious snacks such as *Protein Plus* and *Nutrinuggets* which have been in the commercial market since 1972 and enjoy some degree of government subsidy by way of excise duty exemption.

All of the supplementary foods are claimed by Rao[87] to be highly acceptable. By using locally available products that are compatible with prevailing food habits, there is good market potential through the existing trade channels. Many of the processing techniques in India have been promoted in rural areas employing low-cost, labor-intensive technologies to suit local needs using indigenous resources. These, rather than centralized high technology procedures make extremely good socioeconomic sense in India. An interesting use of traditional technology to improve caloric density by reduction of viscosity by use of malting has been proposed by Desikachar.[87a] Malting of a mixture of finger millet and green gram not only improved functionality but also increased acceptibility.

## Other Products

So far consideration has been given only to the dry food mixes designed to be used as gruels or weaning foods. However, an increasing number of beverages are being produced. They are not complementary protein mixtures as have been discussed above, but are often soya-based and take advantage of the desire for soft drinks throughout the world (Table 11). Their relevance to PEM is that they do contain protein and they are in direct competition with products such as Coca- Cola® and Pepsi-Cola® and their worldwide imitations which contain no protein whatsoever. By far, the most successful is *Vitasoy* in Hong Kong with sales of over 120 million bottles per year. The reasons for this success have been discussed.[21] The product is sold both cold and hot, thus extending the season. The promotion now emphasizes the "thirst-quenching" properties of the drink rather than the child-feeding aspects. Undoubtedly, however, successful sales are due to the provision of a product that meets consumer needs. It seems unfortunate but true, as with the powdered products, that marketing appeal based on the "it's good for you" approach is rarely successful. A quite different approach is exemplified in *Miltone* which started production in the early 1970s. There are currently three plants in India, Bangalore, Ernakulam, and Hyderabad which are in production. Two more plants are planned to be installed with UNICEF assistance, one in Kanpur and the other probably in Calcutta.[87] The product was developed by the CFTRI as a milk extender. The original formulation consisted of buffalo milk, reconstituted groundnut isolate, and glucose syrup together with minerals and vitamins,[21] present formulations[87] use cows milk rather than buffalo milk. Manufacture consists of forming edible groundnut flour, after treatment with alkali acid and centrifugation, into a protein emulsion. The protein emulsion is then mixed with whole milk, sugar-syrup, and a vitamin premix and is either pasteurized or sterilized. The pasteurized milk contains 4% protein, 2% fat, and supplies 54 kcal (225 kJ)/100 g, while the sterilized variety is sweeter, contains 70 kcal/100 g is flavored and is sold commercially as a beverage. The pasteurized product has been widely used in India

Table 11
COUNTRY OF ORIGIN AND COMPOSITION OF SOME PROTEIN
BEVERAGES

| Product | Country | Ingredients | Comments |
|---------|---------|-------------|----------|
| Beanvit | Singapore and Malaysia | Soya milk | Produced since early 1950s; still on a pilot-plant basis |
| *Milpro* | India | Animal milk, groundnut isolate, and vegetable oil | Marketed in Bombay, 1970; sales remain confined to Bombay[24] |
| *Miltone* | India | Milk, groundnut isolate, glucose, minerals, and vitamins | Total production estimated[21] at 365,000 $\ell$/year; two varieties — one pasteurized and used primarily for child feeding, the other sweetened and flavored for use as commercial beverage[87] |
| *Poluk milk* | Thailand | Soya milk, DSM, and butterfat | Sold since 1964; 400,000 bottles per year, but production not increasing; very highly competitive market for soft drinks in Thailand |
| *Puma* | Guyana | Soya isolate with banana flavor | Produced since 1967; high concern with marketing — image of "vigor"; retail sales in excess of 29,000 bottles per year |
| Saci | Brazil | Soya milk, vitamins, and minerals with flavoring | Test marketed in 1968, by Coca-Cola Company; high concern with marketing — image of "health"; test marketing does not appear successful; protein content 3%; production now discontinued but consideration being given to introduction of a new product containing whey powder as protein source[24] |
| Samson | Puerto Rico | Milk whey, vitamins, and minerals | Dry powder for home reconstitution; a product of the same name also marketed in Surinam since 1970; experimental marketing only |
| Vitabean | Singapore and Malaysia | Soya milk | An improved version of Beanvit with minerals and vitamins; satisfactory sales, expansion planned; protein content 2.8% |
| *Vitasoy* | Hong Kong | Soy milk | Production commenced in 1940 and recommended in 1945; sales initially poor, product and "image" improved; plant capacity trebled over years; sales now in excess of 120 million bottles per year; most successful of all protein beverages, protein content, 3% |
| *Yoo-Hoo* | U.S. and Iran | DSM, whey chocolate flavor, minerals, and vitamins; may also contain vegetable protein | Produced under license in Iran (?) sales satisfactory and expansion planned; protein content, 3.5% |

for feeding programs in Karnataka, Kerala, and Andhra Pradesh and can be sold at Rs 1.40/$\ell$ compared to the cost of cows milk used in its production at Rs 1.60/$\ell$. No details of current production figures are given, but 1972 production was estimated as 365,000 $\ell$.[21] While *Vitasoy* production is usually cited as a success story and the production of 120 million bottles per year seems remarkable; however, to put this into perspective, it represents only 4 g of protein per individual per week for a population of 3.5 m in Hong Kong. In the highly unlikely event of the whole production being consumed by the very young, this would still be only some 40 g/week. This assumes further that the money spent on *Vitasoy* would not have been spent on some other food product — if *Vitasoy* replaces Cola or its equivalent, there is a net increase, albeit small, in protein intake, if it replaces bread, it is another story. In view of the current relatively affluent economic situation in Hong Kong and the rarity of PEM in that country, the role of *Vitasoy* in combating infantile malnutrition is probably not of any great consequence. *Miltone* in India may indeed be far more relevant in that it is enabling the extension of use of the limited milk supply at a lower price and is specifically aimed at infant feeding.[87]

## HOMEMADE FEEDING MIXTURES

The complementary effect between proteins occurs whether they are mixed by a manufacturer or by the mother immediately prior to the feeding of an infant. While homemade feeding mixtures may be more properly considered, the province of infant feeding practice and nutrition education rather than of food science and technology, some consideration must be given to this very relevant approach. The concept is, of course, not new and a considerable body of information on appropriate mixtures has been prepared in many local centers on a worldwide basis. The manual by Cameron and Hofvander[8] on feeding infants and young children (now in a second edition[93]), however, puts much of the information together in one place. The manual was designed to give comprehensive information on the preparation of homemade weaning foods so that more efficient use can be made of the locally available staples. The core of the book consists of tables and recipes demonstrating how foods should be mixed together to maximize the protein value. In Table 12, adapted from Cameron and Hofvander,[8] but recalculated by Pellett and Mamarbachi[93a] using the new FAO/WHO 1973[30] scoring system, the amounts of supplementary foods which should be used with various staple foods are shown. All the mixtures have a similar protein value which is at a level suitable for a young child (NDpCal = 7%). The table includes most of the staple foods in common use for human feeding together with some of the major supplements which could be mixed with them. It can be seen, for example, that 100 g of rice needs 15 g of egg to reach an adequate protein value. In contrast, 100 g cassava flour of much poorer protein value needs 45 g of egg, while oats, a superior cereal protein, can reach NDpCal = 7% with the addition of only 5 g of egg. The information in Table 12 only considers the supplementary protein value and pays no attention to bulk or to food energy value. The approximate food energy content (calorie value) of the various mixtures is, however, also shown in the table and appropriate adjustments can be made to meet food energy needs. Some of these mixtures may then be too bulky for young babies to obtain their protein and food energy needs. Adjustments are possible to reduce their bulk. Some of the staple food can be replaced with a little oil, sugar, or a mixture of both. To make allowance for the extra food energy from these sources, a larger proportion of the supplementary protein may be necessary. In Table 13 (adapted from the second edition of the manual[93]), but also recalculated,[93a] using the new FAO/WHO 1973 scoring system,[30] the adjusted proportions of ingredients are shown. The quantities shown are such that each mixture will provide 1470 kJ (350 kcal) of food energy with a protein value of at least NDpCal = 6% when mixed with appropriate quantities of oil and/or sugar.

Triple mixtures can be made by appropriate adjustments of quantities. Legumes are usually the cheapest available supplementary foods and triple mixes will often contain cereal, legume, and one other supplement. Appropriate quantities for replacement can be estimated from the table. The term "multimix" has been used when small amounts of green leaves and other red or yellow vegetables are added to the double or triple mixes and when fruit is given after the meal. In general, the more components there are in a meal, the better the variety of nutrients provided. Small amounts of vegetables and fruits do not provide many calories but they do have vitamins and minerals. They

Table 12

DOUBLE MIXES[a] TO GIVE PROTEIN VALUE NDpCal 7—8%

Staple foods

| Supplement | Oats | Wheat | Rice | Millet | Sorghum | Maize[b] | Potato | Sweet potato | Yam | Taro co-coyam | Banana | Plantain | Cassava flour[c] |
|---|---|---|---|---|---|---|---|---|---|---|---|---|---|
| Egg[d] | 5 | 25 | 15 | 10 | 20 | 20 | 5 | 10 | 5 | 5 | 15 | 15 | 45 |
| DSM[e] | 5 | 10 | 5 | 5 | 10 | 5 | 5 | 5 | 5 | 5 | 5 | 5 | 20 |
| DWM[f] | 5 | 15 | 10 | 5 | 15 | 10 | 5 | 10 | 5 | 5 | 10 | 10 | 35 |
| Fresh fish[g] | 5 | 10 | 10 | 5 | 10 | 5 | 5 | 5 | 5 | 5 | 5 | 10 | 30 |
| Chicken or lean meat | 5 | 15 | 10 | 5 | 10 | 10 | 5 | 5 | 5 | 5 | 10 | 10 | 35 |
| Soybean[h] | 5 | 10 | 5 | 5 | 10 | 5 | 5 | 5 | 5 | 5 | 5 | 10 | 30 |
| Legumes[i] | 10 | 10 | 25 | 25 | 25 | 25 | 25 | 25 | 25 | 25 | 25 | 25 | NA[j] |

| | kcal/100 g | kJ/100 g | | kcal/100 g | kJ/100 g |
|---|---|---|---|---|---|
| Average cereal | 350 | 1460 | Legume | 35 | 145 |
| Potato (Irish) | 75 | 315 | Soybean | 40 | 170 |
| Sweet potato | 115 | 480 | Chicken | 20 | 85 |
| Yam/taro | 105 | 440 | DSM | 35 | 145 |
| Plantain | 130 | 544 | DWM | 50 | 210 |
| Banana | 115 | 480 | Egg | 15 | 63 |
| Cassava flour | 340 | 1420 | Fish | 15 | 63 |

*Note:* When 100 g of staple food is mixed with weight (g) of supplementary food shown, the protein value will be between NDpCal 7-8%. Food energy values of various mixes can be estimated from the approximate values shown above.

a    All weights (g) are given as edible food portions.
b    Cereals absorb water during cooking and bulk increases 2-3 times.
c    For fresh cassava root, quantities given for cassava flour should be doubled. Cassava flour increases in bulk during cooking, fresh root does not.
d    Eggs vary in size thus weights are given. A standard egg without shell weighs approximately 50 g.
e    DSM = dried skim milk.

> DWM = dried whole milk.

ᵍ Fresh fish weights given; for dried fish products use 1/3 quantities.

ʰ 10 g Soybean is equivalent to 60 g soybean curd.

ⁱ Most legumes such as cow pea or kidney bean have poorer value than eggs, meat, or milk. They are thus not able to supplement all staple foods as efficiently as is needed. They must be used in larger quantities. This increases the mixture bulk and makes it more difficult for the infant to digest. Although 10 g will improve the value of wheat or oats, the 25 g quantities shown for the other staples are too large to be practicable; with cassava, it is impossible. In addition, double mixes using legumes should be begun gradually in conjunction with other supplements in appropriate amounts. Legume data from Cameron and Hofvander.[8]

ʲ NA = not applicable.

From Pellett, P. L. and Mamarbachi, D., *Ecol. Food Nutr.*, 7, 219-228, 1979. With permission.

# Table 13
## DOUBLE MIXES[a] ADJUSTED FOR LEAST BULK

### Staple foods

| Supplement | Oats | Wheat | Rice | Millet | Sorghum | Maize[b] | Potato | Sweet potato | Yam | Taro co-coyam | Banana | Plantain | Cassava flour[c] |
|---|---|---|---|---|---|---|---|---|---|---|---|---|---|
| Egg[d] | 65 | 65 | 65 | 65 | 60 | 65 | 310 | 190 | 230 | 200 | 190 | 150 | 55 |
|  | 10 | 25 | 20 | 20 | 30 | 25 | 15 | 35 | 15 | 25 | 40 | 45 | 50 |
| DSM[e] | 65 | 65 | 65 | 65 | 65 | 65 | 290 | 185 | 220 | 200 | 175 | 165 | 60 |
|  | 5 | 15 | 10 | 5 | 10 | 10 | 10 | 5 | 5 | 10 | 15 | 15 | 15 |
| DWM[f] | 60 | 55 | 50 | 55 | 50 | 55 | 230 | 120 | 155 | 145 | 120 | 110 | 40 |
|  | 5 | 15 | 15 | 10 | 15 | 10 | 15 | 20 | 15 | 15 | 20 | 20 | 25 |
| Fresh fish[g] | 70 | 75 | 70 | 70 | 75 | 75 | 320 | 220 | 250 | 230 | 220 | 190 | 75 |
|  | 5 | 15 | 15 | 10 | 15 | 10 | 15 | 25 | 10 | 15 | 25 | 25 | 35 |
| Chicken or lean meat | 70 | 70 | 70 | 70 | 70 | 70 | 320 | 200 | 230 | 205 | 195 | 170 | 65 |
|  | 5 | 15 | 15 | 10 | 15 | 10 | 15 | 20 | 10 | 15 | 25 | 25 | 35 |
| Soybean[h] | 65 | 65 | 60 | 70 | 65 | 55 | 270 | 175 | 195 | 185 | 160 | 145 | 55 |
|  | 5 | 10 | 10 | 5 | 10 | 10 | 15 | 15 | 10 | 10 | 15 | 15 | 20 |

*Note:* Quantities as given when supplemented with 10 g oil or 5 g oil and 10 g sugar or 20 g sugar will provide 350 kcal (1460 kJ) with an adequate protein value for the young child (NDpCal 6-7%). For a child of 12 months, this amount would be suitable for one meal a day to supplement milk feeding.

Triple mixes — Can be made by reducing the quantity of any of the supplements and replacing with an appropriate amount of any other supplement.

Multimixes — Can be made by adding some green, leafy vegetable, a little red or yellow vegetable or tomato to any of the mixes or by giving some fruit with or after the meal.

a   All weights (g) given as edible food portions.
b   Cereals absorb water during cooking and bulk increases 2—3 times. Tubers and starchy roots do not increase in bulk during cooking.
c   For fresh cassava root double quantities for cassava flour.
d   Egg weights given since eggs vary in size. A standard egg without shell weighs 50 g.
e   DSM = dried skim milk.
f   DWM = dried whole milk. If fresh milk available, 10 g DWM equals 80 mℓ fresh milk.
g   Fresh fish weights given, dried fish use 1/3 quantities.
h   10 g Soybean is equivalent to 60 g soybean curd.

From Pellett, P. L. and Mamarbachi, D., *Ecol. Food Nutr.*, 7, 219-228, 1979. With permission.

also add new flavors and do not reduce the protein value. Actual recipes for double, triple and multimixes derived from the tabular data shown are also included in the manual which is intended for professional use by those who have some basic knowledge of nutrition. Simplified versions using local products and local language could easily be prepared and their production has been recommended. These could be made available to nutrition aides who could then educate mothers in making the mixes.

The problems of implementing such a program on a scale large enough to be effective should not be underestimated.* However, the major advantages lie in cost. Even cheap manufactured food mixtures are relatively expensive and can sometimes reduce nutrient availability on a fixed income. Education in mixing normally available foods, allows high quality at minimal cost and eliminates many of the limitations and dangers inherent in the food mixture approach.

The values shown in Tables 12 and 13 were thus derived[93a] using the new FAO/WHO 1973 scoring pattern.[30] Since the first edition of the Cameron and Hofvander Manual was originally published in 1971, the new FAO/WHO 1973 scoring pattern[30] has been adopted and has been shown to be more accurate[11,12] than the earlier scoring systems. In this new pattern, reference values for the four amino acids most likely to be limiting in real dietaries, lysine, threonine, tryptophan, and total sulfur amino acids (SAA = methionine + cystine) have all been changed. Tryptophan and SAA were reduced while lysine and threonine were increased. The net result of these changes is that when protein scoring is performed, mixtures are more likely to appear limiting in lysine and threonine and less likely to appear limiting in tryptophan and SAA.[1,11] The protein scores for the various mixtures would be changed and thus the appropriate quantities of components necessary to give protein values between NDpCal 7 to 8% would also be changed. The new edition of the manual[93a] still, however, uses the earlier scoring system[94] and did not change to the newer recommended scoring procedure.[30] In general, the new values[93a] reported show smaller proportions of the supplementary food in the mixtures and are thus somewhat more economical than the mixtures of Cameron and Hofvander.[8,93] In addition to using the newer scoring system, Pellett and Mamarbachi[93a] have also used later amino acid data for both staples and supplements.

The importance of research upon the food legumes has been emphasized in a complete issue of the PAG Bulletin.[83] This issue not only contains the PAG Statement No. 22 on upgrading human nutrition through the improvement of food legumes,[95] but also contains a symposium on legumes and green, leafy vegetables in the nutrition of the infant and young child. Several of the papers in this symposium are especially relevant to the previous discussion on homemade feeding mixtures. Jelliffe and Jelliffe[96] emphasize the useful role of legumes in domestic multimixes, while Gabr[97] discusses the acceptability and tolerance of legumes and green, leafy vegetables in infant and child nutrition with special consideration to the toxic substances potentially present. A further article[98] presents a synthesis of three short papers concerning studies in India. Information is provided on the amount and manner of consumption of legumes and green, leafy vegetables by young children and the acceptability and tolerance of home-processed and -cooked preparations. The improvement in the nutritional quality of food legumes has been recently reviewed by Bressani.[98a] In this review detailed consideration is given not only to digestibility and the presence of antiphysiological factors, but also to the various supplementary effects between legumes and cereal grains. With diets high in grains and legumes, fiber content is an important consideration and possible guidelines for allowable fiber levels have been suggested.[98b]

* The Harvard School of Public Health and the M.I.T. International Food and Nutrition program have entered into a cooperative agreement with USDA to provide technical assistance to USAID for such programs. This program commenced in June 1981.

## CONCLUSIONS

Much emphasis has been placed by nutrition scientists, by United Nations Agencies, and by governments on low-cost nutritious foods as a means of alleviating the problems of world malnutrition. The scientific interest has been understandable, if only for the fact that a considerable armoury of methodology could be brought to bear on the problem and also that, for a long period, it was a fashionable area for allocation of grants by various funding agencies. The interests of governments and United Nations Agencies was also understandable: protein complementation had the element of "two plus two equals five" and did in theory produce a net increase in the total amount of utilizable protein available. As was indicated earlier, we can now see that the expectations were too high and much of the enthusiasm misplaced.

1. Do these products fill a need and do they still show promise in the fight against world malnutrition?
2. Was the whole emphasis based on misconceptions as to the cause of protein-energy malnutrition and are programs producing harmful consequences?

In 1972, an evaluation of experience with protein-rich food mixtures[21] concluded that the nutritional impact was small and would remain small even if all available capacity was fully utilized for production and all that was produced was consumed by the primary target group. For rural areas without social welfare institutions, the potential use was likely to be particularly limited. This population in many countries comprises the majority of the at-risk children. Urban populations would be more accustomed to purchasing some processed foods and could have access to social welfare institutions when they existed. Distribution through these centers could thus make a useful contribution especially where the urban poor are the major groups experiencing infant malnutrition. However, retail distribution, no matter how desirable, would need a considerable degree of price subsidization in order to reach the very poor. The development of a retail trade has been part of the whole concept throughout and has proved extremely disappointing in its attainment.

The United Nations Agencies are fully aware of these problems and many of the more recent recommendations have been upon marketing and promotion rather than upon the food mixtures themselves. Emphasis has also been placed upon understanding and developing channels for influencing preschool feeding. In Table 14 some of these recommendations are summarized and emphasize the roles of several different levels of workers from the local level worker to the clinician, the availability of resource facilities, and the use of commercial channels and mass media in influencing opinions relating to preschool feeding.

Of the various products introduced, *Incaparina* in Guatemala has been one of the more successful. Surveys[99] have shown wide knowledge of the product and favorable opinions on the price and its acceptability. Despite this, the overall consumption per family was low, only some 3 kg per family per year[66] and the use was primarily that of a "family" product rather than specifically for children. When extrapolation is made from 1970 production of 1184 tons using the INCAP recommended consumption of 75 g per child per day, this represents consumption by only 8% of the population of children between 1 to 3 years.[21] If it could be assumed that the individuals most in need received the product then this would be of value, however, it was shown that only 29% of *Incaparina* consumers were in the lowest income level of under $20.00 per annum.[99] Although 1974 production was estimated at 2000 tons,[24] when allowance is made for population growth, it remains probable that usage by the very poor contin-

**Table 14**
**CHANNELS FOR INFLUENCING PRESCHOOL FEEDING**

| | |
|---|---|
| Basic factors | Personal service to the preschool child is a particular gap since the child is not reached directly through schools or through maternal-infant care activities; the four basic factors involved are (1) food availability including cost, family income, and facilities, (2) custom (cultural practices), (3) individual family experience, attitude, and responsibility, and (4) realistic information provided to the family |
| Channels of communication | In developing areas, changes in knowledge, attitude, and practice depend largely on person-to-person communication; even in the areas reached by the limited mass media, there is only marginal influence on populations which are semiliterate and habitually dependent on the opinion of their family, neighbors, and community leaders; agents of change must work through the following channels |
| The local-level worker | Must be community-knowledgeable, must accept the community, and must be accepted by the community; can be achieved by recruiting agents near area of service and keeping them near during training; function include guidance, influencing gossip, counteracting rumors, with ample opportunity for feedback; reasons for resistance to change of feeding practices must be ascertained; objectives must be limited to making a small number of key changes rather than introduction of rigid detailed feeding schedules; local level workers must be multifunctional; priority functions in many areas related to nutrition education include management of pregnancy and delivery including family planning and disease management; in addition, to formal agents (such as school teachers), community development agents, agricultural extension agents and auxiliary nurse, midwives, and informal agents should also be mobilized; when influential agents are not mobilized, they can be potentially serious negative influences |
| Higher-level workers | Function by supervision and training of local level workers and by referring more complex questions to appropriate laboratory research or information facilities; physicians trained in pediatrics and/or obstetrics should be associated with the program; they may require suitable training in modern principles of nutrition with special reference to regional nutritional problems |
| Clinical contact | The first contact with the preschool child is in the maternity ward where the mother is most receptive to education on the needs of her baby; contact during pregnancy is also significant in influencing fetal and early childhood nutrition; the most common contact with preschool children is during the treatment of illness; here also the mother is receptive to education; in all treatment facilities including hospitals, the health worker must emphasize education of the mother along with treatment of the child; if village-level workers can educate, in addition to offering simple treatment, many nutritional problems can be managed before they require expensive in-patient treatment; nutrition-rehabilitation centers[101] have been designed *inter alia* to perform this function |
| Resource facilities | These take the form of institutions and experts which contribute to the training of workers, for guiding survey work, for laboratory analyses, and for the provision of technical information; these resource facilities should have a defined relationship to service and training units |
| Mobile facilities and transport availability | Efficient use of transport requires careful consideration; mobile facilities are not only expensive, but lack impact on knowledge, attitude, and practice since they do not provide continuity of service and the intimate personal contact required; problems exist also relating to maintenance, lack of roads, and difficulties in following regular schedules |

Table 14 (continued)
## CHANNELS FOR INFLUENCING PRESCHOOL FEEDING

| | |
|---|---|
| Commercial channels and government legislation | Stores are more widely distributed than government health service units; cooperation between nutrition program and commercial production and marketing has much potential; governments can influence marketing policies and operations by providing information and by appropriate legislation; the government can provide enrichment or fortification of foods, promote economic distribution of surplus agricultural products, lower taxes and other tariffs on good quality protein foods, tax nutritionally inappropriate products and, establish and administer laws regulating standards and codes of practice for hygienic processing, packaging, and labeling; governments should consult with nutritionists, pediatricians, and other concerned specialists on these matters before introducing administrative changes |
| Mass media | Mass media may have particular potential for influencing opinion of leaders and for conditioning the public favorably for person-to-person contacts; the radio is often one of the major sources of information; the potential of mass media for public education on health and nutrition has not been properly exploited and much greater efforts should be made to work through these media using responsible production and advertising techniques[102] |
| Distribution | An obstacle to feeding programs in many countries is inadequate government machinery to supervise food distribution; the machinery is likely to be less adequate through health channels than through school channels; until this machinery is strengthened the available help of UNICEF, CARE, AID, The World Food Program, and other sources will have limited application. |
| | The hidden costs that have appeared in distribution programs have raised serious questions about the cost benefits of some distributions; permanent dependence on outside supply is undesirable, distributions need to maximize educational benefits and seek ways of phasing themselves out; collaboration with international donor agencies such as the World Food Program and Food for Peace is desirable |
| Role of schools | The schools ordinarily do not reach the preschool child directly; in some cases, the schools might be used as centers of distribution to mothers and preschool children and of parent education; the greatest potential of schools lies in educating the oncoming generation and in using students to educate their families; the school garden and the school lunch are important for practical education |
| Other channels of communication | Womens clubs and youth clubs can be channels of information and distribution; information can sometimes be channeled through industrial employment; this is of growing importance with rapid urbanization, but there are also rural opportunities such as tea estates where female labor is especially likely to be employed |
| The urban contact | When breast feeding is curtailed, consideration should be given to early supplementary feeding through clinics, day care centers, and home visiting; all staff involved must clearly understand, however, that for the large nonprivileged groups of young infants in developing countries, no substitute will equal breast milk with respect to safety in rearing; day care centers and nurseries for working mothers offer opportunities for improving preschool nutrition; in the towns, besides the greater access to mass media, more food is purchased rather than home grown; thus, greater attention should be given to influencing food market availabilities |
| Homemade weaning foods | The *PAG Manual on Feeding Infants* with special reference to homemade weaning foods[8,93] is highly relevant to improved feeding patterns (see also Section on Homemade Feeding Mixtures and Tables 12 and 13 of this review) |
| Miscellaneous | All information channels have some limitations and more pooling of experience and methodologies used is recommended; priority should be given to influencing agricultural practices, industrial-commercial |

**Table 14 (continued)**
**CHANNELS FOR INFLUENCING PRESCHOOL FEEDING**

modification and other factors that can influence acceptance through availability; a reinforcement of current approaches is also essential in order to have adequate impact; all these efforts will help long-term progress rather than pose dramatic easy solutions

Adapted from **FAO/WHO/UNICEF Protein Advisory Group**, Channels for Influencing Preschool Feeding, Feeding the Preschool Child: Report of a PAG *ad hoc* Working Group, Document 1.14/5, United Nations, New York, 1971, 30-37. With permission.

ues at a minimal level. The *Incaparina* experience in Guatemala has recently been reviewed.[99a,99b] It was concluded by Scrimshaw[99a] that:

"Incaparina can thus be considered a success if viewed as a concept that has proved to be reliable, acceptable, and nutritionally sound. If judged by its effect on protein-calorie malnutrition without either governmental or other subsidy, or improvements in social equity, it is not, could not have been, and was never projected to be the answer. Only political and economic policies that improve the purchasing power of the lowest income groups will enable Incaparina or any other food to make a truly significant contribution to this aim."

With the *Faffa* project in Ethiopia the nutritional goal was to supplement the ordinary diet of an undernourished child with about 100 g *Faffa* per day: some 20 g of protein. Market surveys[66] have shown that *Faffa* products were used irregularly and much below the prescribed quantities, averaging only 3 servings per month. A review on the nutrition protection given to vulnerable groups through protein-rich mixtures also concludes that the impact has not been great.[89] *Faffa* has, however, proved of considerable value in famine relief.[92]

A further evaluation by Elizabeth Orr[24] confirms the very limited role of these products in reaching low-income groups especially through the normal retail trade. This review also notes as significant that the various United Nations Agencies who were major influences in the initial development of these products are now concentrating on other approaches such as the encouragement of homemade weaning foods produced locally[8,93] (Tables 12 and 13). The Protein-Food Development Group, a section of the Food Policy and Nutrition Division of FAO, was disbanded in 1973[24] — a further example of the change in emphasis of FAO.

On the other hand, technology has proved that products of high-nutritive value can be made from vegetable materials and that they can be cheap, though perhaps not cheap enough. In this respect the application of low-cost extrusion cooking (LEC) is an important development. Locally grown crops can be processed using these techniques which are suitable for use in developing countries. Jansen and Harpe[99c] describe techniques and mixture compositions as well as current applications in several countries. In overall economic and energy balance terms, the advantage of mixing vegetable proteins together is real: protein that would have been wasted both directly and also in physiological utilization, is saved: this is a real net gain.

The developed world has been as wasteful in its energy use in food production and distribution as it has been with its personal transport. Yields in farm production in relation to energy input have probably decreased in the U.S. since 1945.[103,104] The implications are that if energy costs continue to rise, the price differentials between animal protein foods and vegetable products will increase and the need for food mixtures which can give good quality protein from low-energy-intensive products may well increase.

A further set of advantages are indirect; for example, the production of soybeans in areas where they were not produced before and publicity about protein-rich foods may have influenced overall nutrition to a greater extent than sales figures would indicate.

With regard to the second question that asked whether the development of the products has been based on misconceptions and whether possible harmful consequences can follow, it is salutary to examine again how fundamental views have changed over the last decade. During development of the various products, concepts as to the types of products required were colored by the conventional wisdom of the time relating to the protein problem. It was widely accepted at that time that protein-energy malnutrition was caused by a low intake of high-quality protein. Thus improvements in protein quality or quantity were the advocated cures. A widespread worldwide deficiency of protein had been assumed as illustrated by the publication in 1968 of the volume *International Action to Avert the Impending Protein Crisis*.[105] Some years before, the PAG of the United Nations had been set up to advise on protein needs and a protein gap became part of the conventional wisdom. Many nutritionists, on the basis of protein requirements and extrapolation from the African kwashiorkor experience, claimed that more protein was needed to solve world malnutrition. This message was received and acted upon by plant breeders, animal nutritionists, food technologists, and others who were able by various means to increase the net amount of utilizable protein. Why should they have questioned the initial premise? Perhaps, however, the extrapolation of African experience to the whole world was incorrect, i.e., kwashiorkor was not the only form of PEM, protein requirements may have been set too high and the whole relationship between energy intake and protein utilization may have been given less importance than it merited. As a result of these alternative views there is now strong advocacy of the concept that a worldwide protein gap is no longer tenable.[1,35,36] A recent comprehensive review, however, by Scrimshaw[106] analyzes the past and present recommended dietary allowances for protein and advises caution in the adoption of the new lower FAO/WHO[30] recommended allowances in that they may now be too low. The pendulum between the extreme views of a protein gap or a food energy gap is still swinging since knowledge of protein requirements and all the factors affecting such requirements remain incomplete.[107] It seems that much infantile malnutrition, especially of the nutritional marasmus type, may not be caused primarily by lack of protein in the diet but more by hygienic and family related factors. This has led to the conclusion by some that protein alone and indeed nutrition alone will not solve the nutritional problems that exist. The formulation of new vegetable protein mixtures as well as the production of fish protein concentrate, the development of single cell protein, and the amino acid fortification of staple foods are all uses of advanced science and technology as attempts to improve the nutritional status of individuals whose problems perhaps lie more in hygienic and socioeconomic factors. Unfortunately, in few fields of human endeavor is there such a distressing gap between know-how and its actual implementation, between research input and output in practical terms, and between a humanitarian intention and its efficiency in the field.

We have in the past been searching for simple solutions to complex problems. Just as there is no single cause there is no single solution. Perhaps we should view malnutrition as somewhat analogous to the concept of protein quality and limiting amino acids. In some instances a single deficiency can be repaired and a dramatic improvement in nutrition will result, in other instances several disparate deficiencies all co-exist and no single improvement can show any benefit, only simultaneous changes in several areas may show progress.[7] The net result, however, is that we are left with a massive investment in protein-rich food schemes. These products have been termed "commerciogenic nutritious foods" by Popkin and Latham,[9] who believe that "the limitations and potential dangers of relying on commercially produced, low-cost nutritious foods to reduce or eliminate malnutrition have neither been adequately investigated nor put in persepctive." The burden of their criticism is upon the place of these foods in a market economy rather than on the foods themselves. They believe that commercially processed foods are not appropriate for the very poor and can in fact contribute to a deterioration rather than an improvement in nutritional status. Energy in some of these foods can cost 8 to 40 times its cost in the normal diet and protein may be 3 to 18 times as expensive. Similar values were reported from Lebanon[108] where commercial weaning foods could cost 20 times as much for energy and 43 times as much for protein as home-produced weaning foods. Popkin and Latham[9] demonstrate that **replacement** of standard dietary items by certain commercial products may have disastrous effects on an individual of fixed purchasing power in that both protein and energy intakes could be reduced. This is not even to consider the other unfortunate effects when breast feeding is replaced by artificial feeding in an unhygienic environment.[3,4,85] A further effect under current discussion[86] emphasizes that abandonment of breast feeding where contraception is not in common use can mean both higher birth rates, because of the now well-established contraceptive effect of breast feeding, as well as the higher death rates for infants. It is emphasized that **both** the fertility and mortality implications must be considered jointly in assessing the overall demographic impact.[86]

The whole role of promotion and advertising in these circumstances is of paramount importance, even fully honest advertising can pull in the wrong direction. Dishonest advertising in these circumstances is criminal. Examples of misleading if not downright dishonest advertising in both developed and developing countries in the promotion of bottle feeding by multinational corporations have been given by Greiner.[110] It is now accepted by the industry that some promotion has been at fault and an international code of marketing ethics has been proposed.[111] A further evaluation of this controversial issue appears in the final issue of the PAG Bulletin where two special articles,[112,113] citing numerous literature references, review both sides of the controversy, one critizing the promotion of bottle feeding while the other defends the industry position. The detailed WHO/UNICEF position on this issue is also available.[5a]

There are, however, some encouraging features of the present situation. The multifactorial cause of malnutrition has become widely accepted at all levels and food mixtures are realized to be merely one facet that should be considered within a national nutrition policy. The failure of the policies expasizing retail outlets for food mixtures has been somewhat compensated by the greater number of social welfare infant and child centers, allowing outlets for government subsidized products. These can certainly benefit the urban poor but leave considerable problems in reaching the widespread rural population.[24] A further encouraging feature is the much greater technological skill available in the developing nations and the realization that capability exists in many instances for the production of products at home using locally available foods rather than the reliance on imported products using limited foreign exchange. India is a prime example of this available technology[87] coupled with the needs for involving some production in village centers.

Nevertheless, despite these encouraging features, it must be emphasized that there is no single solution and overall improvement in the alleviation of protein-energy malnutrition in the developing world can only come in the wider and controversial contexts of economics, politics, and national development.

## ACKNOWLEDGMENTS

Grateful thanks are due to Elizabeth Orr of the Tropical Products Institute, London, for making available a copy of her current manuscript, *A Second Look at Food Mixtures,* before its publication by FAO. Thanks are also due to Dr. D. V. S. K. Rao of

UNICEF South Central Asia Region for sending copies of his most useful report on "Supplementary Foods" in India. Dr. V. H. Potty of CFTRI was also extremely helpful in sending us current information on food mixtures from India. In addition, we are grateful to Dr. J. Mauron of the Nestlé Co., Switzerland, for kindly sending us information on the current status of his company's products in South America. Various other individuals responded to questions despite being extremely busy, and gave us helpful advice on the current situation of food mixtures throughout the world. These included Dr. G. Donoso of WHO, India, Dr. K. O. Herz of FAO, Rome, and Dr. Nesheim of Quaker Oats, U.S.; we are grateful for their help.

## REFERENCES

1. Pellett, P. L., Nutritional problems of the Arab World, *Ecol. Food Nutr.*, 5, 205-215, 1976.
2. McLaren, D. S., Nutrition planning: the poverty of holism, *Nature (London)*, 267, 742, 1977.
3. Jelliffe, D. B., Commerciogenic malnutrition: time for a dialogue, *Food Technol. (Chicago)*, 25, 55-56, 1971.
4. Jelliffe, D. B. and Jelliffe, E. F. P., Human milk, nutrition and the world resource crisis, *Science*, 188, 557-561, 1975.
5. FAO/WHO/UNICEF Protein Advisory Group, Promotion of special foods (formula and processed protein foods) for vulnerable groups, *PAG Statement*, No. 23, 1972.
5a. WHO/UNICEF, Statement and Recommendations of a Joint WHO/UNICEF Meeting on Infant and Young Child Feeding, World Health Organization, Geneva, 1979; see also *Food Nutr. Bull.*, 2(3), 24-31, 1980.
5b. ACC-SCN Consultative Group on Maternal and Young Child Nutrition, Dietary management of young infants who are not adequately breast fed, *Food Nutr. Bull.*, 2(3), 41-50, 1980.
6. FAO/WHO/UNICEF Protein Advisory Group, Recommendations on policies and practices in infant and young child feeding and proposals for action to implement them, *PAG Bull.*, 5(1), 1-5, 1975.
7. Pellett, P. L., Marasmus in a newly rich urbanized society, *Ecol. Food Nutr.*, 6, 53-56, 1977.
8. Cameron, M. and Hofvander, Y., For application in the developing areas of the world, with special reference to the home-made weaning foods, PAG Document No. 1, *Manual on Feeding Infants and Young Children*, 1971, 14-26.
9. Popkin, B. M. and Latham, M. C., The limitations and dangers of commerciogenic nutritious foods, *Am. J. Clin. Nutr.*, 26, 1016-1023, 1973.
10. Bodwell, C. E., Ed., *Evaluation of Proteins for Humans*, AVI, Westport, Conn., 1977.
11. Pellett, P. L., Young, V. R., Eds., *Nutrition Evaluation of Protein Foods*, WHTR/UNUP-129, United Nations University, Tokyo, 1980.
12. Pellett, P. L., Protein evaluation revisited, *Food Technol. (Chicago)*, 30(5), 60-76, 1978.
13. Bressani, R., Amino acid supplementation of cereal grain flours tested in children, in *Amino Acid Fortification of Protein Foods*, Scrimshaw, N. A. and Altschul, A. M., Eds., MIT Press, Cambridge, Mass., 1971, 184-204.
14. Bressani, R., Complementary amino acid patterns, in *Nutrients in Processed Foods - Proteins*, White, P. L. and Fletcher, D. C., Eds., Publishing Sciences Group (for the American Medical Association), Acton, Mass., 1974, 149-166.
15. Bressani, R., Protein supplementation and complementation, in *Evaluation of Proteins for Humans*, Bodwell, C. E., Ed., AVI, Westport, Conn., 1977, 204-232.
16. Tannahill, R., *Food in History*, Stein & Day, New York, 1973.
17. Cowan, J. W. and Pellett, P. L., The development of 'Laubina' — infant food mixtures for the Middle East, in *Protein-Enriched Cereal Foods for World Needs*, Milner, M., Ed., The American Association of Cereal Chemists, St. Paul, Minn., 1969, 305-314.
18. Kapsiotis, G. D., History and status of specific protein-rich foods: FAO/WHO/UNICEF protein food, protein and products, in *Protein-Enriched Cereal Foods for World Needs*, Milner, M., Ed., The American Association of Cereal Chemists, St. Paul, Minn., 1969, 255-265.
19. van Veen, A. G. and van Veen, S., Pioneer work on protein foods, *Nutr. Newsl.*, 11(4), October December 1973.
20. Milner, M., Ed., *Protein-Enriched Cereal Foods for World Needs*, The American Association of Cereal Chemists, St. Paul, Minn., 1969.

21. Orr, E., *The Use of Protein-Rich Foods for the Relief of Malnutrition in Developing Countries: An Analysis of Experience,* Report, Tropical Products Institute, No. G 73 IV, 1972.
22. Pellett, P. L., Role of food mixtures in combatting childhood malnutrition, in *Nutrition in the Community,* McLaren, D. S., Ed., John Wiley & Sons, New York, 1976, 185-202.
23. Bressani, R. and Elias, L. G., Development of new highly nutritious food products, in *Man, Food and Nutrition,* Rechcigl, M., Jr., Ed., CRC Press, Cleveland, Ohio, 1973, 251-274.
24. Orr, E., The contribution of new food mixtures to relief of malnutrition — a second look, *Food Nutr.,* 3, 2-10, 1977.
25. Pimentel, D., Dritschilo, W., Krummel, J., and Kutzman, J., Energy and land constraints in food protein production, *Science,* 190, 754-761, 1975.
26. Pekkarinen, M., World food consumption patterns, in *Man, Food and Nutrition,* Recheigl, M., Jr., Ed., CRC Press, Cleveland, Ohio, 1973, 15-33.
27. FAO, *Amino-Acid Content of Foods and Biological Data on Proteins,* Food and Agricultural Organization of the United Nations, Rome, 1970.
28. Pellett, P. L. and Shadarevian, S., *Food Composition Tables for Use in the Middle East,* American University of Beirut, Beirut, Lebanon, 1970.
29. Hegsted, D. M., Nutritional research on the value of amino acid fortification. Experimental studies in animals, in *Amino Acid Fortification of Protein Foods,* Scrimshaw, N. S. and Altschul, A. M., Eds., MIT Press, Cambridge, Mass., 1971, 157-178.
30. FAO/WHO, Energy and protein requirements, Report of a joint FAO/WHO *Ad hoc* expert committee on energy and protein requirements, *WHO Tech. Rep. Ser.,* No. 522, Geneva, 1973; *FAO Nutr. Rep. Ser.,* No. 52, Rome, 1973.
31. Whitehead, R. G., The protein needs of malnourished children, in *Proteins in Human Nutrition,* Porter, J. W. C. and Rolls, B. A., Eds., Academic Press, New York, 1973, chap. 7.
32. Nicol, B. M., Protein and calorie concentration, *Nutr. Rev.,* 29, 83-88, 1971.
33. Hegsted, D. M. and Neff, R., Efficiency of protein utilization in young rats at various levels of intake, *J. Nutr.,* 100, 1173-1179, 1970.
34. Samonds, K. W. and Hegsted, D. M., Protein requirements of young cebus monkeys, *Am. J. Clin. Nutr.,* 26, 30-40, 1973.
35. McLaren, D. S., The great protein fiasco, *Lancet,* 2, 93-95, 1974.
36. Waterlow, J. C. and Payne, P. R., The protein gap, *Nature (London),* 258, 113-117, 1975.
37. Martorell, R., Lechtig, A., Yarbrough, C., Delgado, H., and Klein, R. E., Energy intake and growth in an energy deficient population, *Ecol. Food Nutr.,* 1978.
38. FAO, *FAO Agricultural Commodity Projections, 1970-1980,* Vols. 1 and 2, Food and Agricultural Organization of the United Nations, Rome, 1971.
39. Liener, I. E., Toxic factors in protein foods, in *Proteins in Human Nutrition,* Porter, J. W. G. and Rolls, B. A., Eds., Academic Press, New York, 1973, chap. 33.
40. Liener, I. E., Protease inhibitors and hemagglutinins of legumes, in *Evaluation of Proteins for Humans,* Bodwell, C. E., Ed., AVI, Westport, Conn., 1977, 284-303.
41. Bressani, R. and Elias, L. G., Processed vegetable protein mixtures for human consumption in developing countries, *Adv. Food Res.,* 16, 126-228, 1968.
42. Rao, S. V., McLaughlan, J. M., and Noel, F. J., quoted in *Amino Acid Content of Foods and Biological Data on Proteins,* Food and Agricultural Organization of the United Nations, Rome, 1970.
43. Sirinit, K., Soliman, A. M., Van Loo, A. T., and King, K. W., Nutritional value of Haitian cereal-legume blends, *J. Nutr.,* 86, 415-423, 1965.
44. Bressani, R., Valiente, A. T., and Tejada, C. E., All vegetable protein mixtures for human feeding. VI. The value of combinations of lime-treated corn and cooked black beans, *J. Food Sci.,* 27, 394-400, 1962.
45. Phansalkar, S. V., Ramachandran, M., and Patwardhan, V. N., Nutritive value of vegetable proteins. I. Protein efficiency ratios of cereals and pulses and the supplementary effect of the addition of a leafy vegetable, *Indian J. Med. Res.,* 45, 611, 1957; FAO, in *Amino Acid Content of Foods and Biological Data on Proteins,* Food and Agricultural Organization of the United Nations, Rome, 1970.
46. Bressani, R. and Valiente, A. T., All-vegetable protein mixtures for human feeding. VII. Protein complementation between polished rice and cooked black beans, *J. Food Sci.,* 27, 401-406, 1962.
47. Daniel, V. A., Leela, R., Rao, S. V., Hariharan, K., Indiramma, K., Swaminathan, M., and Parpia, H. A. B., Mutual and amino acid supplementation of proteins. II. Nutritive value of the proteins of blends of wheat, groundnut, soya bean, Bengal gram, sesame and skim milk powder fortified with limiting essential amino acids, *J. Nutr. Diet,* 1, 293, 1964; FAO, in *Amino Acid Content of Foods and Biological Data on Proteins,* Food and Agricultural Organization of the United Nations, Rome, 1970.

48. de Groot, A. P. and Van Stratum, O. G. C., Biological evaluation of legume proteins in combination with other plant protein sources, *Qual. Plant Mater. Veg.*, 10, 168, 1963; FAO, in *Amino Acid Content of Foods and Biological Data on Proteins,* Food and Agricultural Organization of the United Nations, Rome, 1970.

49. FAO/WHO/UNICEF Protein Advisory Group, PAG guideline on preclinical testing of novel sources of protein, *PAG Guideline,* No. 6, 1972.

50. Carpenter, K. J., Damage to lysine in food processing: its measurement and its significance, *Nutr. Abstr. Rev.,* 43, 424-451, 1973.

51. FAO/WHO/UNICEF Protein Advisory Group, PAG *ad hoc* working group meeting on clinical evaluation and acceptable nucleic acid levels of SCP for human consumption, *PAG Bull.,* 5(3), 17-26, 1975.

52. Sternberg, M., Kim, C., and Schwende, F., Lysinoalanine: presence in foods and food ingredients, *Science,* 190, 992-994, 1975.

53. Samonds, K. W. and Hegsted, D. M., Animal bioassays: a critical evaluation with special reference to assessing nutritive value for the human, in *Evaluation of Proteins for Humans,* Bodwell, C. E., Ed., AVI, Westport, Conn., 1977, 68-80.

54. Hegsted, D. M. and Samonds, K. W., A collaborative study to evaluate four methods of estimating protein quality, in *Nutritional Evaluation of Protein Foods,* WHTR/UNUP-129, United Nations University, Tokyo, 1980.

55. Friedman, M., *Protein Nutritional Quality of Foods and Feeds,* Part I and II, Marcel Dekker, New York, 1975.

56. U.S. Food and Drug Administration, Appraisal of the Safety of Chemicals in Food, Drugs and Cosmetics, Association of Food and Drug Officials of the United States, Austin, Tex., 1959.

57. NAS — Food Protection Committee, *Evaluating the Safety of Food Chemicals,* National Academy of Sciences, Washington, D.C., 1970.

58. FAO/WHO/UNICEF Protein Advisory Group, PAG guideline on human testing of supplementary food mixtures, *PAG Guideline,* No. 11, 1972.

59. FAO/WHO/UNICEF Protein Advisory Group, PAG guideline on sanitary production and use of dry protein foods, *PAG Guideline,* No. 7, 1972.

60. Jelliffe, D. B., *The Assessment of the Nutritional Status of the Community,* WHO Monograph Series No. 53, World Health Organization, Geneva, 1966.

61. Hegsted, D. M., Balance studies, *J. Nutr.,* 106, 307-311, 1976.

62. Young, V. R. and Scrimshaw, N. S., Human protein and amino acid metabolism and requirements in relation to protein quality, in *Evaluation of Proteins for Humans,* Bodwell, C. E., Ed., AVI, Westport, Conn., 1977, 11-54.

63. Bressani, R., Human Assays and Applications, in *Evaluation of Proteins for Humans,* Bodwell, C. E., Ed., AVI, Westport, Conn., 1977, 205-232.

64. Kies, C. V., Techniques in human nitrogen balance studies, in *Evaluation of Proteins for Humans,* Bodwell, C. E., Ed., AVI, Westport, Conn., 1977, 162-176.

65. FAO/WHO/UNICEF Protein Advisory Group, PAG guideline on protein rich mixtures for use as supplementary foods, *PAG Guideline,* No. 8, 1972.

66. FAO/WHO/UNICEF Protein Advisory Group, PAG guideline on the marketing of protein-rich foods in developing countries, *PAG Guideline,* No. 10, 1971.

67. FAO/WHO/UNICEF Protein Advisory Group, Report of a PAG *Ad Hoc* working group, *PAG Guideline on Feeding the Preschool Child,* October 1977.

68. FAO/WHO/UNICEF Protein Advisory Group, Marketing and distribution of protein rich foods, *PAG Statement,* No. 5, 1971.

69. Mauron, J., From pilot plant tests to the commercialization of protein-rich vegetable mixtures, in *Proc. 7th Int. Congr. Nutr.,* Vol. 3, Friedr. Vieweg und Sohn, Braunshweig, Hamburg, 1967, 183-193.

69a. Mauron, J., Personal Communication, Nestlé Products Technical Assistance Co., Ltd., Lausanne, Switzerland, 1977.

70. Bressani, R., Elias, L. G., Aguirre, A., and Scrimshaw, N. S., All-vegetable protein mixtures for human feeding. III. Development of INCAP vegetable mixture nine, *J. Nutr.,* 74, 201-208, 1961.

71. Bressani, R., Aguirre, L. G., Elias, R., Arroyave, R. J., and Scrimshaw, N. S., All-vegetable protein mixtures for human feeding. IV. Biological testing of INCAP vegetable mixture nine in chicks, *J. Nutr.,* 74, 209-216, 1961.

72. Scrimshaw, N. S., Behar, M., Wilson, D., Viteri, F., Arroyave, G., and Bressani, R., All-vegetable protein mixtures for human feeding. V. Clinical trials with INCAP mixture 8 and 9 and with corn and beans, *Am. J. Clin. Nutr.,* 9, 196-205, 1961.

73. Bressani, R. and Elias, L. G., All-vegetable protein mixtures for human feeding. The development of INCAP vegetable mixture 14 based on soybean flour, *J. Food Sci.,* 31, 626-631, 1966.

74. Squibb, R. L., Wyld, M. K., Scrimshaw, N. S., and Bressani, R., All-vegetable protein mixtures for human feeding. I. Use of rats and baby chicks for evaluating corn-based vegetable mixtures, *J. Nutr.*, 69, 343-350, 1961.

74a. Bressani, R., Braham, J. E., and Elias, L. G., Human nutrition and gossypol, *Food Nutr. Bull.*, 2(4), 24-32, 1980.

75. Doraiswamy, T. R., Chandresekhara, M. R., Subbaraya, B. H., Sankaran, A. N., and Subrahman-yan, V., Use of an infant food formula based on groundnut protein isolate and skim milk powder in feeding infants, *Indian J. Pediatr.*, 30, 365-368, 1963.

76. Barja, I., Munoz, P., Solimano, G., Vallejas, E., Rodrigan, M. E., and Tagle, M. A., Infant feeding formula based on chickpea *(Cicer arientinum)*, its use as the sole food in health infants, *Indian J. Nutr. Diet.*, 11(6), 335-341, 1974.

77. Prasannappa, G., Chandrasekhara, H. N., Rani, R. P., Srinivasan, K. S., and Chandrasekhara, M. R., Supplementary foods for preschool children, *Nutr. Rep. Int.*, 18, 71-77, 1976.

78. Tannous, R. I., Cowan, J. W., Rinnu, F., Asfour, R. J., and Sabry, Z. I., Protein-rich food mixtures for feeding infants and preschool children in the Middle East. I. Development of evaluation of Lau-bina mixtures, *Am. J. Clin. Nutr.*, 17, 143-147, 1965.

79. Asfour, R. Y., Tannous, R. I., Sabry, Z. I., and Cowan, J. W., Protein-rich food mixtures for feeding infants and young children in the Middle East. II. Preliminary clinical evaluation with Lau-bina mixtures, *Am. J. Clin. Nutr.*, 17, 148-151, 1965.

80. Matoth, Y., Elian, E., and Gruenberg, G., Evaluation of a protein-rich mixture based on vegetable foods of Middle Eastern countries, *Am. J. Clin. Nutr.*, 21, 226-229, 1968.

81. Dastur, S. K. and Potty, V. H. An avenue for meeting the nutritional needs of the Pre-Balwadi groups in rural areas, personal communication, Central Food Technological Research Institute, My-sore, India, 1977.

82. Graham, G. C. and Baertl, J. M., Nutritional effectiveness of soy cereal foods in undernourished infants, *J. Am. Oil Chem. Soc.*, 51, 152A, 1974.

83. FAO/WHO/UNICEF Protein Advisory Group, Symposium on legumes and green leafy vegetables in the nutrition of the infant and young child, *PAG Bull.*, 3(2), 25-53, 1973.

84. Knapp, J., Barness, L. A., Hill, L. L., Blaltner, R., and Sloan, J. M., Growth and nitrogen balance in infants fed cereal proteins, *Am. J. Clin. Nutr.*, 26, 586-590, 1973.

85. Wade, N., Bottle feeding: adverse effects of a western technology, *Science*, 184, 45-48, 1974.

86. Knodel, J., Breast feeding and population growth, *Science*, 198, 1111-1115, 1977.

87. Rao, D. V. S. K., *Supplementary Foods for Combatting Child Malnutrition in India,* Food & Village Technology UNICEF, South Central Asia Region, New Delhi, November 1977.

87a. Desikachar, H. S. R., Development of weaning foods with high caloric density and low hot-paste viscosity using traditional technologies, *Food Nutr. Bull.*, 2(4), 21-23, 1980.

88. Abrahamson, L., Hambraeus, L., and Vahlquist, B., Swedish emergency food (SEF): an onging applied nutrition research program, Protein-Calorie Advisory Group of the United Nations System, Eds., *PAG Bull.*, 4(4), 26-30, 1974.

89. Agren, G. Y., Hofvander, R., Selinus, and Vahlquist, B., Faffa: a supplementary cereal-based wean-ing food mixtures in Ethiopia, in *Protein-Enriched Cereal Foods for World Needs*, Milner, N., Ed., The American Association of Cereal Chemists, St. Paul, Minn., 1969, 278-287.

90. De Muelenaere, H. J. H., Development production and marketing of high-protein foods, in *Protein-Enriched Cereal Foods for World Needs*, Milner, M., Ed., The American Association of Cereal Chemists, St. Paul, Minn., 1969, 266-277.

91. Stapleton, T., Infant feeding in the People's Republic of China, in *PAG Bull.*, 4(4), 31-33, 1974.

92. Gebre-Medhin, M. and Vahlquist, B., Famine in Ethiopia — the period 1973-75, *Nutr. Rev.*, 35, 194-202, 1977.

93. Cameron, M. and Hofvander, Y., *Manual on Feeding Infants and Young Children,* 2nd ed., Calorie Advisory Group of the United Nations System, United Nations, New York, 1976.

93a. Pellett, P. L. and Mamarbachi, D., Recommended proportions of foods in home-made feeding mix-tures, *Ecol. Food Nutr.*, 7, 219-228, 1979.

94. FAO, Protein requirements, *FAO Nutr. Stud.*, No. 16, 1957.

95. FAO/WHO/UNICEF Protein Advisory Group, PAG Statement No. 22 on upgrading of human nutrition through the improvement of food legumes, *PAG Bull.*, 3(2), 1-24, 1973.

96. Jelliffe, D. B. and Jelliffe, E. F. P., The role of legumes and dark green leafy vegetables in domestic multimixes for the trasitional, *PAG Bull.*, 3(2), 40-45, 1973.

97. Gabr, M., Legumes and green leafy vegetables in infant and young child nutrition, *PAG Bull.*, 3(2), 46-49, 1973.

98. Anon., Use of legumes and green leafy vegetable for infant and young child feeding: summary of results of studies in three different parts of India, *PAG Bull.*, 3(2), 51-53, 1973.

98a. Bressani, R. and Elias, L. G., Improvement of the nutritional quality of food legumes, *Food Nutr. Bull.*, 1(4), 23-34, 1979.

99. Shaw, R. L., *Incaparina* in Central America, in *Protein-Enriched Cereal Foods for World Needs*, Milner, M., Ed., American Association of Cereal chemists, St. Paul, Minn., 1969, 320-333.

99a. Scrimshaw, N. S., A look at the *Incaparina* experience in Guatemala, *Food Nutr. Bull,.* 2(2), 1-2, 1980.

99b. Wise, R. P., The case of *Incaparina* in Guatemala, *Food Nutr. Bull.,* 2(2), 3-8, 1980.

99c. Jansen, G. R. and Harper, J. M., Application of low-cost extrusion cooking to weaning foods in feeding programmes. I. and II, *Food Nutr.,* 6(1), 2-9; 6(2), 15-23, 1980.

100. FAO/WHO/UNICEF Protein Advisory Group, *Channels for Influencing Preschool Feeding. Feeding the Preschool Child:* Report of a PAG *Ad Hoc* Working Group, Document 1.14/5, United Nations, New York, 1971, 30-37.

101. Beghin, I. D., Centres for combatting childhood malnutrition, in *Nutrition in the Community*, McLaren, D. S., Ed., John Wiley Sons, New York, 1976, 169-183.

102. FAO/WHO/UNICEF Protein Calorie Advisory Group of the United Nations, PAG Statement No. 27 on mass communications in nutrition education and symposium on mass communications, *PAG Bull.,* 4(1), 2-18, 1974.

103. Pimentel, D., Hurd, L. E., Bellotti, A. C., Forster, M. J., Oka, I. N., Sholes, O. D., and Whitman, R. J. Food production and the energy crisis, *Science,* 182, 443-449, 1973.

104. Steinhart, J. S. and Steinhart, C. E., Energy use in the U.S. food system, *Science,* 184, 307-316, 1974.

105. United Nations, *International Action to Avert the Impending Protein Crisis*, No. E68 XIII 2, United Nations, New York, 1968.

106. Scrimshaw, N. S., Analysis of past and present recommended dietary allowances for protein in health and disease. I and II, *New Engl. J. Med.,* 294, 136-142 and 198-203, 1976.

107. Scrimshaw, N. S., Through a glass darkly: discerning the practical implications of human dietary protein-energy interrelationships, *Nutr. Rev.,* 35, 321-337, 1977.

108. Pellett, P. L. and McGregor, L., Food as a cause of childhood malnutrition, in *Proc. 6th Symp. Nutr. Health, Near East*, McLaren, D. S. and Dagher, N., Eds., American University of Beirut, Beirut, Lebanon, 1970, 53-64.

109. de Mello, A. V., Chaves, N., de Lucena, M. A. F., Varela, R. M., Costa, T., Teixeira, S. F. G., Salzano, A. C., Martins, G. C., and Monteiro, E. A., The testing of Nutriene V, a plant protein mixture, in the recuperation of undernourished children, *Am. J. Clin. Nutr.,* 26, 1024-1029, 1973.

110. Greiner, T., *The Promotion of Bottle Feeding by Multinational Corporations: How Advertising and the Health Professions Have Contributed*, Cornell International Nutrition Monograph Series No. 2, Cornell University Program on International Nutrition and Development Policy, Ithaca, New York, 1975.

111. Benton, D. A., The role of the infant food industry in promoting desirable policies and practices in feeding of infants and children, *PAG Bull., 5(1)* 20-24, 1975; see also Abbott Laboratories, *Code of Marketing Ethics for Developing Countries*, Abbott Laboratories, Chicago, Ill., 1977.

112. International Council of the Infant Food Industries (ICIFI), Infant feeding in the less developed countries: an industry viewpoint, *PAG Bull.,* 7 (3-4), 62-72, 1977.

113. Margulies, L., A critical essay on the role of promotion in bottle feeding, *PAG Bull.,* 7 (3-4), 73-83, 1977.

114. Graham, G. G., Morales, E., Acevedo, G., Placko, R. P., and Cordano, A., Dietary protein quality in infants and children. IV. A corn soy milk blend, *Am. J. Clin. Nutr.,* 24, 416-421, 1971.

# FOODS IN TIMES OF DISASTER AND FAMINE

## A. Omololu

There are two main types of foods used in times of disaster and famine:

1.  Milks or fluids
2.  Flours, grits and mixtures

Milks are meant for the feeding of infants and young children, to supply extra protein to all groups and, in some special cases, to treat malnutrition. In the last case, it is usually advised that sucrose and oil be added to increase the caloric value of the drinks.

Flours, grits and mixtures can be used in any way that conforms to the traditional eating habits of the people. Thus, flours may be made into different types of bread; grits and mixtures made into thin or thick porridge for drinking or eating with a condiment, while other flours, like the Swedish Formula, may be added to whatever food is eaten to increase the protein content.

Certain characteristics should be common to all these foods. Among these are

1.  **Long shelf-life** — this is ensured by using well-cleaned and pest-free ingredients, by precooking in some cases, and by proper packaging.
2.  **Easy transportation and packaging** — this is why most of the foods are in the forms of powders, flours, or grits because this makes for easy packaging. Ingredients of unequal or large sizes would make the bags uneven and easily punctured.
3.  **Versatility** — the foods must be in a form that can be used in many ways to conform to local, traditional eating habits. Fluids and thin porridges are acceptable all over the world as foods for infants and children. Porridges are used in almost all cultures while in most developing countries, thick porridges are eaten with condiments.
4.  **Easy preparation** — most drinks can be made up by the simple addition of water while some of the foods to be used as porridge are precooked to reduce cooking time.

In most areas where famine and disasters occur, the urgent needs are to feed infants and children and to give high-calorie and/or protein food to all.

Some of the foods described are supplemented with Soya flour to give extra protein. As the addition of sucrose will increase proneness to ant and insect infestation, this is not usually done. Sucrose can, in most cases, be added just before eating. The addition of oils and fats — another good source of calories — leads to early rancidity. Thus, instructions are usually given to add oils and fats during cooking or preparation of the product.

These foods are not meant for full- or long-time feeding of adult populations. They should only be used for a short time and as soon as possible; local or solid foods acceptable to the area added to the diet.

The modes of preparation stated under each food are guidelines (Tables 1 to 22). Local people should be given the opportunity to experiment with ways of cooking acceptable to them.

## Table 1

Name: Nonfat Dry Milk (Fortified with
Vitamins A and D) Skimmed Milk (Fortified
with Vitamins A and D)

**Ingredients and Processes**
  100% Nonfat, dry, spray process
  + Vitamin A
  + Vitamin D

**Nutritional Data**
  Chemical analysis

| | | | |
|---|---|---|---|
| Moisture 3.5 >< 4% | | Fiber = 0 | |
| Protein % = 35.9 | | Ash = 0 | |
| Fat % = 0.8 | | Carbohydrate = 59.8 | |

  Amino acid in mg AA/g protein

| | | | |
|---|---|---|---|
| Isoleucine | 330 | Tyrosine | 311 |
| Leucine | 619 | Threonine | 263 |
| Lysine | 453 | Tryptophan | 89 |
| Methionine & cystine | 220 | Valine | 402 |
| Phenylalanine | 303 | | |

  Protein quality

| | |
|---|---|
| P.E.R. | 2.9 |
| N.P.U. % | 77.4 |
| Utilizable protein | 27.8 |

  Calories
    Megajoules per 100 g of finished product
    Total >1.63 MJ (390 cal)
    From protein 0.600 MJ (143.6 cal)
    From fat 0.030.1 MJ (7.2 cal)
    From carbohydrate 1.00 MJ (239.2 cal)
    25.6 g contains 0.418 MJ (100 cal)
    >9.2 g protein in 0.418 MJ (100 cal)
    >10.7 g protein (adjusted for Casein Equivalent) in 0.418 MJ
      (100 cal)
  Vitamins per 100 g

| | | | |
|---|---|---|---|
| A palmitate (IU) | >2200 | Ergocalciferol (IU) | >440 |
| Thiamine (mg) | 0.4 | | |
| Riboflavine (mg) | 2.0 | | |
| Niacin (mg) | 1.0 | | |
| Ascorbic acid (mg) | 7.0 | | |

  Minerals per 100 g

| | | |
|---|---|---|
| Calcium carbonate | (mg) | 1308 |
| Phosphorus | (mg) | 1016 |
| Iron | (mg) | 1.0 |
| Potassium | (mg) | 1745 |
| Sodium | (mg) | 532 |

**Uses**
  1. As supplement drinks for malnourished and other children, also for
  adults
  2. *NOT* to be used as main feed for infants (without the addition of oil
  or fat)

**Packaging**
  22.5 kg filled multiwall paper sacks with minimum of three walls of
  paper and an inner polyethylene liner

## Table 2

Name:      Whey Soy Drink Mix

### Ingredients and Processes

| | | |
|---|---|---|
| Whey | 41.3 | Sweet Solids |
| Soy flour | 36.5 | Full-fat (toasted), fortified with at least 42% protein |
| Soy bean oil | 12.2 | Refined, deodorized, partially hydrogenated, winterized, bleached, stabilized with BHA, BHT to reduce susceptibility of rancidity; propyl gallate to retain good oil stability and initial flavor; citric acid added to increase density of calories; reduce salt concentration in whey and aid in reconstituting beverage for freshness |
| Corn cereal solids/corn syrup | 9.125 | Aid in freshness when beverage is made; sweetening effect to reduce soy flour flavor; also to reduce salt concentration in whey |
| Vitamin premix | 0.1165 | |
| Mineral premix | 0.7583 | |

### Nutritional Data

#### Chemical analysis

| | | | |
|---|---|---|---|
| Moisture | <5% | Fiber | <1.5 |
| Protein | >19% | Ash | <6.5 |
| Fat | >19% | Carbohydrate | 49% |

#### Amino acid in mg AA/g protein

| | | | |
|---|---|---|---|
| Isoleucine | 67.1 | Phenylalanine | 52.6 |
| Leucine | 96.1 | Tyrosine | 32.0 |
| Lysine | 76.5 | Threonine | 52.8 |
| Methionine | 17.0 | Tryptophan | 16.1 |
| Cystine | 22.4 | Valine | 63.6 |

#### Protein quality

P.E.R. >2.1
N.P.U.% >66.1
Utilizable protein >12.6

#### Calories

Megajoules per 100 g of finished product
Total 1.853 MJ (443 cal)
From protein 0.251 MJ (76 cal)
From fat 0.715 MJ (171 cal)
From carbohydrate 0.820 MJ (196 cal)
22.6 g contains 0.418 MJ (100 cal)
>9.2 g protein in 0.418 MJ (100 cal)
>10.7 g protein (adjusted for Casein Equivalent) in 0.418 MJ (100 cal)

#### Vitamins per 100 g

| | | | |
|---|---|---|---|
| A palmitate | 1929 IU | Cyanocobalamin | 5.0 µg |
| Thiamine | 0.3 mg | Ascorbic acid | 47.0 mg |
| Riboflavine | 0.5 mg | Ergocalciferol | 231.0 IU |
| Niacin | 5.8 mg | α-Tocopherol | 8.7 IU |
| Ca D-pantothenic | 3.2 mg | Folate | 230.0 µg |
| Pyridoxine | 0.2 mg | | |

#### Minerals per 100 g

| | |
|---|---|
| Calcium carbonate | 700.0 mg |
| Iron | 18.0 mg |
| Potassium iodite | 70.0 µg |
| Zinc | 5.0 mg |

Table 2 (continued)

Packaging
   22.5 kg multiwalled paper sacks with five walls of paper and a polyethylene
   liner
Uses
   Make up with suitable quantity of boiled and cooled water and feed as drink

Table 3

Name:          Corn Soya Milk (CSM)

**Ingredients and Processing**

| | | |
|---|---|---|
| Corn meal | 60 | Processed, partially precooked, gelatinized, dehulled, and degermed |
| Soy flour | 17.5 | Defatted (toasted) or full-fat; fortified at least 44% protein |
| Milk powder | 15 | Nonfat, dry, spray process |
| Soy oil | 5.5 | Refined, deodorized, stabilized with BHA, BHT, and citric acid |
| Vitamin premix | 0.1 | |
| Minerals premix | 1.3 | Iron added |
| Calcium phosphate | 0.6 | |

**Nutritional Data**

Chemical analysis

| | | | |
|---|---|---|---|
| Moisture | <10 | Fiber | <2 |
| Protein | >19 | Carbohydrate | 63 |
| Fat | >6 | | |

Amino acid pattern in mg AA/gN

| | | | |
|---|---|---|---|
| Isoleucine | 328 | Phenylalanine | 303 |
| Leucine | 581 | Tyrosine | 259 |
| Lysine | 343 | Threonine | 250 |
| Methionine | 100 | Tryptophan | 75 |
| Cystine | 96 | Valine | 334 |

Protein quality
   P.E.R. =   2.4
   MN.P.U. =  70.3%

Energy values

| | | | |
|---|---|---|---|
| Per 100 g gives | 1.598 | MJ | |
| | 0.318 | MJ | from protein |
| | 0.226 | MJ | from fat |
| | 1.054 | MJ | from carbohydrate |

Vitamins in 100 g

| | | | | | |
|---|---|---|---|---|---|
| A palmitate | 1653 | IU | Cyanocobalamin | 4 | μg |
| Thiamine | 0.3 | mg | Ascorbic acid | 40 | mg |
| Riboflavine | 0.4 | mg | Ergocalciferol | 198 | IU |
| Niacin | 5.0 | mg | α-Tocopherol | 7.5 | IU |
| Ca D-pantothenic | 2.8 | mg | Folate | 190 | μg |
| Pyridoxine | 0.2 | mg | | | |

Minerals in 100 g

| | | | | | |
|---|---|---|---|---|---|
| Calcium carbonate | 600 | mg | Iodine | 4950 | μg |
| Tricalcium phosphate | 600 | mg | Potassium | 800 | mg |
| Phosphorus | 800 | mg | Sodium | 300 | mg |
| Magnesium | 100 | mg | Zinc | 4 | mg |
| Iron | 2 | mg | | | |

Uses
   Thin porridge as drinks: thick porridge to be eaten with
   condiments — must be cooked

## Table 3 (continued)

**Packaging**

22.5 kg filled multiwall paper sacks with five walls of
paper and a polyethylene liner; outer wall of wet strength
and made insect resistant

**Source**

U.S.

## Table 4

**Name:**          Instant Corn Soya Milk

**Ingredients and Processing**

| | | | |
|---|---|---|---|
| Corn meal | | 63 | Fully cooked and completely gelatinized, corn dehulled and degermed |
| Soy flour | 29.2 | | Full-fat |
| or | | 29.2 | |
| Soy flour | 23.7 | | Defatted and toasted — fortified with at least 42% protein |
| Soy oil | 5.5 | | Refined, deodorized, and stabilized with BHA, BHT, and citric acid added |
| Milk powder | 5 | | Nonfat dry, spray process |
| or | | 5 | |
| Modified whey | 5 | | |
| or | | | |
| Dry butter milk | 5 | | Spray process |
| Vitamin premix | | 0.1 | |
| Minerals premix | | 2.7 | Iron added |

**Nutritional Data**

Chemical analysis — same as corn soya milk (CSM)

Amino acid pattern in mg AA/gN

| | | | |
|---|---|---|---|
| Isoleucine | 250 | Phenylalanine and tyrosine | 481 |
| Leucine | 594 | Threonine | 244 |
| Lysine | 363 | Tryptophan | 63 |
| Methionine & cystine | 175 | Valine | 281 |

Protein quality — same as CSM

Energy values — same as CSM

Vitamins in 100 g — same as CSM

Minerals in 100 g

| | | | |
|---|---|---|---|
| Calcium carbonate | 900 mg | Iodine | 4950 μg |
| Tricalcium phosphate | 2000 mg | Potassium | 900 mg |
| Phosphorus | 700 mg | Sodium | 300 mg |
| Magnesium | 100 mg | Zinc | 4 mg |
| Iron | 2 mg | | |

**Uses**

Instant — needs no cooking
  Can be made into thin or thick porridge like CSM

**Packaging**

Same as CSM

**Source**

U.S.

## Table 5

Name: Faffa

**Ingredients and Processes**

| | |
|---|---|
| Whole wheat | 57% |
| Chick peas | 10% |
| Soy flour (defatted) | 18% |
| Dried skim milk | 5% |
| Sugar + iodized salt | 9% |
| Mineral mixture (Ca + Fe) | 1% |
| Vitamin mixture | Added |

**Nutritional Data**

Chemical composition per 100 g

| | | | |
|---|---|---|---|
| Energy | 1.422 MJ | Calcium | 300 mg |
| Protein (N × 6.25) | 21.2 g | Iron | 15 mg |
| Fat | 2.2 g | Thiamine | 0.84 mg |
| Moisture | 8 % | Riboflavine | 0.61 mg |
| Carbohydrate | | Niacin | 9.8 mg |
| (including 1.0 g fiber) | 64.5 g | Ascorbic acid | 31 mg |
| Ash | 4.1 g | Folic acid | 0.68 mg |

Amino acid composition in mg AA / gN

| | | | |
|---|---|---|---|
| Isoleucine | 257 | Tyrosine | 217 |
| Leucine | 565 | Threonine | 233 |
| Lysine | 319 | Tryptophan | 50 |
| Methionine | 100 | Valine | 281 |
| Cystine | 142 | | |
| Phenylalanine | 308 | | |

Protein quality
P.E.R = 2.83

**Packaging**
1. 250 g thick plastic bag for local sale
2. 22.5 kg sack for local relief work in Ethiopia

**Preparation**
Mix with suitable amount of water, add 3 more measures of water
mixing well; boil for 5-10 min stirring constantly;
serve hot as porridge; suitable as drink or food for
children and adults

**Source**
Publication — Faffa by
Ethiopian Nutrition Institute and discussion with
technical producers

## Table 6

**Name: Incaparina**

| | | | |
|---|---|---|---|
| Ground whole corn (rice, sorghum, or other suitable grains or mixtures may be used) | 58 | | Precooked |
| Cotton seed flour | 38% | 19% | Specially processed mature |
| and/or | or | + | seeds , hulled; cooking temper- |
| Soya flour | 38% | 19% | atures are kept low to avoid fixing of gossypol |
| | | | Relatively more oil is left in the pressed cake |
| Torula yeast | 3% | | |
| CaCo₃ | 1% | | |
| Vitamin A IU | 4500 | | |
| Lysine | 0.2% | | As L-lysine HCl |

**Nutritional Data**

Chemical composition per 100 g

| | | | |
|---|---|---|---|
| Protein | 27.5 g | Niacin | 7.8 mg |
| Fat | 4.2 g | Vitamin A | 4500  IU |
| Carbohydrate | 53.8 g | Calcium | 656  m*l* |
| Thiamine | 2.3 m*l* | Iron | 8.4 m*l* |
| Riboflavine | 1.1 m*l* | Sodium | 3.7 meq |
| Calories | 370.0 g | Phosphorus | 698  m*l* |
| | | Potassium | 27.9 meq |

Amino acid pattern in g/100 g

| | | | |
|---|---|---|---|
| Isoleucine | 1.12 | Total sulfur AA | 0.92 |
| Leucine | 2.08 | Threonine | 0.87 |
| Lysine | 1.58 | Tryptophan | 0.24 |
| Phenylalanine | 1.52 | Valine | 1.14 |
| Arginine | 2.34 | Histidine | 1.00 |

Energy Values

Per 100 g gives     1.560 MJ

                27.5% Protein

                4.2% Fat

**Preparation and Uses**

Mix desired amount with water and boil for 5-6 min to make a thin porridge; suitable as drink for children and adults

**Note**

Incaparina is made in many countries of Central and South America using local foods; thus, corn, cotton seed flour, or soya flour may be replaced by other locally available cereal or flour

**Source**

Incaparina; INCAP, Guatemala

## Table 7

Name: Supplementary Enriched Food Swedish Formula (SEF)

**Ingredients and Processes**

| | | |
|---|---|---|
| Wheat flour | 61 | High grade 80% extraction |
| Dry skim milk | 12 | Spray-dried |
| Vegetable oil | 10 | Stabilized mixture of vegetable oil |
| Sugar | 9 | |
| Fish protein concentrate | 7 | Fish protein concentrate, type A; odorless and tasteless |
| Salt minerals and vitamins | 1 | |

**Nutritional Data**

Chemical analysis per 100 g flour

| | |
|---|---|
| Moisture | 11 |
| Protein | 16 |
| Fat | 10 |
| Carbohydrate | 64 |
| Energy | 1.7 MJ (400 kcal) |

Vitamins and minerals

| | | | |
|---|---|---|---|
| Thiamine | 0.6 mg | Vitamin A | 0.4 mg (1300 IU) |
| Riboflavine | 0.7 mg | Vitamin D | 10 µg (400 IU) |
| Niacin | 6.0 mg | Calcium | 640.0 mg |
| Folic acid | 0.3 mg | Iron | 12 mg |
| Vitamin B$_{12}$ | 2.2 mg | Iodine | 100 µg |
| Ascorbic acid | 40.0 mg | | |

Protein quality

P.E.R. = 3.0

N.P.U. = 75

**Uses**

This food is a high-protein food supplement or an addition to traditional foods in areas where there is food shortage or malnutrition

## Table 8

Name:    Superamine

**Ingredients and Processes**

| | |
|---|---|
| Wheat flour | Precooked (blend) |
| Legume flour | Precooked (blend) |
| Dry skim milk | |
| Vitamins | |
| Minerals | |

**Nutritional Data**

Energy Values

Per 100 g gives > 1.422 MJ

20% Protein

3.5% Fat

**Uses**

Mix with suitable quantity of boiled, cooled water and feed as drink or porridge; can be used as weaning food or supplement for children and adults

**Source**

Egypt and North Africa

# Table 9

Name:    Balahar

Ingredients
Whole wheat flour
Defatted peanut flour
Chick pea flour
Vitamins
Minerals

Nutritional Data
Energy Values
Per 100 g gives   1.560 MJ
20 g Protein
4 g Fat

Uses
Roast powder for 2—3 min; add salt to taste;
add water and boil for 5—6 min; and feed as porridge
to children and adults

Source
India

# Table 10

Name:         Special Weaning Food (SWF)

Ingredients and Processes
Cereal flour                                Precooked blend
Soy or other oil seed flours or both        Defatted
Vitamins
Minerals

Nutritional Data
Energy Values
Per 100 g gives   1.560 MJ
15 g Protein
0 Fat

Uses
Mix well with 1/6 part of oil, boiled
and cooled water added with stirring; give as a
drink for weaning infants and children

Source
UNICEF

## Table 11

Name:  Precooked Flour Mixture (PKFM)

Ingredients and Processes
    Maize flour                    Precooked blend
    Soy flour                      Full-fat
    Dry skim milk
    Sucrose
    Vitamins and minerals

Nutritional Data
    Energy Values
        Per 100 g gives   1.673 MJ
                          20 g Protein
                           9 g Fat

Uses
    Mix with boiled cooled water and feed as drink for
    children; can be used for rehabilitating cases of
    P.E.M. *after* acute phase

Source
    UNICEF

## Table 12

Name: Kwashiokor Mixture No. 2 (K Mix 2)

Ingredients
    Calcium caseinate              18
    Dry skim milk                  28
    Sucrose                        54

Processes and Uses
    Vegetable oil *must* be added before being fed; every
    150 g K Mix 2 should be mixed with 60 g oil
    For use for *treatment* of Kwashiorkor or Marasmus in
    acute phase; very frequent feeds — 6-8 times daily
    Mix desired amount of oil with estimated amount of dry
    food mixture for use in a single feed; 1½ to 2 vol
    of boiled water is added to render the
    feeds in form of thick liquid or porridge

Source
    UNICEF

## Table 13

Name: Soy Fortified Bread Flour (12%)

**Ingredients and Processes**

| | | |
|---|---|---|
| Bread wheat flour | 88% | Unbleached |
| Soy flour | 12% | Defatted, lightly toasted, fortified at least 52% protein |
| Sodium stearoyl | 2 | |
| Lactylate (SSL) | 0.5 of total mix | |
| Potassium bromate | 10—40 ppm | |

Minerals
  Calcium        +
  Iron           +

**Nutritional Data**

Chemical analysis
  Moisture      <12.4%
  Protein       >16.2%
  Ash           1.52%
  Carbohydrate  30.2%

Amino acid pattern of protein in mg AA/g

| | | | |
|---|---|---|---|
| Isoleucine | 232 | Phenylalanine | 331 |
| Leucine | 475 | Threonine | 186 |
| Lysine | 174 | Tryptophan | 61 |
| Methionine | 81 | Valine | 258 |
| Cystine | 132 | | |

Protein quality
  P.E.R.              > 1.9 g
  N.P.U.              >63.3%
  Protein             >16.2%
  Utilizable protein  >10.3%

Energy values in 100 g
  Total           0.778 MJ
  From protein    0.273 MJ
  From carbohy-   0.505 MJ
    drate
  0.418 MJ contained in 53.8 g food which gives >8.7 g protein

Vitamins per 100 g
  A palmitate       Between 882 and 1323 IU
  Thiamine          Between 0.4 and 0.6 mg
  Riboflavine       About 0.3 mg
  Niacin            Between 3.5 and 4.4 mg
  Ca D-pantothenic  0.8 mg
  Pyridoxine        0.1 mg
  $\alpha$-tocopherol  1.3 IU
  Folate            0.06 mg

Minerals per 100 g
  Calcium carbonate  Between 165 and 301 mg
  Phosphorus         154 mg
  Magnesium          59 mg
  Iron               Between 3 and 7 mg
  Iodine             0.1 $\mu$g
  Potassium          358 mg
  Sodium             6 mg
  Zinc               1.5 mg

**Uses**

Same as wheat flour

## Table 13 (continued)

Packaging
22.5 kg filled multiwall paper sacks with five walls of paper, a polyethylene liner full-length and outer wall with wet strength and insect resistant

Sources
U.S. through international

## Table 14

Name: Wheat Flour (Fortified with Vitamin A and Calcium Flour All-Purpose or Bread Flour)

Ingredients
| | | |
|---|---|---|
| Wheat flour or bread flour | 100% | |
| Vitamin A palmitate | + | |
| Calcium | + | |

Nutritional Data
Chemical analysis
| | | |
|---|---|---|
| Moisture | <13.5 | |
| Protein | > 9 | All purpose |
| | >11 | Bread flour |
| Ash | 0.81 | |
| Carbohydrate | 76.7 | All purpose |
| | 74.7 | Bread flour |

Amino acid pattern in mg
| | | | |
|---|---|---|---|
| Isoleucine | 262 | Phenylalanine | 322 |
| Leucine | 442 | Tyrosine | 174 |
| Lysine | 126 | Threonine | 174 |
| Methionine | 78 | Tryptophan | 69 |
| Cystine | 114 | Valine | 262 |

Protein quality
| | | |
|---|---|---|
| P.E.R. | 0.8 g | |
| N.P.U. | 47.7% | |
| Protein | > 9% | All purpose |
| | >11% | Bread flour |
| Utilizable Protein | > 4.3 | All purpose |
| | > 5.2 | Bread flour |

Energy supply per 100 g
| | | |
|---|---|---|
| Total calories | 1.435 MJ | |
| From protein | 0.150 | All purpose |
| | 0.184 | Bread flour |
| From carbohydrate | 1.280 | All purpose |
| | 1.250 | Bread flour |

0.418 MJ contained in 29.2 g
0.418 MJ of food gives >2.6 g protein 1 — all purpose
>3.2 g protein — bread flour

Vitamins in 100 g
| | |
|---|---|
| A palmitate | Between 882 and 1323 IU |
| Thiamine | 0.4 mg |
| Riboflavine | 0.3 mg |
| Niacin | 4.0 mg |

Minerals in 100 g
| | |
|---|---|
| Calcium carbonate | Between 110 and 138 mg |
| Phosphorous | 372 mg |
| Iron | 3 mg |

## Table 14 (continued)

| | |
|---|---|
| Potassium | 370 mg |
| Sodium | 3 mg |

**Uses**

Baked as bread, biscuits, and cakes and used for chappatis and other local breads

**Packaging**

22.5 Kg filled woven polypropylene or polyethylene fabric or filled paper sack, give walls

## Table 15

Name: Bulgur or Bulgur wheat

**Ingredients and Processing**

| | | |
|---|---|---|
| Bulgur wheat | 100% | Obtained from clean bulgur wheat; cracked and partially cooked; partially debranned |

**Nutritional Data**

Chemical analysis

| | | | |
|---|---|---|---|
| Moisture | <11.5% | Ash | < 1.8 |
| Protein | >9.3% | Carbohydrate | 75.4% |
| Fiber | <2% | | |

Amino acid pattern in mg AA/gN

| | | | |
|---|---|---|---|
| Isoleucine | 223 | Phenylalanine | 302 |
| Leucine | 415 | Tyrosine | 194 |
| Lysine | 166 | Threonine | 185 |
| Methionine | 94 | Tryptophan | 77 |
| Cystine | 98 | Valine | 271 |

Protein quality

| | |
|---|---|
| P.E.R. | 1.2 |
| N.P.U.% | 53.4 |
| Protein | >9.3 |
| Utilizable protein | >5 |

Energy Values per 100 g

| | |
|---|---|
| Total calories | 1.418 MJ |
| From protein | 156 MJ |
| From carbohydrate | 1.261 MJ |
| 29.5 g of food contain 0.418 MJ | |
| 29.5 g which contain >2.7 g protein | |

Vitamins in 100 g

| | |
|---|---|
| Thiamine | 0.3 mg |
| Riboflavine | 0.1 mg |
| Niacin | 3.5 mg |

Minerals in 100 g

| | |
|---|---|
| Calcium carbonate | 23 mg |
| Phosphorus | 430 mg |
| Iron | 8 mg |
| Potassium | 229 mg |
| Sodium | 0.2 mg |

**Uses**

Cooked or used in place of rice

**Packaging**

22.5 kg filled cotton sack or woven polypropylene fabric or burlap bag

**Source**

U.S.

Table 16

Name: Wheat Soy Blend

**Ingredients and Processing**

| | | |
|---|---|---|
| Wheat fractions Maybe | 73.1 | |
| 1. Bulgar flour | 53.1 | Partially precooked and gelatinized; cracked and grinded |
| + | | |
| Wheat protein concentrate | 20.0 | Heated and milled |
| or | | |
| 2. Straight grade flour | 38.1 | Processed |
| + | | |
| Wheat protein concentrate | 35.0 | |
| Soy flour | 20 | Defatted, toasted, and fortified at least 50% protein |
| Soy oil | 4 | Deodorized, refined, and stabilized with citric acid and BHA |
| Vitamin premix | 0.1 | |
| Mineral premix | 2.8 | Iron added |

**Nutritional Data**

Chemical analysis (%)

| | | | |
|---|---|---|---|
| Moisture | <11 | Fiber | <2.5 |
| Protein | >20 | Ash | <6.6 |
| Fat | >6 | Carbohydrate | 53.9 |

Amino acid pattern in mg AA/gN

| | | | |
|---|---|---|---|
| Isoleucine | 300 | Phenylalanine | 338 |
| Leucine | 506 | Tyrosine | 231 |
| Lysine | 328 | Threonine | 234 |
| Methionine | 125 | Tryptophan | 106 |
| Cystine | 147 | Valine | 343 |

Protein quality

| | |
|---|---|
| P.E.R. | 2.4 |
| N.P.U. | 70.3% |
| Protein | >20% |
| Utilizable protein | >14.1% |

Energy values

Per 100 g gives 1.464 MJ
From protein gives 0.334 MJ
From fat gives 0.226 MJ
From carbohydrate gives 0.902 MJ
28.6 g gives 0.418 MJ
28.6 g give >5.7 g protein

Vitamins per 100 g

| | | | |
|---|---|---|---|
| A palmitate | 1653 IU | Cyanocobalamin | 4 μg |
| Thiamine | 0.3 mg | Ascorbic acid | 40 mg |
| Riboflavine | 0.4 mg | Ergocalciferol | 198 IU |
| Niacin | 5.0 mg | α-tocopherol | 7.5 IU |
| Ca D-pantothenic | 2.8 mg | Folate | 190 μg |
| Pyridoxine | 0.2 mg | | |

Minerals in 100 g

| | | | |
|---|---|---|---|
| Calcium carbonate | 749 mg | Iodine | 5250 μg |
| Tricalcium phosphate | 2000 mg | Potassium | 624 mg |
| Phosphorus | 562 mg | Sodium | 296 mg |
| Magnesium | 202 mg | Zinc | 4 mg |
| Iron | 21 mg | | |

**Uses**

Use as flour or porridge

Table 16 (continued)

Packaging
22.5 kg filled multiwall paper sacks with five walls
of paper and a polyethylene liner; outer wall wet
strength and made insect resistant

Source
U.S.

## Table 17

Name: Soy Fortified Corn Meal

### Ingredients and Processing

| | | |
|---|---|---|
| Corn meal | 85 | Degermed |
| Soy flour | 15 | Defatted (toasted) and fortified at least at 50% protein |
| Vitamins | + | |
| Thiamine | | |
| Riboflavine | | |
| Niacin | | |
| A palmitate | | |
| Minerals | + | |
| Calcium | | |
| Iron | | |

### Nutritional Data

Chemical analysis

| | | | |
|---|---|---|---|
| Moisture | <13% | Fiber | <2% |
| Protein | >13% | Ash | >2.025 |
| Fat | >1.5% | Carbohydrate | 68.5 |

Amino acid pattern in mg AA/gN

| | | | |
|---|---|---|---|
| Isoleucine | 206 | Phenylalanine & tyrosine | 388 |
| Leucine | 575 | Threonine | 194 |
| Lysine | 181 | Tryptophan | 44 |
| Methionine & cystine | 163 | Valine | 244 |

Protein quality

| | |
|---|---|
| P.E.R. | 1.8 |
| N.P.U. | 61.8% |
| Protein | >13 |

Energy values

| | |
|---|---|
| Per 100 g contain | 1.22 MJ |
| From protein | 0.217 MJ |
| From fat | 0.56.5 MJ |
| From carbohydrate | 1.146 MJ |
| 29.4 g contain 0.418 MJ | |

Vitamins in 100 g

| | | | |
|---|---|---|---|
| A palmitate | Between 382 and 1323 IU | Cyanocobalamin | 0.1 $\mu$g |
| Thiamine | Between 0.4 and 0.7 mg | $\alpha$-tocopherol | 1.0 IU |
| Riboflavine | Between 0.3 and 0.4 mg | | |
| Niacin | Between 3.5 and 5.3 mg | | |
| Ca D-pantothenic | 0.7 mg | | |
| Pyridoxine | 0.3 mg | | |

Minerals in 100 g

| | | | |
|---|---|---|---|
| Calcium carbonate | Between 110 and 165 mg | Potassium | 467 mg |
| Phosphorus | 189 mg | Sodium | 13 mg |
| Magnesium | 70 mg | Zinc | 1 mg |
| Iron | Between 3 and 6 mg | | |

### Uses
Thin porridge or thick porridge with condiment

## Table 17 (continued)

**Packaging**
22.5 kg filled multiwall paper sacks with five walls of paper and a polyethylene liner in full-length; outer wall with wet strength and paper made insect

repellant
**Source**
U.S.

## Table 18

**Name: Wheat Soy Blend (WSB)**

**Ingredients and Processes**

| | | |
|---|---|---|
| Bulgur flour | 53.1 | Partially precooked; gelatinized, and |
| | 73.1 | debranned; cracked and grinded |
| Wheat protein concentrate | 20 | Heated to inactivate enzymes; as a result of milling, greater protein and lesser filler relative to wheat |
| or | | flour because of greater amino acid lysine, vitamins, minerals, and fat |
| Straight grade flour | 38.1 | Processed for gelatinization and to inactivate enzymes |
| Wheat protein concentrate | 35.0 | |
| Soy flour | 20.0 | Defatted (toasted); fortified at least at 50% protein |
| Soy oil | 4.0 | Stabilized with citric acid BHA, deodorized, refined; BHA added to reduce susceptibility to rancidity; fat levels were raised to create density of calories and better use of vitamins in the body |
| Vitamin premix | 0.1 | |
| Mineral premix | 2.8 | Iron added to lessen susceptibility to rancidity |

**Nutritional Data**
Chemical analysis

| | | | |
|---|---|---|---|
| Moisture | <11% | Fiber | <2.5% |
| Protein | >20% | Ash | <6.6% |
| Fat | >6% | Carbohydrate | 53.9% |

Amino acid pattern in mg AA/g protein

| | | | |
|---|---|---|---|
| Isoleucine | 300 | Phenylalanine | 338 |
| Leucine | 506 | Tyrosine | 231 |
| Lysine | 328 | Threonine | 234 |
| Methionine | 125 | Tryptophan | 106 |
| Cystine | 147 | Valine | 343 |

## Table 18 (continued)

Protein quality

| | |
|---|---|
| P.E.R. | 2.4 |
| N.P.U.% | 70.3 |
| Protein% | >20 |
| Utilizable Protein | >14.1 |

Megajoules per 100 g of product

| | |
|---|---|
| Total | 1.464 |
| From protein | 0.334 |
| From fat | 0.226 |
| From carbohydrate | 0.902 |

28.6 g of dry food contains 0.418 MJ
>5.7 g protein in 0.418 MJ
>5.5 g protein (adjusted for Casein Equivalents) in 0.418 MJ

Vitamins per 100 g

| | | | |
|---|---|---|---|
| A palmitate | 1653 IU | Cyanocobalamin | 4.0 gmg |
| Thiamine | 0.3 mg | Ascorbic acid | 40.0 mg |
| Riboflavine | 0.4 mg | Ergocalciferol | 198.0 IU |
| Niacin | 5.0 mg | $\alpha$-tocophenol | 7.5 IU |
| Ca D-pantothenic | 2.8 mg | Folate | 190 $\mu$g |
| Pyridoxine | 0.2 mg | | |

Minerals per 100 g

| | | | |
|---|---|---|---|
| Calcium carbonate | 749 mg | Potassium | 624 mg |
| Tricalcium phosphate | 2000 mg | Sodium | 296 mg |
| Phosphorus | 562 mg | Zinc | 4.0 mg |
| Magnesium | 202 mg | | |
| Iron | 21 mg | | |
| Iodine | 5250 $\mu$g | | |

Packaging

22.5 kg filled multiwall paper sacks with five walls of paper
and a polyethylene liner

Uses

Mix with suitable quantity of boiled and cooked water and
feed as a drink; drink supplement for infants,
children, and adults, but
*not* as feeds for infants.

Table 19

Name:  Defatted Soy Flour

**Ingredients and Processing**

| | | |
|---|---|---|
| Soy flour | 100% | Defatted by toasting; fortified with at least 50% protein |

**Nutritional Data**

Chemical analysis

| | | | |
|---|---|---|---|
| Moisture | <10% | Fiber | < 3.7% |
| Protein | >50% | Ash | < 6.7% |
| Fat | < 2% | Carbohydrate | 27.6% |

Amino acid pattern of protein in mg AA/gN
   Same as full-fat soy flour

Protein quality

| | |
|---|---|
| P.E.R. | 1.8 |
| N.P.U. | 61.8% |
| Protein | >50% |
| Utilizable protein | >31% |

Energy values
   Per 100 g contain 1.372 MJ
      Of which protein provide 0.836 MJ
      Of which fat provide 0.075 MJ
      Of which carbohydrate provide 0.462 MJ
   30.5 g of food supply 0.418 MJ
   30.5 g of food contain >15.3 g protein

Vitamins in 100 g

| | |
|---|---|
| A palmitate | 40 IU |
| Thiamine | 1.0 mg |
| Riboflavine | 0.3 mg |
| Niacin | 3.0 mg |

Minerals in 100 g

| | |
|---|---|
| Calcium carbonate | 265 mg |
| Phosphorus | 655 mg |
| Iron | 11 mg |
| Potassium | 1820 mg |
| Sodium | 1 mg |

**Uses**
   Use as ordinary flour or mixed with other foods to increase protein and energy values

**Packaging**
   Same as full-fat soy flour

## Table 20

Name: Soy Flour Full-Fat (FF Soy F)

**Ingredients and Processing**

| | | |
|---|---|---|
| Soy flour | 100% | Full-fat; finely ground cooked soya beans; fortified with at least 42% protein |

**Nutritional Data**

Chemical analysis

| | | | |
|---|---|---|---|
| Moisture | <10% | Fiber | <3% |
| Protein | >42% | Ash | <6% |
| Fat | >20% | Carbohydrate | 19% |

Amino acid pattern of protein in mg AA/gN

| | | | |
|---|---|---|---|
| Isoleucine | 288 | Phenylalanine | 313 |
| Leucine | 488 | Threonine | 244 |
| Lysine | 400 | Tryptophan | 88 |
| Methionine & cystine | 131 | Valine | 288 |

Protein quality

| | |
|---|---|
| P.E.R. | 1.8 |
| N.P.U.% | 61.8 |
| Protein % | >42 |
| Utilizable protein | >26% |

Energy values

| | |
|---|---|
| Per 100 g gives | 1.773 MJ |
| Of which | 0.703 MJ are from protein |
| | 0.753 MJ are from fat |
| | 0.318 MJ are from carbohydrate |

23.6 g contain 0.418 MJ
23.6 g contain >9.9 g protein

Vitamins in 100 g

| | |
|---|---|
| A palmitate | 110 IU |
| Thiamine | 0.9 mg |
| Riboflavine | 0.3 mg |
| Niacin | 2.0 mg |

Minerals in 100 g

| | |
|---|---|
| Calcium carbonate | 199 mg |
| Phosphorus | 558 mg |
| Potassium | 1660 mg |
| Sodium | 1 mg |

**Uses**

Use as ordinary flour or mixed with other foods to increase protein and energy values

**Packaging**

22.5 kg filled multiwall paper sacks with five walls of paper and a polyethylene liner in full-length; outer wall will be wet strength paper made insect resistant

**Source**

U.S.

## Table 21

Name:  Soy Fortified Bulgur Wheat

**Ingredients and Processing**

| | | |
|---|---|---|
| Bulgur wheat | 85% | Cracked, partially cooked, and partially debranned |
| Soy grits | 15% | Defatted, toasted, and fortified at least 50% protein |

**Nutritional Data**

Chemical analysis

| | | | |
|---|---|---|---|
| Moisture | <11.5% | Fiber | <2.3% |
| Protein | >17.3% | Ash | <2.6% |
| Fat | <2.6% | Carbohydrate | 63.7% |

Amino acid pattern in mg AA/gN

| | | | |
|---|---|---|---|
| Isoleucine | 248 | Phenylalanine | 317 |
| Leucine | 441 | Tyrosine | 207 |
| Lysine | 230 | Threonine | 211 |
| Methionine | 96 | Tryptophan | 77 |
| Cystine | 95 | Valine | 334 |

Protein quality

| | |
|---|---|
| P.E.R. | 2.3 |
| N.P.U. | 70% |
| Protein | >17.3% |
| Utilizable protein | >12.1% |

Energy values

| | |
|---|---|
| Per 100 g gives | 1.376 MJ |
| | 0.289 MJ from protein |
| | 0.022 MJ from fat |
| | 1.066 MJ from carbohydrate |
| 30.4 g gives | 0.418 MJ |
| 30.4 g contains >5.3 g protein | |

Vitamins in 100 g

| | | | |
|---|---|---|---|
| Thiamine | 0.3 mm | α-tocopherol | 1.7 IU |
| Riboflavine | 0.1 mg | Folate | 75 μg |
| Niacin | 4.2 mg | | |
| Ca D-pantothenic | 1.0 mg | | |
| Pyridoxine | 0.4 mg | | |

Minerals in 100 g

| | | | |
|---|---|---|---|
| Calcium carbonate | 54 mg | Potassium | 424 mg |
| Phosphorous | 385 mg | Sodium | 0.2 mg |
| Magnesium | 169 mg | Zinc | 5.0 mg |
| Iron | 5 mg | | |
| Iodine | 87 mg | | |

**Uses**

Use like bulgur wheat

**Packaging**

Same as bulgur wheat

**Source**

U.S.

# Table 22

**Name: Soy Fortified Sorghum Grits**

**Ingredients and Processing**

| | | |
|---|---|---|
| Sorghum grits | 85 | Dehulled and degermed |
| Soy grits | 15 | Defatted (toasted); fortified at least at 40% protein |

**Nutritional Data**

Chemical analysis

| | | | |
|---|---|---|---|
| Moisture | <13.5 | Ash | <2.6 |
| Protein | >15 | Carbohydrate | 64.8 |
| Fat | <2 | | |
| Fiber | <2.1 | | |

Amino acid pattern in mg AA/gN

| | | | |
|---|---|---|---|
| Isoleucine | 306 | Phenylalanine & tyrosine | 538 |
| Leucine | 738 | Threonine | 238 |
| Lysine | 256 | Tryptophan | 100 |
| Methionine & cystine | 219 | Valine | 311 |

Protein quality

| | |
|---|---|
| P.E.R. | 2.1 |
| N.P.U.% | 66.1 |

Energy values

Per 100 g gives 1.410 MJ
0.251 MJ from protein
0.075 MJ from fat
1.084 MJ from carbohydrate

Vitamins per 100 g

| | | | |
|---|---|---|---|
| Thiamine | 0.2 mg | Pyridoxine | 0.3 mg |
| Riboflavine | 0.1 mg | Folate | 50 μg |
| Niacin | 1.7 mg | | |
| Ca D-pantothenic | 1.0 mg | | |

Minerals per 100 g

| | | | |
|---|---|---|---|
| Calcium carbonate | 42 mg | Iodine | 30 μg |
| Phosphorus | 180 mg | Potassium | 500 mg |
| Magnesium | 50 mg | Zinc | 1 mg |
| Iron | 3 mg | | |

**Uses**

Use as a thin or thick porridge — needs boiling

**Packaging**

22.5 kg filled multiwall paper sacks with five walls of paper and a polyethylene liner in full-length; outer wall will be wet strength paper made insect resistant

**Source**

U.S.

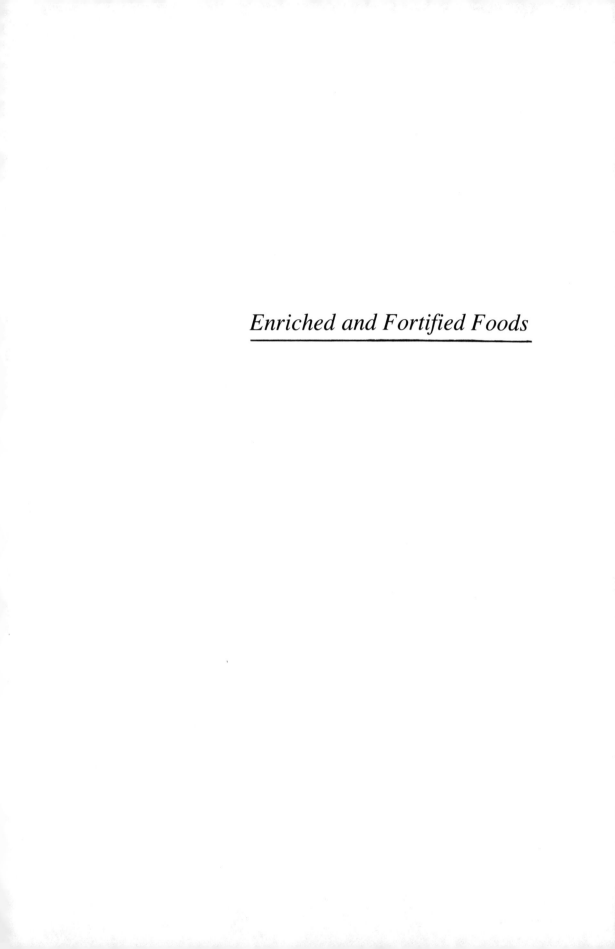

*Enriched and Fortified Foods*

# VITAMIN FORTIFICATION

## H. Mitsuda and A. Yamamoto

Fortification is a public health measure aimed at improving and maintaining the health of individuals in the population through the provision of adequate levels of nutrient intake, e.g., vitamins, minerals, proteins, and amino acids. Various fortification programs have been practiced over the past 40 years in various countries. The Joint FAO/WHO Expert Committee on Nutrition evaluated these programs as follows.[1]

"At the time that many of the programs were instituted, techniques for the evaluation of nutritional status were relatively crude and background data for evaluating the specific effects of the programs were fragmentary. Most of these programs were implemented in developed countries where the prevalence of many of the deficiency diseases was not very high. Their implementation often coincided with a variety of social, economic, agricultural, educational, and public health developments. Although the specific effects of the fortification programs can rarely be identified, improvements in nutritional status did occur. The prevalence of the classical deficiency diseases fell to very low levels, and several were practically eliminated."

Fortification of rice, which is a staple food in Japan, with thiamin, which is often deficient in Japanese diets, is most desirable since this vitamin is indispensable for carbohydrate metabolism. It is thus quite natural to expect a great impact of rice fortification on national nutrition welfare. As a matter of fact, an inverse relationship between the number of deaths from beriberi and annual output of fortified rice has been shown to exist. Beriberi had previously been a major cause of deaths from avitaminosis and malnutrition. After the introduction of rice fortification, beriberi has become a minor cause. This is one of the most significant success stories of fortified foods in Japan.[2]

Within this chapter characteristics of six vitamins to be added, recommended daily intakes of these vitamins, and fortification levels in connection with foods to be used as the vehicle are compiled.* These are some examples of the vitamin fortification programs which are practiced under specific regulations. Technological and economical considerations are hardly included here, while they may be important in designing a fortification program. Further information on these and some different opinions about the relative merits of fortification are presented in the report of the Committee and in other literatures.[1,2]

---

*    Tables 1 to 6 were compiled by H. Mitsuda and A. Yamamoto.

Table 1
VITAMIN A

## I. Characteristics of Vitamin A[1,3-6]

| | |
|---|---|
| Forms: | Vitamin A (retinol), provitamin A ($\alpha,\beta$-carotene, cryptoxanthin) |
| Commercially available forms: | Retinol acetate, retinol palmitate, retinol in oil solutions, emulsions and beadslets, powdered vitamin A, synthetic $\beta$-carotene, and $\beta$-apo-8′-carotenal |
| Function: | Adapt to dim light, promote growth, prevent keratinization of skin and eye, promote resistance to bacterial infection |
| Deficiency disease: | Night blindness, xerophthalmia, hyperkeratosis, poor growth |
| Food sources: | Liver, egg yolk, milk, butter (vitamin A) sweet potatoes, winter squash, greens, carrots, cantaloupe (provitamin A) |
| Toxicity: | Excess vitamin A can create a serious health hazard |
| Units: | Vitamin A in the human diet is derived from preformed vitamin A and from provitamin A carotenoids; provitamin A carotenoids are active only after being converted into retinol during, or subsequent to, absorption through the intestinal wall; vitamin A activity in foods is expressed in international units (IU), 1 IU being equivalent to 0.3 $\mu$g of retinol, 0.344 $\mu$g retinyl acetate, 0.55 $\mu$g of retinyl palmitate, 0.6 $\mu$g of $\beta$-carotene, or 1.2 $\mu$g of provitamin A carotenoids other than $\beta$-carotene |
| Stability and some comments: | (1) Vitamin A is unstable in many applications and antioxidants are necessary to obtain a reasonable shelf life; (2) foods receiving severe heat treatment during processing should preferably be fortified with vitamin A after heating; (3) the vitamin A can be added by spraying an oil/water emulsion onto the surface of the cooked product, e.g., breakfast cereal; (4) stability in oleaginous foods, e.g., margarine, is excellent; (5) stability is good in vegetable oils with antioxidants but not during cooking; and (6) carotene may color products |
| Short history of fortification: | U.S., margarine (1936); U.S., skim and dry milk (1942); Newfoundland, margarine (1945); U.S., milk products (1968); Guatemala sugar (1969); India, tea products; and Philippines, monosodium glutamate |

## II. Recommended Daily Intakes of Vitamin A[7,8]

| World (FAO/WHO)[7] | | Japan[8,b,c] | | U.S.[7,d] | | |
|---|---|---|---|---|---|---|
| Age (years) | $\mu$g RE[a] | Age (years) | IU | Age (years) | $\mu$g RE[a] | IU |
| <1 | 300 | <0.5 | 1300 | 0.5 | 420[e] | 1400 |
| 1—3 | 250 | 0.5—5 | 1000 | 0.5—3 | 400 | 2000 |
| 4—6 | 300 | 6—8 | 1200 | 4—6 | 500 | 2500 |
| 7—9 | 400 | 9—14 | 1500 | 7—10 | 700 | 3300 |
| 10—12 | 575 | >15 | | >11 | | |
| 13—15 | 725 | Male | 2000 | Male | 1000 | 5000 |
| 16—19 | 750 | Female | 1800 | Female | 800 | 4000 |
| >20 | 750 | | | | | |
| Pregnancy[f] | 750 | Pregnancy[f] | +200 | Pregnancy | 1000 | 5000 |
| Lactation[g] | 1200 | Lactation[g] | +1400 | Lactation | 1200 | 6000 |

## Fortification Levels and Type of Foods[1,9,10]

| World (FAO/WHO)[i] | | Japan[9] | | U.S.[10] | |
|---|---|---|---|---|---|
| Dry cereal products | 1500—3000 IU[h] | Miso | | ≥2000 IU[i] | Milk |
| Flour | 4500—6000 | Margarine | | ≥2000[i] | Nonfat dry milk |
| Bread | 2000—4000 | Fish ham | | ≥2000[i] | Lowfat milk |
| Pasta | 2000—4000 | Fish sausage | | ≥2000[i] | Skim milk |
| Milk products | ≥1520[j] | Dry milk for | | 15000[k] | Margarine |

Table 1 (continued)
## VITAMIN A

### I. Characteristics of Vitamin A[1,3-6]

| Margarine | pregnant and | ≥125[l] | Evaporated milk |
| Vegetable oils | lactating women | 4000[h] | Mellorine |

<sup></sup>

- [a]  Retinol equivalents.
- [b]  RDA for persons in light activity.
- [c]  3 IU dietary $\beta$-carotene estimated to be 1 IU vitamin A (retinol).
- [d]  Designed for the maintenance of good nutrition of practically all healthy people in the U.S.
- [e]  Assumed to be all as retinol in milk during the first 6 months of life; all subsequent intakes are assumed to be one half as retinol and one half as $\beta$-carotene when calculated from international units; as retinol equivalents, three-fourths are as retinol and one fourth as $\beta$-carotene.
- [f]  Later half.
- [g]  First 6 months.
- [h]  IU per 100 g.
- [i]  IU/qt.
- [j]  IU per daily intake of the product.
- [k]  IU/lb.
- [l]  IU per fluid ounce; equivalents by volume: 1 qt = 32 fluid oz; equivalents by weight: 1 lb (16 oz) = 453.6 g, 1 oz = 28.35 g.

Table 2
## VITAMIN D

### I. Characteristics of Vitamin D[1,3-5,11]

| | |
|---|---|
| Forms: | Vitamin $D_2$ (ergocalciferol), Vitamin $D_3$ (cholecalciferol) |
| Commercially available forms: | Crystals, standardized oil solutions, emulsions, beadlets |
| Function: | Promote calcium absorption, mineralization of bone, satisfactory growth rate |
| Deficiency disease: | Rickets, osteomalacia |
| Food sources: | Small amounts in eggs, fatty fish, liver, butter |
| Toxicity: | Excess vitamin D can create a harmful condition, hypervitaminosis D |
| Units: | 2.5 g of cholecalciferol are equivalent to 100 IU of vitamin D |
| Stability and some comments: | (1) Vitamins $D_2$ and $D_3$ are susceptible to oxidation and are usually stabilized with antioxidants; vitamin $D_3$ is more stable than vitamin $D_2$; and (2) there are few stability problems with vitamin D in foods |
| Short history of fortification: | Denmark (1909-1920); U.K. (1940); U.S., milk (1932), wheat flour (1943) |

### II. Recommended Daily Intakes of Vitamin D[7,8,11]

| World (FAO/WHO)[7,11] | | | Japan[8,b] | | U.S.[7,c] | |
|---|---|---|---|---|---|---|
| Age (years) | $\mu g^a$ | IU | Age (years) | IU | Age (year) | IU |
| <6 | 10.0 | 400 | <5 | 400 | >0 | 400 |
| >7 | 2.5 | 100 | >6 | 100 | | |
| Pregnancy[d] | 10.0 | 400 | Pregnancy | +300 | Pregnancy | 400 |
| Lactation[e] | 10.0 | 400 | Lactation[e] | +300 | Lactation | 400 |

### III. Fortification Levels and Type of Foods[1,9,10]

| World (FAO/WHO)[1] | | Japan[9] | | U.S.[10] |
|---|---|---|---|---|
| Milk products | ≥ 300 IU[f] | Dry milk for | ≥ 400 IU[g] | Milk |
| Margarines | | pregnant and | 400[g] | Nonfat dry milk |
| Dry cereal products | | lactating women | 400[g,h] | Lowfat milk (optional) |
| Vegetable oils | | | 400[g,h] | Skim milk (optional) |

Table 2 (continued)
## VITAMIN D

| | | |
|---|---|---|
| Fruit drinks | 25[i] | Evaporated milk |
| | 25[h,i] | Concentrated milk (optional) |
| | 250—1000[j] | Corn meal, corn grits, rice |
| | 250—1000[h,j] | Noodle products (optional) |
| | 250—1000[h,j] | Macaroni products (optional) |
| | ⩾ 250[j] | Farina |
| | ⩾ 1500[k] | Margarine |
| | ⩾ 1500[h,k] | Oleomargarine (optional) |

[a]   As cholecalciferol.
[b]   RDA for persons in light activity.
[c]   Designed for the maintenance of good nutrition of practically all healthy people in the U.S.
[d]   Later half.
[e]   First 6 months.
[f]   IU per daily intake of the product.
[g]   IU/qt.
[h]   Optional ingredients.
[i]   IU per fluid ounce.
[j]   USP unit.
[k]   IU/lb.

Table 3
## THIAMINE

### I. Characteristics of Thiamine[1-4,12-15]

| | |
|---|---|
| Form: | Thiamine |
| Commercially available forms: | Thiamine monoitrate, thiamine hydrochloride, coated thiamine, thiamine cetyl sulfate, thiamine thiocyanate, thiamine naphthalene-1,5-disulfonate, thiamine naphthalene-2,6-disulfonate, thiamine phenolphthalate, thiamine laurylsulfate, dibenzoyl-thiamine, dibenzoyl-thiamine -disulfide |
| Function: | Coenzyme in energy metabolism |
| Deficiency disease: | Beriberi |
| Food sources: | Whole grains, organ meats, pork, meats, leafy vegetables, legumes, milk |
| Stability and some comments: | (1) Stable in dry products, low pH fruit drinks, and frozen drink concentrates; (2) degradation during operations requiring heat depends on pH, oxygen content, and other factors; (3) thiamine degradation odors are objectionable in some cereals and almost unnoticeable in others; (4) flavor may be a problem at levels above 4 mg/$l$; (5) heating in solution at pH 5.5—7.0 is undesirable; and (6) with materials like rice, thiamine may be impregnated into or coated on the kernel |
| Short history of fortification: | U.K., wheat flour, bread (1940); U.S., wheat flour (1942); Puerto Rico, polished rice (1951); Philippines, home pounded rice, undermilled rice, milled rice (1952); Japan, polished rice (1952); Canada, cereals, bread (1961) |

### II. Recommended Intakes of Thiamine[7,8]

| World (FAO/WHO)[7] | | Japan[8,a] | | U.S.[7,b] | |
|---|---|---|---|---|---|
| Age (years) | mg | Age (years) | mg | Age (years) | mg |
| <1 | 0.3 | <2 months | 0.2 | <0.5 | 0.3 |
| 1—3 | 0.5 | 2 months | 0.3 | 0.5—1.0 | 0.5 |
| 4—6 | 0.7 | 6 months | 0.35 | 1—3 | 0.7 |
| 7—9 | 0.9 | 1 | 0.4 | 4—6 | 0.9 |
| 10—12 | | 2 | 0.5 | 7—10 | 1.2 |

## Table 3 (continued)
## THIAMINE

| | | | | | | | |
|---|---|---|---|---|---|---|---|
| Male | 1.0 | 4 | 0.6 | | | 11—14 | |
| Female | 0.9 | 6 | 0.7 | | | Male | 1.4 |
| 13—15 | | 9 | 0.8 | | | Female | 1.2 |
| Male | 1.2 | 12 | Male 1.0 | Female 0.9 | | 15—22 | |
| Female | 1.0 | 15 | 1.1 | 0.9 | | Male | 1.5 |
| >16 | | 18 | 1.1 | 0.8 | | Female | 1.1 |
| Male | 1.2 | 20 | 1.0 | 0.8 | | 23—50 | |
| Female | 0.9 | 40 | 0.9 | 0.8 | | Male | 1.4 |
| Pregnancy[c] | +0.1 | 60 | 0.8 | 0.7 | | Female | 1.0 |
| Lactation[d] | +0.2 | 70 | 0.7 | 0.6 | | >51 | |
| | | Pregnancy | +0.1 | | | Male | 1.2 |
| | | Lactation[d] | +0.3 | | | Female | 1.0 |
| | | | | | | Pregnancy | +0.3 |
| | | | | | | Lactation | +0.3 |

## III. Fortification Levels and Type of Foods[1,9,10]

| World (FAO/WHO)[1] | | Japan[9] | | U.S.[10] |
|---|---|---|---|---|
| Dry cereals | 100—150 mg[e] | Rice[f] | 2.9 mg[g] | Self-rising flour |
| Flour | 1.2—1.8 | Pressed barley | 2.0—3.0 | Corn grits, meals |
| Bread | 0.5—0.8 | Wheat flour | 2.0—2.5 | Farina |
| Pasta | 0.3—0.5 | Bread | 2.0—4.0 | Rice |
| Milk products | 0.2—0.4 | Noodles (boiled) | 4.0—5.0 | Macaroni products |
| | 0.5—0.8 | Noodles (dried)[h] | 4.0—5.0 | Nonfat milk macaroni products |
| | 0.5—0.8 | Noodles (instant) | | |
| | 1.2—1.8 | Miso | 1.8 | Bread, rolls, or buns |
| | ≥0.86[i] | Dry milk for pregnant and lactating women | 4.0—5.0 | Noodle products |

[a]    RDA for persons in light activity.
[b]    Designed for the maintenance of good nutrition of practically all healthy people in the U.S.
[c]    Later half.
[d]    First 6 months.
[e]    mg/100 g.
[f]    The rice Kernel premix is added to normal polished rice of an appropriate rate (1:200) to provide the proper nutrient level in the fortified rice.
[g]    Mg/lb.
[h]    Including macaroni and spaghetti.
[i]    Mg per daily intake of the product.

## Table 4
## RIBOFLAVINE

### I. Characteristics of Riboflavine[1-4,12-15]

| | |
|---|---|
| Forms: | Riboflavine |
| Commercially available forms: | Crystalline products, riboflavin-5′-phosphate ester monosodium salt dihydrate, riboflavine butyrate, riboflavine phosphate, sodium riboflavine phosphate, coated riboflavine |
| Function: | Coenzyme in enzyme metabolism |
| Deficiency disease: | Ariboflavinosis |
| Food sources: | Milk and milk products, meat, eggs, fish, leafy vegetables, legumes, nuts, liver |
| Stability and some comments: | (1) Riboflavine is stable in most food applications; and (2) riboflavine may color the food |
| Short history of fortification: | U.S., white rice (1942), wheat flour (1943); Puerto Rico, wheat flour (1948), polished rice (1951); Philippines, home pounded rice, undermilled rice, milled rice (1952); Canada, cereals, bread (1961) |

### II. Recommended Daily Intakes of Riboflavine[7,8]

**World (FAO/WHO)[7]**

| Age (years) | mg |
|---|---|
| < 1 | 0.5 |
| 1—3 | 0.8 |
| 4—6 | 1.1 |
| 7—9 | 1.3 |
| 10—12 | |
| Male | 1.6 |
| Female | 1.4 |
| 13—15 | |
| Male | 1.7 |
| Female | 1.5 |
| 16—19 | |
| Male | 1.8 |
| Female | 1.4 |
| > 20 | |
| Male | 1.8 |
| Female | 1.3 |
| Pregnancy[c] | + 0.2 |
| Lactation[d] | + 0.4 |

**Japan[8,a]**

| Age (years) | mg (Male) | mg (Female) |
|---|---|---|
| < 6 months | 0.3 | |
| 6 months | 0.4 | |
| 1 | 0.5 | |
| 2 | Male 0.7 | Female 0.6 |
| 3 | 0.7 | 0.7 |
| 4 | 0.8 | 0.7 |
| 5 | 0.9 | 0.8 |
| 6 | 1.0 | 0.9 |
| 9 | 1.2 | 1.1 |
| 12 | 1.4 | 1.3 |
| 15 | 1.4 | 1.2 |
| 18 | 1.4 | 1.1 |
| 20 | 1.3 | 1.1 |
| 40 | 1.2 | 1.0 |
| 60 | 1.1 | 0.9 |
| > 70 | 1.0 | 0.8 |
| Pregnancy[e] | | + 0.1 |
| Pregnancy[c] | | + 0.2 |
| Lactation[d] | | + 0.4 |

**U.S.[7,b]**

| Age (years) | mg |
|---|---|
| < 0.5 | 0.4 |
| 0.5—1.0 | 0.6 |
| 1—3 | 0.8 |
| 4—6 | 1.1 |
| 7—10 | 1.2 |
| 11—14 | |
| Male | 1.5 |
| Female | 1.3 |
| 15—18 | |
| Male | 1.8 |
| Female | 1.4 |
| 19—22 | |
| Male | 1.6 |
| Female | 1.4 |
| 23—50 | |
| Male | 1.7 |
| Female | 1.2 |
| 51 | |
| Male | 1.5 |
| Female | 1.1 |
| Pregnancy | + 0.3 |
| Lactation | + 0.5 |

### III. Fortification Levels and Type of Foods[1,9,10]

| World (FAO/WHO)[1] | | Japan[9] | | U.S.[10] |
|---|---|---|---|---|
| Dry cereals | 50—100 mg[f] | Rice | 1.8 mg[g] | Flour |
| Flour | 1.2—1.8 | Pressed barley | 1.8 | Self-rising flour |
| Bread | 0.3—0.5 | Wheat flour | 1.2—1.8 | Corn grits |
| Pasta | 0.2—0.4 | Bread | 1.2—1.8 | Corn meals |
| Milk products | | | 1.2—2.4 | Rice |
| | 0.5—0.8 | Noodles (dried)[h] | 1.7—2.2 | Macaroni products |

## Table 4 (continued)
### RIBOFLAVINE

| 0.5—0.8 | Noodles (instant) | 1.7—2.2 | Nonfat milk |
| 1.5—2.3 | Miso | | macaroni products |
| ≥ 0.76[i] | Dry milk for | 1.7—2.2 | Noodle products |
| | pregnant and | | |
| | lactating | | |
| | women | | |

a   RDA for persons in light activity.
b   Designed for the maintenance of good nutrition of practically all healthy people in the U.S.
c   Later half.
d   First 6 months.
e   First half.
f   Mg/100 g.
g   Mg/lb.
h   Including macaroni and spaghetti.
i   Mg per daily intake of the product.

## Table 5
### NIACIN

### I. Characteristics of Niacin[1-4,12-15]

| Forms: | Niacin, nicotinic acid, niacinamide |
| Commercially available forms: | Nicotinic acid, niacinamide, coated niacinamide |
| Function: | Coenzyme in energy metabolism |
| Deficiency disease: | Pellagra |
| Food sources: | Whole grains, nuts, legumes, lean meats, liver |
| Stability and some comments: | (1) Stability is rarely a problem in foods; and (2) niacinamide is usually preferred to nicotinic acid |
| Short history of fortification: | U.S., white rice (1942), wheat flour (1943); Puerto Rice, polished rice (1951); Philippines, home pounded rice, undermilled rice, milled rice (1952); Canada, grain and bakery products (1961) |

### II. Recommended Daily Intakes of Niacin[7,8]

| World (FAO/WHO)[7] | | Japan[8,a,b] | | | U.S.[7,c] | |
| --- | --- | --- | --- | --- | --- | --- |
| Age (years) | mg | Age (years) | mg | | Age (years) | mg |
| <1 | 5.4 | <2 months | 4 | | <0.5 | 5 |
| 1—3 | 9.0 | 2 months | 5 | | 0.5—1.0 | 8 |
| 4—6 | 12.1 | 6 months | 6 | | 1—3 | 9 |
| 7—9 | 14.5 | 1 Male | 7 | Female 6 | 4—6 | 12 |
| 10—12 | | 2 | 8 | 8 | 7—10 | 16 |
| Male | 17.2 | 3 | 9 | 9 | 11—14 | |
| Female | 15.5 | 4 | 10 | 9 | Male | 18 |
| 13—15 | | 5 | 11 | 10 | Female | 16 |
| Male | 19.1 | 6 | 12 | 11 | 15—18 | |
| Female | 16.4 | 9 | 14 | 13 | Male | 20 |
| 16—19 | | 12 | 17 | 16 | Female | 14 |
| Male | 20.3 | 15 | 18 | 15 | 19—22 | |
| Female | 15.2 | 18 | 18 | 14 | Male | 20 |
| 20 | | 20 | 17 | 13 | Female | 14 |
| Male | 19.8 | 40 | 15 | 13 | 23—50 | |

## Table 5 (continued)
### NIACIN

| | | | | | | |
|---|---|---|---|---|---|---|
| Female | 14.5 | 60 | 13 | 11 | Male | 18 |
| Pregnancy[d] | +2.3 | >70 | 12 | 10 | Female | 13 |
| Lactation[e] | +3.7 | Pregnancy[f] | | +1 | >51 | |
| | | Pregnancy[d] | | +2 | Male | 16 |
| | | Lactation[e] | | +5 | Female | 12 |
| | | | | | Pregnancy | +2 |
| | | | | | Lactation | +4 |

## III. Fortification Levels and Type of Foods[1,9,10]

| World (FAO/WHO)[1] | | Japan[9] | | U.S.[10] | |
|---|---|---|---|---|---|
| Dry cereals | ≥0.29 mg | Dry milk for | 24 mg | Flour | |
| Flour | | pregnant and | 24 | Self-rising flour | |
| Bread | | lactating women | | | |
| Pasta | | | 27—34 | Noodle products | |
| Milk products | | | 27 — 34 | Nonfat milk macaroni | |
| | | | | products | |
| | | | 27—34 | Macaroni products | |
| | | | 16—32 | Rice | |
| | | | 16—20 | Farina | |
| | | | 16—24 | Corn meal | |
| | | | 16—24 | Corn grits | |

[a]   RDA for persons in light activity.

[b]   Niacin equivalents include dietary tryptophan, 60 mg tryptophan represents 1 mg niacin.

[c]   Designed for the maintenance of good nutrition of practically all healthy people in the U.S.

[d]   Later half.

[e]   First 6 months.

[f]   First half.

[g]   Mg/100 g.

[h]   Mg/lb.

## Table 6
## ASCORBIC ACID

### I. Characteristics of Ascorbic Acid[2-5]

| | |
|---|---|
| Forms: | L-Ascorbic acid |
| Commercially available forms: | L-Ascorbic acid, L-ascorbic acid stealate, sodium ascorbate |
| Function: | Form collagen, promote use of calcium in bones and teeth, promote elasticity and strength of capillaries, convert folacin to active form |
| Deficiency disease: | Scurvy |
| Food sources: | Citrus fruits, strawberries, papayas, broccoli, cabbage, tomatoes, potatoes |
| Stability and some comments: | (1) Ascorbic acid is quite unstable in foods, especially under adverse conditions of storage and food preparation; (2) stability in solution depends on pH, copper and iron content, and exposure to oxygen and temperature; (3) ascorbic acid degradation occurs even in frozen storage of foods |
| Short history of fortification: | Ascorbic acid has been added to many products in some countries |

### II. Recommended Daily Intakes of Ascorbic Acid[7,8]

| World (FAO/WHO)[7] | | Japan[8,a] | | U.S.[7,b] | |
|---|---|---|---|---|---|
| Age (years) | mg | Age (years) | mg | Age (years) | mg |
| <12 | 20 | <1 | 35 | <1 | 35 |
| >13 | 30 | 1—11 | 40 | 1—10 | 40 |
| Pregnancy[c] | 30 | >12 | 50 | >11 | 45 |
| Lactation[d] | 30 | Pregnancy | + 10 | Pregnancy | 60 |
| | | Lactation[d] | + 35 | Lactation | 80 |

### III. Fortification Levels and Type of Foods[1,9]

| World (FAO/WHO)[1] | Japan[9] | U.S.[10] |
|---|---|---|
| Canned, frozen, and dried fruit drinks; canned and dried milk products; dry cereal products | | 30—60 mg[e] Tomato, orange, pineapple, grape, apple, and citrus unshiu (canned, bottled, concentrated juice) |

[a] RDA for persons in light activity.
[b] Designed for the maintenance of good nutrition of practically all healthy people in the U.S.
[c] Later half.
[d] First 6 months.
[e] Mg/fluid oz of the finished food amounts.

# REFERENCES

1. Joint FAO/WHO Expert Committee on Nutrition, Food fortification protein-calorie malnutrition, 8th rep., *WHO Tech. Rep. Ser.,* No. 477, 1-33, 1971.
2. Mitsuda, H., New approaches to amino acid and vitamin enrichment in Japan, in *Protein-Enriched Cereal Foods for World Needs,* Milner, M., Ed., The American Association of Cereal Chemists, St. Paul, Minn. 1969, 208-219.
3. Arlin, M., *The Science of Nutrition,* 2nd ed., Macmillan, New York, 1977.
4. Stare, F. J. and McWilliams, M., *Living Nutrition,* 2nd ed., John Wiley & Sons, New York, 1977.
5. Furia, T. E. Ed., *Handbook of Food Additives,* 2nd ed., CRC Press, Cleveland, Ohio, 1972, 92-114.
6. Joint WHO/USAID Meeting, Vitamin A deficiency and xerophthalmia, *WHO Tech. Rep. Ser.,* No. 590, 1976.
7. Anon., Special Report, *Nutr. Rev.,* 33, 147-157, 1975.
8. National Nutrition Council, Recommended Dietary Allowances for Japanese, National Academy of Science, Tokyo, Revised 1975.
9. Public Health Bureau, Ministry of Health and Welfare, Circ. Notice No. 222, *Admission to the Labelling for Special Nutrition Foods,* 1972.
10. Code of Federal Regulations, Title 21, Food and Drugs, Part 100 to 199, Office of the Federal Register, National Archives and Records Service, General Services Administration, Washington, D.C., Revised as of April 1, 1977, 1-333.
11. Joint FAO/WHO Expert Group, Requirements of ascorbic acid, vitamin D, vitamin $B_{12}$, folate, and iron, *WHO Tech. Rep. Ser.,* No. 452, 1970.
12. Republic of the Philippines, Department of Health, Rules and Regulations Governing the Enforcement of Republic Act No. 832, Supplementing Administrative Order No. 8, S-1953, 1953.
13. National Health and Welfare, The Food and Drugs Act and Regulations in Canada (Division 13), 1959.
14. Government of Puerto Rico, Department of Health, Office of the Commissioner, Regulations for the Enforcement of Act No. 430, 1951.
15. The Minister of Agriculture, Fisheries and Food, and the Ministry of Health, Composition-England and Wales, The Food and Drugs Act, The Flour Composition Regulations No. 1183, 1956.

# NUTRIENT FORTIFICATION OF DAIRY PRODUCTS

## Vernal S. Packard

## INTRODUCTION

Dairy products are most commonly fortified with vitamins A and D and skim milk solids. More recently some fluid milk supplies have also been fortified with iron. While milk contains a variety of vitamin and minerals, it is a relatively poor source of vitamin C and iron. Yet, it has rarely been fortified with either of these nutrients, the former largely because of philosophical questions regarding the appropriateness of enriching a natural foodstuff with nutrients not usually associated with it, the other for technical reasons. In this discussion, nutrient fortification of milk and dairy products will be limited to vitamin A, vitamin D, skim milk solids, and iron.

## VITAMIN A

As it comes from the cow, milk is a significant source of vitamin A, but it is a variable source. Depending upon the season, chiefly reflected in different feeding practices, vitamin A content may vary from 500 to 3000 IU/qt. Even within a given season (or feeding regimen), the amount of this nutrient varies widely. Milk produced in winter months may range from 500 to 1000 IU/qt, in summer, with cows on pasture, from 2000 to 3000 IU/qt.[12] The National Dairy Council[4] assigns to whole milk an average vitamin A level of 1272 IU/qt.

In milk, vitamin A value consists of both vitamin A *per se* and various carotenoids, chief of which is beta-carotene.

As in other foods, vitamin A in milk is associated with the fat. For this reason, the level of vitamin A in any given dairy product varies greatly depending upon the fat content. In skim milk products (both fluid and dry skim milk), essentially all of the vitamin A is lost. Thus are these and other lowfat products commonly fortified with this vitamin. Often such fortification is made mandatory, and is legally enforced. In the U.S., vitamin A addition is required in lowfat and fluid skim milk, in vitamin-fortified nonfat dry milk, and evaporated skimmed milk. It may be added optionally to other dairy products. Table 1 provides a complete listing, along with required levels of fortification. Both in fluid milk and nonfat dry milk products this level is standardized at 2000 IU/qt. The U.S. RDA for this nutrient is 5000 IU.

Vitamin A fortification of dairy products is accomplished by direct addition of vitamin A derivatives in concentrate form. Over the years a "haylike" off-flavor has been attributed to this practice as applied to skim milk. The defect occurs spottily and appears to be related both to the kind (or source) of vitamin A and the presence of oxidizing conditions.[12]

## VITAMIN D

Milk is a naturally poor source of vitamin D, normally ranging between 3.1 and 43.8 IU/qt.[11] Being fat soluble, though, the vitamin is concentrated in high-fat dairy products. Butter, at 80% fat, is a reasonably good source. Vitamin D content of milk varies with breed of cattle, season, and feed.

The nutritional advantage of fortifying milk and certain dairy products with vitamin D has long been recognized. As an aid to the absorption and metabolism of both calcium and phosphorus, this vitamin is appropriately added to those foods which are major sources of these two minerals. Particularly, vitamin D is desirable in enhancing the utilization of calcium, a mineral in generally short supply. In the U.S., nearly 75% of the calcium in the diet derives from dairy foods. To make vitamin D available in the same food makes good nutritional sense.

Serious attempts to upgrade vitamin D content of milk were started during the 1930s. The near eradication of rickets in the developed nations of the world would seem to attest to the ultimate success of the fortification program that evolved.

Earlier methods of increasing the vitamin D content of milk involved the use of UV irradiation and the feeding of irradiated yeast to dairy cows. Neither of these practices find significant usage at the present time. Today, the process of choice is the monitoring into fluid milk of vitamin D concentrates. Both vitamin $D_2$ (cholecalciferol) and vitamin $D_3$ (ergocalciferol) are used. The former, vitamin $D_2$, is a naturally occurring form found in the animal kingdom. Vitamin $D_3$, however, is a synthetic prepared mainly by irradiation of ergosterol from plants and fungi.[5] In the fortification process, concentrates of one of the two forms of the vitamin are simply monitored into the liquid dairy products.

Fortification of milk with vitamin D is endorsed by the Committee on Nutrition of the American Academy of Pediatrics and the Council of Foods and Nutrition of the American Medical Association. While its addition to homogenized whole milk is done on a voluntary basis in the U.S., estimates place the level of fortification at 98% of all such milk sold.[8] Fluid milk products (whole milk, lowfat milk, and skim milk) and nonfat dry milk (on a reconstituted basis) are fortified at levels of not less than 400 IU/qt. Evaporated milk and evaporated skimmed milk are both fortified at 25 IU per fluid ounce. See Table 1 for a complete listing of products and levels of fortification of vitamin D.

## IRON

Iron-fortified milk products have seen only very limited use to this point in time, both as a result of philosophical and nutritional issues of need, and also for technical reasons. While there are possible advantages of such fortification for adult populations, the need for infants appears to be more clear-cut. The Committee on Nutrition, American Academy of Pediatrics, is on record as recommending availability of iron-fortified fluid whole milk or evaporated milk for infant feeding.[2] Nevertheless, technical problems exist, including the bioavailability of supplements, their catalytic effect in triggering oxidative flavor defects, and the protection of lipase enzymes, with the potential for lipolysis to occur. Bioavailability is concerned with the degree to which iron components may be absorbed and/or utilized by the body. Oxidative and/or lipolytic changes in milkfat result in rancid flavors unacceptable to most persons. Despite these problems, research and interest continues in fortifying milk products with iron.

Scanlon and Shipe[14] were among the first researchers to demonstrate the susceptibility of multivitamin/mineral-supplemented milk to oxidation. Others[13] showed that lipase(s), the enzyme(s) causing lipolysis, was protected by ferric ammonium citrate during pasteurization at 73.3°C for 16 sec. Edmondson et al.,[7] however, found that this problem, and the resultant development of lipolytic rancidity, could be entirely overcome by pasteurizing at temperatures of 79°C or higher. These authors also observed a reduction in oxidative deterioration, as induced by ferrous forms of iron, by a process of aeration prior to addition of the iron compound. The most feasible method of adding iron, they concluded, was to use ferric ammonium citrate, followed by pasteurization at 81°C.

In a study of both susceptibility to oxidation and bioavailability of iron, Demott[6] observed only minor off-flavor development when ferric pyrophosphate or ferric phos-

## Table 1
### COMMONLY FORTIFIED DAIRY PRODUCTS AND U.S. STANDARDS OF FORTIFICATION

| Product | Vitamin A | | Vitamin D | | Skim milk solids | |
|---|---|---|---|---|---|---|
| | Level of fortification | Legal requirement[a] | Level of fortification | Legal requirement[a] | Level of fortification | Legal requirement[a] |
| Whole milk | Not <2000 IU/qt | Opt. | Not <400 IU/qt | Opt. | — | — |
| Lowfat milk | Not <2000 IU/qt | Man. | Not <400 IU/qt | Opt. | To 10% MSNF[b] | Opt. |
| Skim milk | Not <2000 IU/qt | Man. | Not <400 IU/qt | Opt. | To 10% MSNF[b] | Opt. |
| Evaporated milk | 125 IU/fluid oz | Opt. | 25 IU/fluid oz | Man. | — | — |
| Evaporated skimmed milk | 125 IU/fluid oz | Man. | 25 IU/fluid oz | Man. | — | — |
| Vitamin-fortified nonfat dry milk | 2000 IU/qt[c] | Man. | 400 IU/qt | Man. | — | — |
| Lowfat dry milk | 2000 IU/qt[c] | Man. | 400 IU/qt | Opt. | — | — |
| Dry whole milk | 2000 IU/qt[c] | Opt. | 400 IU/qt | Opt. | — | — |

[a] Optional (Opt.) or mandatory (Man.) addition under U.S. standards.

[b] Total skim milk solids, including amounts naturally present.

[c] On a reconstituted basis.

phate were used as supplements of whole milk or skim milk at levels of 5.2 to 12.6 ppm elemental iron. When fed as the sole ration to weanling rats for 9 weeks, whole milk fortified with these same two forms of iron was found to satisfactorily maintain tooth color, hematocrit, and body weight, though less effectively than a standard dry ration plus water. Other iron compounds investigated in this study included ferrous sulfate, ferric ammonium citrate, ferrous gluconate, and ferrous lactate.

Perhaps one of the more promising methods of adding iron to milk products utilizes an iron-protein powder in which ferripolyphosphate is combined with cottage cheese whey.[3]

As thus far practiced on a commercial basis, iron supplementation of milk ranges in amount from 10 to 12 mg/qt. At these levels an 8 oz glass of milk would provide from 14 to 17% U.S. RDA, a quart 55 to 67% U.S. RDA.

## SKIM MILK SOLIDS

"Milk-solids-not-fat (MSNF)" and "nonfat solids" are two terms used to distinguish the solids content of the skim milk portion of milk. They may be used in reference to both fluid or dry products. In either case, all milk constituents are understood to be included except fat and water; i.e., protein (both casein and whey proteins), lactose (milk sugar), and mineral components.

U.S. standards of identity for whole milk require milkfat to be present to a minimum of 3.25% and skim milk solids to 8.25%. Because there is a general relationship between fat content and skim milk solids in milk, higher levels of fat are usually accompanied by higher levels of MSNF. On an average, herd milk at 3.2 to 3.3% fat will contain between 8.4 and 8.45% nonfat solids. One authority[1] gives the average value of skim milk solids in whole milk in the U.S. as 8.55%. The discrepancy between that and the former figures can be accounted for by a national milk supply averaging somewhat higher than 3.25% fat, thus, a generally higher level of MSNF.

Over the years there developed a general practice in the dairy industry of adding small amounts of MSNF to lowfat fluid milk products. These added solids tended to provide somewhat better body and flavor characteristics. Another advantage, of course, was the enhancement of nutrient content. In practice, the level of fortification varied all the way from 0.5 to about 2.0% added MSNF. Above the upper value, a salty flavor begins to appear and amounts beyond that become to some extent self-limiting. Nevertheless, some milk supplies are commonly raised to a total MSNF content of 10% (or slightly higher), which implies addition of between 1.0 and 2.0% solids. In 1973, a final order was issued by the Food and Drug Administration allowing for use of the term "protein-fortified" for lowfat and skim milk products in which the MSNF content had been raised to a minimum of 10%.[9] But that specific name came under question shortly thereafter. The reason was this: previously the word "fortified" had been restricted to foods containing added nutrient(s) not usually found associated with a given food. "Enriched" was the name applied to foods in which added nutrient(s) were of the kind common to the particular foodstuff. Ultimately, the 1973 order was amended and the term "protein-fortified" prohibited.[10] In its place, the phrase "with added milk solids not fat" was designated. This declaration is allowed only when the product contains not less than 10% of milk-derived nonfat solids.

# REFERENCES

1. Blakeslee, W., Dairymen propose nutritional boost for milk, *Mid Am Reporter,* Mid America Dairymen, Inc., Springfield, Mo., 1977, 10.
2. Iron-deficiency anemia in infants and preschool children, *Dairy Counc. Dig.,* 43(1), 4, 1972.
3. Iron-deficiency anemia in infants and preschool children, *Dairy Counc. Dig.,* 43(1), 5, 1972.
4. Functions and interrelationships of vitamins, *Dairy Counc. Dig.,* 43(5), 26, 1972.
5. Recent developments in Vitamin D, *Dairy Counc. Dig.,* 47(3), 14, 1976.
6. Demott, B. J., Effects on flavor of fortifying milk with iron and absorption of the iron from intestinal tract of rats, *J. Dairy Sci.,* 54(11), 1609-1614, 1971.
7. Edmondson, L. F., Douglas, F. W., Jr., and Avanto, J. K., Enrichment of pasteurized whole milk with iron, *J. Dairy Sci.,* 54(10), 1422-1426, 1971.
8. *Fed. Reg.,* 38(195), 27924, 1973.
9. *Fed. Reg.,* 38(195), 27924-27929, 1973.
10. *Fed. Reg.,* 45(241), 81737, 1980.
11. Henderson, J. L., *The Fluid Milk Industry,* 3rd ed., AVI Publishing, Westport, Conn., 1971, 282.
12. Jenness, R. and Patton, S., *Principles of Dairy Chemistry,* John Wiley & Sons, New York, 1959, 404.
13. Reisfield, R., Harper, W. J., Gould, I. A., The effect of mineral fortification on lipase activity in pasteurized milk, *J. Dairy Sci.,* 38(6), 595-596, 1955.
14. Scanlon, R. A. and Shipe, W. F., Factors effecting the susceptibility of multivitamin mineral milk to oxidation, *J. Dairy Sci.,* 45(12), 1449-1455, 1962.

# PRESENT PUBLIC HEALTH ASPECTS OF SALT FORTIFICATION

Frank W. Lowenstein

## SALT

### Definition

For the purpose of this paper salt is being defined as a mineral, either crude or refined, which contains more than 95% sodium chloride and is used all over the world in the preparation of food. This includes not only cooking, but also salting of certain foods for preservation.

### Is Salt an Essential Nutrient?

Because both sodium and chlorine are essential ions in body fluids which need to be replaced through the food consumed, salt should be considered as an essential nutrient. This, however, does not necessarily imply that salt needs to be added in relatively large quantities to the food consumed as many foods, particularly those of animal origin, contain usually enough sodium and chlorine to satisfy requirements. Only under conditions of severe heat stress where people may lose up to 8$l$ of sweat a day may it become necessary to add relatively large amounts of salt to the diet in order to replace losses.

### Why Does Salt Lend Itself Relatively Easily to Fortification?

Because salt is used almost universally and continuously it lends itself relatively easily to fortification with other essential nutrients some of which may actually have been present in its original form before processing and refining. This is true for iodine and calcium.

## FORTIFICATION WITH IODINE

The fortification of salt with iodine compounds (potassium-iodide or iodate) has been developed around 50 years ago as a successful means for the control and prevention of endemic goiter. This method has been adopted in a number of countries on all continents. In a recent worldwide survey by the World Health Organization (WHO),[1] 106 countries of 150 surveyed provided substantive information on their goiter problem; 59 countries mentioned that they had some legislation and/or regulations regarding the use of iodated salt. This is more than twice the number in 1965 when the author made a similar survey for WHO.[2] The speed of progress has certainly increased since 1965, but there are still a great many countries with a goiter problem which have no goiter control program. One of the main reasons is the relatively low priority assigned by governments to the control and prevention of endemic goiter, a disease with an extremely low mortality in comparison to many other diseases. On the other hand endemic goiter with its more serious, associated conditions cretinism and deaf-mutism is one of the few public health problems that can be relatively easily controlled within a reasonably short time and at a very low cost. As examples of successful programs the experiences in Northern Thailand[3] and Northern India[4] are mentioned. The Swiss experience[5] serves as example of a slow and insufficient iodization program with best results seen in young children and adolescents; the effectiveness of the program diminishes rapidly with age. The Federal Republic of Germany is an example of a highly developed, affluent country where endemic goiter has been known to be a public health problem for almost 100 years, but no salt iodization program exists.[6]

## What Can be Done to Accelerate Progress?

The following steps should be taken to accelerate progress in the control and prevention of endemic goiter, cretinism and deaf-mutism. (1) Those countries where endemic goiter is known to exist, but its magnitude and severity is unknown, should ask for assistance in organizing surveys, usually of school aged children; such assistance can be made available from the WHO. (2) Those countries where the magnitude and severity of the goiter problem is already known should make requests for technical assistance usually from the international organizations such as WHO and UNICEF in the organization of a control program. This will consist in the great majority in the fortification of all salt for human consumption with either potassium-iodide in the cooler climates or iodate in the tropics at a dosage of 1:10.000 to 1:100.000 ppm. It may be feasible to arrive at regional or subregional arrangements whereby, e.g., one country exporting salt to several other countries in the same region would start iodizing its salt and export already iodized salt to those countries in need of it. Such arrangements might become feasible in West and East Africa and in Southeast Asia with the help of such international organizations as WHO on the technical side, UNICEF and UNDP on the financial-managerial side.

## What are Some of the Unsolved Problems?

### Iodine Losses from Salt

Losses of iodine from iodinated salt may be considerable due to oxidation after exposure to air, particularly warm, humid air. In Greece, Voudouris[28] showed that not only the humidity, but also the presence of other minerals such as magnesium and iron in the salt could cause oxidation of iodine and lead to losses of between 15 to 30% after storage over 300 days. Potassium iodide (KI) is less stable than potassium iodate (KIO$_3$). For this reason iodate is usually recommended for use in the humid tropical countries. Stabilizers may be added such as sodium hyposulfite as recommended by the Nutrition Commission of the National Academy of Medicine in France.[7] According to their recommendation, 35 mg of sodium hyposulfite (Na$_2$S$_2$O$_3$) added to 1 kg of salt prevents oxidation and does not present a health hazard.

Iodine excretion levels in the urine of subjects receiving iodinated salt are used as an indicator of the reliability of a program. In Taiwan,[29] urinary levels of iodine in school children rose from very low values to similar levels, as in school children in areas without goiter, with a simultaneous decrease in goiter prevalence of 80%. In New Zealand, Purves[30] used urinary excretion of iodine to show that the iodination level had been too low at 1 part potassium iodide to 250.000 parts salt, and succeeded in having the level raised to 1 in 20.000 parts of salt in 1939. In 1958, the goiter prevalence in school children was down to 0.1% from 15%.

### Control and Inspection of the Manufacturing and Sale of Iodinated Salt

Although control and inspection are an essential part of any iodation program, usually under the supervision of some governmental agency, they encounter many difficulties. Checks of spot samples of salt sold under the label of iodized or iodated salt are revealing that many times these samples do not contain the amount of iodine they are supposed to have. This may be due to faulty processing during the manufacture of the salt or to losses during storage (see Section on Iodine Losses from Salt). More than 50% of samples spot checked in Mexico[8] and six European countries[6] showed significantly lower amounts of iodine than expected.

### Toxicity

Possible toxic effects of iodinated salt have been reported from several countries. In Mendoza, Argentina, prevalences of hyperthyroidism and cancer of the thyroid increased 30% or more after iodization of salt at 1:30.000 started in 1953.[9] A similar experience has been reported from the endemic areas in Austria in regard to thyroid cancer.[10] These cancers usually developed in older women with so-called "hot nodules" of goitrous thyroid tissue which had been present for many years. Observations such as the foregoing are, fortunately, rare and need not deter public health officials from using iodinated salt in endemic goiter areas. However, certain groups with a possible high risk to develop a toxic reaction to increased iodine intake such as older women with nodular goiter should be closely watched for any signs of toxicity so that they can be taken off the iodinated salt before serious signs of toxicity develop.

## FORTIFICATION WITH CALCIUM

In recent years interest has developed in adding minerals other than iodine to salt that are found either too low in customary diets or are needed in increased amounts for specially vulnerable groups.

Calcium is one of those minerals found low in many diets, particularly those based on cereals such as rice. The high-phytate content of cereals may further decrease the amount of calcium actually absorbed because part of it becomes unavailable through the formation of insoluble calcium phytate. In spite of the low intake found in many countries, usually during dietary surveys, clear-cut signs of calcium deficiency are usually lacking. This can be explained through the ability of the human body to adapt to low intakes and establish equilibrium through low excretion. On the other hand, additional sources of calcium usually escaping routine surveys such as betel nut-lime mixtures in India or coca leaf-lime mixtures in Peru that are chewed may raise low dietary levels considerably. Another not infrequent source of calcium in the diet that is often forgotten is water in hard-water areas. There still remain, however, groups of people living in soft water areas and not chewing betel nut or other mixtures who may be in need of additional calcium. In such areas the fortification of salt with a suitable calcium compound such as calcium sulfate and/or phosphate may be of real benefit. When the calcium intake of 16 girls (age 5 to 12 years) in Mysore, India, was raised from 300 to 640 mg/day by the addition of calcium-enriched salt to their otherwise marginal rice-bean diet, these girls showed significantly greater height increments with nonsignificantly greater increments in weight and hemoglobin, and a significantly lower nutritional deficiency score than 16 girls on the same diet, but with ordinary salt over a 5-month period.[11] It appears that based on similar experiences the Indian government may be ready to permit fortification of salt with calcium sulfate at 5% incorporated during the crystallization process. This measure does not present any major technical problems and the calcium-enriched salt is well accepted. Such a salt can be expected to benefit particularly the vulnerable groups, i.e., children and pregnant and lactating women who are in need of extra calcium. Once the Indian experience has become well established, other countries may adopt similar measures. It is to be understood, however, that such a measure should be limited to those areas where the need for additional calcium has been established after thorough investigation of the dietary intake and nutritional status of the people concerned.

## FORTIFICATION WITH IRON

The third mineral receiving attention as a possible additive to salt is iron.

### Why is Additional Iron Needed?

Iron deficiency is widespread and is causing the most frequent type of anemia in the world. Although the reasons for this are not always dietary, i.e., a low supply of iron in the food supply, the addition of a suitable iron compound to the diet is helpful, particularly in the most vulnerable groups (pregnant and lactating women, young children). Iron salts have been added to flour and cereals for many years in this country and Great Britain. One of the first developing countries to fortify salt with iron was Mauritius in the Indian Ocean, East Africa.[12] They used iron pyrophosphate, a relatively insoluble iron salt. The results of this experiment were poor not only because of the use of an unsuitable compound, but also because of poor market control (a lot of unfortified salt was sold as revealed by a survey of the salt sold by retailers which revealed that only 30% had iron).

In India, a group of scientists has researched the problem of fortification of salt with iron over the last 10 years, and after many trials and errors have come up with two compounds which seem to offer solutions.[13] The first compound used ferrous sulfate and orthophosphoric acid as a stabilizer which makes the salt keep well on storage without color development; however, high humidity, as present in many parts of India, affects the bioavailability of the iron in the salt after storage for more than 10 weeks. The second compound used is ferrous phosphate and sodium acid sulfate as promoter of absorption of a less soluble salt. The salt fortified with this compound keeps well without any color development for several months. Bioavailability of iron from this salt was comparable to that from salt enriched with ferrous sulfate, and did not decrease even after storage for 4 to 5 months. Acceptability of this salt tested in families of different socioeconomic background was good. This compound is recommended as the method of choice by Rao and associates[13] for iron enrichment in tropical countries after extensive field trials. The results of such a trial[14] in an urban community in India have recently become available. The salt was fortified with 3500 ppm of ferrous phosphate (available iron equals 1000 ppm) and 5000 ppm of sodium acid sulfate. A total of 1065 children, age 5 to 15 years, was involved. Two schools, one with 390 children, aged 5 to 12 years, and the second with 300 children, aged 12 to 15 years, served as experimental schools and a third with 275 children served as control. All children were fed from a community kitchen and the use of salt could, therefore, be controlled. Before the start of the experiment all schools were supplied with crushed, unfortified salt for 1 month to enable them to get used to the crushed salt. Hemoglobin and hematocrit were determined in all children every 6 months. The mean daily salt intake was 15 g in the 3 schools. The fortified salt provided about 15 mg additional iron to the 25 to 30 mg of iron provided in the daily diet. At the end of 1 year a significant increase in mean hemoglobin was observed in the two experimental schools but not in the control.

### MEAN Hb LEVELS IN 3 SCHOOLS (g/100 m$\ell$)

| Age (years) | Experimental school #1 | | Experimental school #2 | | Control school #3 | |
| --- | --- | --- | --- | --- | --- | --- |
| | Before | After 1 yr. | Before | After 1 yr. | Before | After 1 yr. |
| 5—12 | 11.5 ± 0.98 | 12.9 ± 1.4 | | | 12.4 ± 1.9 | 11.9 ± 1.4 |
| 12—15 | | | 12.6 ± 1.4 | 14.1 ± 1.5 | 12.8 ± 2.0 | 12.2 ± 1.5 |

The prevalence of anemia decreased from 29 to 5% in the 12 to 15 year olds and from 63 to 21% in the 5 to 12 year olds, while it remained essentially unchanged in controls. Because the situation is different in the rural areas, a similar trial in rural communities is under way.

Recently, Rao advocated the use of ferrous sulfate instead of ferrous orthophosphate which would cut the cost of the formula used. He found that a formula consisting of 3200 parts ferrous sulfate, 2200 parts orthophosphoric acid, and 5000 parts sodium acid sulfate per million parts salt gave a percent iron absorption comparable to that from ferrous sulfate tablets.[31]

Another compound has been studied in South Africa by Sayers et al.[15] which looks promising, but has apparently not been field tested as yet. These authors also used ferrous phosphate at the same concentration as the Indians and added 2.5% starch to prevent any discoloration; they also added ascorbic acid at 1.25% to enhance absorption. They found that absorption was similar to that from ferrous sulfate in contrast to previous findings reported by Rao from India[16] and Cook from the U.S.,[17] who found absorption from ferrous sulfate several times better than from ferrous phosphate. The authors ascribe their improvement to the added ascorbic acid which makes the iron available. The salt thus enriched was stable under subtropical conditions for more than 1 year.

In Thailand, Suvanik and co-workers[32] are working with a salt fortified with 5 g ferrous sulfate and 3 g sodium acid sulfate which are dissolved in 15 m$\ell$ of water and to this solution is added 10 m$\ell$ of a stock solution of sodium hexametaphosphate instead of orthophosphoric acid used by Rao in India per kilogram of salt. A spray mixing method is used. This compound gave uniformly good results in regard to minimal iron losses over a 19-month storage period, stability of color, taste, and smell; it was well accepted by consumers and has shown good bioavailability. A field trial involving 1450 persons in a village in Northeastern Thailand is underway. The same workers are also trying to add iodine to this iron-fortified salt.[33] First they added potassium iodate but results were unsatisfactory. Then they used thyroglobulin prepared from hog thyroid in powder form which contains 0.7% of organically bound iodine. This powder was added to the iron-fortified salt at a concentration of 1-part organic iodine to 100,000 parts of salt containing 1 g of iron per kilogram of salt. After storage for 6 months no significant losses of either iron or iodine occurred.

It seems that the major problems encountered in the iron fortification of salt are (1) instability of a soluble and easily available compound such as ferrous sulfate and (2) relative insolubility and lack of availability of a compound such as ferrous phosphate have been overcome, and that iron fortification of salt has become a feasible and effective public health measure in the control and prevention of iron deficiency anemia. It should, however, be limited to areas where the need of additional iron clearly exists. Any chronic overdosage of iron may be harmful and should be avoided.

## FORTIFICATION WITH FLUORINE

Another mineral which has been added successfully to salt is fluorine, a trace mineral like iodine. In Switzerland, a fluorine-whole salt ("Fluor-Vollsalz") is available and being used in increasing amounts. This salt contains 10 mg potassium iodide and 200 mg sodium fluoride per kilogram of salt. According to Wespi[18] in 1967, 76% of the packeted salt was fluoridated in Switzerland; five cantons (states) made the sale of this salt compulsory and in another six cantons more than 90% of the packeted salt is fluoridated. The results of two studies, (one by Marthaler[19] in 1961 in Zurich and the second one by the same author in Wadenswil[20]) in school children showed a reduction in new DMF rates of 22 and 30%, respectively, after 4½ to 5½ years of use of fluoridated salt. From these rather poor results, Wespi[18] concluded that the fluorine content of 90 mg fluorine per kilogram of salt was too low and should be raised to 200 to 250 mg. This would achieve an ingestion of 1 mg of fluorine per day at an average salt consumption of 4 to 5 g/day. Urinary excretion of fluorine from a salt containing 250 mg of fluorine per kilogram was similar to that from water fluoridated at 1 mg/kg. This fact suggests that such a salt would be expected to provide a similar fluorine intake and carries preventing effect as water fluoridation. These authors also found that maximum excretion occurred 2 to 4 hr after test dose, and they recommended that urine samples 2 to 4 hr after the main meal be tested as a control to be sure that there is no potentially toxic intake.

Wespi's recommendations have been successfully applied in two cantons in Switzerland and three other countries (Hungary, Colombia, and Spain). In Switzerland, the canton of Vaud has fluoridated all salt for human consumption with 250 mg fluorine per kilogram of salt since 1970. Comparative studies of school children in three tests (communities in Vaud with children in neighboring cantons) showed a significantly greater decrease in DMF rates in the Vaud children.[34] Much of the salt used in the neighboring cantons has only 90 mg of fluorine per kilogram of salt. Correspondingly, urinary excretion levels of fluorine were significantly higher in the canton of Vaud[35] than their neighboring cantons, and the fluorine content of the dental hard tissues from extracted teeth of young persons in Vaud was significantly greater than that of similar persons in Tessin where salt is not fluoridated.[36]

In Hungary, only domestic salt was fluoridated at 250 mg fluorine per kilogram of salt (excluding salt used by bakeries and the food industry). Toth[37] measured the percentage of caries-free teeth in the experimental and control villages over a 10-year period of fluoridated salt usage. There was a 5- to 10-fold increase in these percentages in the children (age 4 to 14 years) in the experimental villages as compared to those in the control villages where there was little change. There was a corresponding decrease in DMF rates of the children in the experimental villages where these rates remained more or less unchanged in the control children. Urinary excretion levels showed a mean fluorine content of $0.81 \pm 0.02$ mg/$\ell$ of urine for all ages, in children, however, it was always lower. Toth postulates, on the basis of these findings, that the fluorine content of salt needs to be increased to 350 mg/kg in order to approach the optimal level of 1 mg/$\ell$ in the urine obtained with water fluoridated with 1 mg/$\ell$. The lower excretion may be due, in part, to the fact emphasized by Toth that 60% of the salt used in the households in Hungary is discarded.

The study in Colombia was done in four villages comparable as to socioeconomic, dietary, and health conditions.[22,23] Two villages received fluoridated salt, one received fluoridated water at 1 ppm, and the fourth village served as control. Two different compounds were used, namely sodium fluoride and calcium fluoride to which stabilizers were added. Thus a premix was prepared to be added to the salt. The first premix consisted of 1% sodium fluoride and 99% calcium pyrophosphate, the second premix of calcium fluoride (0.93%) and tricalcium phosphate (99.07%). Forty-six grams of the premix was added to 1 kg of salt on an average. This provided 200 mg of fluorine per kilogram of salt or 2 mg/day at mean salt consumption of 10.5 g per person per day. After 8 years from the beginning of the study in 1965, DMF rates in children, age 6 to 14 years, in the four villages showed the following:

| Village | Measure used (compound) | DMF rates | | | Total of children involved |
| --- | --- | --- | --- | --- | --- |
| | | 1964 | 1972 | Difference (%) | |
| Armenia | Calcium fluoride | 6.74 | 3.49 | 48.4 | |
| Montebello | Sodium fluoride | 6.30 | 3.17 | 49.7 | |
| San Pedro | Water fluoride | 6.65 | 2.66 | 60.0 | |
| Don Matias | Control | 8.63 | 8.24 | 4.5 | 27.022 |

The effect of the fluoridated salt was comparable to the effect of fluoridated water, although less marked. The authors consider 200 mg of fluorine per kilogram of salt an optimal dose without risk of fluorosis. Other countries where some fluoridated salt has been used or is becoming available are Spain, Finland, Sweden, and Mexico. In

Spain,[38] salt fluoridated with 2.5 mg of sodium fluoride per kilogram of salt was used in 200 children in a closed institution. Average salt consumption was 10 g/day per child. Observations over a 4-year period (1965 to 1969) showed a significant reduction in DMF rates in these children, age 8 to 13 years. In Finland, fluoridated salt had become available as early as 1952 using the Swiss model. In 1976, 7% of all table salt sold in the retail stores was fluoridated at 90 mg fluorine per kilogram. No information seems to exist on the effect of this salt on DMF rates, although Finland has one of the highest caries rates in Europe.[24] The Pan American Health Organization together with the Ministry of Health of Colombia, the University of Antiochia, and the W. K. Kellogg Foundation held the first international symposium on salt fluoridation in September 1977 in Medellin, Colombia. The report of this meeting is in preparation. It will no doubt present the actual state-of-the-art on salt fluoridation. From the above experiences reviewed briefly it can be said that salt fluoridation is a practical, safe, and more economical alternative to water fluoridation, especially in rural areas without central water supplies where fluoridation of water would not be practical. It needs to be emphasized, however, that such a measure should be applied only in areas where the fluorine content of the water is naturally low (below 1 ppm) and no good dietary sources of fluorine are easily available (such as tea, shellfish, etc.).

## FORTIFICATION WITH OTHER NUTRIENTS

**Vitamin A** — is essential for the health of the eye and where it is in short supply to the most vulnerable groups. Usually very young children are subject to dryness of the conjunctiva which may progress to affect the cornea and, if unchecked, will lead to softening of the cornea (keratomalacia) and blindness. Vitamin A deficiency is the most common cause of blindness among young children in many tropical countries. To help prevent this serious condition, vitamin A is being added to all skim milk powder exported to these countries. The experiments with adding it to salt, however, have shown that besides technical problems such as stability during cooking, the cost would be too high. To add 1500 IU of vitamin A to a person's diet in India per day would add about 7¢ to the price per kilo.

**Vitamin C (ascorbic acid)** — is essential for the health of the supporting structures of the body such as the connective tissues. In Czechoslovakia, ascorbic acid has been added to salt at a level of 0.5% and the effect of this salt on the serum level of ascorbic acid has been studied in young apprentices. After the use of fortified salt for 6 weeks a significant rise of the serum level of ascorbic acid was observed in the experimental group as compared to the control group.[25]

**Lysine** — the essential amino acid, usually the first limiting amino acid in cereals, has been added to salt at levels of 1 and 4%. Additional lysine can improve the nutritional value of cereals and cereal based diets by raising the biological value of the cereal protein. Better growth in experimental animals and in children has shown to be one of the results of such a measure. The experiment in India, however, showed the lysine in salt to be unstable and the salt to develop bad odors after several months of storage. The cost would also be high as the lysine would have to be imported. Unless these difficulties can be overcome, lysine fortification of salt does not appear to be a promising approach to the problem of lysine fortification. The cereals forming the basis of the diet in many countries may be the best vehicles for the addition of lysine and/or other nutrients.

## FACTORS TO CONSIDER FOR SALT FORTIFICATION PROGRAMS

### Production and Trade of Salt

First is the production and trade of salt in a given country. The *Handbook of Salt*

*Resources*[26] contains fairly detailed information on where the main salt deposits are located and what the major sources of salt are in most countries. It also gives production figures usually for 1965. For the purpose of any salt fortification program one needs to know what kind of salt is being used (crude or refined, crushed or in blocks, etc.) and whether it is produced in the country or imported. Optimal conditions are pure grade, low-moisture content, uniform, small-particle size, and packaging in moisture-resistant containers. These conditions, however, usually exist only in the industrialized countries in the temperate zones. According to Bauernfeind[39] there is no known technology for uniformly fortifying the crude salts in most tropical countries like India, Indonesia, etc. Furthermore, one needs to know what the total amount is that is used in the country for human consumption and, if imported, where it comes from.

## Cost

The cost of any salt fortification program is a very important point to be considered. A program may be feasible from the technical point, but if it raises the price of salt so much that the poorest people who may be most in need of the fortified product cannot afford to pay the price it would defeat its purpose. This is not the place to discuss cost in detail, but some general ideas on the cost increases to be expected can be presented.

**Cost of iodization programs** — Iodination of salt for human consumption increases the cost 5% or less of the cost of noniodinated salt after machinery for the addition and mixing of the iodine compound has been installed. The initial investment for the machinery is not high, but depends upon the size of the operation.

**Price of iodized salt** — The actual sales price of iodinated salt in 14 countries in Europe is the same as that of noniodinated salt because the additional cost is borne by the governments; in contrast, the sales price of iodinated salt in some of the Latin American countries is higher as the additional cost is passed on to the consumer by the producers, usually private industry.

**Cost of adding calcium and iron to salt** — The addition of calcium sulfate at a 5% level would increase the individual annual cost of salt in India (5.5 kg per person) by less than 1¢, a negligible amount. Fortification with an iron compound containing 20% at a 0.25% level would increase the cost of the salt thus enriched somewhat more by about 1.5¢ per person per year. At this level of fortification a person consuming 15 g of salt a day would receive 7.5 mg of additional iron. If 1/10 of this is absorbed by the body it will provide 0.75 mg/day to the body or 50 to 75% of the daily requirement.

**Cost of adding vitamin A and lysine** — The cost of adding vitamin A to salt would be high as already mentioned. The same would be true for lysine fortification of salt in a country like India.

## Consumption of Salt

In order to plan for any salt fortification program one needs to know how much salt people use. The amount of the specific nutrient to be added will depend upon the average amount of salt used by people who are to benefit from the fortification. Mean requirements of nutrients are more or less similar all over the world, but mean consumption levels differ greatly for many nutrients including salt. The lower the average amount of salt consumed the more of the nutrient needs to be added in order to arrive at the required level.

Consumption levels differ also according to age groups, socioeconomic status, custom, etc. within a country or ethnic group. Altava et al.[40] found a considerable variability in daily salt consumption between persons in an urban community (it ranged from 1.63 to 13.50 g) and also between urban and rural people (the latter had a consumption ranging from 7.07 to 17.62 g/day per person). Toth et al.[41] determined the daily salt consumption in 242 persons, age 4 months to 85 years, in different parts of Hungary and related the amount consumed to the body weight. He found that younger persons consumed more salt per kilogram body weight than older persons, and men up to age 30 consumed more than women of the same age. Data collected during several Interdepartmental Committee on Nutrition and National Defense (ICNND) surveys have shown that the military consume two to four times as much salt as the civilians in the same country. In regard to socioeconomic groups there seem to be considerable variations; whereas in Viet Nam high-income groups consume two to five times as much salt as low-income groups, in urban Delhi, the monthly per capita consumption of salt is much larger in the lower castes than that of the higher castes, low-income vegetarians consume more salt than high-income nonvegetarians. Very little is known on the differences in salt consumption levels between different age groups. This kind of knowledge is needed, in particular, for the most vulnerable groups, i.e., pre-school children and pregnant and lactating women, who are expected to benefit most from some fortification programs. It would do no good to fortify salt with calcium and/or iron, if, for instance, young children would hardly take any salt in their food in a given country.

## WHAT CAN BE DONE TO GET DATA?

It is not too difficult to get fairly accurate information on salt intake for different age groups by either including salt among the food items recorded during any dietary survey or by doing special surveys on salt intake as was done in India. In this way the great gap in our knowledge could be filled.

## CONCLUSIONS AND RECOMMENDATIONS

1. Because of its almost universal and continuous use, salt lends itself as an excellent vehicle for adding essential nutrients that are either lacking or are in short supply in the diets of many countries.
2. The addition of iodine to salt as either potassium-iodide or iodate is a well-accepted and tested method to reduce the incidence of endemic goiter and allied conditions to such low levels that it ceases to be a public health problem.
3. The addition of other essential minerals such as calcium, iron, and fluorine is still in the experimental stage; it appears that calcium fortified salt is well accepted and is economical in a country like India. It could increase the mean calcium intake which is low in the rice eating areas by 175 mg per person per day and thus benefit the vulnerable groups. The addition of fluorine to salt appears also feasible and could become an effective measure in reducing dental caries, particularly in rural areas where fluoridation of water supplies would be impractical. Fortification of salt with iron could develop into an important public health measure to reduce widespread iron deficiency anemia, provided the results of more field trials in different countries show results which are as good or better than those mentioned in India.
4. The questions whether the addition of other nutrients such as Vitamin A and C and/or essential amino acids to salt may be feasible as a practical public health measure requires further study.
5. While information on salt production, imports and exports is available in most countries, information on salt consumption is usually lacking, particularly when it comes to different age and socioeconomic groups. Such information is essential for planning any salt fortification program and could be collected without great difficulties or costs during all food consumption (dietary) surveys. It is, there-

fore, strongly recommended that salt be included as an item of study in the planning and execution of all dietary surveys. Where such surveys are not planned in the near future, special surveys on salt alone or including some other items such as bread and tea in Delhi, India should be organized.

6. The cost of iodination programs is known and is low enough to make it economical. The same seems to be true for calcium and iron fortification in India. The cost of fortification with other nutrients needs further study.

7. Efforts should be made to stimulate governments particularly in Africa and Southeast Asia to plan and organize iodination programs for the control and prevention of their endemic goiter problem. Ways and means of organizing such programs on an inter-country or regional basis should be explored.

## REFERENCES

1. WHO, *The Control of Endemic Goitre,* World Health Organization, Geneva, 1979.
2. Lowenstein, F. W., Iodized salt in the prevention of endemic goiter: a worldwide survey of present programs, *Am. J. Public Health,* 57, 1815-1823, 1967.
3. Nondasuta, A., Goitre in Thailand, *Proc. 1st Asian Congr. Nutrition,* Nutrition Society of India, 1972; 623-630.
4. Sooch, S. S. et al., Prevention of endemic goitre with iodized salt, *Bull. WHO,* 49, 307-321, 1973.
5. Steck, A. et al., Effects of improved iodine prophylaxis on endemic goitre and iodine metabolism, *Schweiz. Med. Wochenschr.,* 102, 829-837, 1972.
6. Habermann, J. et al., Alimentary iodine deficiency in the Federal Republic of Germany, *Nutr. Metab.,* 21(Suppl. 1), 45-47, 1977.
7. Laroche, G., Sur l'addition d'hyposulfite de sodium au sel "iode", *Bull. Acad. Natl. Med. (Paris),* 154(19), 445, June 1970.
8. Pacheco, M. G. et al., Determinacion quantitativa de Yodato en sal de mesa por Titulacion Volumetrica, *Rev. Invest. Sal. Publ. (Mexico),* 31(3), 144-151, 1971.
9. Perinetti, H., Goiter in Mendoza Province, Argentina, *Environ. Res.,* 3(516), 463, 1970.
10. Riccabona, G. et al., Epidemiology and therapy of hyperthyreoses in an endemic goitre region, *Klin. Wochenschr. (Wiener),* 84(22), 360-363, 1972.
11. Desikachar, H. et al., Level of protein intake and quality of protein. Calcium and phosphorus absorption, *Indian J. Med. Res.,* 37, 85-90, 1949.
12. Foy, H., Fortification of salt with iron. Letter to the editor, *Am. J. Clin. Nutr.,* 29(9), 935-936, 1976.
13. Rao, B. S. N. et al., Fortification of common salt with iron: effect of chemical additives on stability and bioavailability, *Am. J. Clin. Nutr.,* 28, 1395-1401, 1975.
14. NCMR, A Community Trial with Iron Fortified Salt in India, Annual Report for 1976, National Institute of Nutrition, National Council of Medical Research, Hyderabad, 1977, 176-180.
15. Sayers, M. H. et al., The fortification of common salt with ascorbic acid and iron, *Br. J. Haematol.,* 28, 483-495, 1974.
16. Rao, B. S. N. et al., Iron absorption in Indians studied by whole body counting: a comparison of iron compounds used in salt fortification, *Br. J. Haematol.,* 22, 281-286, 1972.
17. Cook, J et al., Absorption of fortification iron in bread *Am. J. Clin. Nutr.,* 26, 861-872, 1973.
18. Wespi, H. J. and Burgi, W., Salt fluoridation and urinary fluoride excretion, *Caries Res.,* 5, 88-95, 1971.
19. Marthaler, T., Zur Frage des Fluorvollsalzes; erste Klinische Resultate, *Schweiz. Monatsschr. Zahnheilk.,* 71, 671-682, 1961.
20. Marthaler, T. and Schenardi, C., Inhibition of caries in children after 5½ years use of fluoridated table salt, *Helv. Odontol., Acta,* 6, 1-6, 1972.
21. Toth, K., Dental Caries, its prevention and fluoridation of table salt, *Fogorv. Sz.,* August 1977.
22. Restrepo, D. et al., Estudio sobre la Fluoruracion de la sal, *Bol. Of. Sanit. Panam.,* 73(5), 418-424, 1972.
23. Mejia, R. et al., Fluoruracion de la sal en quatro Communidades Colombianas. VIII. Resultados obtenidos de 1964 a 1972, *Bol. Of. Sanit. Panam.,* 80(3), 205-218, 1976.
24. Tala, H., Some Aspects of Salt Fluoridation in Finland, 1st Int. Symp. Salt Fluoridation, Medellin, Colombia, 1977.

25. Hejda, S., The effect of the administration of salt fortified with vitamin C, *Cesk. Hyg.*, 6, 2-3, 1961.
26. Lefond, S. J., Ed., *Handbook of World Salt Resources,* Plenum Press, New York, 1969.
27. Moulik, T. K., Consumption Patterns of Salt, Tea and Bread in the Greater Delhi Area, *USAID, India,* May 1968.
28. Voudouris, E., Zur Beständigkeit des jodhaltigen Kochsalzes, *Z. Lebensm. Unters. Forsch.*, 157, 287, 1975.
29. Hsieh, Y. H. et al., Urinary iodine excretion of school children, *J. Formosan Med. Assoc.*, 72, 218, 1973.
30. Purves, H. D., The aetiology & prophylaxis of endemic goitre-cretinism. The New Zealand experience, *N. Z. Med. J.*, 80, 529, 1974.
31. Rao, B. S. and Narasingat Vjayasarathy, C., An alternate formula for the fortification of common salt with iron, *Am. J. Clin. Nutr.*, 31, 1112, 1978.
32. Suvanik, R. et al., Iron and iodine fortification in Thailand, *J. Med. Assoc. Thailand,* 62(Supplement), 1979.
33. Suvanik, R. et al., Letter to the Editor, *J. Med. Assoc. Thailand,* 62, December 1979.
34. Crousaz de Ph. et al., Comparison of various fluoridation methods in Switzerland with particular attention to fluoridated salt use in Vaud, *Schweiz. Monatsschr. Zahnbeilk.,* Special No. 790, September 1, 1980.
35. Peters, G. et al., L'excrétion urinaire de fluorine chez les habitants du canton de Vaud ingerant du sel fluoré/comparée a c'elle d'habitants de communes limitrophes ingerant du sel non-fluoré, *Soz. Praev. Med.,* November 1975.
36. Baumgartner, W. et al., The fluorine-content of teeth in fluoridated salt using areas and controls, *Soz. Praev. Med.,* 21, 153, July 1976.
37. Toth, K., Ten years of fluoridated salt in Hungary, *Acta Paediatr Acad. Sci. Hungary,* 19, 319, 1978.
38. Vines, T. J., Fluorprofilaxis de la caries dental a traves de la sal flururada, *Rev. Clin. Esp.,* 120, 319, 1971.
39. Bauernfeind, T. C., Technical problems in the fortification of salt, *Food Nutr., (Roma),* 6, 10, 1980.
40. Altava, V. T. et al., Profilaxis del ocio endemico, *Anot. Metod. Actual,* 45, 105, February 1975.
41. Toth, K. et al., Über den täglichen, auf das Körpergewicht bezogenen Verbrauch von Speisesalz, *Dtsche. zahnaerztl. Z.,* 30, 231, 1975.

# FORTIFICATION OF SUGAR*

## Juan M. Navia

## BACKGROUND

Sugar (sucrose) is a food ingredient that provides a source of carbohydrates and a desirable sweet taste. It is consumed in all parts of the world as an ingredient of food and beverages to provide energy, to improve their organoleptic qualities, and/or to contribute specific technologic advantages.[42] The sugar generally used for these different purposes is highly refined to yield a pure food ingredient with excellent storage qualities whose only nutritional contribution is energy. Therefore, foods that are made up essentially of sugar as a major ingredient, provide mainly calories. An example of these types of products would be confectionery products that contain 60 to 100% sugar. One of the nutritional problems posed by excessive consumption of high-sugar containing products is that they take the place in the diet of other foods which provide proteins, vitamins, and minerals besides energy. Therefore, since there is a definite number of calories that individuals should consume depending on age, sex, and level of energy expenditure, the excessive intake of high-energy foods, either dilutes the nutritional quality of the diet making it difficult to meet nutritional requirements, or if added as extra calories to the diet, it will result in an undesirable body weight increase. The nutritional consequences of such dietary behavior is easy to recognize and define in its extreme situation, i.e., frequent consumption of large quantities of foods containing considerable amounts of sugar. It is not simple, however, to identify and quantitate human health effects of occasional consumption of a food containing moderate amounts of sugar. Although, the nutritional risk in this latter situation is probably nonexistent, it is still a debatable issue.[43]

More difficult to interpret is the effect of consuming moderate amounts of a sugar containing food on oral health. Sugar[29,45] has been suggested to have a role in the etiology of various human disease, but most claims have been discarded or disproved, except for the role of sugar on oral health, which has been extensively investigated and documented. It is clearly understood today that sugar is not the only etiological agent in dental caries, and that factors such as the pattern and form of sugar consumption, type and virulence of specific bacteria colonizing tooth surfaces, and other factors related to saliva composition, enamel structure, tooth morphology, and fluoride status are important contributors to the expression and severity of the disease. However, numerous clinical and animal studies[11] have shown that under similar conditions, frequent consumption of sugar or sugar-containing foods increases the severity of dental caries. Again, in this case, definition of specific thresholds relative to percent of sugar in foods or number of sugar exposures during the day that are detrimental to oral health are difficult to establish and need to be further investigated.

Sugar disappearance data suggests that consumption in the U.S. has increased steadily in the last 70 years, and since the last 2 decades it has probably stabilized at around 100 lb/year per person. Consumption patterns for sugars in general have changed dramatically in the U.S.[13] The change in the pattern of consumption has been mainly characterized by: (1) increased consumption of other sugars, such as high-fructose corn syrup, (2) sugar replacement of starches and starch-containing foods in the diet, (3) decreased sugar consumption from the bowl, and (4) increased use of sugar in a large number of manufactured foods.

* Supported in part by NIH-NIDR Grants Number DE-07020 and DE-02670.

These characteristics are specially detrimental to oral health when they are combined with a change in dietary habits that has taken place over the last 20 years. Traditionally, most sugar-containing foods have been consumed at the end of a meal as dessert, but now many of these foods are consumed frequently between meals as a snack; thus the U.S. population has changed from being meal eaters to nibblers. Frequent nibbling of sugar-containing foods contributes to implantation, colonization, and metabolic activity of cariogenic microorganisms, and thus, enhances formation of dental plaque and development of plaque dependent diseases such as caries.

Some of the different problems created by this increased and frequent consumption of sugar-containing foods could be partly alleviated by: (1) substituting sugar in food snacks with new synthetic sweeteners, (2) reducing the very high concentrations of sugars in some manufactured foods to a lower level, as well as the frequency with which they are consumed, or (3) supplementing sugar and sugar-containing snacks with vitamins, minerals, and trace elements to improve its nutritional value and/or to reduce its caries potential. Some of the approaches suggested for this latter measure will be reviewed in the following sections.

## NUTRITIONAL FORTIFICATION OF SUGARS

Supplementation of different foods with a variety of nutrients has been done successfully in all parts of the world to fulfill a number of objectives summarized by Harris[23,24] as follows:

1. Restoration of nutrient concentration to natural levels
2. Fortification above the normal concentration
3. Enrichment with various nutrients to fulfill public health objectives
4. Enrichment to equalize the concentrations of nutrients found in interchangeable foods
5. Fortification to make a food nutritionally self-sufficient
6. Addition of nutrients to a food for nonnutritional purposes

Sugar, a staple ingredient consumed all over the world, has been fortified with different nutrients for a variety of reasons. Navia[34] has discussed enrichment of sugar and sugar products, and indicated that of the different philosophies that had been proposed to fortify foods, the one suggesting fortification to make a food nutritionally self-sufficient could be applicable to sugar. Recently, however, nutritional fortification of sugar has been implemented also to take advantage of its broad use as a food ingredient, to deliver specific nutrients to population groups, and thus fulfilling a public health objective.[3] A third aspect of sugar fortification has to do with addition of cariostatic mineral elements which might lower the caries promoting properties of sugar, while at the same time contributing indirectly to the nutrition of the consumer of such fortified sugar products. These three different approaches to sugar fortification have been evaluated and in some cases implemented at a national level.

### Enrichment of Sugar to Improve its Nutritional Value

Fortification of sugar to make it metabolically self-sufficient, is a concept discussed by Navia.[34] It is based on the fact that sugar is a pure carbohydrate and does not contain the co-factors needed for its metabolism. Consumption of a high-sugar containing product displaces other foods which usually are a better source of vitamins and minerals than sugar and, furthermore, make sugar dependent for its metabolism on co-factors, such as thiamine and niacin, provided by foods in the diet. For these reasons, fortification of sugar with thiamine and niacin at concentrations of 0.2 and

4.0 mg, respectively, per 100 g of sucrose could be considered, to make sugar metabolically self-sufficient. The fortification of sugar with other vitamins such as riboflavin, pyridoxine, or biotin does not seem necessary, if this particular philosophy is considered, since these co-factors are involved more in protein and fat metabolism than in carbohydrate metabolism. Fortification with these suggested levels of thiamine and niacin constitute approximately twice the amount of co-factors necessary to metabolize 1000 cal of carbohydrate and represent an improvement of the nutrient density index of sugar and sugar-containing foods.

Some efforts have been made to produce industrially fortified sugar. The Magro Company* has for many years been involved in efforts to produce and market a fortified sugar which has been supplemented with the following vitamins and minerals: vitamin $B_1$, 0.5 mg; vitamin $B_2$, 0.6 mg; niacin, 5.0 mg; iron, 3.0 mg; and iodine, 0.1 mg/100 grams of sugar. Initially production of fortified sugar followed the procedure patented by Carter,[14] but recently other procedures have been developed to manufacture the product and extend its shelf-life. The most serious problems associated with manufacture of fortified sugar have been stability of vitamins, slight discoloration, and odor in the sugar after storage for some time. The producers claim that many of these organoleptic changes have been eliminated and hope to be able to market the product successfully in the future.[51]

### Fortification of Sugar for Public Health Reasons
*Fortification with Iron Compounds*

Iron metabolism is characterized in humans by the fact that limited amounts of dietary iron are available for absorption, and most of the iron absorbed is conserved and not excreted.[21] Absorption is further complicated by presence (or absence) of specific food components that interact with iron to bind it or to change its oxidation status. Because of the limited amount of iron present in the diet of different groups of people around the world, iron deficiency is common, especially in children and women consuming cereal-based diets. In an attempt to increase intake of iron, Disler et al.[17] conducted studies to determine whether cane sugar, a staple ingredient widely consumed, might represent a suitable carrier for a combination of Fe and ascorbic acid. The vitamin was added to the fortification mixture to promote iron absorption.

Two levels of sugar fortification were evaluated, either 100 or 200 mg Fe/kg in various chemical forms. Ascorbic acid additions were made at a concentration of either 1 or 2 g/kg of sugar. The iron-containing compound and/or ascorbic acid were added to sugar by first adding water (1 g/kg) to moisten the sugar, and then, mixing in each supplement, and finally drying with warm air. Sugar fortified in this manner could be stored for up to 2 years without appreciable discoloration. Fortification studies using $FeSO_4 \cdot 7H_2O$ with or without ascorbic acid were not promising, because it was found that this compound produced marked black discoloration after addition of fortified sugar to tea, and therefore, $FePO_4 \cdot H_2O$ was tested in a series of experiments. This latter iron compound did not discolor tea, but its absorption was found to be poor when it was added to cereal porridge after it was prepared. However, if fortified sugar was cooked with porridge, absorption of iron was improved in the presence of adequate amounts of ascorbic acid.

Derman et al.[16] realizing the many problems involved in iron fortification of sugar (i.e., discoloration produced by soluble iron salts and poor absorption of insoluble iron salts added after cooking) have presented data to support their suggestion that fortification of sugar with ascorbic acid alone should be considered. Their study indicated that ascorbic acid does not enhance the absorption of $Fe_2O_3$ or rust from cooking

---

* The Magro Company, 3700 Carew Tower, Cincinnati, Ohio 45202.

utensils made of iron, but there is a marked effect on the absorption of $Fe(OH)_3$, an iron compound which is a common contaminant from soil in foods and unpurified waters. Thus, addition of ascorbic acid fortified sugar to a cereal would not have any organoleptic effects on the diet, and yet, could facilitate the absorption of iron naturally contaminating the food.

Layrisse et al.[27] have also investigated the use of sugar as a vehicle for iron administration to population groups in the Andes. They also recognize that cereal foods such as wheat flour, farina, and even maize inhibited the absorption of iron used in fortifying these foods, but starch, sucrose, and salt did not. Salt has been previously suggested as a carrier for iron. Sayers et al.[41] fortified salt with 0.1% of Fe as ferric orthophosphate and ascorbic acid, and recommended it for people living in areas where a maize-meal porridge is consumed.

Layrisse et al.[27] reported that considering total nonheme iron utilization from both fortified sugar (15 mg Fe) and native food iron in the Andes diet (14.4 mg Fe), iron absorption doubled when fortified sugar was administered with meals, and quadruple, when the same amount of iron from fortified sugar was administered during and between meals. A further increase was noted when ascorbic acid was added to fortified sugar. Several carbonated cola beverages and fruit drinks were tested as a between meal snack to provide iron and no interference was found with its absorption.

Several other ferric and ferrous compounds were added to sugar and tested for absorbability. Among them Fe(III)-EDTA was found to be absorbed as well as ferrous sulfate. It also reacted very slowly with tea tannins and therefore, tea color was not altered.[28] Viteri[50] et al. have also found NaFe-EDTA to be better absorbed with $FeSO_4$, regardless of whether these compounds were given in aqueous solutions (5 mg/Fe) or with a standard meal consisting of beans, tortilla, bread, and coffee which provided also a total of 5 mg Fe. Layrisse et al.[28] also suggested the possibility of using soft drinks containing fortified sugar for prevention of iron deficiency anemia. They estimated that 2 soft drinks per day consumed between meals would provide 0.5 to 1.60 mg of iron, and thus contribute to the iron requirements of a large proportion of women, who could also obtain from the diet approximately 1 mg more. One concern that has been expressed for this chelate of iron with ethylene diaminetetracetate (NaFe-EDTA) is that it may interfere with the bioavailability of other important essential elements such as zinc. Solomons et al.[46] studied the effect of a dose of 15 mg of this chelate which is equivalent to that amount in a cup of coffee sweetened with 15 g of fortified sugar, and also of higher doses (40 mg) which are equivalent to that consumed in a day by rural Guatemalans and did not find a significant depression of zinc uptake. High doses of NaFe-EDTA, outside of this range did impair zinc absorptions, thus suggesting that fortification of sugar with NaFe-EDTA at one part per thousand would not influence zinc nutriture. It seems clear that fortification of sugar with iron, and perhaps, also ascorbic acid would help provide needed iron supplements to diets which are commonly low in iron. Fortification of sugar with iron seems to be more advantageous than fortification of cereals and even salt, however, care should be exercised in the selection of the iron source and the possible changes due to food processing.[30] The disadvantages associated with this delivery system are some possible organoleptic changes of beverages such as tea and coffee sweetened with fortified sugar; individual variability in consumption of soft drinks and sugar containing snacks which would affect iron intake from fortified sugar; possible danger of excessive intake by men who have lower requirements than women, and also by children consuming excessive amounts of foods prepared with iron fortified sugars; and finally, consideration should be given to the impact that such between meal snacking could have on body weight control and dental caries. Fortification of sugar with iron to fulfill a public health need should not be recommended through educational programs suggesting increased consumption between meals of snacks containing fortified sugar, as this would add an additional energy intake, and would stimulate caries developemnt. Such risk/benefit considerations need to be evaluated carefully before implementation of such fortification programs.

*Fortification with Vitamin A*

Sugar has also been used as a carrier for another nutrient, vitamin A. Arroyave[3,4] has described in detail the philosophy and methodology used in fortification of sugar with vitamin A. There is no question that many populations around the world lack dietary sources of vitamin A, and deficient individuals show impaired growth rate, and loss of integrity of their epithelial tissues. The eyes are the organs most affected, and corneal lesions develop which may lead to permanent blindness. Several approaches have been suggested to administer vitamin A to population groups lacking a dietary source for this vitamin such as; (1) oral administration of a massive dose of 90,000 $\mu$g of retinol; (2) fortification with vitamin A of special foods such as prepared infant formulas, milk powder, margarine, and wheat flour, and (3) nutrition education programs emphasizing the use of foods rich in carotene (i.e., palm oil) instead of others devoid of vitamin A.

Fortification of sugar with vitamin A was formulated on the principle of utilizing as a vehicle a dietary ingredient consumed by large numbers of people from all age groups in relatively constant amounts. The sugar used was refined, and fortification was done with a commercial preparation of retinol palmitate (250-SD) with a potency of 250,000 IU/g or with retinol acetate 325 $\ell$.[26] Based on data suggesting an average daily sugar consumption in Central America and also FAO/WHO recommended allowances for vitamin A, it was decided that fortified sugar should have the following potency: 1 g sugar = 20.8 $\mu$g of retinol or 69.5 IU. Cost of such fortification was estimated to be 0.102 $\cent$/lb or about $0.03 per person/year. Arroyave,[3] in his discussion of this approach, indicated that no significant organoleptic changes were noted in foods prepared with fortified sugar, and biological availability was found to be excellent. In a longitudinal evaluation[5] to test the effects of vitamin A fortification of sugar on serum retinol levels from preschool-aged children, was done in five consecutive surveys conducted every 6 months. After 1 year of fortification, 76% of the children experienced an elevation of retinol. Mean values increased significantly particularly for children having serum vitamin A levels below 20 $\mu$g/dl whose levels increased from 16.2 ± 2.9 to 30.2 ± 9.7 $\mu$g/dl. Similar results were obtained after 2 years; thus suggesting the effectiveness of such measures in modifying low-serum retinol levels.

Perhaps one of the most difficult aspects that had to be solved by proponents of this fortification program[18] was obtaining legislation implementing this program at a national level. These efforts have been successful in Central America due to the close collaboration of scientific institutions such as Instituto de Nutrición de Centro América y Panama'(INCAP), governmental agencies, and private industries concerned with sugar and vitamin production. Similar efforts and studies are being done in other parts of the world.[1,2] A report by Toro et al.[48] describing a study conducted in the mountainous region of Arica, Chile added support to the effectiveness of distributing vitamin A fortified sugar to people living in remote villages. In these studies sugar fortified with retinol acetate 325 $\ell$ (5000 IU/40 g of sugar) was administered for a period of 3 months to people living in four Indian villages. The result was a marked increase in serum retinol of children and adults.

Programs involving fortification of sugar with vitamin A offer many benefits. Considering the poor dietary sources of vitamin A in diets of people with low-socioeconomic levels, and the nutritional requirements of male and female, young and old, provision of a moderate amount of vitamin A in sugar represents a definite advantage with practically no risk for the population at large. Arroyave[3] has specifically warned against any type of advertisement or incentive to increase sugar consumption, and no emphasis is made to increase consumption of sugar between meals, consequently there is no threat to oral health or the maintenance of adequate calorie intake. With this fortification program no change in habits are needed, individuals would continue to use sugar in their accustomed manner, and yet, receive the benefit of an increased intake of a needed nutrient. Even in the event that new dietary modifications were to be adopted resulting in a reduction of overall sugar consumption, this can be easily compensated by increasing the concentration of vitamin A in the fortification formula. Thus, fortification of sugar with vitamin A constitutes a worthwhile effort that should be further implemented and monitored.

## FORTIFICATION OF SUGAR TO REDUCE ITS CARIES POTENTIAL

In the last 10 years, there has been growing concern over the prevalence and severity of oral diseases, such as dental caries, among the U.S. population. The National Caries Program of the National Institute of Dental Research has started research efforts to try to find solutions to this problem through investigations on oral hygiene procedures, microbiological changes, and dietary manipulations, which include among other approaches substitution of sugar with synthetic sweeteners.[43]

One of the solutions that have been suggested to reduce the caries potential of sugar-containing foods is to fortify them with cariostatic agents.[25] Fortification to lower caries potential of foods would be limited to those containing carbohydrates, particularly sugars which are readily metabolized by bacterial plaque. This type of fortification, therefore, would be done to fulfill a public health need, rather than a strict nutritional need. Fortification of sugar and sugar-containing foods to fulfill these public health objectives should meet the following criteria:

1. The cariostatic agent should be effective enough to neutralize the caries promoting properties of the food to which it is added, and thus make it essentially non-caries promoting.
2. The agent should be nontoxic and safe when consumed in amounts normally expected for the food it fortifies.
3. It should not change the organoleptic (color, texture, flavor, etc.) properties of the food it fortifies.
4. The agent should be chemically stable under normal conditions of food processing, storage, and use.
5. The agent used to fortify should not interact with nutrients in the food to limit their availability or create an imbalance of essential nutrients.
6. There should be reasonable assurance that excess consumption of the fortified product would not result in a toxic level intake for the agent.
7. The agent and the fortification process should not be unduly expensive, to maintain price of the product at a competitive level in the marketplace.

Complete fulfillment of this criteria is difficult, but it seems essential that an agent to be used in food fortification for a reason, other than for nutritional purposes should meet this criteria.

The food candidates for fortification at this time are mostly sugar-containing snacks which are consumed frequently between meals. Starch and flour products, such as bread, are to some extent also caries promoting, but much less than sweet snacks, and therefore, they are not strong candidates for fortification to reduce their caries potential.

Agents to be used in fortification of sugar and sugar-containing products are generally: (1) compounds which affect the bacteria in dental plaque by affecting adhesion, growth, and/or metabolic activity including acid production; (2) compounds that increase tooth resistance to dental caries;[36] and (3) compounds that affect the flow or composition of saliva to retard or inhibit caries. Some work has been done on the first two approaches, but except for immunological studies, little has been done to investigate what possible modifications could be done to control caries through changes in saliva flow, composition, and buffering capacity.

### Fortification with Fluorides

When nutritional and dietary factors that influence caries are evaluated[35] it is realized that few substances can be considered as agents to fortify sugar and sugar products. Very few fulfill all the criteria outlined previously. Fluorides and phosphates are the most promising because of their strong cariostatic properties, although each has some limitations. Some trace elements are also known to be cariostatic, but they have not been tested sufficiently to be considered as food additives for this purpose.

Fluoride is undoubtedly the most effective cariostatic agent available today. No other element or inorganic compound can produce the decrease in caries seen in people consuming water containing as little as 1 ppm fluoride. Brown and König[12] edited the proceedings of a NIDR-NIH workshop where various mechanisms proposed to explain the cariostatic effect of fluoride were evaluated and discussed. Some of these include fluoride effects on enamel solubility, enhancement of large enamel crystal formation, stimulation of remineralization, and antibacterial and antienzymatic effects on dental plaque bacteria. The numerous studies reported and discussed at this workshop suggest that the beneficial action of fluoride seems to take place at the enamel-plaque interphase, and that posteruptive administration of frequent, small doses of fluoride is most effective in preventing caries. This being the case, there would be an advantage in using small concentrations of fluoride to fortify sugars and sugar-containing snacks, since these low levels, not exceeding 5 to 10 ppm, would exert some protective effect against caries induced by the sugar.[31] Though the cariostatic property of fluoride is unquestionable, the suggestion to use it as an agent to fortify foods has been received without enthusiasm. Two points in the previously stated criteria would have to be documented and studied before attempting to implement such fortification: (1) the cariostatic efficacy of fluoride used to fortify sugar-containing foods would have to be clearly documented in animal tests and clinical trials to demonstrate its ability to reduce caries, and (2) there should be no danger of excessive consumption of snacks containing fluoride, to avoid a high intake of fluoride by children who would be at risk to develop dental fluorosis. Fortification of sugar and sugar-containing foods with fluoride could probably meet with a similar opposition to the one generated against water fluoridation, and therefore, its efficacy and low risk should be carefully tested and documented before attempting to implement such a program. Such programs should be even more carefully evaluated when implemented in population groups where malnutrition is present because fluoride metabolism could be altered in these circumstances.

### Fortification with Phosphates

The other agent that has been considered for fortification of sugar and sugar-containing foods are phosphates. It is important to emphasize that even though phosphates are referred to as a single cariostatic agent, in reality, there are a large number of inorganic and organic phosphate compounds which have distinct and broadly different chemical characteristics and cariostatic properties. Several years ago in a conference held to discuss effects of phosphates on dental caries, Nizel and Harris[37] reviewed the literature on phosphates, and pointed to their differences in cariostatic properties depending on structure, chemical composition, and stage of tooth development or maturity when the phosphate is administered.[35] Several clinical studies have been conducted[9,44,47] using CaHOP$_4$ phosphate which has been shown to have a low cariostatic potential when tested in animals.[37] Within the last years two other clinical studies have been done,[19,20,39] which suggested that addition of dicalcium phosphate dihydrate to chewing gum determined a significant reduction in caries increment in children consuming this product in comparison to those that chewed a sugar gum without phosphate. While the study conducted by Finn and co-workers[19,20] gave positive results, other clinical studies have provided inconsistent results. One of the most recent studies was the one reported by Ashley et al.[6,7] in which effect on caries of boiled sweets fortified with dicalcium phosphate dihydrate (3%) was tested. These investigators conducted a 3 year unsupervised study and reported caries incidence in subjects who were 11 to 12 years old at the beginning of the study. They also reported[7] caries prevalence for younger siblings of children taking part in this investigation to determine possible effects of their consuming also these boiled sweets. No reduction in caries incidence was found when the group consuming sweets with CaHOP$_4 \cdot 2H_2O$ was compared with the group consuming sweets similar to those available commercially.

Several other phosphate compounds such as sucrose phosphate,[15] glycerophosphates,[10,22] and sodium trimetaphosphate[37] have been suggested as possible candidates to be used as food additives to lower the caries potential of sugar. The 3 year study done by Finn et al.[20] on school-age children consuming a chewing gum containing 1.5% sodium trimetaphosphate, indicated that a small, but significant reduction in proximal surface dental caries increments were observed in those children compared to children in a nonchewing gum group. These and several other studies suggest that some phosphates may be useful as sugar additives to reduce its caries potential provided that the appropriate phosphates, time of delivery relative to tooth development, and methods of fortification are used.

Several aspects should be clarified before implementing fortification of sugar and sugar-containing foods with phosphates to reduce their caries phosphate used to fortify a food. The effectiveness would have to be demonstrated in a clinical study after conducting adequate animal experimentation. Secondly, these must be assurances that the structure of the phosphate, which is probably essential to its cariostatic properties is not altered during food processing and distribution. Such precautions would have to be taken with trimetaphosphate, a cyclic phosphate which is changed to a linear structure, tripolyphosphate, if the temperature is raised under acid conditions. Animal studies indicate that tripolyphosphate, pyrophosphate, or orthophosphates are not as cariostatic as trimetaphosphate. Thirdly, there must be assurance that there is no interaction with other elements or that phosphate additions do not induce nutritional imbalances. Phosphates are known to affect the absorption of essential trace elements such as zinc, and also of minerals such as calcium, and assurances must be made that frequent consumption of phosphate containing foods do not produce nutritionally undesirable effects. Lastly, it is important to determine that increased consumption of the fortified product, does not increase the level of phosphate intake in such a way that bone metabolism is affected. Such concern was suggested by Raines Bell et al.,[38] who indicated that high-phosphorus diets are known to cause bone loss in aged animals; and this raises the possibility that excess phosphorus in human dietaries may also contribute to undesirable changes in calcium and phosphorus metabolism, and diseases such as osteoporosis.

## CONCLUSION

Evaluation of the literature concerning food additives[40] indicates that these are a large number of substances that have been added to foods to fulfill different nutritional, organoleptic, and technological purposes.[8,33] Fortification of sugar with nutrients to fulfill public health objectives or to make it metabolically self-sufficient are worthwhile programs, but risk/benefit ratios need to be carefully evaluated before implementing fortification programs of this type on a national or regional level. Determination of which nutrients should be added to the list of acceptable additives should be the concern of consumers, scientists, industry, and the government working in unison.[32]

Sugar is a pure ingredient which has fulfilled a major role in manufactured foods. When consumed in moderate amounts it poses no special threat to health, as human tissues can metabolize this nutrient together with other nutrients provided by food. However, when sugar consumption is misused and abused, sugar becomes a real concern and a threat to oral health. It is under these circumstances that fortification with substances that reduce the caries effect of excessive and frequent consumption of sugar containing snacks should be considered, and then, risk/benefit considerations should also be carefully weighed before implementing these fortification programs.

# REFERENCES

1. Araujo, R. L., Borges, E. L., Silva, J. D. B., Palhares, R. D., and Vieira, E. C., Effect of the intake of vitamin A fortified sugar by pre-school children, *Nutr. Rep. Int.,* 18, 429-436, 1978a.
2. Araujo, R. L., Souza, M. S. L., Mata-Machado, A. J., Mata-Machado, L. T., Mello, M. L., Cruz, T. A. C., Vieira, E. C., Souza, D. W. C., Palhares, R. D., and Borges, E. L., Response of retinol serum levels to the intake of vitamin A fortified sugar by pre-school children, *Nutr. Rep. Int.,* 17, 307-314, 1978b.
3. Arroyave, G., Distribution of vitamin A to population groups, *Proc. West. Hemsph. Nutr. Congr.,* 3, 68-79, 1971.
4. Arroyave, G., Aguilar, J. R., Flores, M., and Guzman, M. A., Evaluation of sugar fortification with vitamin A at the national level, *Sci. Publ. Pan Am. Health Organ.,* 384, 82, 1979.
5. Arroyave, G., Mejia, L. A., and Aguilar, J. R., The effect of vitamin A fortification of sugar on the serum vitamin A levels of preschool Guatemalan children: a longitudinal evaluation, *Am. J. Clin. Nutr.,* 34, 41-49, 1981.
6. Ashley, F. P., Naylor, M, N., and Emslie, R. D., Clinical testing of dicalcium phosphate supplemented sweets. I. 3 Years caries incidence in subjects aged 11 to 15 years, *Br. Dent. J.,* 136, 361-366, 1974a.
7. Ashley, F. P., Naylor, M. N., and Emslie, R. D., Clinical testing of dicalcium phosphate supplemented sweets. II. Caries prevalence in subjects aged 3 to 14 years following a maximum of three years exposure to the sweets, *Br. Dent. J.,* 136, 418-423, 1974b.
8. Austin, J. E., Ed., *Global malnutrition and Cereal Fortification,* Ballinger Publishing, Cambridge, Mass., 1979.
9. Averill, H. M. and Bibby, B. G., A clinical test of additions of phosphate to the diet of children, *J. Dent. Res.,* 43, 1150-1155, 1964.
10. Bowen, W. H., The cariostatic effect of calcium glycerophosphate in monkeys, *Caries Res.,* 6, 43-51, 1972.
11. Bowen, W. H., Role of carbohydrates in dental caries, in *Sweeteners and Dental Caries,* Shaw, J. and Roussos, G., Eds., Information Retrieval Inc., Washington, D.C., 1978, 147-155.
12. Brown, A. and König, K. G., Cariostatic mechanisms of fluorides, *Caries Res.,* 11, (Suppl), 1-137, 1977.
13. Cantor, S. M., Pattern of use of sweeteners, in *Sweeteners and Dental Caries,* Shaw, J. H. and Roussos, G., Eds., Information Retrieval Inc., Washington, D.C., 1978, 111-129.
14. Carter, J. F., Production of Fortified Sugar, U.S. Patent No. 3,607,310, September 21, 1971.
15. Craig, G. G., The use of a calcium sucrose phosphate-calcium ortho-phosphate complex as a cariostatic agent, *Br. Dent. J.,* 138, 25-28, 1975.
16. Derman, D. M., Sayers, M. H., Lynch, S. R., Charlton, R. W., Rothwell, T. H., and Mayet, F., Iron absorption from a cereal-based meal containing sugar fortified with ascorbic acid, *Br. J. Nutr.,* 38, 261-269, 1977.

17. Disler, P. B., Lynch, S. R., Charlton, R. W., Rothwell, T. H., Walker, R. B., and Mayet, F., Studies on the fortification of cane sugar with iron and ascorbic acid, *Br. J. Nutr.*, 34, 141-152, 1975.

18. Dorion, R. C. and Arroyave, G., Control of vitamin A deficiency: fortification of sugar with vitamin A, *Sugar Azucar*, 33-40, August 1977.

19. Finn, S. B. and Jamison, H., The effect of a dicalcium phosphate chewing gum on caries incidence in children: 30 months results, *J. Am. Dent. Assoc.*, 74, 988-995, 1967.

20. Finn, S. B., Frew, R. A., Leibowitz, R., Morse, W., Manson-Hing, L., and Brunelle, J., The effect of sodium trimetaphosphate (TMP) as a chewing gum additive on caries increments in children, *J. Am. Dent. Assoc.*, 96, 651-655, 1978.

21. Green, R., Charlton, R., Seftel, H., Rothwell, T., Mayet, F., Adams, B., Finch, C., and Layrisse, M., Body iron excretion in man: a collaborative study, *Am. J. Med.*, 45, 336-353, 1968.

22. Grenby, T. H. and Bull, J. M., Protection against dental caries in rats by glycerophosphates or calcium salts or mixtures of both, *Arch. Oral Biol.*, 20, 717-724, 1975.

23. Harris, R. S., Supplementation of foods with vitamins, *Agric. Food Chem.*, 1, 88-102, 1959.

24. Harris, R. S., Attitudes and approaches in supplementation of foods and nutrients, *J. Agric Food Chem.*, 16, 184-189, 1968.

25. Harris, R. S., Fortification of foods and food products with anticaries agents, *J. Dent. Res.*, 49, 1340-1344, 1970.

26. INCAP, Fortificación del azucar con vitamina A en Centro América y Panamá, Guatemala Talleres Gráficos, INCAP, Guatemala, 1974.

27. Layrisse, M., Martinez-Torres, C., Renzi, M., Velez, F., and Gonzales, M., Sugar as a vehicle for iron fortification: further studies, *Am. J. Clin. Nutr.*, 29, 274-279, 1976a.

28. Layrisse, M., Martinez-Torres, C., and Renzi, M., Sugar as a vehicle for iron fortification: further studies, *Am. J. Clin. Nutr.*, 29, 274-279, 1976b.

29. Lee, V. A., The nutrition significance of sucrose consumption, 1970-1980, *Crit. Rev. Food Sci. Nutr.*, 14(1), 1-47, 1981.

30. Lee, K. and Clydesdale, F. M., Iron sources used in food fortification and their changes due to food processing, *Crit. Rev. Food Sci. Nutr.*, 11, 117-153, 1978.

31. Menaker, L., Navia, J. M., and Taylor, R. E., Rat molar incorporation and cariostatic effect of fluoride consumed together with sucrose, *Proc. Int. Assoc. Dent. Res.*, No. 146 (Abstr.), A-111, 1978.

32. Miller, S. A., Risk/benefit, no effect levels, and Delaney: is the message getting through?, *Food Technol. (Chicago)*, 32, 93-96, 1978.

33. NAS, Proceedings of a workshop, in *Technology of Fortification of Foods*, National Academy of Sciences, Washington, D.C., 1975.

34. Navia, J. M., Enrichment of sugar and sugar products, *J. Agric. Food Chem.*, 16, 172-176, 1968.

35. Navia, J. M., Evaluation of nutritional and dietary factors that modify animal caries, *J. Dent. Res.*, 49, 1213-1327, 1970.

36. Navia, J. M., Prevention of dental caries: agents which increase tooth resistance to dental caries, *Int. Dent. J.*, 22, 427-440, 1972.

37. Nizel, A. E. and Harris, R. S., The effects of phosphates on experimental dental caries. A literature review, *J. Dent. Res.*, 43, 1123-1136, 1964.

38. Raines Bell, R., Draper, H. H., Tzeng, D. Y. M., Shin, H. K., and Schmidt, G. R., Physiological responses of human adults to foods containing phosphate additives, *J. Nutr.*, 107, 42-50, 1977.

39. Richardson, A. S., Hole, L. W., McCombie, F., and Kolthammer, J., Anticariogenic effect of dicalcium phosphate dihydrate chewing gum: results after two years, *J. Can. Dent. Assoc.*, 6, 213-218, 1972.

40. Sapeika, N., Food additives, *World Rev. Nutr. Health*, 16, 335-362, 1973.

41. Sayers, M. H., Lynch, S. R., Charlton, R. W., Rothwell, H., Walker, R. B., and Mayer, F., The fortification of common salt with ascorbic acid and iron, *Br. J. Hematol.*, 28, 483-495, 1974.

42. Schultz, H. W., Cain, R. F., and Wrolstad, R. W., *Symposium on Foods: Carbohydrates and Their Roles*, AVI Westport, Conn., 1969.

43. Shaw, J. H. and Roussos, G. G., *Sweeteners and Dental Caries*, Abstr. 403, Information Retrival Inc., Washington, D.C., 1978.

44. Ship, I. I. and Mickelsen, O., The effects of calcium acid phosphate on dental caries in children. A controlled clinical trial, *J. Dent. Res.*, 43, 1144-1149, 1964.

45. Sipple, H. L. and McNutt, K. W., *Sugars in Nutrition*, Academic Press, New York, 1974.

46. Solomons, N. W., Jacobs, R. A., Pineda, O., and Viteri, F. E., Studies on the bioavailability of zinc in man: effects of the Guatemalan rural diet and of the iron-fortifying agent, NaFe-EDTA, *J. Nutr.*, 109, 1519-1528, 1979.

47. Stralfors, A., The effect of calcium phosphate on dental caries in school children, *J. Dent. Res.*, 43, 1137-1143, 1964.

48. Toro, O., de Pablo, S., Aguayo, M., Gattan, V., Contreras, I., and Monckeberg, F., Prevention of vitamin A deficiency by fortification of sugar. A field study, *Arch. Latinoamer. Nutr.*, 27, 169-179, 1977.
49. Vecchionacce, L. M. and Setser, C. S., Quality of sugar cookies fortified with liquid cyclone processed cottonseed flour with stabilizing agents, *Cereal Chem.*, 57, 303-306, 1980.
50. Viteri, F. E., Garcia-Ibanez, R., and Torun, B., Sodium iron NaFe-EDTA as an iron fortification compound in Central America. Absorption studies, *Am. J. Clin. Nutr.*, 31, 961-971, 1978.
51. Magro, J. L., personal communication.

# FORTIFICATION OF INFANT FOODS

Ray C. Frodey

## INTRODUCTION

Traditionally, infant foods have been fortified with vitamins and/or minerals in accordance with the purpose they are designed to serve in the infant's diet. There are two general classifications, namely *complete* foods which are designed to be the sole source of nutrients and *supplementary* foods which are designed to provide nutrients in short supply when the volume of milk which can be readily consumed is insufficient to meet increased nutritional needs.

## FORTIFICATION OF COMPLETE FOODS

Breast milk and infant formulas are generally considered to be complete foods. By federal law, infant foods which purport to be a complete or partial substitute for breast milk must provide minimal levels of 28 essential nutrients. These minimum values are not the same as the National Academy of Sciences-National Research Council (NAS-NRC)[1] or the U.S. Recommended Dietary Allowances (RDA).[2] Minimum requirements are expressed as the amount of nutrient per 100 kcal of food, whereas the RDAs are the amounts of nutrients recommended per day. The U.S. labeling regulations for complete foods require that the amount of the specific nutrients present per 100 kcal and per volume usually prepared for consumption be given on the label. Since formulas are normally diluted with water to contain 20 kcal per fluid ounce and the usual daily consumption is 32 fluid ounces per day, manufacturers usually fortify their products to contain 100% or more of U.S. RDA per quart of formula diluted for normal feeding. These levels in most cases exceed the U.S. minimum requirements for infant formulas.

In Table 1 the minimum vitamin and mineral requirements per quart of formula diluted for normal feeding are compared to the U.S. and NRC recommended dietary allowances.

Formula fortification has been carried out by incorporating synthetically prepared forms of vitamins and mineral compounds whose bioavailability has been established. These compounds are listed in Table 2 together with the reference standards specified in the federal regulations.[2]

Complete foods must contain high-biological value protein. The specification that each 100 kcal of formula contain 1.8 g of protein of biological quality equivalent to casein has led manufacturers to fortify certain vegetable protein formulas with amino acids in short supply. For example; methionine has been used for this purpose in certain hypoallergenic soybean based formulas.

Complete infant foods must also contain not less than 30% of the total available kilocalories as fat and 3% of the available kilocalories as linoleate. This latter specification necessitates the use of unsaturated vegetable oils as an ingredient of many formulas.

Of course, a major problem in the fortification of all types of infant foods is the stability of the essential nutrients during preparation and storage prior to use. It is not possible to predict loss of nutrient value during preparation or storage as many variable factors such as heat, light, oxygen, pH, and other reactive components of the foods affect the rate and extent of nutrient loss.

Table 1
COMPARISON OF MINIMUM REQUIREMENTS FOR COMPLETE INFANT
FOODS WITH U.S. AND NATIONAL RESEARCH COUNCIL
RECOMMENDED DIETARY ALLOWANCES

| Nutrient | Units of measurement | Minimum requirement per 100 kcal[a] | Minimum requirement per qt diluted 640 kcal | U.S.-RDA (0—12 months) | NRC-RDA (6—12 months) |
|---|---|---|---|---|---|
| Vitamin A | IU | 250 | 1600 | 1500 | 2000 |
| Vitamin D | IU | 40 | 256 | 400 | 400 |
| Vitamin E | IU | 0.3 | 1.9 | 5 | 4 |
| Ascorbic acid | mg | 8.0 | 51 | 35 | 35 |
| Thiamine | mg | 0.040 | 0.26 | 0.5 | 0.5 |
| Riboflavin | mg | 0.06 | 0.38 | 0.6 | 0.6 |
| Niacin | mg | 0.25 | 1.6 | 8.0 | 8.0 |
| Vitamin $B_6$ | mg | 0.035 | .22 | 0.4 | 0.6 |
| Folacin | μg | 4.0 | 25.6 | 100 | 45 |
| Pantothenic acid | mg | 0.3 | 1.9 | 3 | — |
| Vitamin $B_{12}$ | μg | 0.15 | 0.96 | 2 | 1.5 |
| Biotin | μg | 1.5 | 9.6 | 0.15 | — |
| Vitamin K | μg | 4.0 | 25.6 | — | — |
| Choline | μg | 7.0 | 44.8 | — | — |
| Calcium | mg | 50 | 320 | 600 | 540 |
| Phosphorus | mg | 25 | 160 | 500 | 360 |
| Magnesium | mg | 6 | 38 | 70 | 70 |
| Iron | mg | 0.15 | 0.96 | 15 | 15 |
| Iodine | μg | 5 | 32.0 | 45 | 50 |
| Copper | mg | 0.06 | 0.6 | 0.6 | — |
| Zinc | mg | 0.5 | 3.2 | 5 | 5 |

*Note:* IU-international units; mg-milligram; mg equiv.-milligram equivalents; and μg-microgram.

[a]   From the Infant Formula Act of 1980.

Responsible food manufacturers have carried out extensive studies on nutrient retention in their products under a variety of processing and storage conditions. Use of deaeration, optimum sterilization time and temperature, container size, shape and construction, as well as controlled temperature storage are regularly used to maximize nutrient retention and minimize the overages needed to guarantee label declarations throughout the shelf-life of the food product.

## FORTIFICATION OF SUPPLEMENTARY INFANT FOODS

Calories, iron, thiamine, and vitamin C are the nutrients most likely to be in short supply for the infant who has outgrown the nutrient density of a fluid diet. For this reason infant cereals, whose caloric density is approximately twice that of infant formula when prepared for spoon feeding, are fortified with iron and B vitamins. Fruits and fruit juices have been selected for vitamin C fortification because they are generally considered to be a natural source of vitamin C, and vitamin C retention is enhanced by the acidity and normal components of some, particularly citrus, fruits.

The Food & Drug Administration (FDA) regulations for nutritional labeling specify that conventional foods containing one or more vitamins or minerals added at 50% or more of the U.S. RDA are subject to the dietary supplement regulation as specified in Section 105.85 CFR Title 21.[2] This regulation, in effect, requires minimum levels of a single nutrient or minimum levels of 10 vitamins and/or 5 essential minerals.

## Table 2
## COMPOUNDS USED FOR FORTIFICATION OF INFANT FOODS AND REFERENCE STANDARDS

| Nutrient | | Reference standard |
|---|---|---|
| Vitamin A | | Vitamin A palmitate |
| D | | Vitamin D$_3$, ergocalciferol |
| E | | α-Tocopherol acetate |
| C | L-Ascorbic acid | Ascorbic acid, sodium ascorbate |
| B$_1$ | Thiamine chloride-HCl | Thiamine chloride hydrochloride, thiamine mononitrate |
| B$_2$ | Riboflavin | Riboflavin |
| Niacin | Nicotinic acid | Niacinamide |
| Vitamin B$_6$ | Pyridoxine | Pyridoxine hydrochloride |
| Folacin | Pteroyl-mono-L-glu-tamic acid | Folic acid |
| Panthothenic acid | D-Pantothenic acid | Calcium pantothenate |
| Vitamin B$_{12}$ | Cyanocobalamine | Cyanocobalamine |
| Biotin | D-Biotin | Biotin |
| Vitamin K | | Phytonadione |
| Choline | | Choline chloride |
| Calcium | | Tricalcium phosphate, calcium citrate, calcium carbonate |
| Phosphorous | | Calcium phosphate |
| Magnesium | | Dibasic magnesium phosphate, magnesium chloride |
| Iron | | Ferrous sulfate, electrolytic |
| Iodine | | Potassium iodide |
| Copper | | Cupric sulfate, cupric gluconate |
| Zinc | | Zinc sulfate |
| Manganese | | Manganese sulfate |

Since conventional infant cereals are not suitable carriers for this multivitamin-mineral mixture, nutrient additions have been restricted to less than 50% of the U.S. RDA in infant cereals. The conventional cereal enrichment ingredients are thiamine, riboflavin, niacin, calcium, and iron. The levels used vary depending upon the method for estimating niacin equivalents and the calcium phosphorus ratio in the final product. In the enrichment of infant fruit juices, vitamin C has been restored to 120% of the U.S. RDA per serving. Strained fruits are enriched to the 45% U.S. RDA level. The strained cereals with fruit carry the 45% enrichment of thiamine, riboflavin, niacin, iron, vitamin C, and also vitamin B$_6$.

Calcium additions have been deleted from the wet canned cereals. The level of enrichment of various supplementary infant foods is given in Table 3.

The technological problems of fortifying infant foods are much the same as those with other foods. For example; with vitamin C, exposure to heat, oxygen, copper, xanthocyanin pigments, and elevated pH must be minimized for retention of nutrient value. Thiamine is also quite sensitive to oxidizing agents such as sulfite, particularly at high pH. Thiamine mononitrate has been found to be a more stable form than the hydrochloride in dry products. Riboflavin is less sensitive to these agents but must be protected from light. The naturally occurring pyridoxal form of vitamin B$_6$ is particularly unstable, hence, pyridoxine hydrochloride is universally preferred form for fortification. Due to the relatively minute levels of vitamins used in fortifying foods, suppliers offer vitamin mixtures in a suitable carrier for more facile handling under production conditions. Their vitamin potency is certified by the supplier and checked by the manufacturer customarily in the finished product.

Fortification with iron has offered specific problems in that the bioavailability of the various forms of iron could not be accurately assessed until recently.[3] Some of the

Table 3
LEVEL OF ENRICHMENT FOR INFANT FOODS (% U.S.
RDA PER SERVING)

| Nutrient | Dry cereal (14 g) | Jarred cereals with fruit (4.5 fluid oz) | Jarred strained fruits (4.5 fluid oz) | Jarred fruit juices (4.5 fluid oz) |
|---|---|---|---|---|
| Thiamine | 45 | 45 | — | — |
| Riboflavin | 45 | 45 | — | — |
| Niacin | 25—45 | 45 | — | — |
| Vitamin $B_6$ | — | 45 | — | — |
| Vitamin C | — | 45 | 45 | 120 |
| Calcium | 15—45 | — | — | — |
| Iron | 45 | 15—45 | — | — |

early forms of iron used for food enrichment because they did not cause discoloration or rancidity of fat were later shown to have limited availability to man.[1] At present ferrous sulfate is the compound of choice for the fortification of "wet canned" infant foods or formulas. Electrolytically reduced iron or carbonyl iron is the fortification iron of choice for dry cereal products because their large active surface area increases bioavailability[5] without inducing rancidity or discoloration.

The elimination of salt from supplementary infant foods in 1977 also eliminated their fortification with iodine. Prior to 1977, salt containing potassium iodate at the level of 0.01% I was used in vegetables, meat and vegetable, and meat infant foods at the level of 0.25% NaCl.

## REFERENCES

1. Recommended Dietary Allowances, 9th ed., National Academy of Sciences—National Research Council, Food and Nutrition Board (NAS-NRC-FNB), Washington, D.C., 1980.
2. Code of Federal Regulations Title 21, Chapter 1, Part 105, revised as of April 1, 1977.
3. Cook, J. D. et al., Food iron absorption measured by an extrinsic tag, *J. Clin. Invest.,* 51, 805, 1972.
4. Rios, E., Hunter, R. E., Cook, J. D., Smith, R. J., and Finch, C. A., The absorption of iron as supplements in infant cereal and infant formula, *Pediatrics,* 55, 686, 1975.
5. Bjorn-Rasmussen, E., Hallberg, L., and Rossander, L., Absorption of fortification iron, *Br. J. Nutr.,* 37, 375, 1977.

# Index

# INDEX